Identification and Characterization of Antimicrobial Peptides with Therapeutic Potential

Special Issue Editor

Guangshun Wang

MDPI • Basel • Beijing • Wuhan • Barcelona • Belgrade

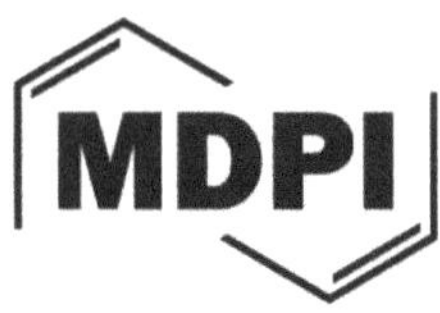

Special Issue Editor
Guangshun Wang
University of Nebraska Medical Center
USA

Editorial Office
MDPI AG
St. Alban-Anlage 66
Basel, Switzerland

This edition is a reprint of Special Issues published online in the open access journal *Pharmaceuticals* (ISSN 1424-8247) from 2014–2015 (available at: http://www.mdpi.com/journal/pharmaceuticals/special_issues/therapeutic-potential; http://www.mdpi.com/journal/pharmaceuticals/special_issues/antimicrobial-peptides2015).

For citation purposes, cite each article independently as indicated on the article page online and as indicated below:

Author 1; Author 2. Article title. *Journal Name* **Year**, *Article number*, page range.

First Edition 2017

ISBN 978-3-03842-462-8 (Pbk)
ISBN 978-3-03842-463-5 (PDF)

Articles in this volume are Open Access and distributed under the Creative Commons Attribution license (CC BY), which allows users to download, copy and build upon published articles even for commercial purposes, as long as the author and publisher are properly credited, which ensures maximum dissemination and a wider impact of our publications. The book taken as a whole is © 2017 MDPI, Basel, Switzerland, distributed under the terms and conditions of the Creative Commons license CC BY-NC-ND (http://creativecommons.org/licenses/by-nc-nd/4.0/).

Table of Contents

Part III: Therapeutic Potential of Antimicrobial Peptides

About the Special Issue Editor

Guangshun Wang is an Associate Professor at the University of Nebraska Medical Center (Omaha, USA). He is interested in developing new compounds to treat human diseases, such as drug-resistant superbugs, viruses and cancer. His laboratory utilizes an integrated approach by combining chemistry, biophysics, bioinformatics, genetics, and structural biology. Two general methods are exploited to identify novel drug candidates. First, his laboratory has constructed the Antimicrobial Peptide Database (http://aps.unmc.edu/AP) to search and screen starting templates. At present, this database contains over 2800 antibacterial, antiviral, antifungal, antiparasitic and anticancer peptides, primarily from natural sources, including bacteria, fungi, protists, plants, and animals. Second, three-dimensional structural information is harnessed to conduct structure-based or rational design. Recently, his laboratory has also combined the library approach with structure-based design to obtain compounds with desire properties. Dr. Wang has edited a book entitled Antimicrobial Peptides: Discovery, Design and Novel Therapeutic Strategies (CABI, 1st version 2010; 2nd version 2017). Dr. Wang has published 90 original articles, invited reviews, and book chapters.

Preface to "Identification and Characterization of Antimicrobial Peptides with Therapeutic Potential"

Antimicrobial peptides are key defense molecules adopted by all life forms. The Antimicrobial peptide field is advancing rapidly as a result of the following: First, the antibiotic resistance issue has caught the attention of politicians, scientists, and the general public. There is the consensus that measures should be taken to curb the growth of antibiotic resistance. Efforts in this direction may range from discovering alternative antimicrobials to exploring different applications of existing antibiotics [1]. Second, there is a great desire to understand the functional roles of antimicrobial peptides in humans, animals, and plants. Studies in this direction will elucidate when and where such peptides are expressed in response to invading pathogens and how they work together with other components in the immune system to maintain a healthy host. Third, it is now appreciated that commensal bacteria play an essential role in human health. An elegant example is human microbiota. A current view is that a loss of beneficial commensal bacteria opens the door to infection by microbial intruders [2]. This view indicates the importance to maintain the homeostasis of our microbiota to prevent related diseases. It also implies that one may try to restore the commensal microbes as a therapeutic option [3]. Whichever the direction may be, the identification and characterization of naturally occurring antimicrobial peptides clearly constitute an important step toward these goals. Consequently, there is an increasing effort in discovering novel antimicrobial peptides from natural resources by genomic mining or proteomic approaches [4]. Identification and Characterization of Antimicrobial Peptides with Therapeutic Potential, an eBook consisting of three parts, is constructed to tell the story of antimicrobial peptides discovered from a variety of kingdoms or classes. These articles were selected from the two Special Issues on antimicrobial peptides originally published in the open access journal Pharmaceuticals during the period 2014–2016.

The first part (Chapter 1) highlights leaps made in peptide discovery, new function, mechanisms of action, and potential applications of antimicrobial peptides. Based on the antimicrobial Peptide Database (APD; http://aps.unmc.edu/AP), roughly 100–300 new peptides with demonstrated antimicrobial activity are discovered each year [5], including unique sequences, which cannot be predicted by modern machine learning algorithms. Then, my research team and I continue to describe new mechanisms for existing antimicrobial peptides that have been known for decades. We propose that multiple functions of antimicrobial peptides are realized by their ability to recognize and interact with different molecular targets or cells. Finally, we discuss various potential applications of antimicrobial peptides, ranging from peptide therapeutics, surface coating, nanoparticle-based drug delivery systems and biosensors to detection devices.

The second part is the main body of this eBook that contains a series of articles on natural antimicrobial peptides from diverse sources. Fungi, as eukaryotes, provide a useful source for antimicrobial peptides. There are well-known examples such as plectasin, eurocin, micasin, and copsin. Among them, plectasin is extensively characterized in terms of structure, activity, and potential applications [6]. In Chapter 2, Shunyi Zhu and colleagues describe the great opportunity to identify many more defensin-like peptides from the sequenced fungal genomes. A sequence similarity search leads to 69 new peptides from 26 fungal species. A recent article from the same lab demonstrates that, however, not all such peptides possess antimicrobial activity, at least based on the in vitro tests of select bacterial strains [7]. It is likely that numerous peptides expressed simultaneously are endowed with distinct functions to maximize the benefits to the host.

Plants constitute another important source for novel antimicrobial peptides (341 entries in the current APD). Many plant antimicrobial peptides comprise disulfide bonds that usually form β-sheet structures. Additionally, disulfide-linked sequences can also form α-helical structures. In Chapter 3, James Tam and colleagues systematically deal with the sequence, structure and activity of these plant peptides. Cyclotides, circular peptides stabilized by three disulfide bonds, are a special class of plant peptides whose antimicrobial activity remains to be tested. Their stable scaffold and recognition of bacterial phosphatidylethanolamine (PE) are outstanding traits for developing antimicrobials with the needed properties.

Animals are diverse and can be broadly separated into invertebrates and vertebrates. Most animals are invertebrates, such as insects, spiders, and scorpions. In Chapter 4, Václav Čeřovský and his associate vividly tell the story of lucifensin, which is believed to be the long-sought-after magic molecule for Maggot therapy. For spiders and scorpions, Xiuqing Wang and I have recently conducted a structural and bioinformatics analysis [8]. While spiders use both glycine-rich and helical peptides for defense, scorpions use only helical peptides. Vertebrates are also versatile, covering fish in water, reptiles on land, and birds in the sky. In Chapter 5, Gill Diamond and his associate discuss a variety of fish antimicrobial peptides that kill both human and fish pathogens. In addition, these peptides also modulate immune responses. Of particular interest is that fish antimicrobial peptides may work at high concentrations of salts or low pH, useful properties for developing the next generation of antimicrobials. In Chapter 6, Michael Conlon and his colleague describe select antimicrobial peptides from skin secretions of frogs (~1000 in the current APD). The authors comment that "the therapeutic potential of frog skin peptides as anti-infective agents has not been realized so that alternative clinical applications as anti-cancer, anti-viral, anti-diabetic, or immunomodulatory drugs are being explored." In Chapter 7, Monique van Hoek discusses antimicrobial peptides from reptiles. Recently, she and her colleagues have proposed an innovative approach that enriches peptides from reptile blood [9]. This method accelerates the discovery of additional reptile peptides. Chapter 8, by Guolong Zhang and his associates, summarizes the biology and therapeutic potential of avian antimicrobial peptides. Structure–activity relationship studies help identify candidates for antimicrobial use or vaccine adjuvants. Dietary additives have been utilized to modulate the expression of antimicrobial peptides to prevent diseases in chicken. In Chapter 9, I describe human antimicrobial peptides, covering discovery, antimicrobial/anticancer activities, mechanisms of action, three-dimensional structure and therapeutic strategies. Provided in Table 1 is a timeline for the discovery of select human antimicrobial peptides (over 100 in the APD). These peptides and proteins can adopt various structural scaffolds to attack pathogens by different mechanisms. These include disruption of membranes, inhibition of metal uptake or cell wall synthesis, and association with ribosomes. Finally, various factors such as isoleucine, sunlight and vitamin D can be utilized to induce the expression of human antimicrobial peptides, opening a new avenue to curb pathogen infection.

The third part of this book highlights the therapeutic potential of antimicrobial peptides. The moonlighting of antimicrobial peptides (i.e., multiple functions) lays the foundation for us to explore their potential uses. Interestingly enough, bacteria also produce antimicrobial peptides (generally called bacteriocins). Several bacterial peptides (e.g., daptomycin, gramicidin, and nisin) are already in use. In Chapter 10, Anne Ulrich and her colleagues report the treatment of patients with root canal infections using gramicidin S. Antiviral effects of antimicrobial peptides are also of high interest considering viral infections such as SARS, Zika, and Ebola in the news. In Chapter 11, Kevan Hartshorn and his colleague describe the role and therapeutic potential of antiviral antimicrobial peptides, including human α-defensins, β-defensins, retrocyclins, LL-37, histones, amyloid peptides, lactoferrin and bacterial/permeability increasing protein (BPI) derived peptides. While intact LL-37 itself lost activity, its central fragment (GI-20) remained effective against a pandemic influenza virus strain H1N1 of 2009. Antimicrobial peptides may also be useful in preventing undesired pregnancies and as anti-HIV microbiocides [10]. In Chapter 12, Nongnuj Tanphaichitr and her colleagues discuss spermicidal AMPs. They propose that human cathelicidin LL-37 is the most promising peptide for this purpose. Many peptides are currently under active development for therapeutic applications [1]. It appears that the potential of these natural peptides is unlimited and remains to be unlocked by the young generation of researchers for the benefit of our biosphere. I hope that this eBook provides a useful introduction to newcomers and refreshes the minds of the veterans. Finally, I would like to take this opportunity to thank all the authors who contributed their insightful work to this eBook and the Pharmaceuticals editorial team for publishing it.

Guangshun Wang
Special Issue Editor

References

1. Mishra, B.; Reiling, S.; Zarena, D.; Wang, G. Host defense antimicrobial peptides as antibiotics: design and application strategies. *Curr. Opin. Chem. Biol.* **2017**, *38*, 87–96.
2. Nakatsuji, T.; Chen, T.H.; Narala, S.; Chun, K.A.; Two, A.M.; Yun, T.; Shafiq, F.; Kotol, P.F.; Bouslimani, A.; Melnik, A.V.; et al. Antimicrobials from human skin commensal bacteria protect against Staphylococcus aureus and are deficient in atopic dermatitis. *Sci. Transl Med.* **2017**, *9*, doi:10.1126/scitranslmed.aah4680.
3. Kommineni, S.; Kristich, C.J.; Salzman, N.H. Harnessing bacteriocin biology as targeted therapy in the GI tract. *Gut Microbes*. **2016**, *7*, 512–517.
4. Wang, G. (Ed.) *Antimicrobial Peptides: Discovery, Design and Novel Therapeutic Strategies*; 2nd Version; CABI: Wallingford, UK, 2017.
5. Wang, G.; Li, X.; Wang, Z. APD3: The antimicrobial peptide database as a tool for research and education. *Nucleic Acids Res.* **2016**, *44*, D1087–D1093.
6. Mygind, P.H.; Fischer, R.L.; Schnorr, K.M.; Hansen, M.T.; Sönksen, C.P.; Ludvigsen, S.; Raventós, D.; Buskov, S.; Christensen, B.; De Maria, L.; et al. Plectasin is a peptide antibiotic with therapeutic potential from a saprophytic fungus. *Nature* **2005**, *437*, 975–980.
7. Wu, Y.; Gao, B.; Zhu, S. New fungal defensin-like peptides provide evidence for fold change of proteins in evolution. *Biosci. Rep.* **2017**, *37*, doi:10.1042/BSR20160438.
8. Wang, X.; Wang, G. Insights into Antimicrobial Peptides from Spiders and Scorpions. *Protein Pept. Lett.* **2016**, *23*, 707–721.
9. Bishop, B.M.; Juba, M.L.; Russo, P.S.; Devine, M.; Barksdale, S.M.; Scott, S.; Settlage, R.; Michalak, P.; Gupta, K.; Vliet, K.; et al. Discovery of Novel Antimicrobial Peptides from Varanus komodoensis (Komodo Dragon) by Large-Scale Analyses and De-Novo-Assisted Sequencing Using Electron-Transfer Dissociation Mass Spectrometry. *J. Proteome Res.* **2017**, *16*, 1470–1482.
10. Wang, G. Database-guided discovery of potent peptides to combat HIV-1 or Superbugs. *Pharmaceuticals* **2013**, *6*, 728–758.

Part I:
Introduction to Antimicrobial Peptides

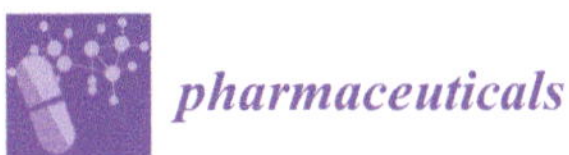

MDPI

Review

Chapter 1:

Antimicrobial Peptides in 2014

Guangshun Wang [1,*], Biswajit Mishra [1], Kyle Lau [1], Tamara Lushnikova [1], Radha Golla [1] and Xiuqing Wang [1,2]

1 Department of Pathology and Microbiology, University of Nebraska Medical Center, 986495 Nebraska Medical Center, Omaha, NE 68198-6495, USA

2 Institute of Clinical Laboratory, Ningxia Medical University, Yinchuan 750004, China

* Author to whom correspondence should be addressed; gwang@unmc.edu; Tel.: +402-559-4176; Fax: +402-559-4077.

Academic Editor: Jean Jacques Vanden Eynde

Received: 11 February 2015; Accepted: 17 March 2015; Published: 23 March 2015

Abstract: This article highlights new members, novel mechanisms of action, new functions, and interesting applications of antimicrobial peptides reported in 2014. As of December 2014, over 100 new peptides were registered into the Antimicrobial Peptide Database, increasing the total number of entries to 2493. Unique antimicrobial peptides have been identified from marine bacteria, fungi, and plants. Environmental conditions clearly influence peptide activity or function. Human α-defensin HD-6 is only antimicrobial under reduced conditions. The pH-dependent oligomerization of human cathelicidin LL-37 is linked to double-stranded RNA delivery to endosomes, where the acidic pH triggers the dissociation of the peptide aggregate to release its cargo. Proline-rich peptides, previously known to bind to heat shock proteins, are shown to inhibit protein synthesis. A model antimicrobial peptide is demonstrated to have multiple hits on bacteria, including surface protein delocalization. While cell surface modification to decrease cationic peptide binding is a recognized resistance mechanism for pathogenic bacteria, it is also used as a survival strategy for commensal bacteria. The year 2014 also witnessed continued efforts in exploiting potential applications of antimicrobial peptides. We highlight 3D structure-based design of peptide antimicrobials and vaccines, surface coating, delivery systems, and microbial detection devices involving antimicrobial peptides. The 2014 results also support that combination therapy is preferred over monotherapy in treating biofilms.

Keywords: antimicrobial peptide; bacterial detection; biofilms; mechanism of action; nanoparticle; peptide discovery; sensors; structure-based design; surface coating

---

1. Introduction

Antimicrobial peptides, or host defense peptides, are important components of innate immune systems. This field is currently moving rapidly. On one hand, there is an urgent demand for novel antimicrobials due to the current trend of reduction in the potency of commonly used antibiotics. On the other hand, our research now pays more attention to innate immune systems where antimicrobial peptides play an essential role. An imbalanced expression of antimicrobial peptides has been implicated in human disease [1–5]. All these research activities around the world led to a substantial increase in the number of scientific papers on antimicrobial peptides. In 2014 alone, a search of the PubMed using "antimicrobial peptides and 2014" returned 7562 publications (~20 articles per day) [6]. About 10% of these publications are review articles. However, a summary in the style of annual report is lacking.

During our regular update of the Antimicrobial Peptide Database (APD) (*http://aps.unmc.edu/AP*) [7–9] in the past years, we noticed new peptides of outstanding interest and created a website for them (*http://aps.unmc.edu/AP/timeline.php*) [10]. We also felt the need to write a story on these interesting molecules. Since the antimicrobial peptide field is rather broad, a detailed report on every aspect of the research is out of the scope of this review. Instead, we chose to highlight the antimicrobial peptide research by focusing on the following topics: (1) Of the new peptides discovered in 2014, are there any unique members that expand our current knowledge of natural antimicrobial peptides? (2) For known peptides, have we uncovered new functions that fill in our knowledge gap? (3) What progress have we made in mechanistic studies? Have any of our existing views been challenged? What about the genetic basis of bacterial resistance? (4) Are there advances in peptide applications? In the following, we discuss these four aspects of the antimicrobial peptide research based on the *new* discoveries made during 2014. We apologize if your important work did not fit into the scope of this article or escaped our attention.

2. New Host Defense Peptides Reported in 2014

This section features new antimicrobial peptides discovered in 2014. Two major methods were utilized for peptide discovery: a combination of chromatographic approaches [11–21] and genomic and proteomic approaches [22–25]. The proteomic approach has the potential of identifying a large number of peptides. However, we only registered peptides into the APD database if they have a known amino acid sequence (usually less than 100 amino acids) and demonstrated antimicrobial activity. In 2014, 104 new antimicrobial peptides were registered in the APD [7,8]. This 2014 total is comparable to those annual totals of peptides (over 100) collected into the APD since 2000 [26]. In the following, we highlight unique peptides from various life kingdoms.

Of the 104 new antimicrobial peptides, 29 bacteriocins (*i.e.*, bacterial antimicrobial peptides) were isolated from the bacterial kingdom. The peptide BacFL31 is unusual in that its N-terminal amino acid sequence contains six hydroxyprolines (X in the sequence GLEESXGHXGQXGPXGPXGAXGP) [11]. Baceridin, a non-ribosomally synthesized circular peptide with only six amino acids (50% D-amino acids), was isolated from a plant-associated Bacillus strain [12]. This peptide can inhibit cell cycle progression and causes apoptosis in cancer cells independent of p53. It is the most hydrophobic peptide (100%) and the shortest circular peptide in the APD (Table 1). Lassomycin was found to be similar to lassos since its aspartic acid 8 forms a bond with the N-terminal glycine. This peptide kills *Mycobacterium tuberculosis* by binding to ATP-dependent protease ClpC1P1P2 [13]. It is exciting that humans have reached organisms deep in the sea. Using transformation-associated recombination (TAR) technology, Yamanaka *et al.* succeeded in cloning and expression of a silent lipopeptide biosynthetic gene cluster from the marine actinomycete *Saccharomonospora* sp. CNQ-490 to produce taromycin A, a daptomycin analog [14]. In addition, several lipopeptides were found from a marine bacterium *Bacillus subtilis*. One of them, gageotetrin A, consists of only leucine and glutamic acid followed by a new fatty acid 3-hydroxy-11-methyltridecanoic acid at the C-terminus [27]. Interestingly, these peptides displayed rather good antibacterial activity (0.01–0.06 μM) against *Staphylococcus aureus, B. subtilis, Salmonella typhimurium, Pseudomonas aeruginosa, Rhizoctonia solani, Colletotrichum acutatum,* and *Botrytis cinera.* Although gageotetrin A is a conjugate, it possesses the shortest peptide sequence (Table 1) in the APD. The structure of anionic gageotetrin A (peptide + fatty acid) is clearly different from synthetic ultra-short lipopeptides (fatty acid + peptide), which are usually cationic to mimic cationic antimicrobial peptides [28]. Gageotetrin A has a simpler molecular design compared to anionic daptomycin, the first lipopeptide antimicrobial approved by FDA in 2003 [29]. Another peptide, sonorensin with broad activity spectrum against both Gram-positive and Gram-negative bacteria, was also identified from a marine bacterium *Bacillus sonorensis* MT93. It possesses a unique amino acid sequence with multiple copies of the CWSCXGHS motif, where X is methionine or alanine (Table 1). Sonorensin is the first characterized bacteriocin from the heterocycloanthracin subfamily [30]. These successful examples prove that it is likely to identify novel antimicrobial peptides from unexplored organisms.

The discovery of new antimicrobial peptides from the fungal kingdom is lagging behind other life kingdoms. In 2014, we collected only one defensin-like peptide from *Coprinopsis cinerea*. Like fungal plectasin and eurocin [31,32], copsin inhibited cell wall synthesis by binding to lipid II [33]. These fungal peptides share the same 3D fold, comprising one α-helix packed with a two-stranded β-sheet. Differing from plectasin and eurocin with three disulfide bonds, however, copsin is stabilized by six disulfide bonds. In addition, the N-terminus of copsin is modified into a pyroglutamate (17 peptides in the APD with such a modification [8]), furthering conferring stability to the peptide against high temperatures and protease digestion. Thus, fungi constitute yet another important kingdom for novel antimicrobial discovery.

In 2014, five new antimicrobial peptides were characterized from the plant kingdom and one of them is quite unique. Different from many disulfide bond stabilized defensins with a β-sheet structure, EcAMP3 is a disulfide-stabilized hairpin-like α-helical peptide. It is the first such peptide that inhibits phytopathogenic bacteria [20]. Hispidalin from winter melon *Benincasa hispida* [34] shows only 31% sequence similarity to tachycitin from horseshoe crabs [35] and amphibian brevinin-1PRb [36] based on sequence alignment in the APD [7]. Since hispidalin is a newly discovered peptide, it has not been trained in the existing programs. Not surprising, several online machine-learning programs were unable to predict it as an antimicrobial peptide [37–39].

Table 1. Select antimicrobial peptides discovered in 2014.

APD ID	Name	Source	Peptide amino acid sequence	Unique features [1]
2381	Gageotetrin A	Bacteria	LE	The shortest lipopeptide
2397	Sonorensin	Bacteria	CWSCMGHSCWSCMGHSC WSCAGHSCWSCMGHSCWSCM GHSCWSCAGHCCGSCWHGGM	Repeating CWSCXGHS motif
2372	Baceridin	Bacteria	WAIVLL	The shortest circular peptide consisting entirely of hydrophobic amino acids
2440	Copsin	Fungi	QNCPTRRGLCVTSGLTACR NHCRSCHRGDVGCVRCSN AQCTGFLGTTCTCINPCPRC	The first fungal defensin with six disulfide bonds
2407	Hispidalin	Plants	SDYLNNNPLFPRYDIGNVEL STAYRSFANQKAPGRLNQN WALTADYTYR	A unique peptide with 31% similarity to known sequences. Not predicted by existing programs
2477	EcAMP3	Plants	GADRCRERCERRHRGD WQGKQRCLMECRRREQEED	The first disulfide-stabilized hairpin-like helical peptide that inhibits phytopathogenic bacteria
2424	Crotalicidin	Animals	KRFKKFFKKVKKSVKK RLKKIFKKPMVIGVTIPF	Rich in lysine (38%)

[1] Additional peptide properties can be found in the APD database (*http://aps.unmc.edu/AP*) [8] using peptide ID in the table. A full list of the 2014 antimicrobial peptides can also be studied there.

Of the 104 antimicrobial peptides found in 2014, 69 originated from animals. This is consistent with the overall picture in the APD that antimicrobial peptides from the animal kingdom dominate [26].

Moreover, amphibians remain a major source for discovering natural antimicrobial peptides, accounting for 35% of the 2014 total (38.8% of the entire database entries). Most of these new sequences resemble the known frog antimicrobial peptides, which are linear and have the potential to form a helical structure [18,19]. Although cathelicidins have been identified from a variety of animals, ranging from birds, fish, and reptiles, to mammals [40], candidates from amphibians were not reported until 2012 [41]. In 2014, two new members appeared [42], leading to a total of six amphibian cathelicidins in the APD (five helical and one glycine-rich). These cathelicidins are quite distinct from the main body of amphibian peptides. For example, cathlicidin RC-1 has a high content of lysines (32%). Crotalicidin [17], a homologous snake cathelicidin, contains an even higher content of lysines (38%) (Table 1).

Also in 2014, some known human peptides or proteins were demonstrated to be antimicrobial. These include human α-defensin 6 (HD-6), β-defensin 120 (DEFB120), chemokine CCL24 (eotaxin-2), CCL26 (eotaxin-3), and human ribonuclease 6 (RNase 6). While HD-6 is active against *Bifidobacterium adolescentis* [43], recombinant DEFB120 is active against *Escherichia coli*, *S. aureus*, and *Candida albicans* [44]. Eotaxin-1 (CCL11), eotaxin-2, and eotaxin-3 are known chemokines, which are also active against the airway pathogens *Streptococcus pneumoniae*, *S. aureus*, *Haemophilus influenzae*, and *P. aeruginosa* [45]. In addition, human RNase 6 is inducible and shows activity against uropathogens, underscoring its defense role in the urinary tract [46]. These characterized members further expand the known reservoir of human host defense peptides and proteins reviewed in 2014 [47].

3. New Light on Known Human Antimicrobial Peptides

Antimicrobial peptides may be constitutively expressed to keep defined loci in a healthy state [1,48]. Compared to neonatal and adult keratinocytes, the corresponding fetal cells express much more human antimicrobial peptides for host defense [49]. Alternatively, these molecules can also be induced upon bacterial invasion. For example, a human cathelicidin peptide is induced in skin fat cells upon *S. aureus* infection, underscoring the significance of adipocytes in host defense [50]. Previously, Gallo and colleagues also found that overexpression of cathelicidin PR-39 protected animals from group A Streptococcus (GAS) infection [51]. Interestingly, the gut possesses both constitutively expressed and induced antimicrobial peptides. While human cathelicidin LL-37 and β-defensins 2-4 (hBD-2 to HBD-4) are induced, human α-defensin 5 (HD-5), HD-6, and β-defensin 1 (hBD-1) are constitutively expressed [52]. These constitutively expressed human peptides also play a special role in host defense. In 2014, HD-5 was shown to be especially potent against the most virulent form of *Clostridium difficile*, thereby preventing its infection of small intestine. This is a significant observation considering that *C. difficile* can evade the action of other host microbicidal peptides and disturb the balance of gut microbiota [53]. Human papillomavirus (HPV) infections can lead to cervical cancer and HD-5 can prevent viral entry [54]. In addition, Wiens and Smith showed that HD-5 directly interferes with a critical host-mediated viral processing step, furin cleavage of L2, at the cell surface [55]. Structurally, HD-5 can form a disulfide bond swapped dimer *in vitro* [56]. It should be interesting to test whether this dimer is linked to host defense *in vivo*.

How HD-6 plays the defense role in human gut has been puzzling for years. Similar to human hBD-1 [57], Schroeder *et al.* found that human Paneth cell HD-6 only exerted antibacterial activity under reduced conditions, establishing it as a bona fide antimicrobial peptide [43]. This reduction may be achieved *in vivo* by the NADPH thioredoxin-reductase system. *In vitro*, removal of the N-terminal two amino acid residues of HD-6 enabled a full reduction by dithiothreitol without influencing its activity. Such a truncated form was isolated previously from ileal neobladder urine [58]. In addition, HD-6 can form neutrophil extracellular traps (NETs) to trap invading microbes [59]. Thus, recent breakthroughs have uncovered two possible mechanisms for HD-6 in host defense.

The importance of environmental conditions for antimicrobial activity is not limited to α-defensins. In 2014, Abou Alaiwa *et al.* showed that the composition of the airway surface liquid is critical for human LL-37 and hBD-3 to kill inhaled and aspirated bacteria. A decrease in pH from 8 to 6.8 in pulmonary airway reduced the activity of both peptides against *S. aureus* as well as synergistic effects between innate immune peptides [60].

It is known that pH modulates the oligomerization state of human LL-37. At acidic pH, LL-37 is monomeric; it aggregates at physiological pH [61]. The mode of oligomerization was also studied in 2014 by using disulfide-linked dimers [62]. NMR studies confirmed this pH-dependent phenomenon [63]. However, the link of this phenomenon to biology was not clear. In 2014, Gao and colleagues reported that LL-37 enhancement of signal transduction by Toll-like receptor 3 (TLR3) is regulated by pH [64]. Upon acidification in endosomes, oligomerized LL-37 dissociates, allowing the release of delivered dsRNA to act as an agonist for TLR3 signaling. In contrast, LL-29, a natural fragment of human LL-37 that lacks the C-terminal portion [65], is unable to do so. Since our previous NMR studies found that nearly all the residues of LL-37 (residues 1-36) are involved in oligomerization [63,66], the C-terminal portion of LL-37 might be involved in the tetramer formation of LL-37. The salt bridges, likely involving R34 and/or E36, can be disrupted at acidic pH, providing a molecular basis for pH-dependent oligomer dissociation and dsRNA release.

All these examples above underscore that environmental conditions are an important mediator of the function of antimicrobial peptides. There are also other mediators that regulate peptide activity, including proteases, metals, salts, and chemical modifications. While 3D triple-resonance NMR studies show that the helical region (residues 2-31) of LL-37 is responsible for both membrane and lipopolysaccharides (LPS) binding [63], citrullination of arginines can reduce its ability in preventing endotoxin-induced sepsis [67]. Likewise, ADP-ribosylation of four out of the five arginines of human LL-37 may regulate this property [68]. A more recent discovery reveals that during *S. aureus* invasion, skin adipocytes can replicate rapidly and produce a cathelicidin peptide longer than LL-37 to prevent infection [50]. Previously, a different form of human cathelicidin, ALL-38, was also isolated from the human reproductive system [69]. Therefore, human proteases at a defined location play an important role in determining the exact molecular form of mature antimicrobial peptides required for host defense [47].

4. Mechanisms of Action of Antimicrobial Peptides and Genetic Basis of Bacterial Resistance

4.1. *Peptide at Work*

Although there are anionic peptides, natural antimicrobial peptides are usually cationic with an average net charge of +3.2 [7,8]. A leading view is that these cationic peptides target negatively charged bacterial membranes. However, other mechanisms are possible [4,5,47,63]. In the case of membrane targeting, how it damages the membranes remains debatable. A variety of possible membrane-weakening mechanisms have been summarized by Vogel [70] and three of them are depicted in Figure 1. These models are helpful and may inspire the design of new experiments to check their validity. In the carpet model [71], antimicrobial peptides are assumed to locate on the membrane surface. Is the peptide flat? In 2014, solid-state NMR studies of piscidins revealed peptide tilting to achieve an optimal interaction. The extent of tilting depends on both peptide sequence and lipid composition. The glycine at position 13 may be important for peptide plasticity [72]. Numerous peptide examples, including human cathelicidin LL-37 [66], possess a similar glycine that may modulate peptide activity against different bacteria. However, there are only a few examples with a defined pore. Structural determination yielded evidence for channel or pore formation. Gramicidin and alamethicin are two known examples [73,74]. Recently, the crystal structure of human dermcidin implies another possible channel [75,76]. In 2014, a C-type lectin is proposed to form a pore in bacterial membranes based on a combined structural determination by X-ray diffraction with electron microscopy data. In this model, six copies of human RegIIIα assemble into a ring structure with a hole in the center [77].

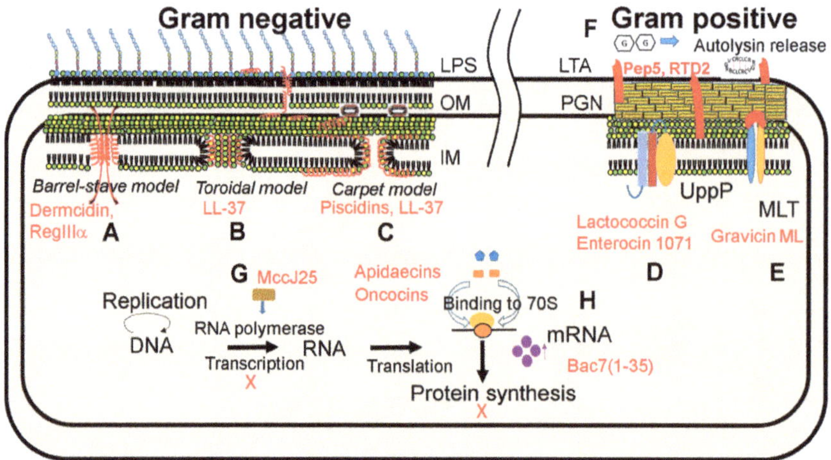

Figure 1. Mechanisms of action of antimicrobial peptides in 2014. Membrane channel formation (**A**) is proposed for dermicidin [76] and transmembrane pore formation for C-type lectin RegIIIα [77]. While human LL-37 [78] may form a toroidal pore (**B**), it started with a carpet model [79] (**C**) where antimicrobial peptides such as piscidins [72] are located on the membrane surface. Receptor mediated binding was observed for Lactococcin G and Enterocin 1071, which bind to UppP, an enzyme involved in cell wall synthesis (**D**) [80]. In addition, Gravicin ML binds to maltose ABC receptors (**E**) [81]. Further, RTD2, as well as lantibiotic Pep5, interacts with membranes causing the release of autolysin (**F**) [82]. Beyond membranes, bacterial MccJ25 could inhibit RNA polymerase (**G**) [83], while apidaecins, oncocins [84] and Bac7 [85] inhibit protein synthesis by binding to ribosomal proteins (**H**). Abbreviations used in the figures are OM, outer membrane; IM, inner membrane; PGN, peptidoglycan; LTA, lipoteichoic acid; MLT, maltose transporter. In addition, refer to the text.

Human α-defensin HNP1 and β-defensin hBD-3 are known to inhibit cell wall synthesis [86,87]. What about θ-defensins [16]? In 2014, Selsted and colleagues asked this question. In collaboration with Sahl, they found that RTD-2 did not bind to lipid II. Rather, it interacted with bacterial membranes in the presence of glucose. In addition, they detected the release of peptidoglycan lytic enzymes (or autolysins) by *S. aureus*. Interestingly, bacterial lantibiotic Pep5 can work in the same manner [82]. There is precedence for such a similarity. Like defensins, it is common for lantibiotics to inhibit cell wall synthesis by binding to lipid II [88]. In addition, some lantibitics and cyclotides share the same phosphatidylethanolamine (PE) lipid target [89,90]. Such a cyclotide binding to PE-rich membrane rafts is proposed to be responsible for activity against cancer and HIV-1 [91]. The similarity between cyclotides and lantibiotics was initially suggested by their similar amino acid composition plots [63]. The mechanistic similarities between thioether bonded lantibiotics and disulfide bonded defensing-like peptides are remarkable (Table 2), supporting a recent universal peptide classification that groups them into one big class: sidechain-sidechain linked peptides [9].

Table 2. Mechanistic similarities between thioether-bonded lantibiotics and disulfide-boned peptides.

Mechanism	Lantibiotic Examples	Disulfide-Linked Examples
Inhibition of cell wall synthesis [1]	Nisin A, lacticin 3147, mersacidin, bovicin HJ50	HNP1, hBD-3, plectasin, lucifensin, eurocin, copsin
Membrane and autolysin release	Pep5	θ-defensins such as RTD-2
Binding to lipid PE	Duramycins, cinnamycin	Kalata B1, cycloviolacin O_2

[1] Selected from the APD [7,8]. A more complete list can be searched in the APD.

For years, proline-rich peptides were proposed to act by binding to heat shock proteins [92]. Two papers published in 2014 challenged this view. Krizsan *et al.* found that insect-derived proline-rich apidaecins and oncocins inhibited bacterial protein translation at the 70S ribosome [84]. Both cationic and hydrophobic amino acids of the peptides were involved in such binding. Interestingly, Mardirossian *et al.* also observed that Bac7(1-35), another proline-rich peptide corresponding to N-terminal 35 residues of bovine cathelicidin Bac7, could accumulate within *E. coli* to a high concentration of 340 μM and inhibits protein synthesis by targeting ribosomal proteins [85]. These studies indicate that the well-documented chaperone DnaK is unlikely the major target for proline-rich peptides. Of note, bacterial lasso peptides such as microcin J25 (MccJ25) can inhibit RNA polymerase [83].

Some antimicrobial peptides can associate with DNA. In 2014, Ghosh *et al.* found that the WW motif of indolicidin is essential for DNA binding. They provided high-resolution structural information for the interaction of indolicidin with duplex DNA [93]. Such a structure can be useful for designing novel antibiotics.

Interestingly, some bacteriocins use receptors as the target. While garvicin ML recognizes a maltose ABC transporter, LsbB uses metallopeptidase as the targets [81]. In 2014, Kjos *et al.* found lactococcin G and enterocin 1071 (two-chain bacteriocins) used UppP as the receptor. UppP is an enzyme involved in cell wall synthesis [80]. Such findings not only enrich our view on the mechanisms of action of antimicrobial peptides, but also open new opportunities for antimicrobial development.

Although it is likely that some antimicrobial peptides mainly utilize one mechanism to inhibit bacteria, a single peptide may also deploy multiple mechanisms, rendering it difficult for pathogens to develop resistance. In 2014, Wenzel *et al.* illustrated this using a model arginine and tryptophan-rich peptide RWRWRW-NH_2 (C-terminal amidation) [94]. The peptide is primarily membrane targeting (e.g., D and L-forms have same activity) and only a very small population can enter the bacterial cell. As a new mechanism, the authors found that multiple surface proteins could be delocalized by the peptide. While the replacement of cytochrome C hinders bacterial energy metabolism, delocalization of MinD interferes with bacterial replication. Another surface protein, MurG, can also be delocalized, leading to impaired bacterial cell wall synthesis. The authors proposed that such bacterial surface protein delocalization by cationic antimicrobial peptides may be a general mechanism. Our own recent findings may provide additional insight into this protein delocalization. Surface attachment is usually mediated by a short amphipathic sequence, which weakly interacts with bacterial membranes [95]. In contrast, cationic antimicrobial peptides are able to better interact with bacterial membranes since they have a broader hydrophobic surface or higher membrane perturbation potential [96]. Such a membrane-binding difference could be one of the fundamental reasons for surface proteins to be replaced by cationic antimicrobial peptides. In addition, membrane binding of short amphipathic sequences requires anionic lipids [95]. When short cationic peptides cause lipid domain formation [94, 97,98], the migration of anionic lipids toward cationic antimicrobial peptides could weaken the attachment of surface proteins to the re-organized membranes, causing protein delocalization and loss of function as demonstrated by Wenzel *et al.* [94].

A single peptide can also possess multiple functions and human cathelicidin LL-37 is a typical example for this [99]. The observation that LL-37 can associate with DNA led to the idea that DNA binding may be part of the bacterial killing mechanism as well. However, Mardirossian *et al.* showed that only 5% of LL-37 inhibited protein synthesis [85]. In agreement, we did not observe a correlation between peptide activity and DNA retardation (Lau, K.; Lushnikova, T.; Wang, G., unpublished results). However, we did observe a correlation between membrane permeation and antimicrobial activity of LL-37 fragments [100]. These results support the existing view that membrane permeation and disruption by the helical region (residues 2-31) is the major mechanism via which LL-37 kills bacteria [78,79,97]. It appears that nucleic acid binding plays a more important role in RNA delivery into endosomes [101] and in stabilizing neutrophil extracellular traps to prevent DNA cleavage [102]. Moreover, human LL-37 can associate with cell receptors to trigger signal transduction [103,104]. Interestingly, LL-37 also modulates innate immunity by promoting macrophages to phagocyte bacteria [105] or influencing neutrophil responses to influenza A virus [106]. In addition, overexpressed LL-37, as an antigen, can be specifically recognized by CD4+ and/or CD8+ T cells in psoriasis [107]. It is clear that the multifunctional roles of human LL-37 are realized by its ability to recognize and interact with different molecular targets and immune cells.

4.2. Resistance Genes for Pathogens and Survival Skills for Commensal Bacteria

It has been appreciated that bacteria have been co-evolving with host defense peptides [108]. Some have learned how to avoid the attack by cationic peptides. The major mechanism appears to alter cell envelope charge and composition. In addition, an ATP-binding cassette (ABC) transporter coupled with an adjacent two-component system (TCS) also constitutes a resistance module against antimicrobial peptides [109,110]. Elucidation of the genetic basis of bacterial resistance may be helpful for the design of more potent antibiotics. In the following sections, we highlight progress made in this direction during 2014.

4.2.1. Gram-Positive Bacteria

One can identify the bacterial genes involved in peptide response by two methods: proteome analysis or genome analysis. Using proteome analysis of bacitracin-treated and untreated cells, Gebhard *et al.* identified an ABC transporter EF2050-2049 of *Enterococcus faecalis* that mediates resistance against bacitracin [109]. To validate this, they transferred the resistance and regulatory pathway to *B. subtilis*, leading to bacitracin resistance. Thus, the ABC transporter and the TCS are indeed required for resistance to antimicrobial peptides. Nevertheless, a previous genomic analysis identified two such ABC transporters [110], which were induced by bacitracin [109]. Based on these results, the authors proposed a model for the bacitracin resistance network of *E. faecalis*. The presence of bacitracin is initially detected by the EF2752-51 ABC transporter, which relays this signal to an adjacent TCS (EF0926-27). Activation of the regulatory domain of the TCS leads to an increase in expression of the EF2050-49 ABC transporter that confers resistance to antimicrobial peptides. This two transporters and one TCS network mechanism [109] differs from those single ABC transporter and TCS cases where the transporter senses the peptide and relays this signal to the adjacent TCS that upregulates the same ABC transporter for resistance [110].

The five-component system GraXSR-VraFG of *S. aureus* is well-established as the major sensing and resistance system [111] that reduces the toxic effect of cationic antimicrobial peptides by upregulating genes such as *mprF* and *dltABCD*. While MprF can put lysines on anionic phophatidylglycerols (PGs), DltABCD can modify the cell wall by transferring of D-alanine into teichoic acids [108,112]. GraSR was found to regulate the *dltABCD* and *mprF* genes [113,114]. In 2014, a loop region of sensor protein GraS was identified to recognize cationic peptides. Cheung *et al.* generated mutants of *graS* from the MRSA strain MW2. Deletion of *graS* (ΔgraS strain) or its 9-amino acid extracellular loop region (ΔEL strain) made the strain more susceptible to daptomycin, polymyxin B, human neutrophil defensin 1 (HNP-1), and RP-1 (a platelet factor 4 derived peptide that retains activity in blood). Meanwhile, these mutants became less infectious *in vivo* in an endocarditis model. Interestingly, a synthetic trimeric loop region EL mimic, *i.e.*, $(DYDFPIDSL)_3$, could protect the parental MW2 strain from killing by those cationic peptides. These results suggest that the acidic residues in the extracellular loop region of GraS can directly interact with cationic peptides for sensing and activation [115].

It has been elucidated that Group A Streptococcus responds to the human antimicrobial peptide LL-37 by upregulating virulence factors controlled by the CsrRS system. In 2014, Velarde *et al.* identified RI-10, the smallest LL-37 fragment required to bind to CsrRS using a series of synthetic LL-37 fragments. RI-10 can directly bind to sensor kinase CsrS to activate the expression of virulence factors [116]. The same peptide was previously found by us to have no antibacterial activity against bacteria [97,98]. Since antimicrobial activity is not required for this recognition by kinase receptor, such a response could occur *in vivo* at a very low level of LL-37, which is not high enough to kill the bacteria. We propose that interfacial cationic residues R23 and K25, which are important for membrane permeation and bacterial killing [100], are also important residues for interaction with the acidic amino acids on the CsrS receptor.

4.2.2. Gram-Negative Bacteria

Different from Gram-positive bacteria, LPS is the major component in the outer membranes of Gram-negative bacteria [66]. Modifications of bacterial LPS provide a general mechanism that confers resistance to cationic antimicrobial peptides [117]. The 2014 research on the genetic basis of bacterial resistance yielded additional support for this. First, pathogenic *Vibrio cholerae* strains can be >100-fold more resistant to polymyxins by modifying LPS (*i.e.*, glycylation). Henderson *et al.* confirmed AlmF as an aminoacyl carrier protein, which is activated by the enzyme AlmE. Interestingly, these proteins in the AlmEFG trio system function in a manner similar to nonribosomal peptide synthetases [118]. Second, the resistance of human pathogen *Neisseria gonorrhoeae* results from phosphoethanolamine (PEA) decoration of lipid A by transferase encoded by the *lptA* gene [119–121]. Kandler *et al.* found that high-frequency mutation in a polynucleotide repeat of the *lptA* gene influences bacterial resistance. An *lptA* mutant is highly susceptible to cationic peptides [122]. In addition, the PEA-modification of lipid A has an immunostimulatory role during infection [123]. Third, in the case of the gastrointestinal pathogen *S. typhimurium*, resistance genes involving both LPS defects and mutation in *phoP* were found from a transposon library in 1992 [124]. The PhoPQ two-component system regulates peptide resistance, bacterial lipid A remodeling, and intracellular survival within acidified phagosomes. In 2014, the PhoPQ system was found to also regulate acidic glycerophospholipid content in the outer membrane [125]. These authors have recently summarized the resistance strategies of *S. typhi* [126,127].

In summary, both Gram-positive and Gram-negative bacteria are able to decorate their cellular surfaces to make them less attractive to cationic antimicrobial peptides. Interestingly, a recent study reveals that gut bacteria can use a similar mechanism by removing a phosphate group from LPS [128]. Here a resistant mechanism for "bad bugs" has become a survival strategy for "good bugs". Therefore, such surface decorations achieved by a different chemistry provide a general mechanism that enables bacteria, for good or bad, to "work under an umbrella" to dodge the "bullets" of the host.

5. Potential Applications of Antimicrobial Peptides

5.1. Toward Therapeutic Uses

There is continued interest in developing therapeutic uses for antimicrobial peptides. Because of molecular simplicity and easy synthesis, linear peptides have been extensively explored for favorable properties. Here we highlight a structure-based design based on the human cathelicidin LL-37. Wang identified a chymotrypsin-resistant template by screening an LL-37 peptide library [129]. This template contains partial D-amino acids and has a novel amphipathic structure [130]. However, it is not active against community-associated methicillin-resistant *S. aureus* (MRSA) USA300. Based on the 3D structure, we enhanced anti-MRSA activity of the peptide by inserting a bulkier hydrophobic group into the structural cavity. One of the peptide analogs, 17BIPHE2, not only eliminated MRSA, but also recruited monocytes to the infection site [129]. In addition, other approaches were explored to make use of LL-37 or hBD-2. Since cathelicidin can reverse intestinal fibrosis in models of colitis [131], this peptide may be used to treat inflammatory bowel disease (IBD) by introducing cathelicidin-overexpressing bacteria. Using an adenoviral vector to deliver the gene of hBD-2, Woo *et al.* found both viral inhibition and clearance for experimental otitis media [132]. In 2014, LL-37-containing vector was electroporated to promote skin wound healing [133]. In addition, 1,25-dihydroxyvitamin D3 (active form) was also used to induce both LL-37 and hBD-2 production in keratinocytes from diabetic foot ulcers, promoting wound healing [134]. UV light or sunlight may be an alternative since hydroxylation of vitamin D can occur [135]. It is notable that traditional practice can also boost our immune systems. While yoga stretching significantly increases human hBD-2 [136], green tea helps the production of lactoferrin in saliva after exercise [137]. Although at the early stage, these positive results on antimicrobial peptides imply that our traditional life styles can be helpful to keep us healthy.

Unlike linear peptides that can be rapidly degraded by proteases in hours, circular peptides have inherent stability. This is because these peptides such as cyclotides comprise three conserved disulfide bonds in addition to a peptide bond that connects the N- and C-termini. Consequently, there is great interest in utilizing these natural templates to engineer useful therapeutics [138,139]. In 2014, Craik and colleagues demonstrated the molecular grafting technology where a desired antigenic peptide was inserted into an exposed loop region of kalata B1 [140]. This technology confers protease stability to the sequence motif, which can otherwise be rapidly degraded when tested alone. MOG3, one out of the seven peptides grafted to loop 5, was used to vaccinate mice and found to display *in vivo* efficacy in an animal model of multiple sclerosis, an inflammatory disease of the central nervous system. Taken together with previous examples [138,139], these authors proved the concept of segment grafting at loops 5 and 6 of cyclotides. It appears that sequence composition rather than length determines whether the grafted segment is tolerated without disrupting the protein fold. To obtain a sufficient amount of material for research, cyclotides were initially isolated from plants [141]. Later, chemical synthesis was established [142]. In 2014, two laboratories reported an alternative approach by using engineered sortase A to make the circular molecule [143,144]. A more efficient synthesis will bring us one step closer to practical use of these interesting templates.

5.2. Peptide Surface Coating

Immobilization of antimicrobial peptides (either covalently or adsorbed) onto solid supports extends their capabilities as surface-active molecules. This direction of research aims at improving biomedical devices, drug delivery systems, bio-sensor and detection, and so on. Recent advances in the field include simplification of the chemistry for surface attachment, development of novel substrate-attaching platforms, including nanomaterial for wider applications, product development with promising proof of concepts and *in vivo* testing in animal models.

Of all the problems related to loss in efficiency of medically implantable medical devices is the development of microbial biofilms. Peptide immobilization has been shown to reduce bacterial colonization and biofilm formation. However, the major challenges that often hinder the immobilization of antimicrobial peptides are the inefficiency of the conjugation chemistries and their inability to achieve a sufficient surface concentration of peptides, along with the limited number of usable biomaterials. A recent study by Lim *et al.* [145] demonstrated a simple dopamine based chemical reaction for the functionalization of antimicrobial peptides onto a commonly used Silicon Foley catheter. Not only did the catheter prototype reduce biofilm formation by common pathogens that caused a urinary tract infection, it was also stable for 21 days. In addition, hLF1-11 immobilized onto titanium [146] has been shown to possess excellent anti-biofilm properties. There have also been improvements in other chemical platforms, including the development of thiolated self-assembled monolayer on a gold surface to which small peptides, temporin-SHf, can be tethered, resulting in broad-spectrum activity [147].

To understand the possible influence of structure and dynamics on immobilized antimicrobial peptides and to apply rational design, molecular dynamics simulation studies were carried out on cecropin P1 immobilized on silane-EG4-maleimide self-assembled monolayers [148]. Other factors governing immobilization reactions, such as spacer chain length, reactant concentration and energy dependence, are demonstrated by Mishra *et al.* [149]. Additional coating strategies can be found in a recent review [150]. Moving toward practical applications, a significant *in vivo* study is presented by Dutta *et al.* [151]. Melimine immobilized eye lenses are not only cytotoxically safe but also possess antibacterial activity after worn as tested in both rabbit and human. In addition, another peptide SESB2V immobilized on titanium surfaces prevents perioperative corneal infection in a rabbit keratitis model [152].

5.3. *Nanoparticle-Based Drug Delivery Systems*

Apart from the anti-biofilm and antibacterial functions, antimicrobial peptides tagged to nanoparticles impart a site-specific targeting and delivery of drug molecules. It can be used in treating a variety of diseases, including cancer. Currently, dermaseptin entrapped chitosan nanoparticles have been shown to possess excellent antitumor activities [153]. Moving one step forward, dual targeting nanoparticles with both blood−brain barrier (BBB) and blood−brain tumor barrier (BBTB) including glioma cell were achieved by functionalizing lactoferrin to the surface of poly(ethylene glycol)−poly(lactic acid) nanoparticles. Administration with tLyP-1, a tumor-homing peptide that mediates tissue penetration through the neuropilin-1-dependent internalization pathway, resulted in deep penetration of the nanoparticle into the glioma parenchyma [154]. It opens a new direction for administration of antitumerogenic drugs with high penetration capability.

Additionally, glutamic acid substitution of basic residues in LL-37, melittin, and bombolitin V linked to lipid nanoparticles could be used for endosomal escape and efficient gene delivery using intravenous injections. These yield expression levels comparable to those obtained using Lipofectamine 2000 and the probable mode of action resembles viruses [155]. Antimicrobial peptides have also been shown to have superb drug releasing properties in PEG-PLGA microparticles [156]. The direct evidence is presented by encapsulating LL-37 in PLGA nanoparticles by Chereddy *et al.* [157]. PLGA-LL-37 nanoparticles as a biodegradable drug delivery system were found to promote wound closure. It functions due to the sustained release of both LL-37 and lactate, and induction of enhanced cell migration without effects on the metabolism and proliferation of keratinocytes. Moreover, peptides as short as dimer conjugated to naphthalene could be used as antimicrobial nanomaterials in eliminating biofilm infections and for drug delivery [158].

5.4. *Biosensors and Detection*

Antimicrobial peptides can also serve as indicators and diagnostic agents. The approach is more cost effective than standard PCR or antibody-based techniques. Detection of bacterial pathogens in a microfluidic chip where antimicrobial peptides are immobilized via cysteine-gold interaction could produce a rapid electrical detection with sufficient sensor signal that allows the detection of pathogens (both Gram-negative and Gram-positive) at a density as low as 10^5 cfu/mL within 25 min [159]. While another platform for the detection of only Gram-positive bacterial strains could reach 10^3 cfu/mL via immobilizing class IIa bacteriocins [160]. In addition, specific detection of fungal *C. albicans* can also be made by using peptide nucleic acid probes [161].

6. Perspectives

It is great news that acquired resistance did not become an issue after decade-long use of antimicrobial peptides such as tyrothricin [162]. Such an observation is encouraging to the current effort in development of antimicrobial peptides into novel therapeutic molecules [63]. From 2000 to 2014, about 100 new antimicrobial peptides were entered into the APD every year [26]. As of December 2014, there were 2493 peptides in this database [7–9]. We anticipate that the important work on the isolation and characterization of novel antimicrobial peptides from new organisms will continue. Scientifically, new peptide sequences will improve our knowledge of natural antimicrobial peptides. As shown in Table 1, the new members can refine the boundary parameters for natural antimicrobial peptides [9]. With the identification of a sufficient number of representative peptide sequences, the APD database will more accurately identify natural peptides most similar to the input sequence. It will facilitate the development of new programs to better predict the likelihood of a new peptide to be antimicrobial. In addition, a unique peptide may directly become a candidate lead for the development of novel antimicrobials to meet the challenge of the antibiotic resistance problem. However, it is important to validate whether a bacteriocin has any undesired virulent property that promotes infection [21].

The 2014 research also enabled us to connect the dots for known human antimicrobial peptides, leading to an improved understanding of their functional roles in innate immunity. Surprisingly, a different form of human cathelicidin peptide can be rapidly expressed by skin fat cells in response to the *S. aureus* invasion, underscoring a direct defense role of human cathelicidin peptides [50]. It is remarkable that a single LL-37 molecule can perform multiple functions by recognizing a variety of molecular partners or receptors on immune cells. In 2014, pH-dependent oligomerization of LL-37 is connected to the delivery of dsRNA into endosomes for subsequent interactions with TLR3 [64]. Although the details are to be elucidated, we propose that the terminal regions of LL-37 contain an important molecular switch based on NMR data [63]. It is demonstrated that local conditions are essential for a proper function of human antimicrobial peptides. While human HD-6, like hBD-1, is active only after disruption of disulfide bonds under reduced conditions [43], many other defensins in the folded form can directly recognize specific lipids in pathogen's membranes [163,164]. During such a molecular recognition process, the flexible residues in the loop regions of these small defense proteins are found to be essential based on several structural studies [163–166].

The 2014 results further expanded our view on the mechanism of action of antimicrobial peptides (summarized in Figure 1). While select antimicrobial peptides are known to inhibit cell wall synthesis, many target bacterial membranes. Surface-binding peptides are shown to be able to replace weakly attached membrane proteins, thereby interfering with bacterial physiology globally [94]. Beyond membranes, bacteriocins can use cell receptors as a target [81]. It has been known for a while that proline-rich peptides interact with heat shock proteins [92]. However, the molecular target has now been traced to ribosomal proteins. The binding of proline-rich peptides leads to inhibition of protein synthesis [84,85].

Although there are few examples, structure-based design has been demonstrated [129,140], leading to antimicrobials or vaccines with desired properties. The overall goal of peptide engineering is to establish or identify a proper peptide template with desired potency, stability, and cell selectivity. In addition, one may also mimic nature's wisdom. Based on the precursor protein construction, one can design pro-peptide forms to minimize potential cytotoxicity and protease degradation. In 2014, Forde *et al.* illustrated this strategy as a potential therapy for cystic fibrosis [167,168]. Nature has created other strategies to circumvent rapid peptide degradation by forming a complex structure. For instance, human LL-37 can oligomerize at physiological pH into nanoparticles to resist the action of proteases [63]. Likewise, LL-37 can bind to DNA to stabilize the entire NETs structure [169]. In 2014, Bachrach and colleagues showed that human LL-37 could also be protected by actin, thereby maintaining its antimicrobial activity *in vivo* [170,171]. There are also natural ways to reduce potential cytotoxicity of antimicrobial peptides. In 2014, Svensson *et al.* discovered that peptide p33 expressed on the surface of various cell types can reduce the potential cytotoxicity of human LL-37 [172]. Moreover, Hiemstra *et al.* discovered the nanoparticle-like vesicles in the human urinary tract [173]. It is predictable that novel functional modes of human innate immune peptides will continue to emerge. All these natural mechanisms may hold the key to future therapeutics.

We anticipate continued efforts in the development of potential applications of antimicrobial peptides, including peptide production methods. Peptide engineering, formulation, and delivery technologies may further expand the horizon of antimicrobial peptides in benefiting human beings [174]. Such applications can vary from medical surface cleaning, water quality monitoring and disinfection, sterile surface materials, to new drugs for infectious diseases [175,176]. Antimicrobial peptides may be included in existing detergent formulation and disinfectants to reduce bacterial biofilms on hospital surfaces [177]. Bovicin HC5 and nisin can be used to treat food-contact surface to reduce bacterial attachment and subsequent biofilm formation [178,179]. It has been demonstrated that injection of an engineered LL-37 peptide or coating peptides to the device surface can prevent biofilm formation [129,145,146]. Importantly, a combined use of antimicrobial peptides with traditional antibiotics can be a more effective strategy to treat bacterial biofilms [180–182]. Finally, molecules that interfere with or even weaken the process of biofilm formation [183–189] can also be combined with antimicrobial peptides to achieve an optimal treatment of bacterial biofilms.

Acknowledgments: This study is supported by the grants from the NIAID/NIH R01AI105147 and the state of Nebraska to GW. We thank Cheryl Putnam for final editing.

Author Contributions: GW conceived the project. GW and BM drafted the manuscript. All authors were involved in literature search, discussion and writing.

Conflicts of Interest: No conflicts of interest was declared.

References

1. Zasloff, M. Antimicrobial peptides of multicellullar organisms. *Nature* **2002**, *415*, 359–365. [CrossRef]
2. Lai, Y.; Gallo, R.L. AMPed up immunity: How antimicrobial peptides have multiple roles in immune defense. *Trends Immunol.* **2009**, *30*, 131–141. [CrossRef] [PubMed]
3. Hancock, R.E.; Lehrer, R. Cationic peptides: A new source of antibiotics. *Trends Biotechnol.* **1998**, *16*, 82–88. [CrossRef] [PubMed]
4. Yeaman, M.R.; Yount, N.Y. Mechanisms of Antimicrobial Peptide Action and Resistance. *Pharmacol. Rev.* **2003**, *55*, 27–55. [CrossRef] [PubMed]
5. Brogden, K.A. Antimicrobial peptides: Pore formers or metabolic inhibitors in bacteria? *Natl. Rev. Microbiol.* **2005**, *3*, 238–250. [CrossRef]
6. NCBI Resource Coordinators. Database resources of the National Center for Biotechnology Information. *Nucleic Acids Res.* **2015**, *43*, D6–D17.
7. Wang, Z.; Wang, G. APD: The antimicrobial peptide database. *Nucleic Acids Res.* **2004**, *32*, D590–D592. [CrossRef] [PubMed]
8. Wang, G.; Li, X.; Wang, Z. The updated antimicrobial peptide database and its application in peptide design. *Nucleic Acids Res.* **2009**, *37*, D933–D937. [CrossRef] [PubMed]
9. Wang, G. Improved methods for classification, prediction, and design of antimicrobial peptides. *Methods Mol. Biol.* **2015**, *1268*, 43–66. [PubMed]
10. Timeline of Antimicrobial Peptide Discovery. http://aps.unmc.edu/AP/timeline.php. Accessed on 16 March 2015.
11. Chakchouk-Mtibaa, A.; Elleuch, L.; Smaoui, S.; Najah, S.; Sellem, I.; Abdelkafi, S.; Mellouli, L. An antilisterial bacteriocin BacFL31 produced by *Enterococcus faecium* FL31 with a novel structure containing hydroxyproline residues. *Anaerobe* **2014**, *27C*, 1–6. [CrossRef] [PubMed]
12. Niggemann, J.; Bozko, P.; Bruns, N.; Wodtke, A.; Gieseler, M.T.; Thomas, K.; Jahns, C.; Nimtz, M.; Reupke, I.; Brüser, T.; *et al.* Baceridin, a cyclic hexapeptide from an epiphytic Bacillus strain, inhibits the proteasome. *Chembiochem* **2014**, *15*, 1021–1029. [CrossRef] [PubMed]
13. Gavrish, E.; Sit, C.S.; Cao, S.; Kandror, O.; Spoering, A.; Peoples, A.; Ling, L.; Fetterman, A.; Hughes, D.; Bissell, A.; *et al.* Lassomycin, a ribosomally synthesized cyclic peptide, kills mycobacterium tuberculosis by targeting the ATP-dependent protease ClpC1P1P2. *Chem. Biol.* **2014**, *21*, 509–518. [CrossRef] [PubMed]
14. Yamanaka, K.; Reynolds, K.A.; Kersten, R.D.; Ryan, K.S.; Gonzalez, D.J.; Nizet, V.; Dorrestein, P.C.; Moore, B.S. Direct cloning and refactoring of a silent lipopeptide biosynthetic gene cluster yields the antibiotic taromycin A. *Proc. Natl. Acad. Sci. U.S.A.* **2014**, *111*, 1957–1962. [CrossRef] [PubMed]
15. Scholz, R.; Vater, J.; Budiharjo, A.; Wang, Z.; He, Y.; Dietel, K.; Schwecke, T.; Herfort, S.; Lasch, P.; Borriss, R. Amylocyclicin, a Novel Circular Bacteriocin Produced by *Bacillus amyloliquefaciens* FZB42. *J. Bacteriol.* **2014**, *196*, 1842–1852. [CrossRef] [PubMed]
16. Tang, Y.Q.; Yuan, J.; Osapay, G.; Osapay, K.; Tran, D.; Miller, C.J.; Ouellette, A.J.; Selsted, M.E. A cyclic antimicrobial peptide produced in primate leukocytes by the ligation of two truncated alpha-defensins. *Science* **1999**, *286*, 498–502. [CrossRef] [PubMed]
17. Falcao, C.B.; de La Torre, B.G.; Pérez-Peinado, C.; Barron, A.E.; Andreu, D.; Rádis-Baptista, G. Vipericidins: a novel family of cathelicidin-related peptides from the venom gland of South American pit vipers. *Amino Acids* **2014**, *46*, 2561–2571. [CrossRef] [PubMed]
18. Conlon, J.M.; Mechkarska, M. Host-defense peptides with therapeutic potential from skin secretions of frogs from the family pipidae. *Pharmaceuticals* **2014**, *7*, 58–77. [CrossRef] [PubMed]

19. Guo, C.; Hu, Y.; Li, J.; Liu, Y.; Li, S.; Yan, K.; Wang, X.; Liu, J.; Wang, H. Identification of multiple peptides with antioxidant and antimicrobial activities from skin and its secretions of *Hylarana taipehensis*, *Amolops lifanensis*, and *Amolops granulosus*. *Biochimie.* **2014**, *105*, 192–201. [CrossRef] [PubMed]
20. Ryazantsev, D.Y.; Rogozhin, E.A.; Dimitrieva, T.V.; Drobyazina, P.E.; Khadeeva, N.V.; Egorov, T.A.; Grishin, E.V.; Zavriev, S.K. A novel hairpin-like antimicrobial peptide from barnyard grass (*Echinochloa crusgalli* L.) seeds: Structure-functional and molecular-genetics characterization. *Biochimie* **2014**, *99*, 63–70. [CrossRef] [PubMed]
21. Li, M.F.; Zhang, B.C.; Li, J.; Sun, L. Sil: A *Streptococcus iniae* bacteriocin with dual role as an antimicrobial and an immunomodulator that inhibits innate immune response and promotes *S. iniae* infection. *PLoS ONE* **2014**, *9*, e96222. [CrossRef] [PubMed]
22. Weisshoff, H.; Hentschel, S.; Zaspel, I.; Jarling, R.; Krause, E.; Pham, T.L. PPZPMs—A novel group of cyclic lipodepsipeptides produced by the Phytophthora alni associated strain Pseudomonas sp. JX090307—The missing link between the viscosin and amphisin group. *Nat. Prod. Commun.* **2014**, *9*, 989–996. [PubMed]
23. Trindade, F.; Amado, F.; Pinto da Costa, J.; Ferreira, R.; Maia, C.; Henriques, I.; Colaco, B.; Vitorino, R. Salivary peptidomic as a tool to disclose new potential antimicrobial peptides. *J. Proteomics* **2014**, *115C*, 49–57. [CrossRef] [PubMed]
24. Bouzid, W.; Verdenaud, M.; Klopp, C.; Ducancel, F.; Noirot, C.; Vetillard, A. *de novo* sequencing and transcriptome analysis for tetramorium bicarinatum: A comprehensive venom gland transcriptome analysis from an ant species. *BMC Genomics* **2014**, *15*, 987. [CrossRef] [PubMed]
25. Capriotti, A.L.; Cavaliere, C.; Foglia, P.; Piovesana, S.; Samperi, R.; Zenezini Chiozzi, R.; Lagana, A. Development of an analytical strategy for the identification of potential bioactive peptides generated by *in vitro* tryptic digestion of fish muscle proteins. *Anal. Bioanal. Chem.* **2015**, *407*, 845–854. [CrossRef] [PubMed]
26. Wang, G. Database-guided discovery of potent peptides to combat HIV-1 or superbugs. *Pharmaceuticals* **2013**, *6*, 728–758. [CrossRef] [PubMed]
27. Tareq, F.S.; Lee, M.A.; Lee, H.S.; Lee, Y.J.; Lee, J.S.; Hasan, C.M.; Islam, M.T.; Shin, H.J. Gageotetrins A-C, Noncytotoxic antimicrobial linear lipopeptides from a marine bacterium *Bacillus subtilis*. *Org. Lett.* **2014**, *16*, 928–931. [CrossRef] [PubMed]
28. Makovitzki, A.; Avrahami, D.; Shai, Y. Ultrashort antibacterial and antifungal lipopeptides. *Proc. Natl. Acad. Sci. U.S.A.* **2006**, *103*, 15997–16002. [CrossRef] [PubMed]
29. First in a New Class of Antibiotics. *FDA Consum* **2003**, *37*, 4.
30. Chopra, L.; Singh, G.; Choudhary, V.; Sahoo, D.K. Sonorensin: an antimicrobial peptide, belonging to the heterocycloanthracin subfamily of bacteriocins, from a new marine isolate, Bacillus sonorensis MT93. *Appl. Environ. Microbiol.* **2014**, *80*, 2981–2990. [CrossRef] [PubMed]
31. Mygind, P.H.; Fischer, R.L.; Schnorr, K.M.; Hansen, M.T.; Sonksen, C.P.; Ludvigsen, S.; Raventos, D.; Buskov, S.; Christensen, B.; De Maria, L.; *et al.* Plectasin is a peptide antibiotic with therapeutic potential from a saprophytic fungus. *Nature* **2005**, *437*, 975–980. [CrossRef] [PubMed]
32. Oeemig, J.S.; Lynggaard, C.; Knudsen, D.H.; Hansen, F.T.; Norgaard, K.D.; Schneider, T.; Vad, B.S.; Sandvang, D.H.; Nielsen, L.A.; Neve, S.; *et al.* Eurocin, a new fungal defensin: structure, lipid binding, and its mode of action. *J. Biol. Chem.* **2012**, *287*, 42361–42372. [CrossRef] [PubMed]
33. Essig, A.; Hofmann, D.; Munch, D.; Gayathri, S.; Kunzler, M.; Kallio, P.T.; Sahl, H.G.; Wider, G.; Schneider, T.; Aebi, M. Copsin, a novel peptide-based fungal antibiotic interfering with the peptidoglycan synthesis. *J. Biol. Chem.* **2014**, *289*, 34953–34964. [CrossRef] [PubMed]
34. Sharma, S.; Verma, H.N.; Sharma, N.K. Cationic bioactive peptide from the seeds of *Benincasa hispida*. *Int. J. Pept.* **2014**, *2014*, 156060. [CrossRef] [PubMed]
35. Kawabata, S.; Nagayama, R.; Hirata, M.; Shigenaga, T.; Agarwala, K.L.; Saito, T.; Cho, J.; Nakajima, H.; Takagi, T.; Iwanaga, S. Tachycitin, a small granular component in horseshoe crab hemocytes, is an antimicrobial protein with chitin-binding activity. *J. Biochem.* **1996**, *120*, 1253–1260. [CrossRef] [PubMed]
36. Conlon, J.M.; Mechkarska, M.; Emanahmed Coquet, L.; Jouenne, T.; Jérômeleprince Vaudry, H.; Hayes, M.P.; Padgett-Flohr, G. Host defense peptides in skin secretions of the Oregon spotted frog Ranapretiosa: Implications for species resistance to chytridiomycosis. *Dev. Comp. Immunol.* **2011**, *35*, 644–649. [CrossRef] [PubMed]
37. Thomas, S.; Karnik, S.; Barai, R.S.; Jayaraman, V.K.; Idicula-Thomas, S. CAMP: A useful resource for research on antimicrobial peptides. *Nucleic Acids Res.* **2010**, *38*, D774–D780. [CrossRef] [PubMed]

38. Lata, S.; Mishra, N.K.; Raghava, G.P. AntiBP2: Improved version of antibacterial peptide prediction. *BMC Bioinformatics* **2010**, *11*, S19. [CrossRef] [PubMed]
39. Xiao, X.; Wang, P.; Lin, W.Z.; Jia, J.H.; Chou, K.C. iAMP-2L: A two-level multi-label classifier for identifying antimicrobial peptides and their functional types. *Anal. Biochem.* **2013**, *436*, 168–177. [CrossRef] [PubMed]
40. Zanetti, M. The role of cathelicidins in the innate host defenses of mammals. *Curr. Issues Mol. Biol.* **2005**, *7*, 179–196. [PubMed]
41. Hao, X.; Yang, H.; Wei, L.; Yang, S.; Zhu, W.; Ma, D.; Yu, H.; Lai, R. Amphibian cathelicidin fills the evolutionary gap of cathelicidin in vertebrate. *Amino acids* **2012**, *43*, 677–685. [CrossRef] [PubMed]
42. Ling, G.; Gao, J.; Zhang, S.; Xie, Z.; Wei, L.; Yu, H.; Wang, Y. Cathelicidins from the bullfrog Rana catesbeiana provides novel template for peptide antibiotic design. *PLoS ONE* **2014**, *9*, e93216. [CrossRef] [PubMed]
43. Schroeder, B.O.; Ehmann, D.; Precht, J.C.; Castillo, P.A.; Kuchler, R.; Berger, J.; Schaller, M.; Stange, E.F.; Wehkamp, J. Paneth Cell Alpha-defensin 6 (HD-6) is an antimicrobial peptide. *Mucosal Immunol.* **2014**. [CrossRef]
44. Liu, H.; Yu, H.; Xin, A.; Shi, H.; Gu, Y.; Zhang, Y.; Diao, H.; Lin, D. Production and characterization of recombinant human beta-defensin DEFB120. *J. Pept. Sci.* **2014**, *20*, 251–257. [CrossRef] [PubMed]
45. Gela, A.; Kasetty, G.; Jovic, S.; Ekoff, M.; Nilsson, G.; Morgelin, M.; Kjellstrom, S.; Pease, J.E.; Schmidtchen, A.; Egesten, A. Eotaxin-3 (CCL26) Exerts innate host defense activities that are modulated by mast cell proteases. *Allergy* **2015**, *70*, 161–170. [CrossRef] [PubMed]
46. Becknell, B.; Eichler, T.E.; Beceiro, S.; Li, B.; Easterling, R.S.; Carpenter, A.R.; James, C.L.; McHugh, K.M.; Hains, D.S.; Partida-Sanchez, S.; *et al.* Ribonucleases 6 and 7 have antimicrobial function in the human and murine urinary tract. *Kidney Int.* **2015**, *87*, 151–161. [CrossRef] [PubMed]
47. Wang, G. Human antimicrobial peptides and proteins. *Pharmaceuticals* **2014**, *7*, 545–594. [CrossRef] [PubMed]
48. Boman, H.G. Antibacterial peptides: Basic facts and emerging concepts. *J. Inter. Med.* **2003**, *254*, 197–215. [CrossRef]
49. Gschwandtner, M.; Zhong, S.; Tschachler, A.; Mlitz, V.; Karner, S.; Elbe-Bürger, A.; Mildner, M. Fetal human keratinocytes produce large amounts of antimicrobial peptides: Involvement of histone-methylation processes. *J. Invest Dermatol.* **2014**, *134*, 2192–2201. [CrossRef] [PubMed]
50. Zhang, L.J.; Guerrero-Juarez, C.F.; Hata, T.; Bapat, S.P.; Ramos, R.; Plikus, M.V.; Gallo, R.L. Innate immunity. Dermal adipocytes protect against invasive *Staphylococcus aureus* skin infection. *Science* **2015**, *347*, 67–71.
51. Lee, P.H.; Ohtake, T.; Zaiou, M.; Murakami, M.; Rudisill, J.A.; Lin, K.H.; Gallo, R.L. Expression of an additional cathelicidin antimicrobial peptide protects against bacterial skin infection. *Proc. Natl. Acad. Sci. U.S.A.* **2005**, *102*, 3750–3755. [CrossRef] [PubMed]
52. Zhao, C.; Wang, I.; Lehrer, R.I. Widespread expression of beta-defensin hBD-1 in human secretory glands and epithelial cells. *FEBS Lett.* **1996**, *396*, 319–322. [CrossRef] [PubMed]
53. Furci, L.; Baldan, R.; Bianchini, V.; Trovato, A.; Ossi, C.; Cichero, P.; Cirillo, D.M. A new role for human alpha-defensin 5 in the fight against *Clostridium difficile* hypervirulent strains. *Infect. Immun.* **2015**, *83*, 986–995. [CrossRef] [PubMed]
54. Hubert, P.; Herman, L.; Roncarati, P.; Maillard, C.; Renoux, V.; Demoulin, S.; Erpicum, C.; Foidart, J.M.; Boniver, J.; Noel, A.; *et al.* Altered alpha-defensin 5 expression in cervical squamocolumnar junction: implication in the formation of a viral/tumour-permissive microenvironment. *J. Pathol.* **2014**, *234*, 464–477. [CrossRef] [PubMed]
55. Wiens, M.E.; Smith, J.G. Alpha-Defensin HD5 Inhibits Furin Cleavage of HPV16 L2 to Block Infection. *J. Virol.* **2014**, *89*, 2866–2874.
56. Wommack, A.J.; Ziarek, J.J.; Tomaras, J.; Chileveru, H.R.; Zhang, Y.; Wagner, G.; Nolan, E.M. Discovery and characterization of a disulfide-locked C(2)-symmetric defensin peptide. *J. Am. Chem. Soc.* **2014**, *136*, 13494–13497. [CrossRef] [PubMed]
57. Schroeder, B.O.; Wu, Z.; Nuding, S.; Groscurth, S.; Marcinowski, M.; Beisner, J.; Buchner, J.; Schaller, M.; Stange, E.F.; Wehkamp, J. Reduction of disulphide bonds unmasks potent antimicrobial activity of human beta-defensin 1. *Nature* **2011**, *469*, 419–423. [CrossRef] [PubMed]
58. Porter, E.M.; Poles, M.A.; Lee, J.S.; Naitoh, J.; Bevins, C.L.; Ganz, T. Isolation of human intestinal defensins from ileal neobladder urine. *FEBS Lett.* **1998**, *434*, 272–276. [CrossRef] [PubMed]

59. Chu, H.; Pazgier, M.; Jung, G.; Nuccio, S.P.; Castillo, P.A.; de Jong, M.F.; Winter, M.G.; Winter, S.E.; Wehkamp, J.; Shen, B.; *et al.* Human Alpha-Defensin 6 Promotes mucosal innate immunity through self-assembled peptide nanonets. *Science* **2012**, *337*, 477–481. [CrossRef] [PubMed]
60. Abou Alaiwa, M.H.; Reznikov, L.R.; Gansemer, N.D.; Sheets, K.A.; Horswill, A.R.; Stoltz, D.A.; Zabner, J.; Welsh, M.J. PH Modulates the activity and synergism of the airway surface liquid antimicrobials beta-defensin-3 and LL-37. *Proc. Natl. Acad. Sci. U.S.A.* **2014**, *111*, 18703–18708. [CrossRef] [PubMed]
61. Johansson, J.; Gudmundsson, G.H.; Rottenberg, M.E.; Berndt, K.D.; Agerberth, B. Conformation-dependent antibacterial activity of the naturally occurring human peptide LL-37. *J. Biol. Chem.* **1998**, *273*, 3718–3724. [CrossRef] [PubMed]
62. Xhindoli, D.; Pacor, S.; Guida, F.; Antcheva, N.; Tossi, A. Native oligomerization determines the mode of action and biological activities of human cathelicidin LL-37. *Biochem. J.* **2014**, *457*, 263–275. [CrossRef] [PubMed]
63. Wang, G. *Antimicrobial Peptides: Discovery, Design and Novel Therapeutic Strategies*; CABI: Wallingford, UK, 2010.
64. Singh, D.; Vaughan, R.; Kao, C.C. LL-37 peptide enhancement of signal transduction by toll-like receptor 3 is regulated by pH: identification of a peptide antagonist of LL-37. *J. Biol. Chem.* **2014**, *289*, 27614–27624. [CrossRef] [PubMed]
65. Yamasaki, K.; Schauber, J.; Coda, A.; Lin, H.; Dorschner, R.A.; Schechter, N.M.; Bonnart, C.; Descargues, P.; Hovnanian, A.; Gallo, R.L. Kallikrein-mediated proteolysis regulates the antimicrobial effects of cathelicidins in skin. *FASEB J.* **2006**, *20*, 2068–2080. [CrossRef] [PubMed]
66. Wang, G.; Mishra, B.; Epand, R.F.; Epand, R.M. High-quality 3D structures shine light on antibacterial, anti-biofilm and antiviral activities of human cathelicidin LL-37 and its fragments. *Biochim. Biophys. Acta* **2014**, *1838*, 2160–2172. [CrossRef] [PubMed]
67. Koziel, J.; Bryzek, D.; Sroka, A.; Maresz, K.; Glowczyk, I.; Bielecka, E.; Kantyka, T.; Pyrc, K.; Svoboda, P.; Pohl, J.; *et al.* Citrullination alters immunomodulatory function of ll-37 essential for prevention of endotoxin-induced sepsis. *J. Immunol.* **2014**, *192*, 5363–5372. [CrossRef] [PubMed]
68. Picchianti, M.; Russo, C.; Castagnini, M.; Biagini, M.; Soldaini, E.; Balducci, E. NAD-Dependent ADP-ribosylation of the human antimicrobial and immune-modulatory peptide LL-37 by ADP-ribosyltransferase-1. *Innate Immun.* **2015**, *21*, 314–321. [CrossRef] [PubMed]
69. Sørensen, O.E.; Gram, L.; Johnsen, A.H.; Andersson, E.; Bangsbøll, S.; Tjabringa, G.S.; Hiemstra, P.S.; Malm, J.; Egesten, A.; Borregaard, N. Processing of seminal plasma hCAP-18 to ALL-38 by gastricsin: A novel mechanism of generating antimicrobial peptides in vagina. *J. Biol. Chem.* **2003**, *278*, 28540–28546. [CrossRef] [PubMed]
70. Nguyen, L.T.; Haney, E.F.; Vogel, H.J. The expanding scope of antimicrobial peptide structures and their modes of action. *Trends Biotechnol.* **2011**, *29*, 464–472. [CrossRef] [PubMed]
71. Gazit, E.; Miller, I.R.; Biggin, P.C.; Sansom, M.S.; Shai, Y. Structure and orientation of the mammalian antibacterial peptide cecropin p1 within phospholipid membranes. *J. Mol. Biol.* **1996**, *258*, 860–870. [CrossRef] [PubMed]
72. Perrin, B.S., Jr.; Tian, Y.; Fu, R.; Grant, C.V.; Chekmenev, E.Y.; Wieczorek, W.E.; Dao, A.E.; Hayden, R.M.; Burzynski, C.M.; Venable, R.M.; *et al.* High-resolution structures and orientations of antimicrobial peptides piscidin 1 and piscidin 3 in fluid bilayers reveal tilting, kinking, and bilayer immersion. *J. Am. Chem. Soc.* **2014**, *136*, 3491–3504. [CrossRef] [PubMed]
73. Fox, R.O., Jr.; Richards, F.M. A voltage-gated ion channel model inferred from the crystal structure of alamethicin at 1.5-Å resolution. *Nature* **1982**, *300*, 325–330. [CrossRef] [PubMed]
74. Kovacs, F.; Quine, J.; Cross, T.A. Validation of the single-stranded channel conformation of gramicidin A by solid-state NMR. *Proc. Natl. Acad. Sci. U.S.A.* **1999**, *96*, 7910–7915. [CrossRef] [PubMed]
75. Burian, M.; Schittek, B. The secrets of dermcidin action. *Int. J. Med. Microbiol.* **2015**, *305*, 283–286. [CrossRef] [PubMed]
76. Song, C.; Weichbrodt, C.; Salnikov, E.S.; Dynowski, M.; Forsberg, B.O.; Bechinger, B.; Steinem, C.; de Groot, B.L.; Zachariae, U.; Zeth, K. Crystal structure and functional mechanism of a human antimicrobial membrane channel. *Proc. Natl. Acad. Sci. U.S.A.* **2013**, *110*, 4586–4591. [CrossRef] [PubMed]
77. Mukherjee, S.; Zheng, H.; Derebe, M.G.; Callenberg, K.M.; Partch, C.L.; Rollins, D.; Propheter, D.C.; Rizo, J.; Grabe, M.; Jiang, Q.X.; *et al.* Antibacterial membrane attack by a pore-forming intestinal c-type lectin. *Nature* **2014**, *505*, 103–107. [CrossRef] [PubMed]

78. Henzler Wildman, K.A.; Lee, D.K.; Ramamoorthy, A. Mechanism of lipid bilayer disruption by the human antimicrobial peptide, LL-37. *Biochemistry* **2003**, *42*, 6545–6558. [CrossRef] [PubMed]
79. Oren, Z.; Lerman, J.C.; Gudmundsson, G.H.; Agerberth, B.; Shai, Y. Structure and organization of the human antimicrobial peptide LL-37 in phospholipid membranes: Relevance to the molecular basis for its non-cell-selective activity. *Biochem. J.* **1999**, *341 (Pt 3)*, 501–513. [CrossRef] [PubMed]
80. Kjos, M.; Oppegard, C.; Diep, D.B.; Nes, I.F.; Veening, J.W.; Nissen-Meyer, J.; Kristensen, T. Sensitivity to the two-peptide bacteriocin lactococcin G is dependent on UppP, an enzyme involved in cell-wall synthesis. *Mol. Microbiol.* **2014**, *92*, 1177–1187. [CrossRef] [PubMed]
81. Cotter, P.D. An 'Upp'-turn in bacteriocin receptor identification. *Mol. Microbiol.* **2014**, *92*, 1159–1163. [CrossRef] [PubMed]
82. Wilmes, M.; Stockem, M.; Bierbaum, G.; Schlag, M.; Gotz, F.; Tran, D.Q.; Schaal, J.B.; Ouellette, A.J.; Selsted, M.E.; Sahl, H.G. Killing of staphylococci by theta-defensins involves membrane impairment and activation of autolytic enzymes. *Antibiotics (Basel)* **2014**, *3*, 617–631. [CrossRef]
83. Mukhopadhyay, J.; Sineva, E.; Knight, J.; Levy, R.M.; Ebright, R.H. Antibacterial peptide microcin J25 inhibits transcription by binding within and obstructing the RNA polymerase secondary channel. *Mol. Cell* **2004**, *14*, 739–751. [CrossRef] [PubMed]
84. Krizsan, A.; Volke, D.; Weinert, S.; Strater, N.; Knappe, D.; Hoffmann, R. Insect-derived proline-rich antimicrobial peptides kill bacteria by inhibiting bacterial protein translation at the 70S ribosome. *Angew. Chem. Int. Ed. Engl.* **2014**, *53*, 12236–12239. [CrossRef] [PubMed]
85. Mardirossian, M.; Grzela, R.; Giglione, C.; Meinnel, T.; Gennaro, R.; Mergaert, P.; Scocchi, M. The Host antimicrobial peptide Bac7(1–35) binds to bacterial ribosomal proteins and inhibits protein synthesis. *Chem. Biol.* **2014**, *21*, 1639–1647. [CrossRef] [PubMed]
86. De Leeuw, E.; Li, C.; Zeng, P.; Li, C.; Diepeveen-de Buin, M.; Lu, W.Y.; Breukink, E.; Lu, W. Functional interaction of human neutrophil peptide-1 with the cell wall precursor lipid II. *FEBS Lett.* **2010**, *584*, 1543–1548. [CrossRef] [PubMed]
87. Sass, V.; Schneider, T.; Wilmes, M.; Körner, C.; Tossi, A.; Novikova, N.; Shamova, O.; Sahl, H.G. Human beta-defensin 3 inhibits cell wall biosynthesis in *Staphylococci*. *Infect. Immun.* **2010**, *78*, 2793–2800. [CrossRef] [PubMed]
88. Bierbaum, G.; Sahl, H.G. Lantibiotics: Mode of action, biosynthesis and bioengineering. *Curr. Pharm. Biotechnol.* **2009**, *10*, 2–18. [CrossRef] [PubMed]
89. Iwamoto, K.; Hayakawa, T.; Murate, M.; Makino, A.; Ito, K.; Fujisawa, T.; Kobayashi, T. Curvature-dependent recognition of ethanolamine phospholipids by duramycin and cinnamycin. *Biophys. J.* **2007**, *93*, 1608–1619. [CrossRef] [PubMed]
90. Henriques, S.T.; Huang, Y.H.; Castanho, M.A.; Bagatolli, L.A.; Sonza, S.; Tachedjian, G.; Daly, N.L.; Craik, D.J. phosphatidylethanolamine binding is a conserved feature of cyclotide-membrane interactions. *J. Biol. Chem.* **2012**, *287*, 33629–33643. [CrossRef] [PubMed]
91. Troeira Henriques, S.; Huang, Y.H.; Chaousis, S.; Wang, C.K.; Craik, D.J. Anticancer and toxic properties of cyclotides are dependent on phosphatidylethanolamine phospholipid targeting. *Chembiochem* **2014**, *15*, 1956–1965. [CrossRef] [PubMed]
92. Otvos, L., Jr.; Insug, O.; Rogers, M.E.; Consolvo, P.J.; Condie, B.A.; Lovas, S.; Bulet, P.; Blaszczyk-Thurin, M. Interaction between heat shock proteins and antimicrobial peptides. *Biochemistry* **2000**, *39*, 14150–14159. [CrossRef] [PubMed]
93. Ghosh, A.; Kar, R.K.; Jana, J.; Saha, A.; Jana, B.; Krishnamoorthy, J.; Kumar, D.; Ghosh, S.; Chatterjee, S.; Bhunia, A. Indolicidin targets duplex DNA: Structural and mechanistic insight through a combination of spectroscopy and microscopy. *ChemMedChem* **2014**, *9*, 2052–2058. [CrossRef] [PubMed]
94. Wenzel, M.; Chiriac, A.I.; Otto, A.; Zweytick, D.; May, C.; Schumacher, C.; Gust, R.; Albada, H.B.; Penkova, M.; Kramer, U.; *et al.* Small cationic antimicrobial peptides delocalize peripheral membrane proteins. *Proc. Natl. Acad. Sci. U.S.A.* **2014**, *111*, E1409–E1418. [CrossRef] [PubMed]
95. Wang, G.; Peterkofsky, A.; Clore, G.M. A novel membrane anchor function for the N-terminal amphipathic sequence of the signal-transducing protein $IIA^{glucose}$ of the *Escherichia coli* phosphotransferase system. *J. Biol. Chem.* **2000**, *275*, 39811–39814. [CrossRef] [PubMed]

96. Wang, G.; Li, Y.; Li, X. Correlation of three-dimensional structures with the antibacterial activity of a group of peptides designed based on a nontoxic bacterial membrane anchor. *J. Biol. Chem.* **2005**, *280*, 5803–5811. [CrossRef] [PubMed]
97. Wang, G. Structures of human host defense cathelicidin LL-37 and its smallest antimicrobial peptide KR-12 in lipid micelles. *J. Biol. Chem.* **2008**, *283*, 32637–32643. [CrossRef] [PubMed]
98. Epand, RF; Wang, G.; Berno, B.; Epand, R.M. Lipid segregation explains selective toxicity of a series of fragments derived from the human cathelicidin LL-37. *Antimicrob. Agents Chemother.* **2009**, *53*, 3705–3714. [CrossRef] [PubMed]
99. Bals, R.; Wilson, J.M. Cathelicidins—A family of multifunctional antimicrobial peptides. *Cell. Mol. Life Sci.* **2003**, *60*, 711–720. [CrossRef] [PubMed]
100. Wang, G.; Epand, R.F.; Mishra, B.; Lushnikova, T.; Thomas, V.C.; Bayles, K.W.; Epand, R.M. Decoding the functional roles of cationic side chains of the major antimicrobial region of human cathelicidin LL-37. *Antimicrob. Agents Chemother.* **2012**, *56*, 845–856. [CrossRef] [PubMed]
101. Nakagawa, Y.; Gallo, R.L. Endogenous intracellular cathelicidin enhances TLR9 activation in dendritic cells and macrophages. *J. Immunol.* **2015**, *194*, 1274–1284. [CrossRef] [PubMed]
102. Neumann, A.; Berends, E.T.; Nerlich, A.; Molhoek, E.M.; Gallo, R.L.; Meerloo, T.; Nizet, V.; Naim, H.Y.; von Kockritz-Blickwede, M. The antimicrobial peptide LL-37 facilitates the formation of neutrophil extracellular traps. *Biochem. J.* **2014**, *464*, 3–11. [CrossRef] [PubMed]
103. Yang, D.; Chen, Q.; Schmidt, A.P.; Anderson, G.M.; Wang, J.M.; Wooters, J.; Oppenheim, J.J.; Chertov, O. LL-37, the neutrophil granule- and epithelial cell-derived cathelicidin, utilizes formyl peptide receptor-like 1 (FPRL1) as a receptor to chemoattract human peripheral blood neutrophils, monocytes, and T cells. *J. Exp. Med.* **2000**, *192*, 1069–1074. [CrossRef] [PubMed]
104. Elssner, A.; Duncan, M.; Gavrilin, M.; Wewers, M.D. A novel P2X7 receptor activator, the human cathelicidin-derived peptide LL37, induces IL-1 beta processing and release. *J. Immunol.* **2004**, *172*, 4987–4994. [CrossRef] [PubMed]
105. Wan, M.; van der Does, A.M.; Tang, X.; Lindbom, L.; Agerberth, B.; Haeggstrom, J.Z. Antimicrobial peptide LL-37 promotes bacterial phagocytosis by human macrophages. *J. Leukoc. Biol.* **2014**, *95*, 971–981. [CrossRef] [PubMed]
106. Tripathi, S.; Verma, A.; Kim, E.J.; White, M.R.; Hartshorn, K.L. LL-37 modulates human neutrophil responses to influenza a virus. *J. Leukoc. Biol.* **2014**, *96*, 931–938. [CrossRef] [PubMed]
107. Lande, R.; Botti, E.; Jandus, C.; Dojcinovic, D.; Fanelli, G.; Conrad, C.; Chamilos, G.; Feldmeyer, L.; Marinari, B.; Chon, S.; *et al.* The antimicrobial peptide LL37 is a T-Cell autoantigen in psoriasis. *Nat. Commun.* **2014**, *5*, 5621. [CrossRef]
108. Peschel, A. How do bacteria resist human antimicrobial peptides? *Trends Microbiol.* **2002**, *10*, 179–186. [CrossRef] [PubMed]
109. Gebhard, S.; Fang, C.; Shaaly, A.; Leslie, D.J.; Weimar, M.R.; Kalamorz, F.; Carne, A.; Cook, G.M. Identification and characterization of a bacitracin resistance network in *Enterococcus faecalis*. *Antimicrob. Agents Chemother.* **2014**, *58*, 1425–1433. [CrossRef] [PubMed]
110. Dintner, S.; Staron, A.; Berchtold, E.; Petri, T.; Mascher, T.; Gebhard, S. Coevolution of ABC transporters and two-component regulatory systems as resistance modules against antimicrobial peptides in Firmicutes Bacteria. *J. Bacteriol.* **2011**, *193*, 3851–3862. [CrossRef] [PubMed]
111. Falord, M.; Karimova, G.; Hiron, A.; Msadek, T. GraXSR proteins interact with the VraFG ABC transporter to form a five-component system required for cationic antimicrobial peptide sensing and resistance in *Staphylococcus aureus*. *Antimicrob. Agents Chemother.* **2012**, *56*, 1047–1058. [CrossRef] [PubMed]
112. Weidenmaier, C.; Peschel, A.; Kempf, V.A.; Lucindo, N.; Yeaman, M.R.; Bayer, A.S. DltABCD- and mprF-mediated cell envelope modifications of *Staphylococcus aureus* confer resistance to platelet microbicidal proteins and contribute to virulence in a rabbit endocarditis model. *Infect. Immun.* **2005**, *73*, 8033–8038. [CrossRef] [PubMed]
113. Li, M; Cha, D.J.; Lai, Y.; Villaruz, A.E.; Sturdevant, D.E.; Otto, M. The antimicrobial peptide-sensing system *aps* of *Staphylococcus aureus*. *Mol. Microbiol.* **2007**, *66*, 1136–1147. [CrossRef] [PubMed]
114. Yang, S.-J.; Bayer, A.S.; Mishra, N.N.; Meehl, M.; Ledala, N.; Yeaman, M.R.; Xiong, Y.Q.; Cheung, A.L. The *Staphylococcus aureus* two-component regulatory system, GraRS, senses and confers resistance to selected cationic antimicrobial peptides. *Infect. Immun.* **2012**, *80*, 74–81. [CrossRef] [PubMed]

115. Cheung, A.L.; Bayer, A.S.; Yeaman, M.R.; Xiong, Y.Q.; Waring, A.J.; Memmi, G.; Donegan, N.; Chaili, S.; Yang, S.J. Site-specific mutation of the sensor kinase GraS in *Staphylococcus aureus* alters the adaptive response to distinct cationic antimicrobial peptides. *Infect. Immun.* **2014**, *82*, 5336–5345. [CrossRef] [PubMed]
116. Velarde, J.J.; Ashbaugh, M.; Wessels, M.R. The human antimicrobial peptide LL-37 binds directly to CsrS, a sensor histidine kinase of group A Streptococcus, to activate expression of virulence factors. *J. Biol. Chem.* **2014**, *289*, 36315–36324. [CrossRef] [PubMed]
117. Chen, H.D.; Groisman, E.A. The biology of the PmrA/PmrB two-component system: The major regulator of lipopolysaccharide modifications. *Annu. Rev. Microbiol.* **2013**, *67*, 83–112. [CrossRef] [PubMed]
118. Henderson, J.C.; Fage, C.D.; Cannon, J.R.; Brodbelt, J.S.; Keatinge-Clay, A.T.; Trent, M.S. Antimicrobial peptide resistance of *Vibrio cholerae* results from an lps modification pathway related to nonribosomal peptide synthetases. *ACS Chem. Biol.* **2014**, *9*, 2382–2392. [CrossRef] [PubMed]
119. Tzeng, Y.L.; Ambrose, K.D.; Zughaier, S.; Zhou, X.; Miller, Y.K.; Shafer, W.M.; Stephens, D.S. Cationic antimicrobial peptide resistance in Neisseria meningitidis. *J. Bacteriol.* **2005**, *187*, 5387–5396. [CrossRef] [PubMed]
120. Balthazar, J.T.; Gusa, A.; Martin, L.E.; Choudhury, B.; Carlson, R.; Shafer, W.M. Lipooligosaccharide structure is an important determinant in the resistance of *Neisseria gonorrhoeae* to antimicrobial agents of innate host defense. *Front. Microbiol.* **2011**, *2*, 30. [CrossRef] [PubMed]
121. Handing, J.W.; Criss, A.K. The lipooligosaccharide-modifying enzyme LptA enhances gonococcal defence against human neutrophils. *Cell. Microbiol.* **2014**. [CrossRef]
122. Kandler, J.L.; Joseph, S.J.; Balthazar, J.T.; Dhulipala, V.; Read, T.D.; Jerse, A.E.; Shafer, W.M. Phase-variable expression of *lpta* modulates the resistance of *Neisseria gonorrhoeae* to cationic antimicrobial peptides. *Antimicrob. Agents Chemother.* **2014**, *58*, 4230–4233. [CrossRef] [PubMed]
123. Packiam, M.; Yedery, R.D.; Begum, A.A.; Carlson, R.W.; Ganguly, J.; Sempowski, G.D.; Ventevogel, M.S.; Shafer, W.M.; Jerse, A.E. Phosphoethanolamine decoration of *Neisseria gonorrhoeae* lipid a plays a dual immunostimulatory and protective role during experimental genital tract infection. *Infect. Immun.* **2014**, *82*, 2170–2179. [CrossRef] [PubMed]
124. Groisman, E.A.; Parra-Lopez, C.; Salcedo, M.; Lipps, C.J.; Heffron, F. Resistance to host antimicrobial peptides is necessary for Salmonella virulence. *Proc. Natl. Acad. Sci. U.S.A.* **1992**, *89*, 11939–11943. [CrossRef] [PubMed]
125. Dalebroux, Z.D.; Matamouros, S.; Whittington, D.; Bishop, R.E.; Miller, S.I. PhoPQ regulates acidic glycerophospholipid content of the *Salmonella typhimurium* outer membrane. *Proc. Natl. Acad. Sci. U.S.A.* **2014**, *111*, 1963–1968. [CrossRef] [PubMed]
126. Matamouros, S.; Miller, S.I. *S. Typhimurium* strategies to resist killing by cationic antimicrobial peptides. *Biochim. Biophys. Acta* **2015**. [CrossRef]
127. Dalebroux, Z.D.; Miller, S.I. Salmonellae PhoPQ regulation of the outer membrane to resist innate immunity. *Curr Opin Microbiol.* **2014**, *17*, 106–113. [CrossRef] [PubMed]
128. Cullen, T.W.; Schofield, W.B.; Barry, N.A.; Putnam, E.E.; Rundell, E.A.; Trent, M.S.; Degnan, P.H.; Booth, C.J.; Yu, H.; Goodman, A.L. Gut Microbiota. Antimicrobial peptide resistance mediates resilience of prominent gut commensals during inflammation. *Science* **2015**, *347*, 170–175. [CrossRef] [PubMed]
129. Wang, G.; Hanke, M.L.; Mishra, B.; Lushnikova, T.; Heim, C.E.; Chittezham Thomas, V.; Bayles, K.W.; Kielian, T. Transformation of human cathelicidin LL-37 into selective, stable, and potent antimicrobial compounds. *ACS Chem. Biol.* **2014**, *9*, 1997–2002. [CrossRef] [PubMed]
130. Li, X.; Li, Y.; Han, H.; Miller, D.W.; Wang, G. Solution structures of human LL-37 fragments and NMR-based identification of a minimal membrane-targeting antimicrobial and anticancer region. *J. Am. Chem. Soc.* **2006**, *128*, 5776–5785. [CrossRef] [PubMed]
131. Leake, I. IBD: cathelicidin can reverse intestinal fibrosis in models of colitis. *Nat. Rev. Gastroenterol. Hepatol.* **2015**, *12*, 3. [PubMed]
132. Steinstraesser, L.; Lam, M.C.; Jacobsen, F.; Porporato, P.E.; Chereddy, K.K.; Becerikli, M.; Stricker, I.; Hancock, R.E.; Lehnhardt, M.; Sonveaux, P.; *et al.* Skin electroporation of a plasmid encoding hCAP-18/LL-37 host defense peptide promotes wound healing. *Mol. Ther.* **2014**, *22*, 734–742. [CrossRef] [PubMed]
133. Woo, J.I.; Kil, S.H.; Brough, D.E.; Lee, Y.J.; Lim, D.J.; Moon, S.K. Therapeutic potential of adenovirus-mediated delivery of beta-defensin 2 for experimental otitis media. *Innate Immun.* **2015**, *21*, 215–224. [CrossRef] [PubMed]

134. Gonzalez-Curiel, I.; Trujillo, V.; Montoya-Rosales, A.; Rincon, K.; Rivas-Calderon, B.; deHaro-Acosta, J.; Marin-Luevano, P.; Lozano-Lopez, D.; Enciso-Moreno, J.A.; Rivas-Santiago, B. 1,25-Dihydroxyvitamin D3 induces LL-37 and HBD-2 production in keratinocytes from diabetic foot ulcers promoting wound healing: An *in vitro* model. *PLoS ONE* **2014**, *9*, e111355. [CrossRef] [PubMed]
135. Mallbris, L.; Edstrom, D.W.; Sundblad, L.; Granath, F.; Stahle, M. UVB upregulates the antimicrobial protein hCAP18 mRNA in human skin. *J. Invest. Dermatol.* **2005**, *125*, 1072–1074. [CrossRef] [PubMed]
136. Eda, N.; Shimizu, K.; Suzuki, S.; Tanabe, Y.; Lee, E.; Akama, T. Effects of yoga exercise on salivary beta-defensin 2. *Eur. J. Appl. Physiol.* **2013**, *113*, 2621–2627. [CrossRef] [PubMed]
137. Lin, S.P.; Li, C.Y.; Suzuki, K.; Chang, C.K.; Chou, K.M.; Fang, S.H. Green tea consumption after intense taekwondo training enhances salivary defense factors and antibacterial capacity. *PLoS ONE* **2014**, *9*, e87580. [CrossRef] [PubMed]
138. Aboye, T.L.; Ha, H.; Majumder, S.; Christ, F.; Debyser, Z.; Shekhtman, A.; Neamati, N.; Camarero, J.A. Design of a novel cyclotide-based CXCR4 antagonist with anti-human immunodeficiency virus (HIV)-1 activity. *J. Med. Chem.* **2012**, *55*, 10729–10734. [CrossRef] [PubMed]
139. Gunasekera, S.; Foley, F.M.; Clark, R.J.; Sando, L.; Fabri, L.J.; Craik, D.J.; Daly, N.L. Engineering stabilized vascular endothelial growth factor-a antagonists: synthesis, structural characterization, and bioactivity of grafted analogues of cyclotides. *J. Med. Chem.* **2008**, *51*, 7697–7704. [CrossRef] [PubMed]
140. Wang, C.K.; Gruber, C.W.; Cemazar, M.; Siatskas, C.; Tagore, P.; Payne, N.; Sun, G.; Wang, S.; Bernard, C.C.; Craik, D.J. Molecular grafting onto a stable framework yields novel cyclic peptides for the treatment of multiple sclerosis. *ACS Chem. Biol.* **2014**, *9*, 156–163. [CrossRef] [PubMed]
141. Craik, D.J.; Henriques, S.T.; Mylne, J.S.; Wang, C.K. Cyclotide isolation and characterization. *Methods Enzymol.* **2012**, *516*, 37–62. [PubMed]
142. Gunasekera, S.; Daly, N.L.; Anderson, M.A.; Craik, D.J. Chemical synthesis and biosynthesis of the cyclotide family of circular proteins. *IUBMB Life* **2006**, *58*, 515–524. [CrossRef] [PubMed]
143. Jia, X.; Kwon, S.; Wang, C.I.; Huang, Y.H.; Chan, L.Y.; Tan, C.C.; Rosengren, K.J.; Mulvenna, J.P.; Schroeder, C.I.; Craik, D.J. Semienzymatic cyclization of disulfide-rich peptides using sortase A. *J. Biol. Chem.* **2014**, *289*, 6627–6638. [CrossRef] [PubMed]
144. Stanger, K.; Maurer, T.; Kaluarachchi, H.; Coons, M.; Franke, Y.; Hannoush, R.N. Backbone cyclization of a recombinant cystine-knot peptide by engineered sortase A. *FEBS Lett.* **2014**, *588*, 4487–4496. [CrossRef] [PubMed]
145. Lim, K.; Chua, R.R.; Ho, B.; Tambyah, P.A.; Hadinoto, K.; Leong, S.S. Development of a catheter functionalized by a polydopamine peptide coating with antimicrobial and antibiofilm properties. *Acta Biomater.* **2014**, *15*, 127–138. [CrossRef] [PubMed]
146. Godoy-Gallardo, M.; Mas-Moruno, C.; Fernandez-Calderon, M.C.; Perez-Giraldo, C.; Manero, J.M.; Albericio, F.; Gil, F.J.; Rodriguez, D. Covalent immobilization of hLf1-11 peptide on a titanium surface reduces bacterial adhesion and biofilm formation. *Acta Biomater.* **2014**, *10*, 3522–3534. [CrossRef] [PubMed]
147. Lombana, A.; Raja, Z.; Casale, S.; Pradier, C.M.; Foulon, T.; Ladram, A.; Humblot, V. Temporin-SHa peptides grafted on gold surfaces display antibacterial activity. *J. Pept. Sci.* **2014**, *20*, 563–569. [CrossRef] [PubMed]
148. Wang, Z.; Han, X.; He, N.; Chen, Z.; Brooks, C.L., 3rd. Molecular structures of C- and N-terminus cysteine modified cecropin P1 chemically immobilized onto maleimide-terminated self-assembled monolayers investigated by molecular dynamics simulation. *J. Phys. Chem. B* **2014**, *118*, 5670–5680. [CrossRef] [PubMed]
149. Mishra, B.; Basu, A.; Chua, R.R.Y.; Saravanan, R.; Tambyah, P.P.; Ho, B.; Chang, M.W.; Leong, S.S.J. Site specific immobilization of a potent antimicrobial peptide onto silicone catheters: evaluation against urinary tract infection pathogens. *J. Mater. Chem. B* **2014**, *2*, 1706–1716. [CrossRef]
150. Salwiczek, M.; Qu, Y.; Gardiner, J.; Strugnell, R.A.; Lithgow, T.; McLean, K.M.; Thissen, H. Emerging rules for effective antimicrobial coatings. *Trends Biotechnol.* **2014**, *32*, 82–90. [CrossRef] [PubMed]
151. Dutta, D.; Ozkan, J.; Willcox, M.D. Biocompatibility of antimicrobial melimine lenses: Rabbit and human studies. *Optom. Vis. Sci.* **2014**, *91*, 570–581. [CrossRef] [PubMed]
152. Tan, X.W.; Goh, T.W.; Saraswathi, P.; Nyein, C.L.; Setiawan, M.; Riau, A.; Lakshminarayanan, R.; Liu, S.; Tan, D.; Beuerman, R.W.; *et al.* Effectiveness of antimicrobial peptide immobilization for preventing perioperative cornea implant-associated bacterial infection. *Antimicrob. Agents Chemother.* **2014**, *58*, 5229–5238. [CrossRef] [PubMed]

153. Medeiros, K.A.; Joanitti, G.A.; Silva, L.P. Chitosan nanoparticles for dermaseptin peptide delivery toward tumor cells *in vitro*. *Anticancer Drugs* **2014**, *25*, 323–331. [CrossRef] [PubMed]
154. Miao, D.; Jiang, M.; Liu, Z.; Gu, G.; Hu, Q.; Kang, T.; Song, Q.; Yao, L.; Li, W.; Gao, X.; *et al.* Co-administration of dual-targeting nanoparticles with penetration enhancement peptide for antiglioblastoma therapy. *Mol. Pharm.* **2014**, *11*, 90–101. [CrossRef] [PubMed]
155. Ahmad, A.; Ranjan, S.; Zhang, W.; Zou, J.; Pyykko, I.; Kinnunen, P.K. Novel endosomolytic peptides for enhancing gene delivery in nanoparticles. *Biochim. Biophys. Acta* **2015**, *1848*, 544–553. [CrossRef] [PubMed]
156. Keohane, K.; Brennan, D.; Galvin, P.; Griffin, B.T. Silicon microfluidic flow focusing devices for the production of size-controlled PLGA based drug loaded microparticles. *Int. J. Pharm.* **2014**, *467*, 60–69. [CrossRef] [PubMed]
157. Chereddy, K.K.; Her, C.H.; Comune, M.; Moia, C.; Lopes, A.; Porporato, P.E.; Vanacker, J.; Lam, M.C.; Steinstraesser, L.; Sonveaux, P.; *et al.* PLGA Nanoparticles loaded with host defense peptide ll37 promote wound healing. *J. Control. Release* **2014**, *194*, 138–147. [CrossRef] [PubMed]
158. Laverty, G.; McCloskey, A.P.; Gilmore, B.F.; Jones, D.S.; Zhou, J.; Xu, B. Ultrashort cationic naphthalene-derived self-assembled peptides as antimicrobial nanomaterials. *Biomacromolecules* **2014**, *15*, 3429–3439. [CrossRef] [PubMed]
159. Lillehoj, P.B.; Kaplan, C.W.; He, J.; Shi, W.; Ho, C.M. Rapid, electrical impedance detection of bacterial pathogens using immobilized antimicrobial peptides. *J. Lab. Autom.* **2014**, *19*, 42–49. [CrossRef] [PubMed]
160. Etayash, H.; Jiang, K.; Thundat, T.; Kaur, K. Impedimetric detection of pathogenic gram-positive bacteria using an antimicrobial peptide from class IIa bacteriocins. *Anal. Chem.* **2014**, *86*, 1693–1700. [CrossRef] [PubMed]
161. Kim, H.J.; Brehm-Stecher, B.F. Design and evaluation of peptide nucleic acid probes for specific identification of *Candida albicans*. *J. Clin. Microbiol.* **2015**, *53*, 511–521. [CrossRef] [PubMed]
162. Strauss-Grabo, M.; Atiyem, S.; Le, T.; Kretschmar, M. Decade-long use of the antimicrobial peptide combination tyrothricin does not pose a major risk of acquired resistance with gram-positive bacteria and *Candida* spp. *Pharmazie* **2014**, *69*, 838–841.
163. Shenkarev, Z.O.; Gizatullina, A.K.; Finkina, E.I.; Alekseeva, E.A.; Balandin, S.V.; Mineev, K.S.; Arseniev, A.S.; Ovchinnikova, T.V. Heterologous expression and solution structure of defensin from lentil *Lens culinaris*. *Biochem. Biophys. Res. Commun.* **2014**, *451*, 252–257. [CrossRef] [PubMed]
164. De Medeiros, L.N.; Angeli, R.; Sarzedas, C.G.; Barreto-Bergter, E.; Valente, A.P.; Kurtenbach, E.; Almeida, F.C. Backbone dynamics of the antifungal Psd1 pea defensin and its correlation with membrane interaction by NMR spectroscopy. *Biochim. Biophys. Acta* **2010**, *1798*, 105–113. [CrossRef] [PubMed]
165. Neves de Medeiros, L.; Domitrovic, T.; Cavalcante de Andrade, P.; Faria, J.; Barreto Bergter, E.; Weissmüller, G.; Kurtenbach, E. Psd1 binding affinity toward fungal membrane components as assessed by SPR: The role of glucosylceramide in fungal recognition and entry. *Biopolymers* **2014**, *102*, 456–464. [CrossRef] [PubMed]
166. De Paula, V.S.; Pomin, V.H.; Valente, A.P. Unique properties of human β-defensin 6 (hBD6) and glycosaminoglycan complex: sandwich-like dimerization and competition with the chemokine receptor 2 (CCR2) binding site. *J. Biol. Chem.* **2014**, *289*, 22969–22979. [CrossRef] [PubMed]
167. Forde, E.; Humphreys, H.; Greene, C.M.; Fitzgerald-Hughes, D.; Devocelle, M. Potential of host defense peptide prodrugs as neutrophil elastase-dependent anti-infective agents for cystic fibrosis. *Antimicrob. Agents Chemother.* **2014**, *58*, 978–985. [CrossRef] [PubMed]
168. Forde, E.; Devocelle, M. Pro-moieties of antimicrobial peptide prodrugs. *Molecules* **2015**, *20*, 1210–1227. [CrossRef] [PubMed]
169. Neumann, A.; Völlger, L.; Berends, E.T.; Molhoek, E.M.; Stapels, D.A.; Midon, M.; Friães, A.; Pingoud, A.; Rooijakkers, S.H.; Gallo, R.L.; *et al.* Novel role of the antimicrobial peptide LL-37 in the protection of neutrophil extracellular traps against degradation by bacterial nucleases. *J. Innate Immun.* **2014**, *6*, 860–868. [CrossRef] [PubMed]
170. Sol, A.; Skvirsky, Y.; Nashef, R.; Zelentsova, K.; Burstyn-Cohen, T.; Blotnick, E.; Muhlrad, A.; Bachrach, G. Actin enables the antimicrobial action of LL-37 peptide in the presence of microbial proteases. *J. Biol. Chem.* **2014**, *289*, 22926–22941. [CrossRef] [PubMed]
171. Sol, A.; Wang, G.; Blotnick, E.; Golla, R.; Bachrach, G. Interaction of the core fragments of the LL-37 host defense peptide with actin. *RSC Adv.* **2015**, *5*, 9361–9367. [CrossRef]

172. Svensson, D.; Westman, J.; Wickstrom, C.; Jonsson, D.; Herwald, H.; Nilsson, B.O. Human Endogenous Peptide p33 Inhibits Detrimental Effects of LL-37 on Osteoblast Viability. *J. Periodontal. Res.* **2015**, *50*, 80–88. [CrossRef] [PubMed]
173. Hiemstra, T.F.; Charles, P.D.; Gracia, T.; Hester, S.S.; Gatto, L.; Al-Lamki, R.; Floto, R.A.; Su, Y.; Skepper, J.N.; Lilley, K.S.; *et al.* Human Urinary Exosomes as Innate Immune Effectors. *J. Am. Soc. Nephrol.* **2014**, *50*, 80–88.
174. Carmona-Ribeiro, A.M.; de Melo Carrasco, L.D. Novel formulations for antimicrobial peptides. *Int. J. Mol. Sci.* **2014**, *15*, 18040–18083. [CrossRef] [PubMed]
175. Pina, A.S.; Batalha, I.L.; Fernandes, C.S.; Aoki, M.A.; Roque, A.C. Exploring the potential of magnetic antimicrobial agents for water disinfection. *Water Res.* **2014**, *66*, 160–168. [CrossRef] [PubMed]
176. Silva, R.R.; Avelino, K.Y.; Ribeiro, K.L.; Franco, O.L.; Oliveira, M.D.; Andrade, C.A. Optical and dielectric sensors based on antimicrobial peptides for microorganism diagnosis. *Front. Microbiol.* **2014**, *5*, 443. [PubMed]
177. Otter, J.A.; Vickery, K.; Walker, J.T.; deLancey Pulcini, E.; Stoodley, P.; Goldenberg, S.D.; Salkeld, J.A.; Chewins, J.; Yezli, S.; Edgeworth, J.D. Surface-attached cells, biofilms and biocide susceptibility: implications for hospital cleaning and disinfection. *J. Hosp. Infect.* **2015**, *89*, 16–27. [CrossRef] [PubMed]
178. Pimentel-Filho Nde, J.; Martins, M.C.; Nogueira, G.B.; Mantovani, H.C.; Vanetti, M.C. Bovicin HC5 and nisin reduce *Staphylococcus aureus* adhesion to polystyrene and change the hydrophobicity profile and gibbs free energy of adhesion. *Int. J. Food Microbiol.* **2014**, *190*, 1–8. [CrossRef] [PubMed]
179. Dong, X.; McCoy, E.; Zhang, M.; Yang, L. Inhibitory effects of nisin-coated multi-walled carbon nanotube sheet on biofilm formation from *Bacillus anthracis* spores. *J. Environ. Sci. (China)* **2014**, *26*, 2526–2534. [CrossRef]
180. Singh, A.P.; Preet, S.; Rishi, P. Nisin/β-Lactam adjunct therapy against Salmonella enterica serovar Typhimurium: a mechanistic approach. *J. Antimicrob. Chemother.* **2014**, *69*, 1877–1887. [CrossRef] [PubMed]
181. Dosler, S.; Karaaslan, E. Inhibition and destruction of *Pseudomonas aeruginosa* biofilms by antibiotics and antimicrobial peptides. *Peptides* **2014**, *62*, 32–37. [CrossRef] [PubMed]
182. Maiti, S.; Patro, S.; Purohit, S.; Jain, S.; Senapati, S.; Dey, N. Effective control of Salmonella infections by employing combinations of recombinant antimicrobial human β-defensins hBD-1 and hBD-2. *Antimicrob Agents Chemother.* **2014**, *58*, 6896–6903. [CrossRef] [PubMed]
183. Donelli, G.; Francolini, I.; Romoli, D.; Guaglianone, E.; Piozzi, A.; Ragunath, C.; Kaplan, J.B. Synergistic activity of dispersin B and cefamandole nafate in inhibition of staphylococcal biofilm growth on polyurethanes. *Antimicrob Agents Chemother.* **2007**, *51*, 2733–2740. [CrossRef] [PubMed]
184. Tong, Z.; Zhang, L.; Ling, J.; Jian, Y.; Huang, L.; Deng, D. An *in vitro* study on the effect of free amino acids alone or in combination with nisin on biofilms as well as on planktonic bacteria of *Streptococcus mutans*. *PLoS ONE* **2014**, *9*, e99513. [CrossRef] [PubMed]
185. De la Fuente-Nunez, C.; Reffuveille, F.; Haney, E.F.; Straus, S.K.; Hancock, R.E. Broad-Spectrum anti-biofilm peptide that targets a cellular stress response. *PLoS Pathog.* **2014**, *10*, e1004152. [CrossRef] [PubMed]
186. Bommarius, B.; Anyanful, A.; Izrayelit, Y.; Bhatt, S.; Cartwright, E.; Wang, W.; Swimm, A.I.; Benian, G.M.; Schroeder, F.C.; Kalman, D. A family of indoles regulate virulence and Shiga toxin production in pathogenic *E. coli*. *PLoS ONE* **2013**, *8*, e54456. [CrossRef] [PubMed]
187. Scopel, M.; Abraham, W.R.; Antunes, A.L.; Henriques, A.T.; Macedo, A.J. Mevalonolactone: an inhibitor of *Staphylococcus epidermidis* adherence and biofilm formation. *Med. Chem.* **2014**, *10*, 246–251. [CrossRef] [PubMed]
188. Liaqat, I.; Bachmann, R.T.; Edyvean, R.G. Type 2 quorum sensing monitoring, inhibition and biofilm formation in marine microrganisms. *Curr. Microbiol.* **2014**, *68*, 342–351. [CrossRef] [PubMed]
189. Pereira, U.A.; Barbosa, L.C.; Maltha, C.R.; Demuner, A.J.; Masood, M.A.; Pimenta, A.L. γ-Alkylidene-γ-lactones and isobutylpyrrol-2(5H)-ones analogues to rubrolides as inhibitors of biofilm formation by gram-positive and gram-negative bacteria. *Bioorg. Med. Chem. Lett.* **2014**, *24*, 1052–1056. [CrossRef] [PubMed]

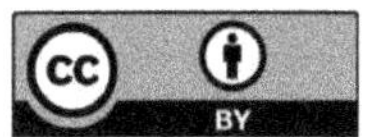

© 2015 by the authors. Licensee MDPI, Basel, Switzerland. This article is an open access article distributed under the terms and conditions of the Creative Commons Attribution (CC BY) license (http://creativecommons.org/licenses/by/4.0/).

Part II:
Antimicrobial Peptides Are Widespread in Nature

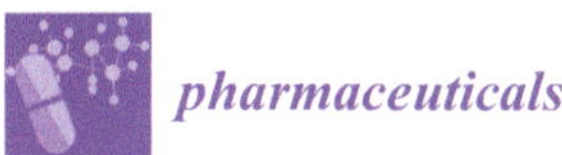

MDPI

Review

Chapter 2:

The Fungal Defensin Family Enlarged

Jiajia Wu, Bin Gao and Shunyi Zhu *

Group of Animal Innate Immunity, State Key Laboratory of Integrated Management of Pest Insects and Rodents, Institute of Zoology, Chinese Academy of Sciences, 1 Beichen West Road, Chaoyang District, Beijing 100101, China

* Author to whom correspondence should be addressed; Zhusy@ioz.ac.cn.

Received: 5 June 2014; in revised form: 5 August 2014; Accepted: 8 August 2014; Published: 18 August 2014

Abstract: Fungi are an emerging source of peptide antibiotics. With the availability of a large number of model fungal genome sequences, we can expect that more and more fungal defensin-like peptides (fDLPs) will be discovered by sequence similarity search. Here, we report a total of 69 new fDLPs encoded by 63 genes, in which a group of fDLPs derived from dermatophytes are defined as a new family (fDEF8) according to sequence and phylogenetic analyses. In the oleaginous fungus *Mortierella alpine*, fDLPs have undergone extensive gene expansion. Our work further enlarges the fungal defensin family and will help characterize new peptide antibiotics with therapeutic potential.

Keywords: peptide antibiotic; gene duplication; exon-intron structure; cysteine-stabilized α-helical and β-sheet motif

---

1. Introduction

Fungal defensin-like peptides (fDLPs) are emerging as attractive anti-infective agents due to their therapeutic efficacy, low toxicity and high serum stability [1,2]. On the basis of a combined analyses of sequence, structural, and phylogenetic data, we has identified seven fDLP families [2,3], in which three members (plectasin, micasin and eurocin), classified as ancient invertebrate-type defensins (AITDs) [1,2,4,5], have been structurally and functionally characterized. These fDLPs exhibit activity against several antibiotic-resistant clinical isolates with significant therapeutic potential [1,2,5,6]. Some efforts have been taken to improve antimicrobial efficacy and to reduce undesirable side effects of fDLPs. For example, an improved mutant of plectasin (NZ2114) is superior to two conventional antibiotics (vancomycin and daptomycin) in inhibiting methicillin-resistant *Staphylococcus aureus* (MRSA) with even more enhanced serum stability and extended *in vivo* half-life [7–9]. In this work, we describe 69 new fDLPs in terms of their sequences, structural characteristics, and phylogenetic relationship. This provides an array of candidates for development of new anti-infective agents against antibiotic-resistant human pathogens.

2. Discovery of New fDLPs

The database search strategy used here has been described previously [3]. Through an exhaustive search of 26 fungal species, we retrieved a total of 69 new fDLPs. As previously stated, overall this class of molecules exhibits a taxa-specific distribution pattern in the fungus kingdom, of which 21 fDLPs are derived from *Ascomycota*, 39 from *Zygomycota*, eight from *Basidiomycota* and one from *Glomeromycota*. In the basal fungi (*Microsporidia* and *Chytridiomycota*), no typical fDLP has been identified (Figure 1). The general features of these peptides are listed in Tables 1 and 2. They can be grouped into six families based on sequence similarity, five of which are classified into the previously known families (fDEF1, fDEF2, fDEF3, fDEF4, and fDEF6) [3] (Figures 2 and 3). This grouping is consistent with the phylogenetic analysis supported by high bootstrap values (Figure 4).

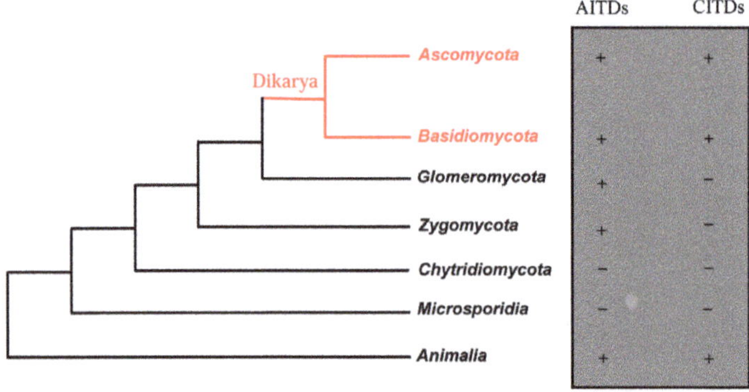

Figure 1. Phylogenetic distribution of fDLPs. The left: A parsimony tree of fungal species, animalia is used as an outgroup. This tree is a modification of the SSU and LSU r-RNA analyses of Lutzoni *et al.* for the fungal kingdom [10]. The right: "+" means presence and "−" means absence.

All the fDLPs characterized here have a signal peptide located in the N-terminus. In comparison with fDEF1 and fDEF2 that possess a propeptide located between signal and mature peptides, fDEF6 and fDEF8 lack a propeptide. Five precursors (maglosin, beauvesin2, manisin, pochlasin2 and asosin) could release two defensins from a single precursor after the removal of a spacer propeptide (Figure 5). The malpisin family from *Mortierella alpine* exhibits two types of precursor organization: (1) the first type contains 10 members, all having a propeptides identified by its acidic feature and single or two basic amino acids at their ends as putative cleavage site of proprotein convertase [11]; (2) the second type contains 14 members that lack a propeptide and thus no further processing step is needed (Figure S1).

Table 1. Sources and characteristics of newly discovered non-*Mortierella* fDLPs.

Name I Accession No.	Class	Species (phylum: subphylum: class)	Size	MW	NC
Pyronesin1 I CATG01000243 (G)		*Pyronema omphalodes* (Ascomycota: Pezizomycotina: Pezizomycetes)	40	4317	+1.2
Pyronesin2 I CATG01000243 (G)		*P. omphalodes*	40	4402	+0.2
Pyronesin3 I CATG01000243 (G)		*P. omphalodes*	40	4389	+1.2
Pyronesin4 I CATG01000243 (G)		*P. omphalodes*	40	4416	+2.2
Pyronesin5 I CATG01000243 (G)	fDEF1	*P. omphalodes*	40	4375	+1.2
Pyronesin6 I CATG01000243 (G)		*P. omphalodes*	40	4291	+2.4
Abisin1 I AEOK01000166 (G)		*Agaricus bisporus* (Basidiomycota: Agaricomycotina: Agaricomycetes)	40	4097	-3.8
Abisin2 I AEOK01000166 (G)		*A. bisporus*	40	4097	-3.8
Abisin3 I AEOK01000166		*A. bisporus*	39	3926	-2.8
Beauvesin1 I ADAH01000714 (G)		*Beauveria bassiana* (Ascomycota: Pezizomycotina: Sordariomycetes)	52	5475	+2.9
Pyrelysin I GAJI01023341 (T)		*Pyrenochaeta lycopersici* (Ascomycota: Pezizomycotina: Dothideomycetes)	55	5858	+5.4
Risin I JAQX01005622		*Rhizophagus irregularis* (Glomeromycota: Glomeromycetes)	55	5972	+6.1
Trimensin I FG132536 (E)		*Trichophyton mentagrophytes* (Ascomycota: Pezizomycotina: Eurotiomycetes)	38	4156	+2.2
Lecasin I AWYC01000479		*Lecanosticta acicola* (Ascomycota: Pezizomycotina: Dothideomycetes)	42	4314	−4.8

Table 1. *Cont.*

Name I Accession No.	Class	Species (phylum: subphylum: class)	Size	MW	NC
Pochlasin1 I AOSW01002431	fDEF2	*Pochonia chlamydosporia* (Ascomycota: Pezizomycotina: Sordariomycetes)	43	4339	−3.5
Perisin I AFRD01000258		*Periglandula ipomoeae* (Ascomycota: Pezizomycotina: Sordariomycetes)	43	4080	−1.5
Masysin I CANK01000016		*Malassezia sympodialis* (Basidiomycota: Ustilaginomycotina: Exobasidiomycetes)	35	3432	+2.2
Maglosin1N I AAYY01000039 (G)	fDEF3	*Malassezia globosa* (Basidiomycota: Ustilaginomycotina: Exobasidiomycetes)	40	3980	+1.2
Maglosin2N I AAYY01000024 (G)		*M. globosa*	40	4022	+0.2
Maglosin1C I AAYY01000039 (G)		*M. globosa*	41	3910	+2.7
Maglosin2C I AAYY01000024 (G)		*M. globosa*	40	3835	+2.7
Beauvesin2C I ADAH01000123 (G)		*B. bassiana*	41	4243	+0.9
ManisinC I ADNJ01000735		*Metarhizium anisopliae* (Ascomycota: Pezizomycotina: Sordariomycetes)	41	4211	−0.1
Pochlasin2C I AOSW01005877		*P. chlamydosporia*	41	4381	+0.2
AsosinC I BACA01000303		*Aspergillus sojae* (Ascomycota: Pezizomycotina: Eurotiomycetes)	38	4002	−1.0
Beauvesin2N I ADAH01000123 (G)	fDEF4	*B. bassiana*	48	5067	+2.9
ManisinN I ADNJ01000735		*M. anisopliae*	46	4921	+0.2
Pochlasin2N I AOSW01005877		*P. chlamydosporia*	49	5185	+2.9
AsosinN I BACA01000303		*A. sojae*	49	5140	−1.1
Rhimisin1 I ANKS01000620	fDEF6	*Rhizopus microsporus* (Zygomycota: Mucoromycotina: Mucorales)	45	4867	+10.0
Rhimisin2 I ANKS01000620		*R. microsporus*	44	4638	+3.4
Rhimisin3 I ANKS01001486		*R. microsporus*	44	4768	+1.5
Rhimisin4 I ANKS01001486		*R. microsporus*	45	4811	+8.0
Rhidesin1 I AACW02000043		*Rhizopus delemar* (Zygomycota: Mucoromycotina: Mucorales)	55	5885	+10.4
Rhidesin2 I AACW02000259		*R. delemar*	48	5270	+0.5
Mirresin I AZYI01000143		*Mucor irregularis* (Zygomycota: Mucoromycotina: Mucorales)	60	6424	+13.4
Mucisin I AOCY01001156 (G)		*Mucor circinelloides* (Zygomycota: Mucoromycotina: Mucorales)	53	5548	+2.2
Phycomysin I EX863311 (E)		*Phycomyces blakesleeanus* (Zygomycota: Mucoromycotina: Mucorales)	50	5342	+9.4
TritoDLP I ACPI01000196 (G)	fDEF8	*Trichophyton tonsurans* (Ascomycota: Pezizomycotina: Eurotiomycetes)	41	4323	+3.7
TrequiDLP I ABWI01000729 (G)		*Trichophyton equinum* (Ascomycota: Pezizomycotina: Eurotiomycetes)	41	4323	+3.7
TriveDLP I ACYE01000402		*Trichophyton verrucosum* (Ascomycota: Pezizomycotina: Eurotiomycetes)	42	4403	+4.7
ArgyDLP I ABQE01000293		*Arthroderma gypseum* (Ascomycota: Pezizomycotina: Eurotiomycetes)	41	4247	+3.7
ArbeDLP I ABSU01000004		*Arthroderma benhamiae* (Ascomycota: Pezizomycotina: Eurotiomycetes)	42	4493	+4.7
TriruDLP I ACPH01000567 (G)		*Trichophyton rubrum* (Ascomycota: Pezizomycotina: Eurotiomycetes)	42	4479	+4.7
MicaDLP I ABVF01000093		*Arthroderma otae* (Ascomycota: Pezizomycotina: Eurotiomycetes)	43	4745	+3.2

Note: MW: molecular weight; NC (net charge) is estimated at pH 7.0 with protein calculation V3.4. "E" means peptides from the Expressed Sequence Tags (EST) database and "T" means peptides from the Transcriptome Shotgun Assembly (TSA) database. "G" means proteins currently annotated in the GenBank database as hypothetical proteins (http://www.ncbi.nlm.nih.gov/) [12].

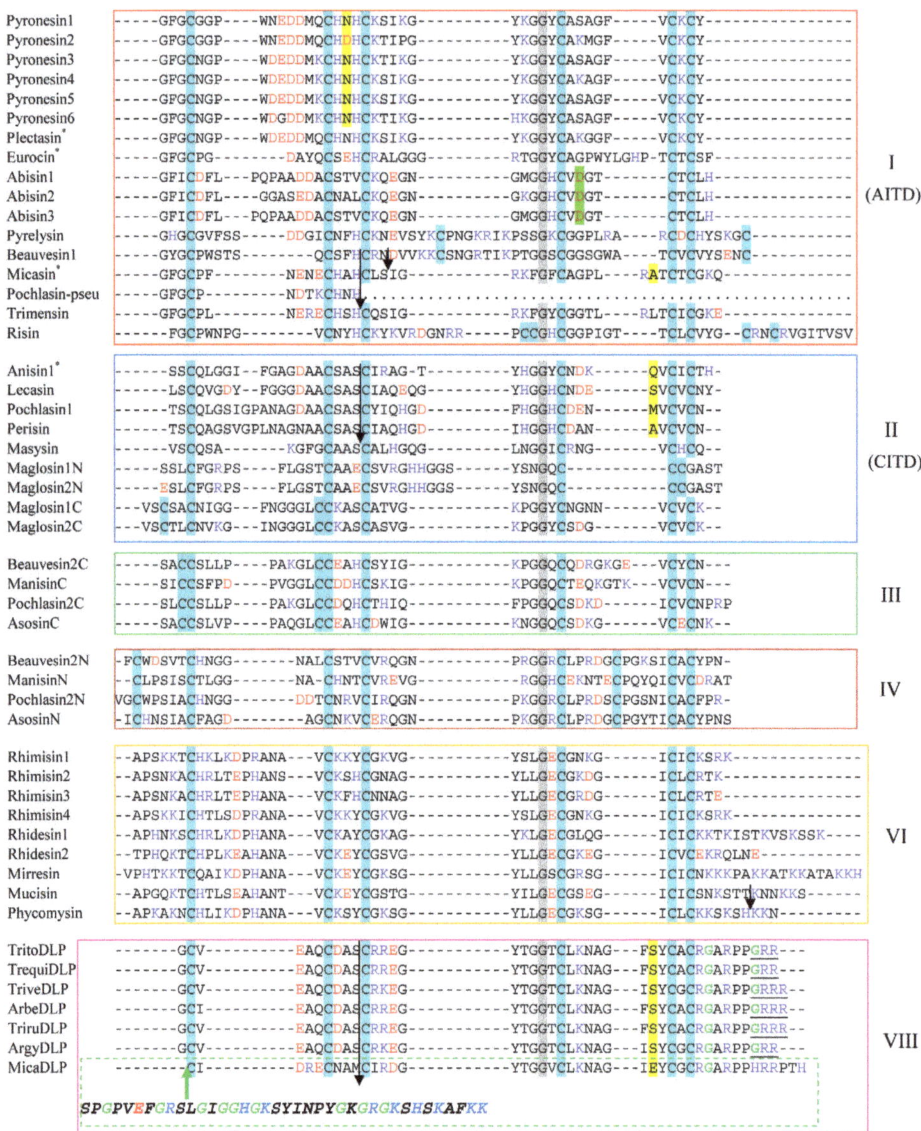

Figure 2. Multiple sequence alignment of fDLPs. Cysteines are shadowed in cyan. Conserved glycines are highlighted in grey. Negatively (D and E) and positively (R, K and H) charged residues are boldfaced in red and blue, respectively. Introns are shown by arrows (phase 0) or small boxes (green: phase 1, yellow: phase 2). Functionally characterized fDLPs were indicated by "*". The N-terminal extension sequence in micaDLP belonging to the family fDEF8 is italicized. Defensins from *Pyronema omphalodes* have been predicted and investigated by RNA-seq [13]. Extra residues for C-terminal amidation are underlined once.

Table 2. Sources and characteristics of the malpisin family.

Name I Accession No.	Organism	Scaffold (Contig)	Range	Size	MW	NC
Malpisin1-1 I AZCI01001104			55070–55405	41	4048	−0.0
Malpisin1-2 I AZCI01001104			55870–56127	48	5166	−3.3
Malpisin1-3 I AZCI01001104		jtg7180000084593 f_7180000084594f	56393–56635	45	5047	+0.7
Malpisin1-4 I AZCI01001104			63869–64117	39	4117	−1.0
Malpisin1-5 I AZCI01000882	*Mortierella alpina* B6842		22045–22248	37	4259	-2.8
Malpisin1-6 I AZCI01000882			25851–26051	39	4543	−3.5
Malpisin1-7 I AZCI01000882		Contig 7180000084767	42456–42677	33	3624	−1.0
Malpisin1-8 I AZCI01000882			43573–43800	47	5078	+1.7
Malpisin1-9 I AZCI01000882			45037–45261	48	5203	+3.0
Malpisin1-10 I AZCI01000882			45559–45738	35	3914	−0.0
Malpisin1-11 I AZCI01000882			46707–46913	43	4941	+5.4
Malpisin1-12 I AZCI01001135		jtg7180000084204f_7 180000084205f_7180000084206f	135437–135676	44	4722	−0.0
Malpisin1-13 I AZCI01001084		jtg7180000084699f_7180000084700f	362415–362627	47	4919	−1.8
Malpisin1-14 I AZCI01001006		jtg7180000084769f_7180000084770f_7 180000084771f_7 180000084772f	179488–179673	38	4188	+0.2
Malpisin2-1 I ADAG01001070			9785–10114	39	4105	+1.0
Malpisin2-2 I ADAG01001070		Contig 1070	10532–10792	48	5187	−2.3
Malpisin2-3 I ADAG01001070			11052–11297	44	4783	−0.0
Malpisin2-4 I ADAG01001070	*Mortierella alpina* ATCC 32222		11773–12021	39	4052	−1.8
Malpisin2-5 I ADAG01000791		Contig 791	4894–5097	37	4259	−2.8
Malpisin2-7 I ADAG01000903			13145–13357	33	3899	+1.2
Malpisin2-8 I ADAG01000903		Contig 903	14223–14450	47	5065	+1.7
Malpisin2-9 I ADAG01000903			15634–15852	45	4917	+4.0
Malpisin2-10 I ADAG01000903			16158–16337	35	3937	+0.2
Malpisin2-11 I ADAG01000903			17264–17446	39	4531	+5.0

```
Micasin*       -----------GFGCPF-NENECHAHCLSIG-RKFGFCAGPL----RATCTCGKQ--------   100
Malpisin1-14   -----------GFGCPD-DERACNDHCKSIN-RNGGYCGGFL----WHTCKCNQS--------   50
Malpisin1-5    -----------GHGCWVFDASECNAFCKEYF-EKPGHCGGFF----YQTCYCE----------   38
Malpisin2-5    -----------GHGCWIFDASECNAFCKEYF-EKPGHCGGFF----YQTCYCD----------   38
Malpisin1-10   -----------NHGCP--FAIFCDEYCKSIN-RSGGYCT------WITTCNCNPT--------   37
Malpisin2-10   -----------NHGCP--LAFFCDEYCKSIH-RSGGYCT------WITTCNCNPT--------   34
Malpisin1-4    -----------NNGCPS-NF-PCNSYCSDRG-FAGGYCSVEDG--ATHRCLCYGP--------   32
Malpisin1-6    -----------GHDCWTFDSTECDRFCREELHRGGGHCAGLF----NQECQCWN---------   30
Malpisin2-4    -----------DYGCPS-NP-PCSLHCEDSG-YAGGYCSVKDG--TIHKCLCYGG--------   29
Malpisin2-1    -------------GCP--NISSCFSTCRGLK-FGRGSCAGDG----HLQCVCYNRPEDA----   20
Malpisin1-1    -------------GCP--NSSSCVSACFGFK-FNGGGCSGDG------QCVCYNHPTPAPTPV   17
Malpisin1-13   -------------GCPE-NVQECSQKCQTEK-RGGGHCSG-------KDCICAKGL-------   28
Malpisin2-11   -----------RISCTP---DVCMERCLLRG-HTQGMCTGRN----RWYCRCYGAPKN-----   20
Malpisin1-11   -----------IRICTP---DACMERCLARG-HAHGICSGRN----RWYCHCLGRPNTKQNF-   18
Malpisin1-8    -----------ISSCPG-TTERCMQACLVRG-FPDGYCTPITIGILRSWCVCSAKMKGEN---   18
Malpisin2-8    -----------LSFCPG-TSEMCMQTCTAKG-FPGGFCTPITLGFLRSWCICKSTETSKN---   18
Malpisin2-2    VASLTNSNDIPDAYCP--NISSCFSHCYYLH-FSHGACAGGG----HLTCYCYDL--------   17
Malpisin1-2    VAPPTAPDDIPDAYCP--NISSCRSHCFYLH-FSHGACVGEG----HLTCSCYDI--------   15
Malpisin1-12   ---SESVVPGGSYGCPG-TSLQCREKCHSIK-WDNGYCDG-------PQCKCVNFS-------   28
Malpisin1-3    ---AELILRDSTYGCPD-TSLQCREKCISLKLWTTGYCNG-------AQCKCMTTF-------   23
Malpisin2-3    ---TELTLTGGSYGCPG-QSEPCRQACHALK-WDNGYCNG-------EKCKCANFF-------   21
Malpisin2-9    ------TMPPLTPSCP--SRSACFQHCVSKN-FYTGRCSGPRN----SRCVCVTQDQA-----   20
Malpisin1-9    ------TIFPSDPSCP--SRPACLRQCVAQN-FHVGRCTGARN----SKCVCLSKEQVEAI--   13

Malpisin1-7    -------------LCP----GGCQKYCQGLG-YADGDCSLFP----WTHCVCYIQ--------   24
Malpisin2-7    -------------FCH----RDCQSFCQKLG-FKDGGCSWFP----WTHCVCYSQ--------   24
```

Figure 3. Multiple sequence alignment of malpisins. Color codes and symbol notes used here are the same as those in Figure 2. Pink box indicates the N-terminus of DLPs with variable length. Sequence identity (%) to micasin is shown on the right.

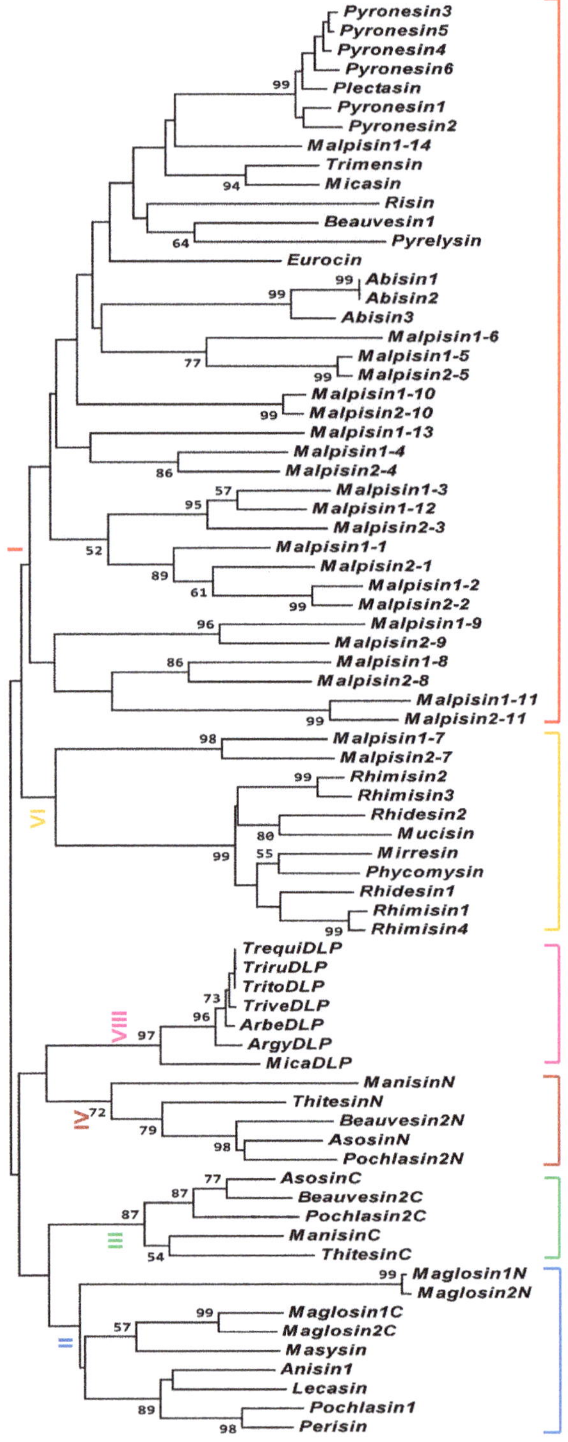

Figure 4. Phylogenetic tree of fDLPs. The tree was constructed from the aligned amino acid sequences presented in Figures 2 and 3 with the neighbor-joining method. The numbers on nodes represent bootstrap values, and only values ≥50% are shown.

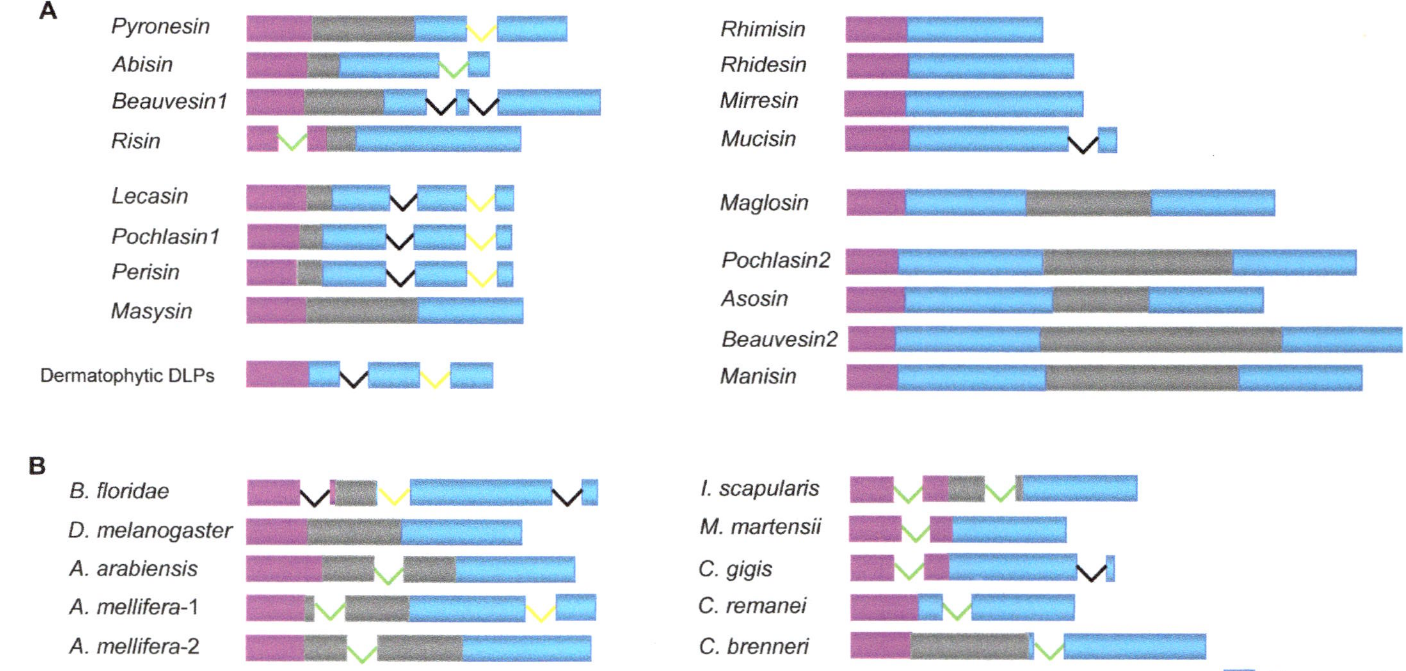

Figure 5. Comparison of precursor organization and exon-intron structures between fDLPs and animal defensins. (**A**) fDLPs; (**B**) Animal defensins. Signal, pro- and mature peptides are shown in pink, grey and blue, respectively. Intron phases are shown in the same colors as Figure 2. Representative animal defensins are derived from *Branchiostoma floridae*, *Drosophila melanogaster*, *Anopheles arabiensis*, *Apis mellifera*, *Ixodes scapularis*, *M. martensii*, *Crassostrea gigas*, *Caenorhabditis remanei*, and *C. brenneri*.

Peptides in fDEF8, all derived from dermatophytes, are characterized as a new family with a short N-terminus and an extra C-terminal extension rich in arginines, prolines and glycines (Figure 2). The C-terminal extension has been considered as a common mechanism for the complexity increase of some invertebrate antimicrobial peptides (AMPs). For example, the hymenopteran defensin-1 subfamily has an extended C-terminus relative to its ancestral defensin-2 subfamily by a so-called intron exonization-mediated mechanism [14,15]. It thus appears that fungal and invertebrate defensins both convergently evolved their C-termini. The extension of a C-terminal sequence via convergent evolution was also recently observed in interleukin 6 (IL-6), a class-I helical cytokine, of two leporids (*Oryctolagus* and *Pentalagus*) [16]. The presence of C-terminal Gly-Arg or Gly-Arg-Arg in some dermatophyte-derived fDLPs suggest that they may be amidated, as previously observed in some animal toxins, e.g., the *Mesobuthus* α-toxins [17]. Interestingly, the mature peptide of micaDLP is larger in size than that of other members in this family, as identified by an N-terminal extension of 38 amino acids (Figure 2). High content of glycines together with a cationic characteristic hints a putative antimicrobial role of this extended unit.

M. alpine is a saprophytic species of *Mucoromycotina*, known as an oleaginous fungus [18]. The draft genome sequences of two *M. alpina* isolates (B6842 and ATCC 32222) [18,19] provide a possibility to undertake comparative study of their fDLPs. We found that the *M. alpine* B6842 genome encodes 14 fDLPs (Figure 3) but only 10 were found in *M. alpine* ATCC 32222. The failure to detect the four homologs (*i.e.*, malpisin1-6, 1-12, 1-13, 1-14) in *M. alpine* ATCC 32222 could be due to the incompletely-assembled genome sequences. Our phylogenetic analysis divides all malpisins into fDEF1 and fDEF6 (Figure 4). Some malpisin members of fDEF1 extended their N-termini with diverse sequences and variable lengths (Figure 3).

3. Gene Duplication of fDLPs

Gene duplication extensively occurs in antimicrobial peptides from insects to humans [15,20,21]. In fungi, initial annotation of defense molecules of *Pyronema omphalodes* also identified gene duplication as a minor multigene family of fDLPs (herein termed pyronesin1 to pyronesin6) [13]. These fDLPs are highly similar to plectasin (Figure 6A). Our studies revealed new gene duplication event in other fungal species. Malpisin is a representative example of gene duplication. As mentioned previously, there are 14 and 10 members in *M. alpine* B6842 and *M. alpine* ATCC 32222, respectively. Malpisin1-1, 1-2, 1-3 and 1-4 are tandem located on one contig (jtg7180000084593f_7180000084594f), and malpisin1-5 to malpisin1-11 on another contig (Contig 7180000084767). In addition, malpisin1-12, malpisin 1-13 and malpisin 1-14 reside on other three contigs, as shown in Figure 6B. In *M. alpine* ATCC 32222, malpisin2-1 to malpisin2-4 are located on contig 1070 and malpisin2-7 to malpisin2-11 on contig 903. Only malpisin2-5 is located on contig 791.

In the widely cultivated mushroom *Agaricus bisporus*, there are three paralogous fDLPs (abisin1 to abisin3) (Figure 6C), two of which (abisin1 and abisin3) share completely identical amino acid sequences in the mature peptide region but exhibit four synonymous substitutions at the nucleotide level. In the *Pochonia chlamydosporia* paralogues, pochlasin1 is highly similar to CITDs and pochlasin2 possesses two defensin-domains. In addition, a putative pseudogene (herein named pochlasin-pseu) was also identified in scaffold 1191 and assigned to AITDs in view of its high sequence similarity to micasin in the first exon. Pochlasin1 and pochlasin-pseu share a conserved phase 0 intron within the α-helical region. The loss of the last two exons (2 and 3) results in the lack the last four cysteines involved in the CSαβ folding of a mature peptide (Figure 2).

Gene duplication also occurs in the *Mucorales*-derived fDLPs, which leads to four and two gene copies in *Rhizopus microsporus* (Figure 6D) and *R. delemar*, respectively. In a Neighbor-Joining (NJ) tree, rhimisin1 and rhimisin4 (*R. microsporus*) constitutes a single clade clustering with the other three fDLPs (rhidesin1 from *R. delemar*, phycomycin from *Phycomyces blakesleeanus* and mirresin from *Mucor irregularis*) whereas rhimisin2 and rhimisin3 (*R. microsporus*) cluster with rhidesin2 (*R. delemar*) and mucisin (*M. circinelloides*) (Figure 4), suggesting that the gene duplication event could have occurred in the ancestor of the *Mucorales* prior to their speciation.

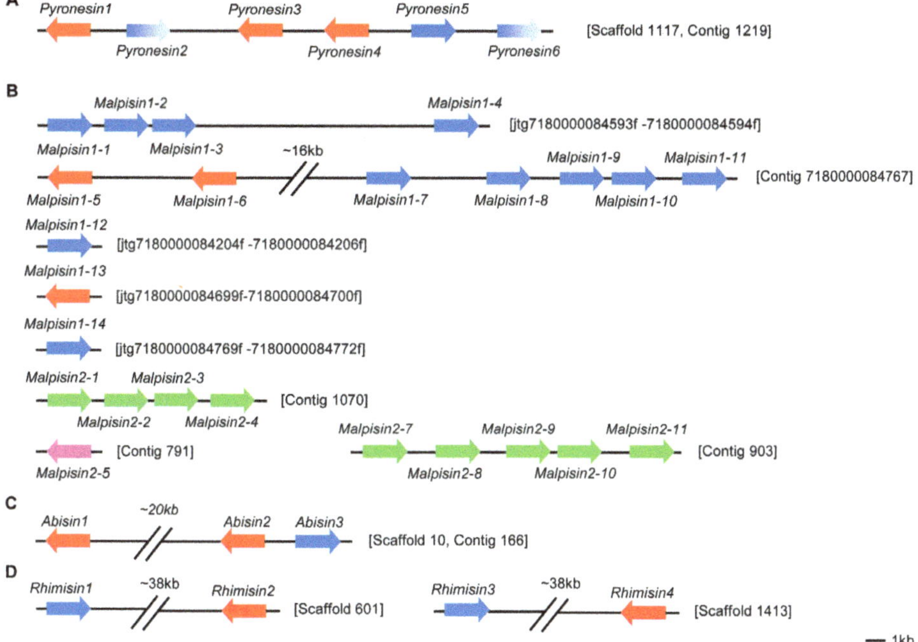

Figure 6. The arrangement of defensin genes in chromosomes. Color arrows refer to different orientation of the genes. **A** to **D** represent the genome location of defensins in four species: *Pyronema omphalodes*, *Mortierella alpine*, *Agaricus bisporus* and *Rhizopus microsporus*. Malpisins in *M. alpine* B6842 is indicated in red and blue while in pink and green in *M. alpine* ATCC 32222. Pseudogenes of pyronesins are shown in gradient blue.

4. Variable Gene Structures of fDLPs

Analysis of the exon-intron structures of the newly-discovered fDLPs revealed their variability that can be described as follows: (1) all the fDLPs retain the integrity of the signal peptide except risin (*Rhizophagus irregularis*) and malpisin1-1 (or malpisin2-1) that have a phase 1 or phase 0 intron disrupting their signal peptides; (2) all of the genes in fDEF8 and three genes in fDEF2 (*i.e.*, lecasin, pochlasin1 and perisin) have the same gene organization as previously identified dermatophytic defensins (micasin, arbesin, trivesin, tritosin and trirusin) and they contain two introns: the first intron (phase 0) disrupting the α-helical region; the second intron (phase 2) disrupting the c-loop; (3) the pyronesin and abisin multi-gene family in fDEF1 have only one intron disrupting either the α-helical or the c-loop region; (4) In addition to these intron-containing fDLP genes, there are some members without introns (Figures 2 and 5).

The highly variable gene structures in fDLPs are reminiscent of invertebrate defensins that also exhibit diverse gene structures [22,23] (Figure 5 and Figure S2). Compared with invertebrate defensins of 5'-biased intron positions, introns of fDLPs occur preferentially in the 3'-end of the precursor-coded sequences. Because all eukaryotic CSαβ-type defensins are hypothesized to be originated from a common bacterial ancestor [24], it is reasonable to infer that considerable intron gains might have occurred in defensins from some eukaryotic lineages, and later they differentially lost in some specific species. Such a dynamic intron evolution thus shapes the biased intron location pattern between fDLPs and animal DLPs after the animal-fungi split. It is also worth mentioning that some recognizable orthologues of defensins in *Branchiostoma floridae* [25,26], the basal chordate amphioxus, also contain a phase 0 intron located in their c-loop (Figure 5 and Figure S2). Given a remote evolutionary distance between fungi and amphioxus, their intron position conservation could be a consequence of convergent insertion in a similar position due to the existence of "protosplice sites" [27,28]. However, the evolution via ancestral origin can be not completely ruled out in the case of the lack of gene structure information in many animal defensins from different lineages.

5. Conclusions

It is estimated that there are as many as 1.5 million species of fungi in this world. However, only a small fraction has been described and even fewer have been sequenced. To date, only about six hundred genomes were being sequenced or completely sequenced. Fungal genome project (FGP) allows us to systematically exploit peptide antibiotics instead of accidental discovery or complicated biochemical screening. This work sheds light on the persistent discovery of fDLPs from model fungal genome data. Despite this, in the lack of experimental data, it cannot be stated that all these fDLPs possess antibacterial function because in fact a classical insect-type fungal defensing - pechrysin was found to lack antibacterial activity [29] likely due to the absence of cationic residues on its molecular surface. In addition, anisin1, a DLP from *Aspergillus giganteus*, was found to be involved in the fitness of the species by linking stress signaling with developmental regulation [30]. Recent studies have also shown that although some peptides of fungal origin contain a similar defensin structure, they exhibit diverse or alternative biological functions beyond antimicrobial activity. An interesting overview is given by Hegedüs and Marx [31]. Therefore, further biochemical characterization of these newly-discovered fDLPs will help evaluate their potential as human medicines.

Acknowledgments: This work was supported by the National Basic Research Program of China (2010CB945300), the National Natural Science Foundation of China (31221091), and the State Key Laboratory of Integrated Management of Pest Insects and Rodents (Grant No. ChineseIPM1307).

Author Contributions: J.W. and S.Z. discovered all fDLP genes described here. J.W. and S.Z. wrote the paper. B.G. revised the paper.

Conflicts of Interest: The authors declare no conflict of interest.

References

1. Mygind, P.H.; Fischer, R.L.; Schnorr, K.M.; Hansen, M.T.; Sonksen, C.P.; Ludvigsen, S.; Raventos, D.; Buskov, S.; Christensen, B.; De Maria, L.; *et al.* Plectasin is a peptide antibiotic with therapeutic potential from a saprophytic fungus. *Nature* **2005**, *437*, 975–980. [CrossRef]
2. Zhu, S.; Gao, B.; Harvey, P.J.; Craik, D.J. Dermatophytic defensin with antiinfective potential. *Proc. Natl. Acad. Sci. USA* **2012**, *109*, 8495–8500. [CrossRef]
3. Zhu, S. Discovery of six families of fungal defensin-like peptides provides insights into origin and evolution of the CSαβ defensins. *Mol. Immunol.* **2008**, *45*, 828–838. [CrossRef]
4. Schneider, T.; Kruse, T.; Wimmer, R.; Wiedemann, I.; Sass, V.; Pag, U.; Jansen, A.; Nielsen, A.K.; Mygind, P.H.; Raventos, D.S.; *et al.* Plectasin, a fungal defensin, targets the bacterial cell wall precursor Lipid II. *Science* **2010**, *328*, 1168–1172. [CrossRef]
5. Oeemig, J.S.; Lynggaard, C.; Knudsen, D.H.; Hansen, F.T.; Norgaard, K.D.; Schneider, T.; Vad, B.S.; Sandvang, D.H.; Nielsen, L.A.; Neve, S.; *et al.* Eurocin, a new fungal defensin: Structure, lipid binding, and its mode of action. *J. Biol. Chem.* **2012**, *287*, 42361–42372. [CrossRef]
6. Hara, S.; Mukae, H.; Sakamoto, N.; Ishimoto, H.; Amenomori, M.; Fujita, H.; Ishimatsu, Y.; Yanagihara, K.; Kohno, S. Plectasin has antibacterial activity and no affect on cell viability or IL-8 production. *Biochem. Biophys. Res. Commun.* **2008**, *374*, 709–713. [CrossRef]

7. Xiong, Y.Q.; Hady, W.A.; Deslandes, A.; Rey, A.; Fraisse, L.; Kristensen, H.H.; Yeaman, M.R.; Bayer, A.S. Efficacy of NZ2114, a novel plectasin-derived cationic antimicrobial peptide antibiotic, in experimental endocarditis due to methicillin-resistant *Staphylococcus aureus*. *Antimicrob. Agents Chemother.* **2011**, *55*, 5325–5330. [CrossRef]
8. Ostergaard, C.; Sandvang, D.; Frimodt-Moller, N.; Kristensen, H.H. High cerebrospinal fluid (CSF) penetration and potent bactericidal activity in CSF of NZ2114, a novel plectasin variant, during experimental pneumococcal meningitis. *Antimicrob. Agents Chemother.* **2009**, *53*, 1581–1585. [CrossRef]
9. Andes, D.; Craig, W.; Nielsen, L.A.; Kristensen, H.H. *In vivo* pharmacodynamic characterization of a novel plectasin antibiotic, NZ2114, in a murine infection model. *Antimicrob. Agents Chemother.* **2009**, *53*, 3003–3009. [CrossRef]
10. Lutzoni, F.; Kauff, F.; Cox, C.J.; McLaughlin, D.; Celio, G.; Dentinger, B.; Padamsee, M.; Hibbett, D.; James, T.Y.; Baloch, E.; *et al.* Assembling the fungal tree of life: Progress, classification, and evolution of subcellular traits. *Am. J. Bot.* **2004**, *91*, 1446–1480. [CrossRef]
11. Seidah, N.G.; Chrétien, M. Proprotein and prohormone convertases: A family of subtilases generating diverse bioactive polypeptides. *Brain Res.* **1999**, *848*, 45–62.
12. Benson, D.A.; Karsch-Mizrachi, I.; Lipman, D.J.; Ostell, J.; Wheeler, D.L. GenBank. *Nucleic Acids Res.* **2008**, *36*, D25–30. [CrossRef]
13. Traeger, S.; Altegoer, F.; Freitag, M.; Gabaldon, T.; Kempken, F.; Kumar, A.; Marcet-Houben, M.; Poggeler, S.; Stajich, J.E.; Nowrousian, M. The genome and development-dependent transcriptomes of *Pyronema confluens*: A window into fungal evolution. *PLoS Genet.* **2013**, *9*, e1003820. [CrossRef]
14. Tian, C.; Gao, B.; Fang, Q.; Ye, G.; Zhu, S. Antimicrobial peptide-like genes in *Nasonia vitripennis*: A genomic perspective. *BMC Genomics* **2010**, *11*, 187. [CrossRef]
15. Zhang, Z.; Zhu, S. Comparative genomics analysis of five families of antimicrobial peptide-like genes in seven ant species. *Dev. Comp. Immunol.* **2012**, *38*, 262–274. [CrossRef]
16. Neves, F.; Abrantes, J.; Pinheiro, A.; Almeida, T.; Costa, P.P.; Esteves, P.J. Convergent evolution of IL-6 in two leporids (*Oryctolagus* and *Pentalagus*) originated an extended protein. *Immunogenetics* **2014**. [CrossRef]
17. Zhu, S.; Peigneur, S.; Gao, B.; Lu, X.; Cao, C.; Tytgat, J. Evolutionary diversification of *Mesobuthus* α-scorpion toxins affecting sodium channels. *Mol. Cell. Proteomics* **2012**. [CrossRef]
18. Wang, L.; Chen, W.; Feng, Y.; Ren, Y.; Gu, Z.; Chen, H.; Wang, H.; Thomas, M.J.; Zhang, B.; Berquin, I.M.; *et al.* Genome characterization of the oleaginous fungus *Mortierella alpina*. *PLoS ONE* **2011**, *6*, e28319. [CrossRef]
19. Etienne, K.A.; Chibucos, M.C.; Su, Q.; Orvis, J.; Daugherty, S.; Ott, S.; Sengamalay, N.A.; Fraser, C.M.; Lockhart, S.R.; Bruno, V.M. Draft genome sequence of *Mortierella alpina* isolate CDC-B6842. *Genome Announc.* **2014**, *2*, e01180-13.
20. Schutte, B.C.; Mitros, J.P.; Bartlett, J.A.; Walters, J.D.; Jia, H.P.; Welsh, M.J.; Casavant, T.L.; McCray, P.B., Jr. Discovery of five conserved β-defensin gene clusters using a computational search strategy. *Proc. Natl. Acad. Sci. USA* **2002**, *99*, 2129–2133. [CrossRef]
21. Semple, C.A.; Rolfe, M.; Dorin, J.R. Duplication and selection in the evolution of primate β-defensin genes. *Genome Biol.* **2003**, *4*, R31. [CrossRef]
22. Froy, O.; Gurevitz, M. Arthropod and mollusk defensins - evolution by exon-shuffling. *Trends Genet.* **2003**, *19*, 684–687. [CrossRef]
23. Rodriguez de la Vega, R.C.; Possani, L.D. On the evolution of invertebrate defensins. *Trends Genet.* **2005**, *21*, 330–332. [CrossRef]
24. Gao, B.; Rodriguez Mdel, C.; Lanz-Mendoza, H.; Zhu, S. AdDLP, a bacterial defensin-like peptide, exhibits anti-*Plasmodium* activity. *Biochem. Biophys. Res. Commun.* **2009**, *387*, 393–398. [CrossRef]
25. Yu, J.K.; Wang, M.C.; Shin-I, T.; Kohara, Y.; Holland, L.; Satoh, N.; Satou, Y. A cDNA resource for the cephalochordate amphioxus *Branchiostoma floridae*. *Dev. Genes Evol.* **2008**, *218*, 723–727. [CrossRef]
26. Zhu, S.; Peigneur, S.; Gao, B.; Umetsu, Y.; Ohki, S.; Tytgat, J. Experimental conversion of a defensin into a neurotoxin: implications for origin of toxic function. *Mol. Biol. Evol.* **2014**, *31*, 546–559. [CrossRef]
27. Sverdlov, A.V.; Rogozin, I.B.; Babenko, V.N.; Koonin, E.V. Reconstruction of ancestral protosplice sites. *Curr. Biol.* **2004**, *14*, 1505–1508. [CrossRef]
28. Rogozin, I.B.; Sverdlov, A.V.; Babenko, V.N.; Koonin, E.V. Analysis of evolution of exon-intron structure of eukaryotic genes. *Brief. Bioinformatics* **2005**, *6*, 118–134. [CrossRef]

29. Wu, Y.; Gao, B.; Zhu, S. Fungal defensins, an emerging source of anti-infective drugs. *Chin. Sci. Bull.* **2014**, *59*, 931–935. [CrossRef]
30. Eigentler, A.; Pocsi, I.; Marx, F. The anisin1 gene encodes a defensin-like protein and supports the fitness of *Aspergillus nidulans*. *Arch. Microbiol.* **2012**, *194*, 427–437. [CrossRef]
31. Hegedus, N.; Marx, F. Antifungal proteins: more than antimicrobials? *Fungal Biol. Rev.* **2013**, *26*, 132–145. [CrossRef]

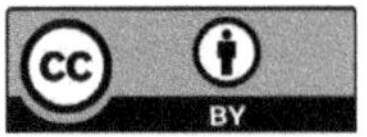

© 2014 by the authors. Licensee MDPI, Basel, Switzerland. This article is an open access article distributed under the terms and conditions of the Creative Commons Attribution (CC BY) license (http://creativecommons.org/licenses/by/4.0/).

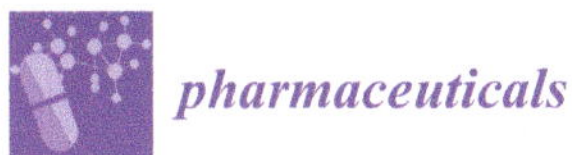

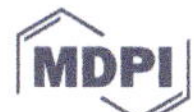

Review

Chapter 3: Antimicrobial Peptides from Plants

James P. Tam [1,*], Shujing Wang [1,2], Ka H. Wong [1] and Wei Liang Tan [1]

1. School of Biological Sciences, Nanyang Technological University, Singapore, Singapore; wangshujing@mail.tsinghua.edu.cn (S.W.); hwka@ntu.edu.sg (K.H.W.); TANW0209@e.ntu.edu.sg (W.L.T.)
2. Department of Pharmacology and Pharmaceutical Sciences, School of Medicine, Tsinghua University, Beijing 100084, China

* Author to whom correspondence should be addressed; jptam@ntu.edu.sg; Tel.: +65-63162863.

Academic Editor: Guangshun Wang
Received: 16 July 2015; Accepted: 1 September 2015; Published: 16 November 2015

Abstract: Plant antimicrobial peptides (AMPs) have evolved differently from AMPs from other life forms. They are generally rich in cysteine residues which form multiple disulfides. In turn, the disulfides cross-braced plant AMPs as cystine-rich peptides to confer them with extraordinary high chemical, thermal and proteolytic stability. The cystine-rich or commonly known as cysteine-rich peptides (CRPs) of plant AMPs are classified into families based on their sequence similarity, cysteine motifs that determine their distinctive disulfide bond patterns and tertiary structure fold. Cystine-rich plant AMP families include thionins, defensins, hevein-like peptides, knottin-type peptides (linear and cyclic), lipid transfer proteins, α-hairpinin and snakins family. In addition, there are AMPs which are rich in other amino acids. The ability of plant AMPs to organize into specific families with conserved structural folds that enable sequence variation of non-Cys residues encased in the same scaffold within a particular family to play multiple functions. Furthermore, the ability of plant AMPs to tolerate hypervariable sequences using a conserved scaffold provides diversity to recognize different targets by varying the sequence of the non-cysteine residues. These properties bode well for developing plant AMPs as potential therapeutics and for protection of crops through transgenic methods. This review provides an overview of the major families of plant AMPs, including their structures, functions, and putative mechanisms.

Keywords: plant antimicrobial peptides; cysteine-rich peptides; cystine knot; thionin; defensin; hevein; knottin

---

1. Introduction

Higher plants have a broad range of defense mechanisms to counter physical, chemical and biological stress such as drought, cold, heavy metal, pollutants and pathogen attacks from fungi, bacteria and viruses. In response to infection by a variety of pathogens, plants display up-regulation of a set of genes associated with systemic acquired resistance [1]. General resistance is accomplished by the release of secondary metabolites like phytoalexins, tannins and polyphenolic compounds, and the generation of pathogenesis-related (PR) proteins. PR proteins were first discovered in the early 1970s in tobacco leaves in response totobacco mosaic virus infections and were later defined as the induced proteins that are released during pathogenic attacks [2,3]. According to a recent review, there are at least 17 families that have been detected and isolated that possess a wide range of defense-related properties, including antibacterial, antifungal, antiviral, anti-oxidative activity, chitinase and proteinase inhibitory activities [1–4]. This review will focus on peptides which possess antimicrobial activity, namely thionin (PR-13 family), defensin (PR-12 family), hevein-like peptide, knottin, α-hairpinin, lipid transfer protein (PR-14 family) and snakin.

Antimicrobial peptides (AMPs) are ubiquitous and found as host defenses against pathogens and pests in diverse organisms ranging from microbes to animals [5]. AMPs exist in different molecular forms, although the majority of them are linear peptides from insects, animals, and plants. Nevertheless, bacteria produce polycyclic peptides such as lantibiotics, and all major forms of life produce circular peptides which include bacteriocins from bacteria, cyclotides from plants and theta-defensins from animals [6–9]. In plants, the majority of AMPs are Cys-rich [10], a feature that enables the formation of multiple disulfide bonds (usually two to six) that contribute to a compact structure and resistance to chemical and proteolytic degradation.

In general, plant AMPs share several common characteristics with those from microbes, insects and animals. They include features such as their molecular forms, positive charge and amphipathic nature, all of which are primarily related to their defensive role(s) as membrane-active antifungals, antibacterials, and antivirals. These features, in addition to being Cys-rich, are well represented by two plant AMP families, thionins and plant defensins. Other families of plant AMPs act on pathogens differently from animal AMPs. For example, hevein-like peptides bind chitins, knottin-type peptides inhibit enzymes such as proteases, and lipid transfer proteins bind lipids to disrupt microbial penetration into cell membranes.

Classification of plant AMP families is largely based on their Cys motifs which exhibit a characteristic Cys pattern with a defined number of non-Cys residues between the two neighboring Cys. Currently, the number of AMPs isolated from a limited number of plants already exceeds a thousand and is likely to increase in the future. Sequence analysis and genomic data mining using these Cys motifs have revealed that Cys-rich peptides (CRPs) with AMP characteristics are under-predicted [11]. In model plants, such as rice and *Arabidopsis*, CRPs may account for about 3% of the expressed proteins.

Like animal AMPs, AMP expression in plants is constitutive or induced and often tissue-specific. Moreover, plant AMPs are evolvable with hypervariable sequences encased in a particular scaffold characteristic of a given family of AMPs, which is analogous, but to a much lesser extent, to the molecular diversity of vertebrate immunoglobulin-based immunity.

This review aims to provide a general overview of the major families of plant AMPs, including their structures, functions, and putative mechanisms of defense. Additional details on plant AMPs can be found in a number of excellent previous reviews [12–25]. Furthermore, information on AMPs from diverse organisms can be accessed through several databases, such as APD, APD2 [26,27], YADAMP [28], DAMPD [29], and PhytAMP (specific for plant AMPs) [10].

2. Classification and Characteristics

Plant AMPs are divided into families based on their sequence similarity, Cys motifs, and distinctive disulfide bond patterns which, in turn, determine their tertiary structure folding. Table 1 lists the major families of plant AMPs based on these criteria; families include thionins, defensins, hevein-like peptides, knottin-type peptides (linear and cyclic), lipid transfer proteins, α-hairpinin families, snakins, and unclassified CRP-AMPs. In addition, non-CRP AMPs, which may be rich in other amino acids, are also described in this review, including the Gly-rich peptide (GRP) Pg-AMP1, the Gly- and His-rich peptide shepherins, and peptides of less than 10 amino acids (aa), such as Cn-AMP1 and Cr-ACP1. The following defining features are found in plant AMPs:

1. Mostly characterized as moderate-size (MW of 2–6 kDa), basic, CRPs with two to six intra-molecular disulfide bonds.
2. Members within a family are classified based on Cys motif, sequence similarity and are conserved in secondary and tertiary structure.

3. One or two additional disulfide bonds are found in members of thionins, defensins, and hevein-like peptides. These additional bonds bolster structural stability without affecting the general scaffold. Because the varying number of Cys residues can create confusion, we refer to AMPs within a family based on the number of Cys when necessary throughout this review (e.g., 6C-thionins contain six Cys and 8C-thionins have eight Cys).
4. In addition to being antimicrobial, AMPs also display "peptide promiscuity", which refers to the multiple functions displayed by a single peptide.
5. All are ribosomally derived and bioprocessed from precursors, which often contain three domains: N- and C-terminal pro-domains and a mature AMP domain. Mature sequences are often hypervariable and display more variation than the conserved terminal domains in the preproprotein to give sequence diversity for adaptation.
6. Because of cross-bracing by multiple disulfide bonds, most CRP-AMPs with a molecular weight (MW) of 2–6 kDa are structurally compact with high thermal, chemical, and enzymatic stability.

Table 1. Major families of plant AMPs.

Peptide	S-S No.	Representative Member			Structural Motif
		Name	AA No.	Disulfide Motif	
6C-Thionin	3	Crambin	46	2-C-0-C-11-C-8-C-5-C-7-C-6	Gamma (Γ) fold
8C-Thionin	4	β-Purothionin	45	2-C-0-C-7-C-3-C-8-C-3-C-1-C-7-C-6	β1-α1-α2-β2-coil motif
8C-Defensin	4	NaD1	47	2-C-10-C-5-C-3-C-9-C-6-C-1-C-3-C	CSαβ motif
10C-Defensin	5	PhD1	47	2-C-3-C-6-C-5-C-2-C-0-C-9-C-6-C-1-C-3-C	β1-coil-α-β2-β3
6C-Hevein	3	Ac-AMP1	29	3-C-4-C-4-C-0-C-5-C-6-C-1	Gly & Cys rich Central β
8C-Hevein	4	Hevein	43	2-C-8-C-4-C-0-C-5-C-6-C-5-C-3-C-2	strands & (short helical)
10C-Hevein	5	EAFP1	41	2-C-3-C-3-C-4-C-0-C-5-C-6-C-5-C-1-C-1-C-2	side coils
Knottin	3	PAFP-S	38	2-C-6-C-8-C-0-C-3-C-10-C-3	Cystine knot Short β
Cyclic Knottin	3	Kalata B1	29	4-C-3-C-4-C-4-C-1-C-4-C-3	strand & coil
α-Hairpinin	2	Ec-AMP1	37	6-C-3-C-13-C-3-C-8	α1-turn-α2
LTP	4	Maize LTP1	93	3-C-9-C-14-C-0-C-19-C-1-C-22-C-13-C-4	Hydrophobic cavity
LTP	4	Wheat LTP2	67	1-C-7-C-13-C-0-C-8-C-1-C-23-C-6-C	α1-α2-α3-α4-coil
Snakin *	6	Snakin-1	63	4-C-3-C-3-C-8-C-3-C-2-CC-2-C-1-C-11-C-1-C-12-C-1	α -helices

* The disulfide and structural motif of Snakin-1 is predicted based on homology modelling.

2.1. Thionins

α-/β-Thionins are the prototypic plant AMP; they are cationic peptides of 45–48 aa with three or four disulfide bonds [12]. Initially, they were known as plant toxins because of their toxicity towards bacteria [30], fungi [31], plant and animal cells [32], as well as insect larvae [33]. The prototypic thionin with antimicrobial activity, α-purothionin, was isolated in the endosperm of wheat [30,34]. Following the discovery of α-purothionin, subsequent thionins isolated from other plants are labeled with descending letters of the Greek alphabet in the order of their discovery (e.g., α-thionins, β-thionins, and γ1/γ1-thionins).

Classification of thionins is largely based on α-purothionin and includes the α-/β-thinoins of crambin, viscotoxins, phoratoxin A, hordothionins, and purothinoins. However, γ-thionins are considered part of the plant defensin family based on structural considerations. Thus, α-/β-thionins share a similar structural fold different from that of γ-thionins. For convenience, α/β-thionins with eight Cys residues will be hereafter referred to as 8C-thionins and those with six Cys designated 6C-thionins (Figure 1A,B).

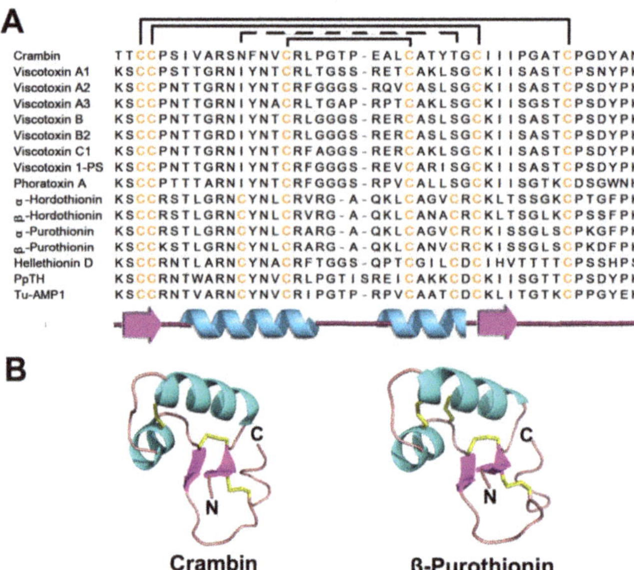

Figure 1. Sequences (**A**) and structures (**B**) of representative thionins. The secondary structure is represented by different colors: cyan-α helix; magenta-β strand; pink-random coil and yellow-disulfide bonds.

2.1.1. Occurrences, Distribution, and Biosynthesis

Thionins have been identified from monocots and dicots and are expressed in different tissues, such as seeds, leaves, and roots [35–37]. The expression of thionins can be induced by infection with various microbes [38,39] and has been shown to be related to the release of the hormone methyl jasmonate upon plant wounding or microorganism invasion [38,40,41]. Thionins are ribosomally derived and expressed as prepropoteins, wherein the prothionin domain is flanked by two conserved sequences, the N-terminal signaling peptide and C-terminal acidic domain [35,38,42]. Mature thionin sequences display more variation than the conserved terminal domains in the prepropotein due to evolutionary pressure [43]. The three-domain precursor of plant AMPs in CRP families is typical and found in other CRP families, including defensins, hevein-like peptides, and knottin-type peptides.

2.1.2. Structure

From the limited number of members identified thus far, thionins have relatively conserved amino acid sequences compared to other plant defense peptides (Figure 1A). They also share a conserved β1-α1-α2-β2-coil secondary structural motif, which forms a gamma (Γ) fold, a special turn consists of three amino acid residues with the first and third residue connected by a hydrogen bond in the tertiary structure (Figure 1A,B).

Thionins can be loosely classified as pseudocyclics because of an end-to-end disulfide bond linking the N- and C-termini, conferring a circular structural topology. They are, however, not true pseudocyclics because there are additional non-cysteine amino acids located at both the N- and C-termini. 8C-Thionins contain four conserved stabilizing disulfide bonds between CysI-CysVIII (Cys numbering in Roman numerals from N-to-C-termini) linking β1 to the C-terminal coil, CysII-CysVII linking the end of β1 with the beginning of β2, CysIII-CysVI linking α1 and the loop after α2, and CysIV-CysV linking α1 and α2. The 6C-thionins have the same Cys pairing as 8C-thionins except for the absence of the CysII-CysVII disulfide bond. The structure of 8C-thionins, including α-/β-purothionins, α-/β-hordothionin, and hellethionin D, are similar to that of 6C-thionins with the Γ-shape but with minor differences in the C-terminal coil region [44–46]. The long arm of the Γ fold comprises the α1-α2 region, and the short arm consists of β1 and the β2-coil. The large groove between the two arms is proposed to be important for the interaction between thionins and membrane lipids [43]. Most hydrophobic side chains cluster around the outer surface of the long arm, while the hydrophilic chains are located on the surface within the groove or outer face of the short arm (Figure 2A).

2.1.3. Structure-Function Relationship

The 6C-thionins with three disulfide bonds include crambin, viscotoxins, and phoratoxin A. Most 6C-thionins are highly basic, amphipathic, and toxic, with the exception of crambin. Crambin is a neutral, hydrophobic, non-toxic peptide identified from *Crambe abyssinica* with two isomers, P22/L25 and S22/I25 [47,48]. High resolution structures of crambin have been determined by NMR and X-ray/neutron crystallography in both water and detergent [47,49–53]. Viscotoxins (including A1, A2, A3, B, B2, C1, and 1-PS) and phoratoxins from the mistletoes share a similar Γ-shape with β1-α1-α2-β2-coil motif [54–60].

8C-Thionins with four disulfide bonds include α-/β-purothionins, α-/β-hordothionins, hellethionin-D, *Pyrularia Pubera* thionin (PpTH), and *Tulipa gensneriana* bulb-purified AMPs (Tu-AMPs). The monomeric conformation of the 45-aa α-hordothionin isolated from barley [61,62] was previously determined by NMR [62], while X-ray crystallography revealed a dimeric structure [61]. A study by Vila-Perello showed that removal of one disulfide bond from PpTH is sufficient to significantly alter its folding [63]. A 45% size-reduced form of PpTH was synthesized, which only contains residues 7–32 with the two antiparallel α-helices stabilized by two disulfide bonds. Size-reduced PpTH appeared to display the same antimicrobial activity and mechanism of action as intact PpTH in selected test microorganisms [64].

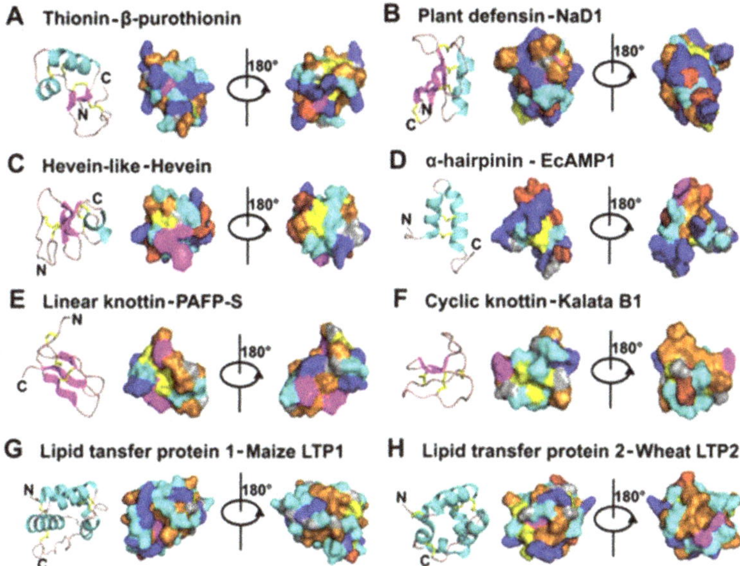

Figure 2. Cartoon illustration and surface plot of representative members of different antimicrobial peptides. The orientation of surface plot (left) of each representative member is the same as the cartoon illustration, while that of the right one is evolved from the left one by 180° turn around the y axis. Color representation rules for different amino acids are as follows: blue-positively charged (R, K & H), red-negatively charged (D & E), orange-hydrophobic (I, L, V, A, P & M), cyan-hydrophilic (S, T, E & Q), magenta-aromatic (F, Y & W), yellow-cysteine (C) and gray-glycine (G).

Tu-AMP1 and Tu-AMP2 are antibacterial, antifungal, and can reversibly bind chitin, a key constituent of the cell wall of fungi and exoskeletons of invertebrates, such as insects, anthropods, and nematodes. Initially, they were suggested to be thionin-like peptides, although Tu-AMP2 is a heterodimer of two chains joined by disulfide bonds [65]. However, it is worthwhile to point out that in our review of plant CRPs, the occurrence of heterodimer is exceedingly rare. In our view, it remains to be determined whether the heterodimeric formation occurs during the isolation process.

2.1.4. Mechanism of Action

Thionins are hydrophobic and likely elicit their toxicity to bacteria, fungi, and animal and plant cells via membrane interactions with their hydrophobic residues or/and positive surface charge [12, 13,18,66–68]. The proposed mechanism of toxicity is attributed to lysis of cell membranes, but it is still under investigation [30,39,68–70]. Stec proposed a structural model of the thionin-phospholipid interaction to explain the solubilization and lysis of cell membranes [43].

Thionins are known to directly interact with membrane lipids apart from protein receptors [67, 71,72]. *Pyrularia* thionin from the nuts of *Pyrularia pubera* mediates the influx of Ca^{2+} during certain cellular responses, while Tyr iodination reduces its hemolysis, phospholipase A2 activation, and cytotoxicity [32]. Structure-function studies have demonstrated that Lys1 and Tyr13 in thionins are highly conserved and proposed to be crucial to their toxicity, with the exception of non-toxic, non-lytic crambin. Instead, crambin contains Thr1 and Phe13 residues [32,43,73,74]. Furthermore, Arg10 is suggested to be important to the folding stability of all thionins, as it is an abundant source of hydrogen bonds between $\beta 1$, $\alpha 1$, and the C-terminal coil [75].

2.2. *Plant Defensins*

Plant defensins are the best known, and likely most abundant, of all plant AMPs with membranolytic functions, according to data mining of selected plant genomes. They are cationic peptides of 45–54 aa with four to five disulfide bonds [76]. Plant defensins have diverse biological functions which include antifungal [77–81], antibacterial [82,83], and α-amylase and trypsin inhibitory activity [84,85]. In addition to being antimicrobial, plant defensins are also involved in the biotic stress response, as well as plant growth and development.

Plant defensins were first identified as γ-thionins, γ1-hordothionin, and γ1-/γ2-purothionins from wheat and barley grains [86,87]. Thus, they were initially classified as γ-thionins due to their limited sequence identity (25%) with α-/β-thionins. Later, they were found to be unrelated to thionins based on structural features [88]. In 1995, they were grouped as plant defensins based on their sequence, structure, and function similarities with mammalian and insect defensins [76,78,88,89].

2.2.1. Occurrences, Distribution, and Biosynthesis

Plant defensins include over 100 members from a wide range of plants, including wheat, barley, tobacco, radish, mustard, turnip, arabidopsis, potato, sorghum, soybean, cowpea, and spinach, among others [15,90]. They have been identified in multiple tissues, tubers [79,91], leaves [79], pods [92], and flowers [93–95], with the majority identified from seeds and roots [96]. Two types of precursors have been identified in plant defensins, wherein the dominant group is composed of the N-terminal signal peptide and a mature plant defensin domain [97], while the minor group is composed of an extra C-terminal acidic pro-domain of 33 aa reportedly associated with the vacuolar sorting mechanism since defensins with this domain were found in vacuoles and those without were found in the outer cell layers [16,79,95].

2.2.2. Structures

Plant defensins are generally characterized by four conserved disulfide bonds (except for PhDs, a 10C-plant defensin isolated from *Petunia hydrida*) with the outer disulfide pair as an end-to-end inner disulfide bridge and the inner three pairs of disulfide bonds forming a cystine knot (see knottins).

A secondary structure characteristic of plant defensins is a Cys-stabilized αβ (CSαβ) motif of the cysteine knot. The CSαβ motif was first characterized in charybdotoxin, a K^+ channel blocker isolated from scorpions [98] and named by Cornet *et al.* [99]. This motif forms a β1-coil-α-β2-β3 pattern in the secondary structure, where the α-helix is parallel to three antiparallel β-strands (Figure 3A,B). The CSαβ scaffold is stabilized and characterized by: (1) two disulfide bonds between the CXXXC motif from the α-helix and the CXC motif in the central β3 strand; (2) one disulfide bond between the β2 strand and the first loop before the α-helix; and (3) an end-to-end disulfide bond between the N- and C-termini, a disulfide connective similar to thionins. However, plant defensins (γ-thionins) differ greatly from α-/β-thinoins in their secondary and tertiary structures. In the secondary structure, α-/β-thionins show a typical β1-α1-α2-β2-coil motif, whereas γ-thionins display a β1-coil-α-β2-β3 motif. At the tertiary structural level, β1 and β2 orient antiparallel in α-/β-thinoins, whereas the corresponding β1and β3 in γ-thionins are oriented in parallel.

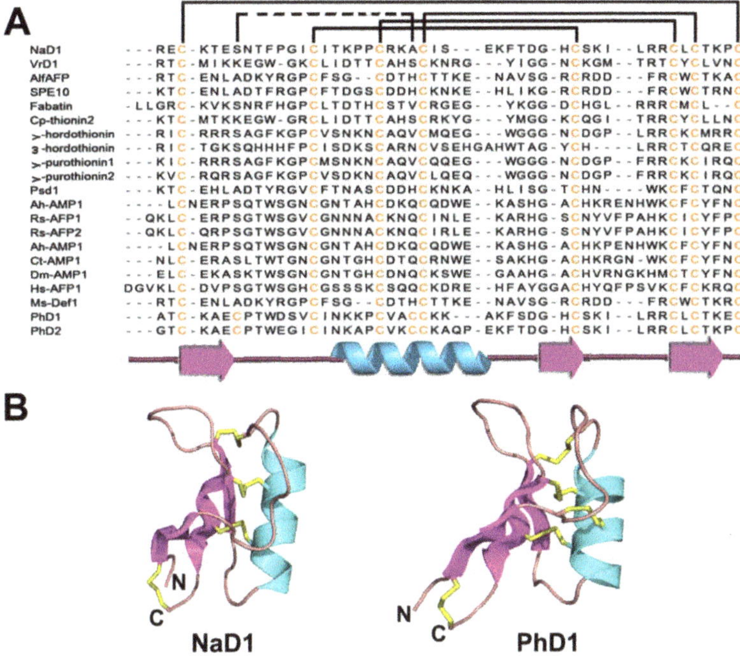

Figure 3. Sequences (**A**) and structures (**B**) of representative plant defensins. The secondary structure is represented by different colors: cyan-α helix; magenta-β strand; pink-random coil and yellow-disulfide bonds.

Similar to thionins, plant defensins are pseudocyclics (see thionins), with conservation of the disulfide bond between the first and last Cys, conferring a circular structural topology by connecting the side chains of the N- and C- termini.

Plant defensins have been reported to be stable in harsh conditions that mimic the digestive system and decoction process, including high temperature (~85 °C), low pH (~2.0), and oxidative and proteolytic environments [100–102]. Although defensins show conservation of the CSαβ motif, there are variations in the number of disulfide bonds, primary sequences, and tertiary structures [89,103,104]. It has been shown that Ala substitutions of non-Cys residues on VrD1 are tolerated in the CSαβ motif although the structural stability and inhibitory effects vary among the mutants [105].

2.2.3. Structure-Function Relationship

Based on the number of Cys, plant defensins are further divided into 8C-plant defensins with four disulfides and 10C-plant defensins with five disulfide bonds.

The 8C-plant defensins include NaD1, VrD1, AlfAFP, ω-hordothionin, Cp-thionin II, Rs-AFPs, Psd1, Fabatins, and Ms-Def1 (Figure 3A,B). NaD1 (47 aa) was identified from the outer cell layers of different flower parts of the ornamental tobacco *Nicotiana alata*. Its distribution is consistent with its protective roles in reproductive organs. *In vitro* results showed that NaD1 inhibits the growth of plant pathogens *Botrytis cinerea* and *Fusarium oxysporus* [95,106]. VrD1 (46 aa) from the mung bean *Vigna radiata* not only inhibits protein synthesis, but is also antimicrobial and insect (bruchids)-resistant [107, 108]. ω-Hordothionin (48 aa) purified from barley endosperm inhibits translational activity in both eukaryotic and prokaryotic cell-free systems [109]. The crystal structure of SPE10, identified from *Pachyrrhizus erosus* seeds [110], shows a dimer with each unit adopting the typical CSαβ motif [111]. Based on structural analysis and mutation studies, the dimeric conformation of SPE10 was suggested to be associated with its function, while the hydrophobic patch on the molecular head is necessary for its antifungal activity.

AlfAFP from *Medicago sativa* seeds is an antifungal peptide that provides robust resistance to the fungal pathogen *Verticillium dahliae* in transgenic potato plants [77,106]. Rs-AFPs (51 aa) purified from *Raphanus sativus* radish seeds are highly basic oligomeric proteins with an N-terminal pyroglutamic acid. They have a broad antifungal spectrum with an IC_{50} = 0.3–100 μg/mL [78,79,81]. Rs-AFPs are abundant in near-mature and mature seeds and released to create a fungal-suppressing microenvironment after disruption of the seed coat [79]. Ms-Def1 from *Medicago sativa* seeds strongly inhibits the fungal growth of *Fusarium graminearum in vitro* [112]; the inhibitory effect is reduced in the presence of Ca^{2+} ions. Homologous antifungal peptides were also reported from seeds of *Aesculus hippocastanum*, *Clitoria ternatea* (Ct-AMP1), *Dahlia merckii* (Dm-AMP1), *Lens culinaris* (Lc-def) and *Heuchera sanguine* (Hs-AFP1) [80,97,113].

Cp-thionin II (47 aa) was identified from *Vigna unguiculata* cowpea seeds and is antibacterial against both Gram-positive and Gram-negative bacteria such as *Staphylococcus aureus*, *Escherichia coli*, and *Pseudomonas syringae* with minimal inhibitory concentrations of 128, 64, and 42 μg/mL, respectively [90]. Psd1, a 46 aa peptide identified from seeds of the pea *Pisum sativum*, is antibacterial and acts as a K^+ channel inhibitor based on a surface charge distribution analysis [114]. Fabatins isolated from the broad bean *Vicia faba* are active against both Gram-positive and Gram-negative bacteria, but inactive against the yeasts *Saccharomyces cerevisiae* and *Candida albicans* [115].

PhDs are 10C-plant defensins. From flowers of *Petunia* hybrids, Lay *et al.* reported two AMPs with antifungal activity, PhD1 (47 aa) and PhD2 (49 aa) [95]. A fifth disulfide bond exists between the α-helix and the loop after β1 within these defensins that do not alter the typical CSαβ topology [108]. The fifth disulfide bond appears only to change the corresponding hydrophobic interaction and hydrogen bond, as in 8C-plant defensins, to a covalent disulfide bond in PhD1 without altering the side-chain orientation of substituted residues.

The γ-thionins which have been reclassified as defensins, γ-hordothionin and ω-hordothionin from *Hordeum vulgare*, were shown to inhibit protein translation in rabbit reticulocytes and mouse liver extracts [87]. However, this inhibitory effect was not observed on plants, such as *Triticum aestivum*, *Cucumis sativus*, *Vicea sativa* and *H. vulgare*, and which may indicate a certain specificity in its mechanism of action. Similarly, no direct interaction was observed between the plant defensins and nucleic acids, which is the proposed mechanism of the inhibitory activity of protein synthesis by the plant thionin family [116]. Instead of protein translation, Mendez *et al.* suggested that ω-hordothionin may act on protein synthesis at the initiation and elongation step [109].

Defensins isolated from the seeds of *Sorghum bicolor*, $S1\alpha_1$, $S1\alpha_2$ and $S1\alpha_3$, were demonstrated to display inhibitory activity against α-amylase activity [84]. They are able to inhibit α-amylase obtained from the gut of the insects *Periplaneta americana* and *Locusta migratoria migratorioides*, and weakly inhibit the α-amylase from human saliva. Defensins from *Vigna unguiculata* and ω-hordothionin, from *H.*

vulgare, also exhibit similar inhibitory activity against insect α-amylase [109,117,118], however, no significant inhibitory effect was observed on porcine α-amylase by plant defensins [119]. Several plant defensins exhibit the ability to inhibit ion channels. Kushmerick *et al.* showed that γ1-zeathionin and γ2-zeathionin from maize kernels block voltage-gated Na^+ channels reversibly in intact mammalian GH3 cells using the patch-clamp technique [120]. These authors postulated that the ion channel inhibitory effect of defensins may be related to the similar 3D structure with scorpion neurotoxin, a well-known Na^+ channel blocker. Plant defensins were also shown to inhibit Ca^{2+} channels [112]. However, no significant inhibitory effect was observed on K^+ channels by plant defensins [119].

Two homologous peptides that display high sequence similarity to plant defensins were isolated from the plant *Cassia fistula*, denoted 5459 and 5144 according to their molecular weight [85]. The 5459 defensin was demonstrated to exhibit trypsin inhibitory activity, whereas no inhibitory effect was observed by the 5144 defensin. Another defensin peptide, Cp-thionin from *V. uguiculata* seeds, was reported to display inhibitory activity against pancreatic bovine trypsin [121].

An enzymatic activity was attributed to a plant defensin. Huang *et al.* cloned the defensin SPD1 from the roots of Ipomoea batatas and showed that it has the ability to regenerate dehydroascorbate (DHA) to ascorbic acid (AsA) in the presence of glutathione [122]. The peptide is also able to convert monodehydroascrobate (MDA) to AsA in the presence of NADH, functioning as a glutathione-dependent dehydroascorbate reductase. SPD1 is likely to function as a regulator of the redox state of AsA, which has been implicated in the response of the plant cell to reactive oxidative stress [123].

2.2.4. Mechanism of Action

The structure-function relationship of plant defensins has been suggested to correlate with their positive charge and amphipathic nature, as illustrated by the structure-surface plot of NaD1 in Figure 2B. Thus, plant defensins could initially bind to microbial membranes through interactions with specific binding sites ("receptors"), as reported for Rs-AFP2, Hs-AFP1, and Dm-AMP1 [16,124,125]. Binding of plant defensins, such as Rs-AFP2 and Dm-AMP1, to the cell membrane results in the influx and efflux of positive ions like Ca^{2+} and K^+ [126,127]. Lastly, Ms-Def1 is able to block the Ca^{2+} channel in a manner similar to the Ca^{2+} channel blocker KP4 [112]. Van der Weerden *et al.* demonstrated that NaD1 does not cause membranes permeabilization via a canonical mechanism which involves nonspecific insertion into membranes [128] but rather a cell wall dependent process, likely requiring a specific receptor. The mechanism of the fungicidal action of NaD1 is likely through permeabilization of the hyphae of *Fusarium oxysporum*, entering into the cytoplasm of the cell and inducing ROS oxidative stress [129]. Hayes *et al.* reported that the high-osmolarity glycerol (HOG) pathway is involved in the protection of the cell against NaD1 [130], indicating that the inhibition of the HOG pathway increases the activity of antimicrobial peptides against *Candida albicans*. Several reviews have discussed in detail the plant defensin mechanism of action [16,101,131,132].

2.3. *Hevein-Like Peptides*

Hevein-like peptides are basic peptides of 29–45 aa with three to five disulfide bonds. They are rich in Gly and contain conserved aromatic residues found in the hevein domain of lectins. Hevein domains bind to chitin [133–135], which is their primary target.

Hevein was first identified as the most abundant protein component from the latex of the rubber tree *Hevea brasiliensis* and displays strong antifungal activity *in vitro* [136,137]. It was also reported to be a major allergen from latex involved in human latex-fruit syndrome [138,139]. Similar to hevein, hevein-like peptides inhibit the growth of chitin-containing fungi and defend plants against attack from a wide range of fungal pathogens [133,140].

2.3.1. Occurrences, Distribution and Biosynthesis

As a chitin-binding domain, the hevein domain is found in several plant lectins, natural variants of heveins (pseudo-hevein, wheat germ agglutinin, *Urtica dioica* agglutinin), and AMPs [134,141,142].

Similar to other families of CRP-AMPs, the hevein-like peptide is processed from a three-domain precursor. For example, the cDNA of the Ar-AMP precursor comprises a 25 aa N-terminal signal sequence, 30 aa mature peptide, and 34 aa C-terminal region which is cleaved during post-translational processing [143]. In 10C-hevein (hevein-like peptide containing 10 cysteine residues), there are two different precursor peptide structures in the C-terminal prodomain. The WAMP 10C-hevein from *Triticum kiharae* have precursor similar to other families CRP-AMPs, with a 45aa C-terminal region [144], while Ee-CBP 10C-hevein from *Euonymus europaeus* is produced as a chimeric precursor consisting of the mature peptide domain linked to a long C-terminal chitinase-like domain [145]. Andreev *et al.* [144] also showed that the WAMP-1 and WAMP-2 gene may have originated from ancestral chitinase genes and that a frame-shift deletion of the coding region for the catalytic domain led to the WAMP gene formation.

2.3.2. Structure

Hevein-like peptides share conserved Cys, Gly, and several aromatic amino acid residues. They vary substantially in their primary sequences and number of disulfide bonds (from three to five; Figure 4A,B). Thus, hevein-like peptides can be divided into 6C-, 8C-, and 10C-hevein-like peptide subgroups based on the number of Cys they contain. All hevein-like peptides has a cysteine knot motif (see knottins). The solid-state and solution structures of the hevein domain, as determined by X-ray crystallography and NMR, respectively [142,146,147], provide the basis for analyzing the carbohydrate binding ability of this domain. Generally, hevein-like peptides contain a coil-β1-β2-coil-β3 secondary structural motif with variations based on the presence of short turns in the two long coils and β3 strand. Antiparallel β-strands form the central β-sheet of the hevein motif with the two long coils located on each side stabilized by disulfide bonds.

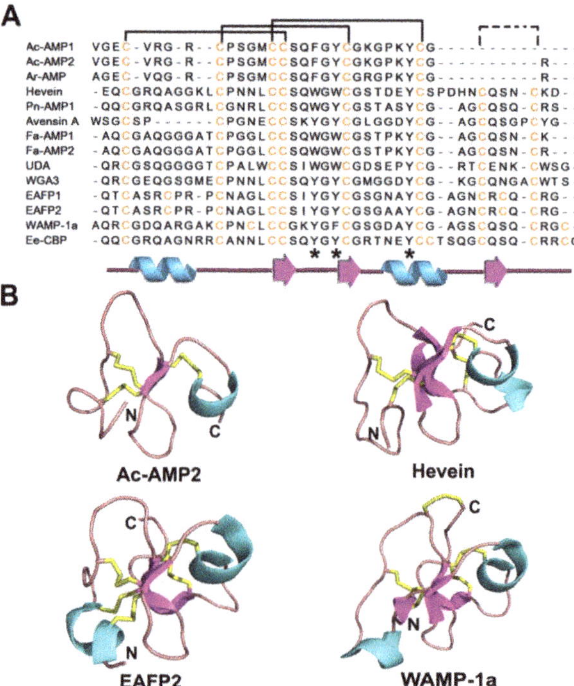

Figure 4. Sequences (**A**) and structures (**B**) of representative hevein-like peptides. The secondary structure is represented by different colors: cyan-α helix; magenta-β strand; pink-random coil and yellow-disulfide bonds.

2.3.3. Structure-Function Study

6C-Hevein-like peptides Ac-AMP1 and Ac-AMP2 isolated from *Amaranthus caudatus* seeds exhibit antimicrobial activity against both Gram-positive bacteria and plant pathogenic fungi with an IC_{50} 2–10 μg/mL [148]. Interestingly, their antimicrobial activity is antagonized by cations. Both Ac-AMP1 and Ac-AMP2 are similar to chitin-binding proteins and known to reversibly bind chitin in the C-terminal truncated fold of hevein [149]. This structure consists of a β-sheet with two antiparallel β-strands as the main central element, an N-terminal coil region, and C-terminal helical turn. The N-terminal coil region is linked to the two central β-strands by two disulfide bonds, while the C-terminal helical coil is connected to the first β-strand through a third disulfide bond. Ar-AMP (30 aa) purified from the seeds of amaranth (*Amaranthus retroflexus*) is another 6C-hevein-like peptide with antifungal activity [143].

Compared to Ac-AMPs, most hevein-like AMPs, including hevein, are 8C-hevein-like peptides with an additional C-terminal sequence containing the fourth disulfide bond. Thus, 8C-hevein contains a central β-sheet of three antiparallel β-stands, wherein the last β-strand is formed from the additional C-terminal sequences and oriented parallel to the fourth disulfide bond. The 6C-hevein32, a truncated form of hevein with the N-terminal 32 aa of hevein similar to Ac-AMP2, is defined as the minimum hevein domain since it presents comparable binding affinity for chito-oligosaccharides as native hevein [150]. Pn-AMP1 and Pn-AMP2 from seeds of the morning glory *Pharbitis nil* are highly basic (pI 12.02) and thermally stable. They exhibit potent antifungal activity against both chitin-containing and non-chitin-containing fungi with an IC_{50} 0.6–75 μg/mL, but lose their antifungal activity in acidic (pH 2.0) or reducing conditions [151]. As the first hevein-like peptides reported antifungal activity similar to thionins, Pn-AMPs have been successfully cloned into tomato and tobacco plants, endowing these transgenic plants with potent antifungal activities [152,153]. Fa-AMP1 and Fa-AMP2 from seeds of the buckwheat *Fagopyrum esculentum,* have antifungal and antibacterial activities with an IC_{50} of 11–36 μg/mL [82]. Avesin A from seeds of the oat *Avena sativa* represents another chitin-binding peptide with weak to moderate antifungal properties [154].

Several hevein-like AMPs contain five disulfide bonds (10C-hevein-like peptides), although the location of the fifth disulfide bond varies by peptide. For example, EAFP1 and EAFP2, each 41 aa long, were purified from the bark of the olive *Eucommia ulmoides Oliv* with an N-terminal pyroglutamic acid [155]. These peptides show inhibitory effects on both chitin-containing and chitin-free fungi with an IC_{50} 18–155 μg/mL and can be antagonized by Ca^{2+}. Both solution and crystal structures indicate that EAFPs contain a chitin-binding domain similar to hevein-like peptides with a distinct Cys7-Cys37 fifth disulfide bond bridging the N-terminal coiled region with the third β-strand [156,157]. In contrast, the fifth disulfide bond within WAMP-1a isolated from the wheat *Triticum kiharae* connects the C-terminus to the central region of the structure [158,159]. Similarly, Ee-CBP from the bark of the spindle tree *Euonymus europaeus* is a potent antifungal peptide with an IC_{50} 1 μg/mL for the fungus *Botrytis cinerea* [160]. Ee-CBP has a primary sequence similar to other hevein-like peptides but with the fifth disulfide bond at the C-terminus.

2.3.4. Mechanism of Action

As a chitin-binding domain, hevein is an excellent model for studying the carbohydrate-peptide interaction, which is reportedly mediated by hydrogen bonding and van der Waals forces. The carbohydrate-induced conformational change to the hevein domain is small based on NMR investigations of pseudo-hevein, a wheat germ agglutinin and truncated hevein mutant [142,161,162]. The interaction between the hydrophobic C-H groups of carbohydrates and the π-electron systems of aromatic amino acids (Trp21, Trp23, and Tyr30 in hevein; Figures 3A and 8C) of hevein-like peptides appear to play an important role in chitin binding, as observed in Ac-AMP synthetic mutants, hevein, and a truncated form of hevein (hevein32) at key interacting positions [150,161,163,164]. Studies on Pn-AMPs showed that they rapidly penetrate fungal hyphae, leading to hyphal tip bursting, which disrupts the fungal membrane causing leakage of cytoplasmic materials [151].

In addition to the chitin binding function of hevein, Slavokhotova *et al.* showed an alternative function in which hevein plays a role in the plant defense against fungal infection [165]. WAMPs which contains an additional Ser at position 36 is able to inhibit the proteolytic activity of the secreted fungal protease fungalysin (Fv-cmp), a Zn-metalloproteinase, isolated from *Fusarium verticillioides*. This protease is able to truncate corn and Arabidopsis class IV chitinases by cleaving within the Gly-Cys site located in the chitin-binding domain of the plant chitinase. The presence of Ser36 prevents WAMP from being digested by Fv-cmp, allowing it to bind to fungalysin, and displace the plant chitinase, thus enabling the chitinase to remain intact and active [165].

2.4. *Knottin-Type Peptides*

Plant knottins belong to a superfamily, with members containing approximately 30 aa. They include inhibitors of α-amylase, trypsin and carboxypeptidase families as well as cyclotides. In general, they are among the smallest in size, but most diverse in functions of plant CRP-AMPs. Knottins typically comprise six Cys residues with conserved disulfide bonds between CysI-CysIV, CysII-CysV, and CysIII-CysVI, forming a cystine knot, but their Cys motifs differ among different subfamilies. Both plant defensins and hevein-like peptides also contain a cysteine-knot motif but they differ in their cysteine spacing.

One characteristic of this family is that they display a very broad range of bioactive functions which include hormone-like functions as well as enzyme-inhibitory, cytotoxic, antimicrobial, insecticidal, and anti-HIV activities [166]. Certain cystine-knot (CK) peptides with identical scaffold structures involved in multiple biological functions has been viewed as "peptide promiscuity" [167].

Historically, the knottin-type peptides were discovered as protease inhibitors sharing in common only in a cystine knot motif, and they are named collectively as cystine-knot inhibitor peptides, knottins. The prototypic knottin scaffold was first discovered in the subfamily of potato carboxypeptidase inhibitor (PCI) in 1982 [168]. The use of knottins also distinguishes the CK-CRPs from those initially described in the structures of the protein growth factors found in animals [169]. As a superfamily, they are believed to be the largest group of plant peptides associated with AMPs, surpassing defensins in the number of molecular forms and sequence diversity.

Knottins in the cyclotide and trypsin inhibitor families are found in two molecular forms, cyclic and linear, based on the presence or absence of backbone (head-to-tail) cyclization. In literature, cyclic knottins of the squash trypsin subfamily are often included in the cyclotide subfamily. Apart from their Cys residues, cyclic knottins and cyclotides share little sequence identity. Currently, both linear (acyclotides) and cyclic (cyclotides) forms of the cyclotide subfamily are found in plants.

2.4.1. Occurrences, Distribution, and Biosynthesis

Linear knottins are found not only in plants, but also in other biological sources, including fungi, insects, and spiders. Thus, CK peptides with identical or related scaffold structures found in diverse life forms provide an example of parallel evolution of protein structures. Cyclotides and their acyclic variants are found only in plants, from the dicot plants of the *Rubiaceae*, *Violaceae*, *Cucurbitaceae*, *Fabaceae*, and *Solanaceae* families to a monocot plant of the *Poaceae* family, with predicted wide and abundant distribution [170–177].

Cyclotides and certain members of cyclic knottins of the squash family are produced from precursor proteins encoding one or more cyclotide domains. The precursor is composed of an endoplasmic reticulum signal region, pro-domain, one (or more) mature cyclotide domain(s), and a short C-terminal tail [172]. However, there are variations in their biosynthesis. A recent report on cyclotides such as cliotides (cT1-cT12) identified from *Clitoria ternatea* showed that they originate from chimeric precursors consisting of Albumin-1 chain A and cyclotide domains [173]. Studies have shown that an asparaginyl endoproteinase could be involved in the backbone cyclization of cyclotides [178–181]. Our laboratory has isolated one of the bioprocessing enzymes responsible for the backbone cyclization process from *C. ternatea*, butelase 1 [181]. Butelase 1 acts as a transamidase, cyclase and ligase and is C-terminal specific to produce Asx-Xaa bonds, with Xaa being a diverse group of residues. Butelase 1 cyclizes various peptides of plant and animal origin efficiently and is the fastest peptide ligase known. Linear variants of cyclotides share high sequence identity and contain a similar knottin scaffold but are biosynthetically unable to cyclize from their precursors [173,182]. Violacin A, a naturally occurring linear cyclotide from *Viola odorata*, lacks the essential bioprocessing signal, the C-terminal Asn residue required for cyclization due to the presence of a stop codon earlier in the C-terminal sequence [177].

Cystine knot α-amylase inhibitors (CKAIs) are plant-derived α-amylase inhibitors originally isolated from *Amaranthus hypocondriacus* [183]. They are the smallest family of proteinacous α-amylase inhibitors among the seven known families [184]. Unlike other knottins, these peptides are rich in proline residues, with at least one of them existing in a *cis*- configuration [185]. In recent studies, Nguyen *et al.* have isolated an additional three members of CKAIs from the leaves and flowers of *Wrightia religiosa* [186] and another five members from the leaves of *Allamanda cathartica* [187]. These CKAIs contain 30 residues, two residues shorter than AAI, and share high sequence homology to each other.

2.4.2. Structure

A common knottin structural motif was initially defined in 1994 as a CK and triple-stranded β-sheet with a long loop connecting the first and second β-strand [166]. The first two disulfide bonds (between CysI-CysIV and CysII-CysV), together with their connecting backbone, form an embedded ring that is penetrated by the third disulfide bond (between CysIII-CysVI). Studies on the subfamily of squash trypsin inhibitors and PCIs showed that only two disulfide bonds (between CysII-CysV and CysIII-CysVI) in the knottin scaffold are highly conserved and sufficient to maintain the Cys-stabilized β-sheet motif [188,189]. It is worthwhile to point out that cystine-knot motifs appear to be common occurrence in plant CRP-AMPs. They are found, at the primary structure level, in plant defensins and heveins. However, they differ in the secondary and tertiary structure levels.

Despite the common knottin motif, knottin-type peptides have hypervariable sequences, differing by their amino acid sequences, the length between CysIII-CysIV and CysIV-CysV, and the linear and cyclic nature of the peptide backbone (Figures 4 and 5). Owing to the high sequence tolerance of the knottin scaffold and its diverse biological functions, the knottin scaffold has been used as a template for drug design. Knottins engineered by substitution of individual or several consecutive amino acids and/or insertion of additional amino acids without changing the structural integrity have been shown to provide novel bioactivity or increase stability [190].

Plant knottin-type peptides, particularly the subfamily of cyclotides, have been reported to possess high thermal, chemical, and enzymatic stability [186,191,192]. Cyclotides are also resistant to gastrointestinal proteases like trypsin, chymotrypsin, pepsin, or elastase [191,193], and certain members of cyclotide family can even penetrate the intestinal mucosa excised from rats [194,195]. Disulfide bonds in the knottin scaffold are crucial to its chemical and enzymatic stability based on studies of various members of cyclotides such as violacin A, kalata B1, and kalata B2 [177,191], whereas the cyclized backbone is important for exopeptidase resistance. For example, stability tests show that acyclic vilacin A is resistant to endopeptidase, trypsin, and thermolysin, comparable to cyclotides. The exoprotease aminopeptidase M cleaves the first two N-terminal residues of violacin A but leaves the third and fourth residues intact due to their proximity to the disulfide bond. Although no large differences are observed in the structure and flexibility between cyclotides and their corresponding linear analogs under standard conditions, simulation studies of linear and circular squash inhibitors revealed that cyclization increases resistance to high temperatures by limiting structure unfolding [192].

CKAIs exhibit another method in which these peptides are able to maintain stability against exopeptidases without a cyclic backbone structure, a pseudocyclic structure [186]. In wrightides, CKAIs isolated from the plant *W. religiosa*, the N-terminus and C-terminus are protected by the formation of disulfide bonds at the ultimate or penultimate residues. Structural analysis showed that this arrangement allows the termini to loop back to the peptide chain via the disulfide bonds especially at the N-terminal, forming a pseudocyclic structure. Allotides, CKAIs from *A. cathartica*, and AAI also exhibit similar structural features [183,187].

2.4.3. Structure-Function Relationship

With the exception of the cyclotide subfamily, the majority of knottins, are linear. They include the subfamilies of PAFP-S, Mj-AMPs, insect α-amylase inhibitor, squash trypsin inhibitor CMTI-1 and carboxypeptidase A inhibitor, as well as several linear homology analogs of cyclotides (violacin A and panitide L2; Figure 5A,B). Several knottin-type peptides were identified as plant AMPs, such as PAFP-S, Mj-AMPs, and Psacotheasin (Ps). PAFP-S was identified from seeds of *Phytolacca americana* and models the typical knottin structure of antifungal peptides [196]. Mj-AMP1 and Mj-AMP2 extracted from *Mirabilis jalapa* seeds have a broad spectrum of antimicrobial activity, being active against all 13 tested fungal pathogens and two tested Gram-positive bacteria but inactive against Gram-negative bacteria and cultured human cells. Reduced and non-reduced SDS-PAGE results suggest that Mj-AMP1 and Mj-AMP2 exist as dimers in their native form [197]. Ps from *Psacothea hilaris* is a 34 aa antibacterial peptide with a minimal inhibitory concentration of 12.5–25 μM [198].

Knottin-type peptides act as α-amylase or protease (carboxypeptidase A or trypsin) inhibitors (Figure 5A,B) and propagate plant defense mechanisms by conferring resistance to insects, pests, and pathogens [199]. The α-amylase inhibitor identified from *A. cathartica* and *W. religiosa* are the smallest peptide inhibitor of α-amylase activity (30 aa) [186,187]. Wr-AI1 and Wr-AI2, CKAIs from the plant *W. religiosa*, have been demonstrated to inhibit the α-amylase activity isolated from *Tenebrio molitor* (yellow mealworm), but no inhibitory was observed in fungal or mammalian α-amylase. Similar α-amylase inhibitory activity was observed from allotide Ac4. However, it was found that allotides interact with TMA differently from AAI and wrightides due to variation in the N-terminal sequences and high content of *cis*-proline. AAI confers pest resistance to plants by targeting insect α-amylase, but does not interfere with α-amylase from mammalian digestive systems, suggesting that amaranth seed AAI could be an attractive candidate to endow pest resistance to transgenic plants.

Squash trypsin inhibitors are 27–32 aa knottin-type peptides (e.g., CMTI-II of both pumpkin *Cucurbita maxima* and fig leaf gourd *Cucurbita ficifolia* seeds) [200]. The first squash inhibitor containing the knottin scaffold was reported from the seeds from squash of the *Cucurbitaceae* family [201]. Most squash trypsin inhibitors have linear backbones, except for MCoTI-I and MCoTI-II. However, not all the protease inhibitor peptides are knottin-type, such as sun flower trypsin inhibitor, a 14 aa cyclic peptide braced by a central disulfide bond [202]. Another type of knottin with protease inhibitory function includes carboxypeptidase inhibitors from potatoes [145] and tomatoes [203]. Potato carboxypeptidase inhibitor (PCI) (39 aa) has long loops instead of the typical β-strands observed in other knottin-type peptides. It binds the active site of carboxypeptidase A with the C-terminal tail as an active fragment binding to protease in a stopper-like manner and uses some aromatic residues as secondary binding sites [204,205].

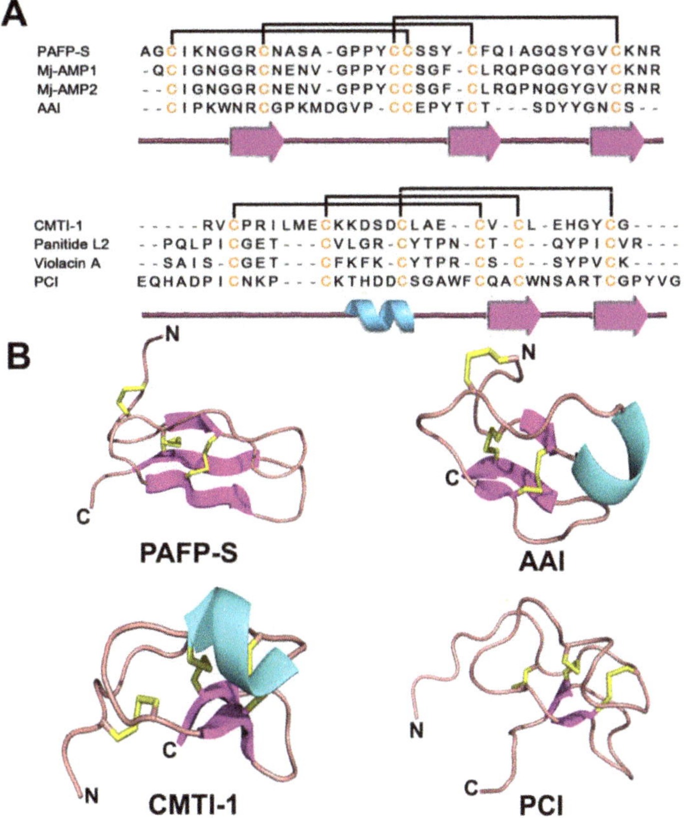

Figure 5. Sequences (**A**) and structures (**B**) of representative linear knottin-type peptides. The secondary structure is represented by different colors: cyan-α helix; magenta-β strand; pink-random coil and yellow-disulfide bonds.

A few linear variants of cyclotides have also been identified from the monocot rice plant *Panicum laxum* of the *Poaceae* family as Panitide L1-12 [175]. Several Panitides are active against *Escherichia coli* and cytotoxic to HeLa cells. The other subgroup of knottin-type peptides is cyclotides, including typical cyclotides and cyclic knotttins such as MCoTIs (Figure 6A,B). Cyclotides are 29–37 aa in length with a CK arrangement of three disulfide bonds which are widely involved in plant defense, as deduced from their activity against insects, nematodes, and mollusks [206–208]. The first cyclotide was identified in 1973 as an uterotonic agent from the African plant *Oldenlandia affinis*, a main component of medicinal tea used to accelerate childbirth [209]. Cyclotides have potential pharmacological functions, considering their antimicrobial, anti-HIV, anti-tumor, and neurotensin activities [22]. Cyclotides are found mainly in *Rubiaceae* (coffee), Violaceae (violet) and families. They are highly variable in sequence, but conserved in structure, and are divided into two types: Möbius and bracelet. Möbius types contain one *cis*-Pro in loop 5 and a twist in the cyclic backbone, while the bracelet type does not [210]. Yet, both types do not significantly differ from one another in the general scaffold structure.

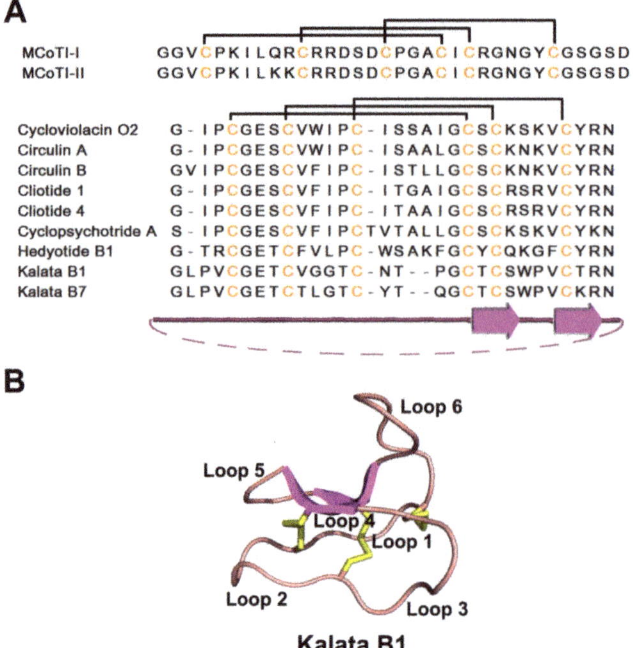

Figure 6. Sequences (**A**) and structures (**B**) of representative cyclic knottin-type peptides. The secondary structure is represented by different colors: magenta-β strand; pink-random coil and yellow-disulfide bonds.

Antimicrobial activity of cyclotides was first reported for four synthetically produced cyclotides isolated from coffee plants, kalata B1, circulin A, circulin B, and cyclopsychotride [211]. Subsequently, more cyclotides were reported to have antimicrobial activity. Cyclotides kalata B1 and B7 (29 aa each) from the tropical plant *Oldenlandia affinis* display antibiotic effects both in salt and salt-free medium [212]. While the 30 aa cycloviolacin O2 from *Viola odorata* is resistant to Gram-negative bacteria [213], cliotides cT1 and cT4 from *Clitoria ternatea* show antimicrobial activity against Gram-negative bacteria and cytotoxicity to HeLa cells [173]. Hedyotide B1, on the other hand, is a positively charged bracelet cyclotide from *Hedyotis biflora*, rich in aromatic residues and active against both Gram-positive and Gram-negative bacteria [214].

MCoTI-I and MCoTI-II are two squash trypsin inhibitors from *Momordica cochinchinensis* that contain a cyclized backbone [215] and have large sequences differences from typical cyclotides, as discussed above (Figure 6A). The C- to N-cyclization in MCoTI-II has no significant impact on the protein structure, though cyclized squash inhibitors are postulated to be less sensitive to exopeptidases [216]. Based on structural studies of MCoTI-II in free and complex forms, Heitz revealed that the cyclization and active site loops of MCoTI-II are flexible in solution, but converge into a single, well-defined conformation upon binding trypsin [217]. Compared to previously defined cyclotides, such as kalata B1 or circulin A, MCoTI-I and MCoTI-II share similar motifs wherein two disulfide bonds stabilize the β-sheet but differ greatly in their amino acid sequences and in loops 3 and 6 [217]. Furthermore, MCoTIs have an entirely charged surface *versus* the amphipathic nature of circulin A. These differences may explain functional disparities such as squash inhibitor MCoTIs having no antibacterial activity, unlike circulins and kalata B1.

2.4.4. Mechanism of Action

Generally, knottin-type peptides with membranolytic functions are amphipathic in nature like other AMPs, a characteristic necessary for membrane interactions which implement their antimicrobial effects. For example, the surface plots of PAFP-S and kalata B1 show hydrophobic patches surrounded by several hydrophilic residues (Figure 2E,F). However, in contrast the strongly cationic-charged thionins and plant defensins, most cyclotides are unlikely to have a strong electrostatic interaction with membranes since they are normally weakly positive or neutral at physiological pH (Figure 2F) [218]. The interaction of cyclotides with membranes has been previously investigated *in vitro* using the detergent dodecylphosphocholine [219]. In this study, the structure of kalata B1 was not significantly altered upon binding the detergent; binding was largely mediated by the strong hydrophobic interactions between cyclotide loops and lipid tails of the detergent, as well as favored by the weak interactions between positively charged kalata B1 and the polar head of the detergent However, similar studies on kalata B2 and cycloviolacin O2 suggest that different cyclotides have different membrane binding modalities because of the varied location of hydrophobic patches in cyclotides [220].

2.4.5. Knottin Scaffold in Pharmaceutical Engineering

The knottin scaffold is an excellent candidate for peptide-based pharmaceutical engineering [221] as a result of several features: (1) remarkable proteolytic, thermal, and chemical stability due to the CK and backbone cyclization of cyclotides; (2) feasibility of chemical synthesis due to small size; and (3) excellent sequence tolerance due to sequence variation in loop regions.

Synthesis of cyclotides and cyclic knottins. To exploit cyclotides and cyclic knottins for agricultural and medical use, it is necessary to develop efficient methods for their production. Methods employed to date include solid phase peptide synthesis [9,211,222–227], as well as chemo-enzymatic and biological methods using modified inteins [210–213] and Asn-endoprotease such as butelase-1 [228–231].

Irrespective of the means of its preparation, a linear precursor containing a macrocycle sequence is first generated, followed by a macrocyclizaion step to give a head-to-tail backbone-cyclized compound. The head-to-tail cyclization poses a substantial hurdle and challenge because it is highly entropy-disfavored due to the great distance between the N- and C-termini, but has been solved elegantly by the discovery of the thia zip cyclization reaction in 1997 [232]. Thia zip cyclization is an entropic reaction, characterized by a series of entropic ring expansion by making use of the multiple Cys residues in a CRP-linear precursor functionalized with an N-terminal Cys and a C-terminal thioester. This construct enables a thiol-thioester to form a thiolactone and then thiol-thiolactone exchange reactions in tandem, ending with a head-to-tail thiolactone which spontaneously forms a peptide bond through an S, N-acyl shift. In 1997, the first report on both Möbius and bracelet cyclotides have been synthesized by the thia zip reaction and regio-selective disulfide bond formation to guarantee the correct knottin scaffold [225]. Since then, many successful syntheses of cyclic CRPs based on thia zip cyclization have been reported. We have recently reviewed the progress of macrocyclization relevant to cyclotides and cyclic knottins [9]. Since 2012, new advances based on amide-to-amide transpeptidation reaction have made preparation of cyclotides, cyclic knottins and other macrocycles possible through chemical or biological means [181].

2.5. α-Hairpinin Family

The α-hairpinin family is composed of Lys/Arg-rich plant defense peptides. α-Hairpinin AMPs share a characteristic C1XXXC2-(X)n-C3XXXC4 motif in their primary sequence and, more importantly, a helix-loop-helix secondary structure (Figure 7A,B). The helix-loop-helix or α1-turn-α2 motif has both α-helices oriented antiparallel and is stabilized by two disulfide bonds in the tertiary structure. This structure is a surprise finding in plant CRPs, and the α-hairpinin family is structurally distinguished from the β-strand decorated CRP-AMPs, such as thionins, defensins, and knottin-type peptides.

Thus far, only a limited number of α-hairpinin AMPs have been reported, including MBP-1, MiAMP2s, Ec-AMP1, Luffin P1, VhT1, BWI-2c, Tk-AMP-Xs, and Sm-AMP-X. MBP-1, a 33 aa peptide isolated from the maize kernel, inhibits spore germination and hyphal enlongation of several plant pathogenic fungi and bacteria *in vitro* [233]. MiAMP2 peptides (50 aa) isolated from the nut kernel of *Macadamia integrifolia* inhibit various plant pathogenic fungi *in vitro* [234]. They are produced from a 666 aa precursor protein homologous to vicilin 7S globulin. Ec-AMP1 from the seeds of the baryard grass *Echinochloa crus-gali* was reported to have antifungal activity against several phytopathogenic fungi with an IC_{50} = 1–10 μM. A confocal microscopy study showed that Ec-AMP1 binds the fungal conidia surface and then internalizes and accumulates in the cytoplasm without disturbing membrane integrity [235].

Tk-AMP-X1 and Tk-AMP-X2 extracted from the wheat *Triticum kiharae* and Sm-AMP-X from seeds of the chickweed *Stellaria media* are another two α-hairpinin members with antifungal activity [236,237]. Both are produced from multimodular precursor proteins. The Tk-AMP-X-related sequences have been shown to be widespread in crops such as barley, rice, and maize, which suggest the importance of this type of plant defense peptide. VhT1 from the seeds of *Veronica hederifolia* and BWI-2c from seeds of the buckwheat *Fagopyrum esculentum* represent a new family of trypsin inhibitors with an α-hairpinin structure and act as defensive peptides in plants [238,239]. Luffin P1, extracted from the seeds of the sponge gourd *Luffa cylindrical*, has been shown to have anti-HIV-1 activity in HIV-1-infected C8166 T-cell lines *in vitro* [240]. This study proposed that Luffin P1 displays a novel inhibitory mechanism owing to its charge complementation with viral and cellular proteins.

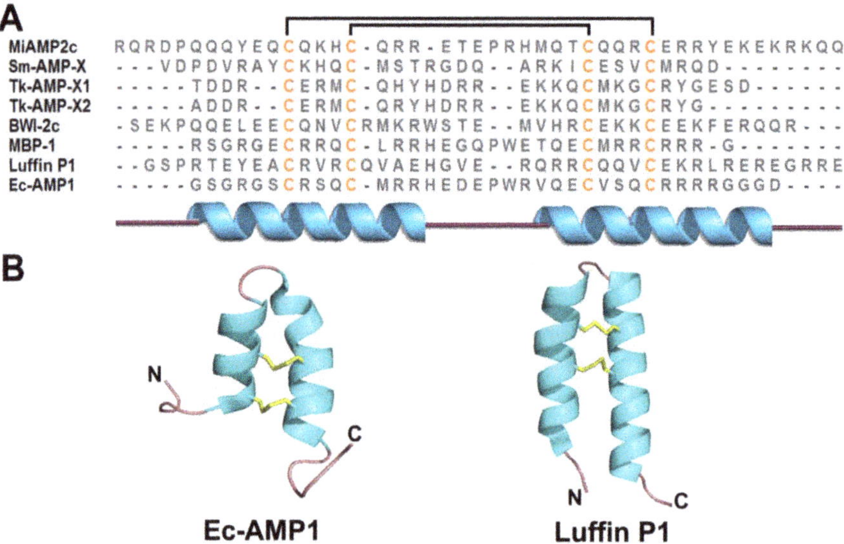

Figure 7. Sequences (**A**) and structures (**B**) of representative α-hairpinins. The secondary structure is represented by different colors: cyan-α helix; pink-random coil and yellow-disulfide bonds.

2.6. Lipid Transfer Proteins

Plant lipid transfer proteins (LTPs) and snakins (described in the following section) are two families of CRP-AMPs with MW >7 kDa, and are considered proteins. LTPs are cationic proteins of approximately 70 and 90 aa with eight Cys residues. They are distinguished from other CRP-AMPs by their lipid transfer activity, in which they bind a wide range of lipids including fatty acids (C10–C14), phospholipids, prostaglandin B2, lyso-derivatives, and acyl-coenzyme A. Consequently, they are also called non-specific LTPs [4,241,242]. LTPs can inhibit growth of fungus and some bacterial pathogens and are involved in the plant defense system. LTPs are subdivided into LTP1s (MW = 9 kDa) and LTP2s (MW = 7 kDa) based on their molecular mass.

2.6.1. Occurrences, Distribution, and Biosynthesis

Plant LTPs have been identified in various species, such as seeds of the radish, barley, maize, *Arabidopsis*, spinach, grapevine, wheat, and onion [4,241–246]. They are synthesized as precursors containing a signal peptide of 20–25 aa and a mature protein with eight Cys [247].

2.6.2. Structure

Although LTPs vary in their primary sequence, they share a defining structural feature, a conserved inner hydrophobic cavity surrounded by α-helices (Figure 8A,B). Surface plots of LTP1 and LTP2 representatives are illustrated in Figure 2G, H. LTP1s and LTP2s share the same Cys signature and similar tertiary fold, but vary in amino acid sequence and disulfide bonding at the CXC motif [248,249]. LTP1 contains four α-helices stabilized by four disulfide bonds (between CysI-CysVI, CysII-CysIII, CysIV-CysVII, and CysV-CysVIII) and a flexible C-terminal coil. In contrast to LTP1, LTP2 contains three extended helices, two single-turn helices, and four disulfide bonds between CysI-CysV, CysII-CysIII, CysIV-CysVII, and CysVI-CysVIII (Figure 8A) [249,250]. The helices in LTP1 and LTP2 form a hydrophobic cavity which accommodates a variety of lipids [251–254].

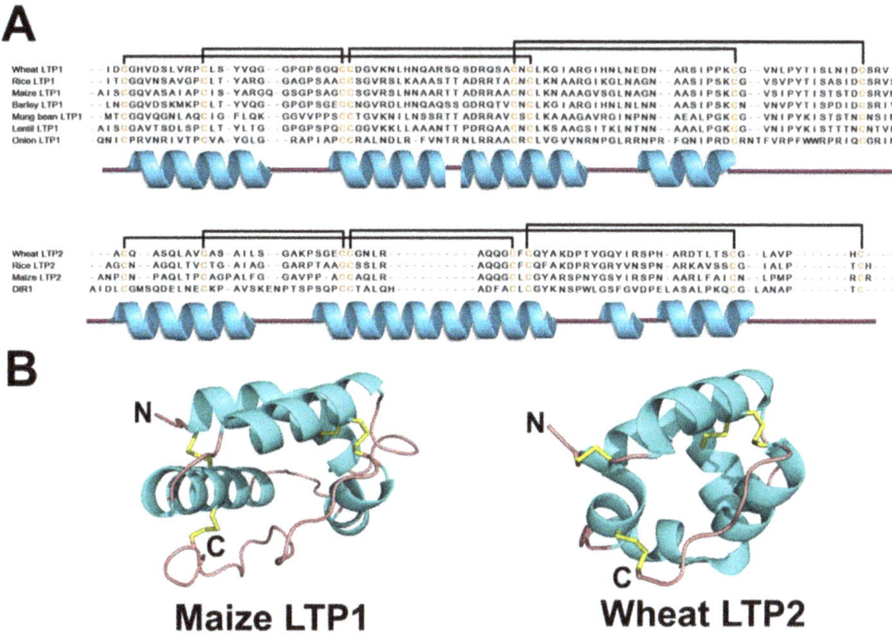

Figure 8. Sequences (**A**) and structures (**B**) of representative lipid transfer proteins. The secondary structure is represented by different colors: cyan-α helix; pink-random coil and yellow-disulfide bonds.

LTP1s and LTP2s have a conserved structure reported in rice [253,255,256], wheat [257,258], barley [259,260], maize [261,262], lentils [263], and mung beans [264]. Their lipid-binding properties can be modulated by subtle changes in their conserved global structure, as evidenced by structural and functional differences of LTP1s in tobacco, wheat, and maize [265]. Mutagenesis studies have revealed that different residues forming the hydrophobic cavity of LTP2 play various roles in maintaining structure and conferring function [266]. Although LTP2 is found to have a similar but smaller hydrophobic cavity compared to LTP1 [249,250,253,254,259], it is quite flexible and can accommodate voluminous sterol molecules [267].

2.6.3. Structure-Function Relationship

Plant LTPs inhibit the growth of bacterial and fungal pathogens to different degrees [243,246,268]. Transgenic expression of barley LTP2 in tobacco and *Arabidopsis thaliana* leaves endows higher tolerance to bacterial pathogens [269]. The antifungal activity of LTPs from *Brassica* and mung beans is found to be thermally, pH-, and pepsin/trypsin treatment-stable [268].

Ace-AMP1 (onion LTP1; Figure 8A) isolated from onion seeds, exhibits a higher antimicrobial activity than the LTP extracted from radish seeds [89,243]. Ace-AMP1 shares a similar global fold as LTP1s, but does not possess a continuous cavity for lipid binding nor does it bind fluorescently labeled phospholipids in solution [252]. In addition, Ace-AMP1 does not exhibit characteristic LTP behavior, such as transferring lipids between membranes *in vitro*. While DIR1 from *Arabidopsis thaliana* shares similar structural and lipid binding properties with plant LTP2, it is distinguished by its acidic pI and ability to bind two long-chain fatty acid derivatives in its cavity, suggesting DIR1 could be a new type of plant LTP [270]. The functions of plant LTPs, such as defensive signaling, cuticle deposition and plant defense, have been previously reviewed by Yeats and Rose [271].

2.6.4. Mechanism of Action

Initially, LTPs were reported to facilitate lipid transfer between membranes of vesicles or organelles *in vitro* [272,273]. However, later discoveries have shown that LTP1s are extracellular cell wall proteins, making *in vivo* intracellular lipid transfer activity unlikely [274,275]. Thus, LTPs promote membrane permeabilization in pathogens rather than host cells [246,276]. Although structural studies have shown that LTPs can "cage" lipid molecules in their hydrophobic cavity, a detailed mechanism of antimicrobial activity mediated by lipid transport remains unclear [271].

2.7. Snakins

Snakin-1 (63 aa) and snakin-2 (66 aa) are AMPs with 12 Cys isolated from potato tubers (*Solanum tuberosum*) [277,278] found to be active against fungal and bacterial pathogens at 1–20 μM. Snakins induce the aggregation of both Gram-positive and Gram-negative bacteria and therefore, are recognized as components of constitutive and inducible plant defense barriers. The structure of snakin is predicted to have two long α-helices with disulfide bonds between CysI-CysIX, CysII-CysVII, CysIII-CysIV, CysV-CysXI, CysVI-CysXII, and CysVIII-CysX, which demonstrates a small degree of structural similarity to thionins and α-hairpinins [279].

A 64 aa homolog of snakin-2, also containing 12 Cys, was identified from the French bean to be a domain of a 42 kDa Pro-rich protein with chitin-binding ability that is involved in plant-pathogen interactions [280]. Snakin-Z (31 aa), identified from the fruit of *Zizyphus jujuba*, contains a sequence similar to the C-terminal region of Snakin-2. It has antimicrobial activity against different bacterial and fungal strains at minimal concentrations (7.65–28.8 μg/mL) [281].

2.8. Other Plant CRP-AMPs

In addition to the different classes of CRP-AMPs mentioned above, there are several unclassified Cys-containing AMPs, such as Ps-AFP1, Ib-AMPs, Pp-AMPs, ToAMPs, and MiAMP1 that contain two to eight Cys. Ps-AFP1 (38 aa) from the pea *Pisum sativum* root contains two disulfide bonds between CysI-CysII and CysIII-CysIV, has been proposed to adopt a novel αβ-trumpet fold, and is capable of binding the cell wall of fungi [282]. Ib-AMPs1-4, purified from the seed of *Impatiens balsamina*, are four basic 20 aa peptides encoded by a single transcript. Ib-AMPs represent a novel class of AMPs that lack homology to other peptides [283,284]. They contain four Cys which share a common CC and CXXXC sequence motif and form two disulfide bonds between CysI-CysIII and CysII-CysIV. The structure of Ib-AMP1 is well-defined, with loops and turns stabilized by two disulfide bonds [285]. Ib-AMPs can inhibit the growth of a range of fungi and Gram-positive bacteria but is not cytotoxic to most Gram-negative bacteria or cultured human cells. Studies of Ib-AMP1 analogs without disulfide bonds have shown these bonds are not essential for its antimicrobial activity, and that Ib-AMP1 targets intracellular components instead of bacterial cell membranes [286].

Pp-AMP1 and Pp-AMP2 are two chitin-binding AMPs from the shoots of the Japanese bamboo *Phyllostachys pubescens* that have antimicrobial activity against pathogenic bacteria and fungi [287]. Pp-AMP1 contains four Cys in its 44 aa sequence, while Pp-AMP2 (45 aa) is composed of six Cys. Although they share relatively high sequence homology with thionins, especially the N-terminal continuous CC motif, their differences in the C-terminal sequence and Cys distribution pattern do not suggest Pp-AMPs are thionins. ToAMPs1-4 are four basic 38–44 aa AMPs identified from *Taraxacum officinale* flowers that have antifungal and antibacterial activity [288,289]. Sequence analysis has shown that ToAMP1, ToAMP2, and ToAMP4 possess a novel peptide motif of six Cys with a –CC– motif between CysII and CysIII, while ToAMP3 has eight Cys with a –CC– motif between CysVI and CysVII.

MiAMP1 is a 76 aa basic AMP identified from the nut kernel of *Macadamia integrifolia*. MiAMP1 inhibits several plant microbial pathogens *in vitro* [290], yet presents no sequence homology with other plant AMPs and has a β-barrelin structure. The β-barrelins contain eight β-strands forming two Greek key motifs that are stabilized by three disulfide bonds. MiAMP1 has a structure similar to that of a yeast killer toxin from *Williopsis mrakii*, which inhibits β-glucan synthesis and thereby disturbs the cell wall of yeast. The structural similarity between these two peptides suggests a similar antimicrobial mode of action.

2.9. Non-CRP Plant AMPs

Although the majority of known plant AMPs are stabilized by multiple disulfide bonds, exceptions include Cn-AMPs, Cr-ACP1, as well as GRPs Pg-AMP1 and shepherins. All of these plant AMPs either do not contain Cys or contain only one and thus, possess high structural flexibility. Cn-AMP1 is a 9 aa Cys-free AMP identified from green coconut (*Cocos nucifera*) water with "promiscuous" activity, as it is antibacterial, antifungal, and immune stimulatory [291]. Cr-ACP1 is a 9 aa AMP from the seeds of *Cycas revoluta* with pro-apoptotic and antimicrobial activities [292]. A previous bioinformatics study suggests that these Cr-AMP1 activities are likely mediated by hydrogen bond-mediated DNA binding within cells.

Pg-AMP1 is a 55 aa GRP extracted from seeds of the guava *Psidium guajava*. It contains 14 Gly and only one Cys [293] and inhibits the growth of both Gram-positive and Gram-negative bacteria, pathogens involved in urinary and gastro-intestinal infections [294]. Shepherins I and II are Gly- and His-rich AMPs identified from the roots of Shepherd's Purse, *Capsella bursa-pastoris* [295]. Shepherin I (28 aa) and shepherin II (38 aa) are produced from a single 120 aa propeptide precursor composed of an N-terminal signal peptide, shepherin I, a linker dipeptide, shepherin II, and a C-terminal peptide. Both exhibit antimicrobial activity against Gram-negative bacteria and fungi with an IC_{50} of 2.5–8 μg/mL.

2.10. Mechanism of AMP Action

AMPs are generally moderate-to-large size, positively charged, amphipathic CRPs. Structurally, AMPs fall into diverse and distinct groups (Table 1; Figure 2), including α-helical peptides (α-hairpinin family and lipid transfer proteins), β-sheet peptides (hevein and knottin-type peptides) as well as mixed α-helical and β-sheet peptides (thionins and plant defensins). Generally, the mechanism of AMP interaction with microbes is believed to be associated with cell lysis due to membrane disruption and/or peptide penetration of lipid membranes followed by attack of intracellular targets [14]. Various mechanistic models have been proposed, such as the barrel-stave model, toroidal pore model, and carpet model, in previous reviews by Barbosa, Rahnamaeian, and Nawrot [14,296,297]. Besides perturbing the lipid membrane, AMPs can also form ion channels, which can induce ion leakage (e.g., K^+) in addition to other intracellular contents [298,299]. All of these actions lead to inhibition of microbial cell growth and cell death.

3. Conclusions and Perspective

A striking feature of plant AMPs is that the majority are families of CRPs, with each family sharing a characteristic motif. In turn, these cysteinyl motifs enable plant AMPs to organize into specific families with conserved structural folds that enable sequence variation of non-Cys residues encased in the same scaffold within a particular family to play multiple functions. This evolvable phenomenon is particularly evident in the family of knottins, and to a lesser extent, in the defensins. Knottins are known to play diverse roles, being antimicrobial, insecticidal, enzyme inhibitory, and agonistic/antagonistic to hormones. The ability of plant AMPs to tolerate hypervariable sequences using a conserved scaffold mimic is, in certain respects, similar to that of immunoglobulins, which recognize diverse targets by varying the sequence of complementary binding regions.

The presence of multiple disulfide bonds in a particular CRP family gives plant AMPs a compact structure and a specific scaffold. In turn, they confer stability against thermal and chemical denaturation and enzymatic degradation. These properties bode well for developing plant AMPs as potential therapeutics and for protection of crops through transgenic methods [300,301]. A cystine-stabilized structure opens the possibility to use it as a stable scaffold for grafting biological active peptides sequences to intracellular targets. Specifically, the backbone portions between cysteine residues can be modified to incorporate bioactive peptides which are normally unstable against digestive enzymes and other physiological conditions [302,303]. This technique has successfully been applied to graft bradykinin B1 antagonists onto kalata B1 as an orally active analgesic [221], human kallikrein-related peptidase 4 inhibitor onto sunflower trypsin inhibitor-1 [228], angiogenic peptides, laminin and osteopontin, onto *Momordica cochinca cochinchinensis* trypsin inhibitor-II [304] and melanocortin onto kalata B1 [305]. More importantly, these grafted peptides have been shown to possess the same biological property with similar potency as compared with the original bioactive peptides, as well as resistance to digestive enzymes due to the robust scaffold. In addition, plants AMPs, in particular defensin, have been shown to protect transgenic plants against microorganism infection. Expression of alfalfa antifungal peptide defensin, from the seeds of *Medicago sativa*, in transgenic potato plants has been found to provide resistance against phyto-pathogen *Verticillium dahilae* [77,306].

AMPs offer several advantages as compared to current antibiotic drugs as they represent a naturally occurring defense mechanism that has been used by plants for thousands of years in combating external pathogenic challenges. Most of the recent studies included in this review were focused on the anti-fungal and anti-bacterial effect of AMPs, while the anti-viral property of AMPs was still under-explored. Further investigation in tackling this issue is urgently warranted. Since plant AMPs have been identified in only a small fraction of plants, it is anticipated that many more plant AMPs, both in molecular form and sequence, will be forthcoming.

Acknowledgments: This work was supported in part by the Singapore National Research Foundation grant NRF-CRP8-2011-05.

Author Contributions: All the authors contributed to manuscript preparation.

Conflicts of Interest: The authors declare no conflict of interest.

References

1. Stintzi, A.; Heitz, T.; Prasad, V.; Wiedemann-Merdinoglu, S.; Kauffmann, S.; Geoffroy, P.; Legrand, M.; Fritig, B. Plant "pathogenesis-related" proteins and their role in defense against pathogens. *Biochimie* **1993**, *75*, 687–706. [CrossRef]
2. Sinha, M.; Singh, R.P.; Kushwaha, G.S.; Iqbal, N.; Singh, A.; Kaushik, S.; Kaur, P.; Sharma, S.; Singh, T.P. Current overview of allergens of plant pathogenesis related protein families. *Sci. World J.* **2014**, *2014*, 543195.

3. Ebrahim, S.; Usha, K.; Singh, B. Pathogenesis related (pr) proteins in plant defense mechanism. *Sci. Against Microb. Pathog.* **2011**, *2*, 1043–1054.
4. Sels, J.; Mathys, J.; De Coninck, B.M.; Cammue, B.P.; De Bolle, M.F. Plant pathogenesis-related (pr) proteins: A focus on pr peptides. *Plant Physiol. Biochem.* **2008**, *46*, 941–950. [CrossRef] [PubMed]
5. Egorov, T.A.; Odintsova, T.I.; Pukhalsky, V.A.; Grishin, E.V. Diversity of wheat anti-microbial peptides. *Peptides* **2005**, *26*, 2064–2073. [CrossRef] [PubMed]
6. Rao, A.G. Antimicrobial peptides. *Mol. Plant Microbe Interact.* **1995**, *8*, 6–13. [CrossRef] [PubMed]
7. Reddy, K.V.; Yedery, R.D.; Aranha, C. Antimicrobial peptides: Premises and promises. *Int. J. Antimicrob. Agents* **2004**, *24*, 536–547. [CrossRef] [PubMed]
8. Montalban-Lopez, M.; Sanchez-Hidalgo, M.; Cebrian, R.; Maqueda, M. Discovering the bacterial circular proteins: Bacteriocins, cyanobactins, and pilins. *J. Biol. Chem.* **2012**, *287*, 27007–27013. [CrossRef] [PubMed]
9. Tam, J.P.; Wong, C.T. Chemical synthesis of circular proteins. *J. Biol. Chem.* **2012**, *287*, 27020–27025. [CrossRef] [PubMed]
10. Hammami, R.; Ben Hamida, J.; Vergoten, G.; Fliss, I. Phytamp: A database dedicated to antimicrobial plant peptides. *Nucleic Acids Res.* **2009**, *37*, D963–D968. [CrossRef] [PubMed]
11. Silverstein, K.A.; Moskal, W.A., Jr.; Wu, H.C.; Underwood, B.A.; Graham, M.A.; Town, C.D.; VandenBosch, K.A. Small cysteine-rich peptides resembling antimicrobial peptides have been under-predicted in plants. *Plant. J.* **2007**, *51*, 262–280. [CrossRef] [PubMed]
12. Stec, B. Plant thionins–the structural perspective. *Cell. Mol. Life Sci.* **2006**, *63*, 1370–1385. [CrossRef] [PubMed]
13. Garcia-Olmedo, F.; Molina, A.; Alamillo, J.M.; Rodriguez-Palenzuela, P. Plant defense peptides. *Biopolymers* **1998**, *47*, 479–491. [CrossRef]
14. Nawrot, R.; Barylski, J.; Nowicki, G.; Broniarczyk, J.; Buchwald, W.; Gozdzicka-Jozefiak, A. Plant antimicrobial peptides. *Folia Microbiol. (Praha)* **2013**, *59*, 181–196. [CrossRef] [PubMed]
15. Padovan, L.; Scocchi, M.; Tossi, A. Structural aspects of plant antimicrobial peptides. *Curr. Protein Pept. Sci.* **2010**, *11*, 210–219. [CrossRef] [PubMed]
16. Lay, F.T.; Anderson, M.A. Defensins–components of the innate immune system in plants. *Curr. Protein Pept. Sci.* **2005**, *6*, 85–101. [CrossRef] [PubMed]
17. Das, S.N.; Madhuprakash, J.; Sarma, P.V.; Purushotham, P.; Suma, K.; Manjeet, K.; Rambabu, S.; Gueddari, N.E.; Moerschbacher, B.M.; Podile, A.R. Biotechnological approaches for field applications of chitooligosaccharides (cos) to induce innate immunity in plants. *Crit. Rev. Biotechnol.* **2013**, *35*, 29–43. [CrossRef] [PubMed]
18. Mander, L.N.; Liu, H.-W. *Comprehensive Natural Products ii Chemistry and Biology*; Elsevier Science: Oxford, England, 2010; p. 1.
19. Tavares, L.S.; Santos Mde, O.; Viccini, L.F.; Moreira, J.S.; Miller, R.N.; Franco, O.L. Biotechnological potential of antimicrobial peptides from flowers. *Peptides* **2008**, *29*, 1842–1851. [CrossRef] [PubMed]
20. De Lucca, A.J.; Cleveland, T.E.; Wedge, D.E. Plant-derived antifungal proteins and peptides. *Can. J. Microbiol.* **2005**, *51*, 1001–1014. [CrossRef] [PubMed]
21. Gruber, C.W.; Cemazar, M.; Anderson, M.A.; Craik, D.J. Insecticidal plant cyclotides and related cystine knot toxins. *Toxicon* **2007**, *49*, 561–575. [CrossRef] [PubMed]
22. Craik, D.J. Host-defense activities of cyclotides. *Toxins (Basel)* **2012**, *4*, 139–156. [CrossRef] [PubMed]
23. van der Weerden, N.L.; Bleackley, M.R.; Anderson, M.A. Properties and mechanisms of action of naturally occurring antifungal peptides. *Cell. Mol. Life Sci.* **2013**, *70*, 3545–3570. [CrossRef] [PubMed]
24. Ng, T.B. Antifungal proteins and peptides of leguminous and non-leguminous origins. *Peptides* **2004**, *25*, 1215–1222. [CrossRef] [PubMed]
25. Harris, F.; Dennison, S.R.; Phoenix, D.A. Anionic antimicrobial peptides from eukaryotic organisms. *Curr. Protein Pept. Sci.* **2009**, *10*, 585–606. [CrossRef] [PubMed]
26. Wang, G.S.; Li, X.; Wang, Z. Apd2: The updated antimicrobial peptide database and its application in peptide design. *Nucleic Acids Res.* **2009**, *37*, D933–D937. [CrossRef] [PubMed]
27. Wang, Z.; Wang, G.S. Apd: The antimicrobial peptide database. *Nucleic Acids Res.* **2004**, *32*, D590–D592. [CrossRef] [PubMed]
28. Piotto, S.P.; Sessa, L.; Concilio, S.; Iannelli, P. Yadamp: Yet another database of antimicrobial peptides. *Int. J. Antimicrob. Agents* **2012**, *39*, 346–351. [CrossRef] [PubMed]

29. Sundararajan, V.S.; Gabere, M.N.; Pretorius, A.; Adam, S.; Christoffels, A.; Lehvaslaiho, M.; Archer, J.A.C.; Bajic, V.B. Dampd: A manually curated antimicrobial peptide database. *Nucleic Acids Res.* **2012**, *40*, D1108–D1112. [CrossRef] [PubMed]
30. Fernandez de Caleya, R.; Gonzalez-Pascual, B.; Garcia-Olmedo, F.; Carbonero, P. Susceptibility of phytopathogenic bacteria to wheat purothionins *in vitro*. *Appl. Microbiol.* **1972**, *23*, 998–1000. [PubMed]
31. Ebrahimnesbat, F.; Behnke, S.; Kleinhofs, A.; Apel, K. Cultivar-related differences in the distribution of cell-wall-bound thionins in compatible and incompatible interactions between barley and powdery mildew. *Planta* **1989**, *179*, 203–210. [CrossRef] [PubMed]
32. Evans, J.; Wang, Y.D.; Shaw, K.P.; Vernon, L.P. Cellular responses to pyrularia thionin are mediated by Ca^{2+} influx and phospholipase a2 activation and are inhibited by thionin tyrosine iodination. *Proc. Natl. Acad. Sci. USA* **1989**, *86*, 5849–5853. [CrossRef] [PubMed]
33. Kramer, K.J.; Klassen, L.W.; Jones, B.L.; Speirs, R.D.; Kammer, A.E. Toxicity of purothionin and its homologues to the tobacco hornworm, manduca sexta (l.) (lepidoptera:Sphingidae). *Toxicol. Appl. Pharmacol.* **1979**, *48*, 179–183. [CrossRef]
34. Balls, A.K.; Hale, W.S.; Harris, T.H. A crystalline protein obtained from a lipoprotein of wheat flour. *Cereal Chem.* **1942**, *19*, 951–961.
35. Ponz, F.; Paz-Ares, J.; Hernandez-Lucas, C.; Carbonero, P.; Garcia-Olmedo, F. Synthesis and processing of thionin precursors in developing endosperm from barley (hordeum vulgare l.). *EMBO J.* **1983**, *2*, 1035–1040. [PubMed]
36. Steinmuller, K.; Batschauer, A.; Apel, K. Tissue-specific and light-dependent changes of chromatin organization in barley (hordeum vulgare). *Eur. J. Biochem.* **1986**, *158*, 519–525. [CrossRef] [PubMed]
37. Gausing, K. Thionin genes specifically expressed in barley leaves. *Planta* **1987**, *171*, 241–246. [CrossRef] [PubMed]
38. Epple, P.; Apel, K.; Bohlmann, H. An arabidopsis-thaliana thionin gene is inducible via a signal-transduction pathway different from that for pathogenesis-related proteins. *Plant. Physiol.* **1995**, *109*, 813–820. [CrossRef] [PubMed]
39. Bohlmann, H.; Clausen, S.; Behnke, S.; Giese, H.; Hiller, C.; Reimann-Philipp, U.; Schrader, G.; Barkholt, V.; Apel, K. Leaf-specific thionins of barley-a novel class of cell wall proteins toxic to plant-pathogenic fungi and possibly involved in the defence mechanism of plants. *EMBO J.* **1988**, *7*, 1559–1565. [PubMed]
40. Andresen, I.; Becker, W.; Schluter, K.; Burges, J.; Parthier, B.; Apel, K. The identification of leaf thionin as one of the main jasmonate-induced proteins of barley (hordeum vulgare). *Plant. Mol. Biol.* **1992**, *19*, 193–204. [CrossRef] [PubMed]
41. Penninckx, I.A.; Eggermont, K.; Terras, F.R.; Thomma, B.P.; De Samblanx, G.W.; Buchala, A.; Metraux, J.P.; Manners, J.M.; Broekaert, W.F. Pathogen-induced systemic activation of a plant defensin gene in arabidopsis follows a salicylic acid-independent pathway. *Plant Cell.* **1996**, *8*, 2309–2323. [CrossRef] [PubMed]
42. Castagnaro, A.; Marana, C.; Carbonero, P.; Garciaolmedo, F. Extreme divergence of a novel wheat thionin generated by a mutational burst specifically affecting the mature protein domain of the precursor. *J. Mol. Biol.* **1992**, *224*, 1003–1009. [CrossRef]
43. Stec, B.; Markman, O.; Rao, U.; Heffron, G.; Henderson, S.; Vernon, L.P.; Brumfeld, V.; Teeter, M.M. Proposal for molecular mechanism of thionins deduced from physico-chemical studies of plant toxins. *J. Pept. Res.* **2004**, *64*, 210–224. [CrossRef] [PubMed]
44. Rao, U.; Stec, B.; Teeter, M.M. Refinement of purothionins reveals solute particles important for lattice formation and toxicity. Part 1: Alpha1-purothionin revisited. *Acta Crystallogr. D Biol. Crystallogr.* **1995**, *51*, 904–913. [CrossRef] [PubMed]
45. Stec, B.; Rao, U.; Teeter, M.M. Refinement of purothionins reveals solute particles important for lattice formation and toxicity. Part 2: Structure of beta-purothionin at 1.7 a resolution. *Acta Crystallogr. D Biol. Crystallogr.* **1995**, *51*, 914–924. [CrossRef] [PubMed]
46. Milbradt, A.G.; Kerek, F.; Moroder, L.; Renner, C. Structural characterization of hellethionins from helleborus purpurascens. *Biochemistry* **2003**, *42*, 2404–2411. [CrossRef] [PubMed]
47. Yamano, A.; Heo, N.H.; Teeter, M.M. Crystal structure of ser-22/ile-25 form crambin confirms solvent, side chain substate correlations. *J. Biol. Chem.* **1997**, *272*, 9597–9600. [PubMed]
48. Yamano, A.; Teeter, M.M. Correlated disorder of the pure pro22/leu25 form of crambin at 150 k refined to 1.05-a resolution. *J. Biol. Chem.* **1994**, *269*, 13956–13965. [PubMed]

49. Hendrickson, W.A.; Teeter, M.M. Structure of the hydrophobic protein crambin determined directly from the anomalous scattering of sulfur. *Nature* **1981**, *290*, 107–113. [CrossRef]
50. Ahn, H.C.; Juranic, N.; Macura, S.; Markley, J.L. Three-dimensional structure of the water-insoluble protein crambin in dodecylphosphocholine micelles and its minimal solvent-exposed surface. *J. Am. Chem. Soc.* **2006**, *128*, 4398–4404. [CrossRef] [PubMed]
51. Schmidt, A.; Teeter, M.; Weckert, E.; Lamzin, V.S. Crystal structure of small protein crambin at 0.48 a resolution. *Acta Crystallogr. Sect. F Struct. Biol. Cryst. Commun.* **2010**, *67*, 424–428. [CrossRef] [PubMed]
52. Chen, J.C.; Hanson, B.L.; Fisher, S.Z.; Langan, P.; Kovalevsky, A.Y. Direct observation of hydrogen atom dynamics and interactions by ultrahigh resolution neutron protein crystallography. *Proc. Natl. Acad. Sci. USA* **2012**, *109*, 15301–15306. [CrossRef] [PubMed]
53. Jelsch, C.; Teeter, M.M.; Lamzin, V.; Pichon-Pesme, V.; Blessing, R.H.; Lecomte, C. Accurate protein crystallography at ultra-high resolution: Valence electron distribution in crambin. *Proc. Natl. Acad. Sci. USA* **2000**, *97*, 3171–3176. [CrossRef] [PubMed]
54. Pal, A.; Debreczeni, J.E.; Sevvana, M.; Gruene, T.; Kahle, B.; Zeeck, A.; Sheldrick, G.M. Structures of viscotoxins a1 and b2 from european mistletoe solved using native data alone. *Acta Crystallogr. D Biol. Crystallogr.* **2008**, *64*, 985–992. [CrossRef] [PubMed]
55. Romagnoli, S.; Fogolari, F.; Catalano, M.; Zetta, L.; Schaller, G.; Urech, K.; Giannattasio, M.; Ragona, L.; Molinari, H. Nmr solution structure of viscotoxin c1 from viscum album species coloratum ohwi: Toward a structure-function analysis of viscotoxins. *Biochemistry* **2003**, *42*, 12503–12510. [CrossRef] [PubMed]
56. Coulon, A.; Mosbah, A.; Lopez, A.; Sautereau, A.M.; Schaller, G.; Urech, K.; Rouge, P.; Darbon, H. Comparative membrane interaction study of viscotoxins a3, a2 and b from mistletoe (viscum album) and connections with their structures. *Biochem. J.* **2003**, *374*, 71–78. [CrossRef] [PubMed]
57. Romagnoli, S.; Ugolini, R.; Fogolari, F.; Schaller, G.; Urech, K.; Giannattasio, M.; Ragona, L.; Molinari, H. Nmr structural determination of viscotoxin a3 from viscum album l. *Biochem. J.* **2000**, *350 (Pt. 2)*, 569–577. [CrossRef] [PubMed]
58. Debreczeni, J.E.; Girmann, B.; Zeeck, A.; Kratzner, R.; Sheldrick, G.M. Structure of viscotoxin a3: Disulfide location from weak sad data. *Acta Crystallogr. D Biol. Crystallogr.* **2003**, *59*, 2125–2132. [CrossRef] [PubMed]
59. Clore, G.M.; Sukumaran, D.K.; Nilges, M.; Gronenborn, A.M. 3-dimensional structure of phoratoxin in solution - combined use of nuclear-magnetic-resonance, distance geometry, and restrained molecular-dynamics. *Biochemistry* **1987**, *26*, 1732–1745. [CrossRef]
60. Mellstra, S.T.; Samuelss, G. Phoratoxin, a toxic protein from mistletoe phoradendron-tomentosum subsp. Macrophyllum (loranthaceae) - improvements in isolation procedure and further studies on properties. *Eur. J. Biochem.* **1973**, *32*, 143–147. [CrossRef]
61. Johnson, K.A.; Kim, E.; Teeter, M.M.; Suh, S.W.; Stec, B. Crystal structure of alpha-hordothionin at 1.9 angstrom resolution. *FEBS Lett.* **2005**, *579*, 2301–2306. [CrossRef] [PubMed]
62. Han, K.H.; Park, K.H.; Yoo, H.J.; Cha, H.; Suh, S.W.; Thomas, F.; Moon, T.S.; Kim, S.M. Determination of the three-dimensional structure of hordothionin-alpha by nuclear magnetic resonance. *Biochem. J.* **1996**, *313 (Pt. 3)*, 885–892. [CrossRef] [PubMed]
63. Vila-Perello, M.; Andreu, D. Characterization and structural role of disulfide bonds in a highly knotted thionin from pyrularia pubera. *Biopolymers* **2005**, *80*, 697–707. [CrossRef] [PubMed]
64. Vila-Perello, M.; Sanchez-Vallet, A.; Garcia-Olmedo, F.; Molina, A.; Andreu, D. Structural dissection of a highly knotted peptide reveals minimal motif with antimicrobial activity. *J. Biol. Chem.* **2005**, *280*, 1661–1668. [CrossRef] [PubMed]
65. Fujimura, M.; Ideguchi, M.; Minami, Y.; Watanabe, K.; Tadera, K. Purification, characterization, and sequencing of novel antimicrobial peptides, tu-amp 1 and tu-amp 2, from bulbs of tulip (tulipa gesneriana l.). *Biosci. Biotechnol. Biochem.* **2004**, *68*, 571–577. [CrossRef] [PubMed]
66. Florack, D.E.; Stiekema, W.J. Thionins: Properties, possible biological roles and mechanisms of action. *Plant Mol. Biol.* **1994**, *26*, 25–37. [CrossRef] [PubMed]
67. Osorio e Castro, V.R.; Vernon, L.P. Hemolytic activity of thionin from pyrularia pubera nuts and snake venom toxins of naja naja species: Pyrularia thionin and snake venom cardiotoxin compete for the same membrane site. *Toxicon* **1989**, *27*, 511–517. [CrossRef]
68. Hughes, P.; Dennis, E.; Whitecross, M.; Llewellyn, D.; Gage, P. The cytotoxic plant protein, beta-purothionin, forms ion channels in lipid membranes. *J. Biol. Chem.* **2000**, *275*, 823–827. [CrossRef] [PubMed]

69. Carrasco, L.; Vazquez, D.; Hernandez-Lucas, C.; Carbonero, P.; Garcia-Olmedo, F. Thionins: Plant peptides that modify membrane permeability in cultured mammalian cells. *Eur. J. Biochem.* **1981**, *116*, 185–189. [CrossRef] [PubMed]
70. Oka, T.; Murata, Y.; Nakanishi, T.; Yoshizumi, H.; Hayashida, H.; Ohtsuki, Y.; Toyoshima, K.; Hakura, A. Similarity, in molecular-structure and function, between the plant toxin purothionin and the mammalian pore-forming proteins. *Mol. Biol. Evol.* **1992**, *9*, 707–715. [PubMed]
71. Richard, J.A.; Kelly, I.; Marion, D.; Pezolet, M.; Auger, M. Interaction between beta-purothionin and dimyristoylphosphatidylglycerol: A p-31-nmr and infrared spectroscopic study. *Biophysic. J.* **2002**, *83*, 2074–2083. [CrossRef]
72. Richard, J.A.; Kelly, I.; Marion, D.; Auger, M.; Pezolet, M. Structure of beta-purothionin in membranes: A two-dimensional infrared correlation spectroscopy study. *Biochemistry* **2005**, *44*, 52–61. [CrossRef] [PubMed]
73. Wada, K.; Ozaki, Y.; Matsubara, H.; Yoshizumi, H. Studies on purothionin by chemical modifications. *J. Biochem.* **1982**, *91*, 257–263. [PubMed]
74. Fracki, W.S.; Li, D.; Owen, N.; Perry, C.; Naisbitt, G.H.; Vernon, L.P. Role of tyr and trp in membrane responses of pyrularia thionin determined by optical and nmr spectra following tyr iodination and trp modification. *Toxicon* **1992**, *30*, 1427–1440. [CrossRef]
75. Rao, A.G.; Hassan, M.; Hempel, J. Validation of the structure-function properties of alpha-hordothionin and derivatives through protein modeling. *Protein Eng.* **1993**, *6*, 117–117.
76. Pelegrini, P.B.; Franco, O.L. Plant gamma-thionins: Novel insights on the mechanism of action of a multi-functional class of defense proteins. *Int. J. Biochem. Cell. Biol.* **2005**, *37*, 2239–2253. [CrossRef] [PubMed]
77. Gao, A.G.; Hakimi, S.M.; Mittanck, C.A.; Wu, Y.; Woerner, B.M.; Stark, D.M.; Shah, D.M.; Liang, J.; Rommens, C.M. Fungal pathogen protection in potato by expression of a plant defensin peptide. *Nat. Biotechnol.* **2000**, *18*, 1307–1310. [PubMed]
78. Terras, F.R.; Schoofs, H.M.; De Bolle, M.F.; Van Leuven, F.; Rees, S.B.; Vanderleyden, J.; Cammue, B.P.; Broekaert, W.F. Analysis of two novel classes of plant antifungal proteins from radish (raphanus sativus l.) seeds. *J. Biol. Chem.* **1992**, *267*, 15301–15309. [PubMed]
79. Terras, F.R.; Eggermont, K.; Kovaleva, V.; Raikhel, N.V.; Osborn, R.W.; Kester, A.; Rees, S.B.; Torrekens, S.; Van Leuven, F.; Vanderleyden, J.; *et al.* Small cysteine-rich antifungal proteins from radish: Their role in host defense. *Plant Cell.* **1995**, *7*, 573–588. [CrossRef] [PubMed]
80. Fant, F.; Vranken, W.F.; Borremans, F.A. The three-dimensional solution structure of aesculus hippocastanum antimicrobial protein 1 determined by 1h nuclear magnetic resonance. *Proteins* **1999**, *37*, 388–403. [CrossRef]
81. Fant, F.; Vranken, W.; Broekaert, W.; Borremans, F. Determination of the three-dimensional solution structure of raphanus sativus antifungal protein 1 by 1h nmr. *J. Mol. Biol.* **1998**, *279*, 257–270. [CrossRef] [PubMed]
82. Fujimura, M.; Minami, Y.; Watanabe, K.; Tadera, K. Purification, characterization, and sequencing of a novel type of antimicrobial peptides, fa-amp1 and fa-amp2, from seeds of buckwheat (*Fagopyrum esculentum* Moench.). *Biosci. Biotechnol. Biochem.* **2003**, *67*, 1636–1642. [CrossRef] [PubMed]
83. Sitaram, N. Antimicrobial peptides with unusual amino acid compositions and unusual structures. *Curr. Med. Chem.* **2006**, *13*, 679–696. [CrossRef] [PubMed]
84. Bloch, C., Jr.; Richardson, M. A new family of small (5 kda) protein inhibitors of insect alpha-amylases from seeds or sorghum (*Sorghum bicolar* (L.) Moench.) have sequence homologies with wheat gamma-purothionins. *FEBS Lett.* **1991**, *279*, 101–104. [CrossRef]
85. Wijaya, R.; Neumann, G.M.; Condron, R.; Hughes, A.B.; Polya, G.M. Defense proteins from seed of cassia fistula include a lipid transfer protein homologue and a protease inhibitory plant defensin. *Plant Sci.* **2000**, *159*, 243–255. [CrossRef]
86. Colilla, F.J.; Rocher, A.; Mendez, E. Gamma-purothionins: Amino acid sequence of two polypeptides of a new family of thionins from wheat endosperm. *FEBS Lett.* **1990**, *270*, 191–194. [CrossRef]
87. Mendez, E.; Moreno, A.; Colilla, F.; Pelaez, F.; Limas, G.G.; Mendez, R.; Soriano, F.; Salinas, M.; de Haro, C. Primary structure and inhibition of protein synthesis in eukaryotic cell-free system of a novel thionin, gamma-hordothionin, from barley endosperm. *Eur. J. Biochem.* **1990**, *194*, 533–539. [CrossRef] [PubMed]
88. Bruix, M.; Jimenez, M.A.; Santoro, J.; Gonzalez, C.; Colilla, F.J.; Mendez, E.; Rico, M. Solution structure of gamma 1-h and gamma 1-p thionins from barley and wheat endosperm determined by 1h-nmr: A structural motif common to toxic arthropod proteins. *Biochemistry* **1993**, *32*, 715–724. [CrossRef] [PubMed]

89. Broekaert, W.F.; Terras, F.R.G.; Cammue, B.P.A.; Osborn, R.W. Plant defensins - novel antimicrobial peptides as components of the host-defense system. *Plant Physiol.* **1995**, *108*, 1353–1358. [CrossRef] [PubMed]
90. Franco, O.L.; Murad, A.M.; Leite, J.R.; Mendes, P.A.; Prates, M.V.; Bloch, C., Jr. Identification of a cowpea gamma-thionin with bactericidal activity. *FEBS J.* **2006**, *273*, 3489–3497. [CrossRef] [PubMed]
91. Moreno, M.; Segura, A.; Garcia-Olmedo, F. Pseudothionin-st1, a potato peptide active against potato pathogens. *Eur. J. Biochem.* **1994**, *223*, 135–139. [CrossRef] [PubMed]
92. Chiang, C.C.; Hadwiger, L.A. The fusarium solani-induced expression of a pea gene family encoding high cysteine content proteins. *Mol. Plant Microbe Interact.* **1991**, *4*, 324–331. [CrossRef] [PubMed]
93. Park, H.C.; Kang, Y.H.; Chun, H.J.; Koo, J.C.; Cheong, Y.H.; Kim, C.Y.; Kim, M.C.; Chung, W.S.; Kim, J.C.; Yoo, J.H.; *et al.* Characterization of a stamen-specific cdna encoding a novel plant defensin in chinese cabbage. *Plant Mol. Biol.* **2002**, *50*, 59–69. [CrossRef] [PubMed]
94. Milligan, S.B.; Gasser, C.S. Nature and regulation of pistil-expressed genes in tomato. *Plant Mol. Biol.* **1995**, *28*, 691–711. [CrossRef] [PubMed]
95. Lay, F.T.; Brugliera, F.; Anderson, M.A. Isolation and properties of floral defensins from ornamental tobacco and petunia. *Plant Physiol.* **2003**, *131*, 1283–1293. [CrossRef] [PubMed]
96. Sharma, P.; Lonneborg, A. Isolation and characterization of a cdna encoding a plant defensin-like protein from roots of norway spruce. *Plant Mol. Biol.* **1996**, *31*, 707–712. [CrossRef] [PubMed]
97. Finkina, E.I.; Shramova, E.I.; Tagaev, A.A.; Ovchinnikova, T.V. A novel defensin from the lentil lens culinaris seeds. *Biochem. Biophys. Res. Commun.* **2008**, *371*, 860–865. [CrossRef] [PubMed]
98. Bontems, F.; Roumestand, C.; Boyot, P.; Gilquin, B.; Doljansky, Y.; Menez, A.; Toma, F. Three-dimensional structure of natural charybdotoxin in aqueous solution by 1h-nmr. Charybdotoxin possesses a structural motif found in other scorpion toxins. *Eur. J. Biochem.* **1991**, *196*, 19–28. [CrossRef] [PubMed]
99. Cornet, B.; Bonmatin, J.M.; Hetru, C.; Hoffmann, J.A.; Ptak, M.; Vovelle, F. Refined three-dimensional solution structure of insect defensin A. *Structure* **1995**, *3*, 435–448. [CrossRef]
100. Broekaert, W.F.; Cammue, B.P.A.; DeBolle, M.F.C.; Thevissen, K.; DeSamblanx, G.W.; Osborn, R.W. Antimicrobial peptides from plants. *Crit. Rev. Plant. Sci.* **1997**, *16*, 297–323. [CrossRef]
101. Thomma, B.P.; Cammue, B.P.; Thevissen, K. Plant defensins. *Planta* **2002**, *216*, 193–202. [CrossRef] [PubMed]
102. Raj, P.A.; Dentino, A.R. Current status of defensins and their role in innate and adaptive immunity. *FEMS Microbiol. Lett.* **2002**, *206*, 9–18. [CrossRef] [PubMed]
103. Bulet, P.; Hetru, C.; Dimarcq, J.L.; Hoffmann, D. Antimicrobial peptides in insects; structure and function. *Dev. Comp. Immunol.* **1999**, *23*, 329–344. [CrossRef]
104. Carvalho Ade, O.; Gomes, V.M. Plant defensins and defensin-like peptides - biological activities and biotechnological applications. *Curr. Pharm. Des.* **2011**, *17*, 4270–4293. [CrossRef] [PubMed]
105. Yang, Y.F.; Cheng, K.C.; Tsai, P.H.; Liu, C.C.; Lee, T.R.; Lyu, P.C. Alanine substitutions of noncysteine residues in the cysteine-stabilized alphabeta motif. *Protein Sci.* **2009**, *18*, 1498–1506. [CrossRef] [PubMed]
106. Lay, F.T.; Schirra, H.J.; Scanlon, M.J.; Anderson, M.A.; Craik, D.J. The three-dimensional solution structure of nad1, a new floral defensin from nicotiana alata and its application to a homology model of the crop defense protein alfafp. *J. Mol. Biol.* **2003**, *325*, 175–188. [CrossRef]
107. Chen, K.C.; Lin, C.Y.; Kuan, C.C.; Sung, H.Y.; Chen, C.S. A novel defensin encoded by a mungbean cdna exhibits insecticidal activity against bruchid. *J. Agric. Food Chem.* **2002**, *50*, 7258–7263. [CrossRef] [PubMed]
108. Janssen, B.J.; Schirra, H.J.; Lay, F.T.; Anderson, M.A.; Craik, D.J. Structure of petunia hybrida defensin 1, a novel plant defensin with five disulfide bonds. *Biochemistry* **2003**, *42*, 8214–8222. [CrossRef] [PubMed]
109. Mendez, E.; Rocher, A.; Calero, M.; Girbes, T.; Citores, L.; Soriano, F. Primary structure of omega-hordothionin, a member of a novel family of thionins from barley endosperm, and its inhibition of protein synthesis in eukaryotic and prokaryotic cell-free systems. *Eur. J. Biochem.* **1996**, *239*, 67–73. [CrossRef] [PubMed]
110. Song, X.; Zhou, Z.; Wang, J.; Wu, F.; Gong, W. Purification, characterization and preliminary crystallographic studies of a novel plant defensin from pachyrrhizus erosus seeds. *Acta Crystallogr. D Biol. Crystallogr.* **2004**, *60*, 1121–1124. [CrossRef] [PubMed]
111. Song, X.; Zhang, M.; Zhou, Z.; Gong, W. Ultra-high resolution crystal structure of a dimeric defensin spe10. *FEBS Lett.* **2011**, *585*, 300–306. [CrossRef] [PubMed]

112. Spelbrink, R.G.; Dilmac, N.; Allen, A.; Smith, T.J.; Shah, D.M.; Hockerman, G.H. Differential antifungal and calcium channel-blocking activity among structurally related plant defensins. *Plant Physiol.* **2004**, *135*, 2055–2067. [CrossRef] [PubMed]
113. Osborn, R.W.; De Samblanx, G.W.; Thevissen, K.; Goderis, I.; Torrekens, S.; Van Leuven, F.; Attenborough, S.; Rees, S.B.; Broekaert, W.F. Isolation and characterisation of plant defensins from seeds of asteraceae, fabaceae, hippocastanaceae and saxifragaceae. *FEBS Lett.* **1995**, *368*, 257–262. [CrossRef]
114. Almeida, M.S.; Cabral, K.M.; Kurtenbach, E.; Almeida, F.C.; Valente, A.P. Solution structure of pisum sativum defensin 1 by high resolution nmr: Plant defensins, identical backbone with different mechanisms of action. *J. Mol. Biol.* **2002**, *315*, 749–757. [CrossRef] [PubMed]
115. Zhang, Y.; Lewis, K. Fabatins: New antimicrobial plant peptides. *FEMS Microbiol. Lett.* **1997**, *149*, 59–64. [CrossRef] [PubMed]
116. Garciaolmedo, F.; Carbonero, P.; Hernandezlucas, C.; Pazares, J.; Ponz, F.; Vicente, O.; Sierra, J.M. Inhibition of eukaryotic cell-free protein-synthesis by thionins from wheat endosperm. *Biochim. Biophys. Acta* **1983**, *740*, 52–56. [CrossRef]
117. Pelegrini, P.B.; Lay, F.T.; Murad, A.M.; Anderson, M.A.; Franco, O.L. Novel insights on the mechanism of action of alpha-amylase inhibitors from the plant defensin family. *Proteins* **2008**, *73*, 719–729. [CrossRef] [PubMed]
118. Dos Santos, I.S.; Carvalho Ade, O.; de Souza-Filho, G.A.; do Nascimento, V.V.; Machado, O.L.; Gomes, V.M. Purification of a defensin isolated from vigna unguiculata seeds, its functional expression in escherichia coli, and assessment of its insect alpha-amylase inhibitory activity. *Protein Expr. Purif.* **2010**, *71*, 8–15. [CrossRef] [PubMed]
119. Carvalho Ade, O.; Gomes, V.M. Plant defensins–prospects for the biological functions and biotechnological properties. *Peptides* **2009**, *30*, 1007–1020. [CrossRef] [PubMed]
120. Kushmerick, C.; de Souza Castro, M.; Santos Cruz, J.; Bloch, C., Jr.; Beirao, P.S. Functional and structural features of gamma-zeathionins, a new class of sodium channel blockers. *FEBS Lett.* **1998**, *440*, 302–306. [CrossRef]
121. Melo, F.R.; Rigden, D.J.; Franco, O.L.; Mello, L.V.; Ary, M.B.; Grossi de Sa, M.F.; Bloch, C., Jr. Inhibition of trypsin by cowpea thionin: Characterization, molecular modeling, and docking. *Proteins* **2002**, *48*, 311–319. [CrossRef] [PubMed]
122. Huang, G.J.; Lai, H.C.; Chang, Y.S.; Sheu, M.J.; Lu, T.L.; Huang, S.S.; Lin, Y.H. Antimicrobial, dehydroascorbate reductase, and monodehydroascorbate reductase activities of defensin from sweet potato [ipomoea batatas (l.) lam. 'Tainong 57'] storage roots. *J. Agric. Food Chem.* **2008**, *56*, 2989–2995. [CrossRef] [PubMed]
123. Chen, Z.; Gallie, D.R. Dehydroascorbate reductase affects leaf growth, development, and function. *Plant Physiol.* **2006**, *142*, 775–787. [CrossRef] [PubMed]
124. Thevissen, K.; Osborn, R.W.; Acland, D.P.; Broekaert, W.F. Specific binding sites for an antifungal plant defensin from dahlia (dahlia merckii) on fungal cells are required for antifungal activity. *Mol. Plant Microbe Interact.* **2000**, *13*, 54–61. [CrossRef] [PubMed]
125. Thevissen, K.; Warnecke, D.C.; Francois, I.E.; Leipelt, M.; Heinz, E.; Ott, C.; Zahringer, U.; Thomma, B.P.; Ferket, K.K.; Cammue, B.P. Defensins from insects and plants interact with fungal glucosylceramides. *J. Biol. Chem.* **2004**, *279*, 3900–3905. [CrossRef] [PubMed]
126. Thevissen, K.; Ghazi, A.; De Samblanx, G.W.; Brownlee, C.; Osborn, R.W.; Broekaert, W.F. Fungal membrane responses induced by plant defensins and thionins. *J. Biol. Chem.* **1996**, *271*, 15018–15025. [PubMed]
127. Thevissen, K.; Terras, F.R.; Broekaert, W.F. Permeabilization of fungal membranes by plant defensins inhibits fungal growth. *Appl. Environ. Microbiol.* **1999**, *65*, 5451–5458. [PubMed]
128. Van der Weerden, N.L.; Hancock, R.E.; Anderson, M.A. Permeabilization of fungal hyphae by the plant defensin nad1 occurs through a cell wall-dependent process. *J. Biol. Chem.* **2010**, *285*, 37513–37520. [CrossRef] [PubMed]
129. Van der Weerden, N.L.; Lay, F.T.; Anderson, M.A. The plant defensin, nad1, enters the cytoplasm of fusarium oxysporum hyphae. *J. Biol. Chem.* **2008**, *283*, 14445–14452. [CrossRef] [PubMed]
130. Hayes, B.M.; Bleackley, M.R.; Wiltshire, J.L.; Anderson, M.A.; Traven, A.; van der Weerden, N.L. Identification and mechanism of action of the plant defensin nad1 as a new member of the antifungal drug arsenal against candida albicans. *Antimicrob. Agents Chemother.* **2013**, *57*, 3667–3675. [CrossRef] [PubMed]

131. De Coninck, B.; Cammue, B.P.A.; Thevissen, K. Modes of antifungal action and in planta functions of plant defensins and defensin-like peptides. *Fungal Biol. Rev.* **2013**, *26*, 109–120. [CrossRef]
132. Gachomo, E.W.; Jimenez-Lopez, J.C.; Kayode, A.P.; Baba-Moussa, L.; Kotchoni, S.O. Structural characterization of plant defensin protein superfamily. *Mol. Biol. Rep.* **2012**, *39*, 4461–4469. [CrossRef] [PubMed]
133. Beintema, J.J. Structural features of plant chitinases and chitin-binding proteins. *FEBS Lett.* **1994**, *350*, 159–163. [CrossRef]
134. Jimenez-Barbero, J.; Javier Canada, F.; Asensio, J.L.; Aboitiz, N.; Vidal, P.; Canales, A.; Groves, P.; Gabius, H.J.; Siebert, H.C. Hevein domains: An attractive model to study carbohydrate-protein interactions at atomic resolution. *Adv. Carbohydr. Chem. Biochem.* **2006**, *60*, 303–354. [PubMed]
135. Kini, S.G.; Nguyen, P.Q.; Weissbach, S.; Mallagaray, A.; Shin, J.; Yoon, H.S.; Tam, J.P. Studies on the chitin binding property of novel cysteine-rich peptides from alternanthera sessilis. *Biochemistry* **2015**, *54*, 6639–6649. [CrossRef] [PubMed]
136. Archer, B.L. The proteins of hevea brasiliensis latex. 4. Isolation and characterization of crystalline hevein. *Biochem. J.* **1960**, *75*, 236–240. [CrossRef] [PubMed]
137. Van Parijs, J.; Broekaert, W.F.; Goldstein, I.J.; Peumans, W.J. Hevein: An antifungal protein from rubber-tree (*Hevea brasiliensis*) latex. *Planta* **1991**, *183*, 258–264. [CrossRef] [PubMed]
138. Diaz-Perales, A.; Collada, C.; Blanco, C.; Sanchez-Monge, R.; Carrillo, T.; Aragoncillo, C.; Salcedo, G. Cross-reactions in the latex-fruit syndrome: A relevant role of chitinases but not of complex asparagine-linked glycans. *J. Allergy Clin. Immunol.* **1999**, *104*, 681–687. [CrossRef]
139. Blanco, C.; Diaz-Perales, A.; Collada, C.; Sanchez-Monge, R.; Aragoncillo, C.; Castillo, R.; Ortega, N.; Alvarez, M.; Carrillo, T.; Salcedo, G. Class i chitinases as potential panallergens involved in the latex-fruit syndrome. *J. Allergy Clin. Immunol.* **1999**, *103*, 507–513. [CrossRef]
140. Gidrol, X.; Chrestin, H.; Tan, H.L.; Kush, A. Hevein, a lectin-like protein from hevea brasiliensis (rubber tree) is involved in the coagulation of latex. *J. Biol. Chem.* **1994**, *269*, 9278–9283. [PubMed]
141. Peumans, W.J.; Van Damme, E.J. Plant lectins: Specific tools for the identification, isolation, and characterization of o-linked glycans. *Crit. Rev. Biochem. Mol. Biol.* **1998**, *33*, 209–258. [PubMed]
142. Asensio, J.L.; Siebert, H.C.; von Der Lieth, C.W.; Laynez, J.; Bruix, M.; Soedjanaamadja, U.M.; Beintema, J.J.; Canada, F.J.; Gabius, H.J.; Jimenez-Barbero, J. Nmr investigations of protein-carbohydrate interactions: Studies on the relevance of trp/tyr variations in lectin binding sites as deduced from titration microcalorimetry and nmr studies on hevein domains. Determination of the nmr structure of the complex between pseudohevein and n,n',n''-triacetylchitotriose. *Proteins* **2000**, *40*, 218–236. [PubMed]
143. Lipkin, A.; Anisimova, V.; Nikonorova, A.; Babakov, A.; Krause, E.; Bienert, M.; Grishin, E.; Egorov, T. An antimicrobial peptide ar-amp from amaranth (*Amaranthus retroflexus* L.) seeds. *Phytochemistry* **2005**, *66*, 2426–2431. [CrossRef] [PubMed]
144. Andreev, Y.A.; Korostyleva, T.V.; Slavokhotova, A.A.; Rogozhin, E.A.; Utkina, L.L.; Vassilevski, A.A.; Grishin, E.V.; Egorov, T.A.; Odintsova, T.I. Genes encoding hevein-like defense peptides in wheat: Distribution, evolution, and role in stress response. *Biochimie* **2012**, *94*, 1009–1016. [CrossRef] [PubMed]
145. Van den Bergh, K.P.; Rouge, P.; Proost, P.; Coosemans, J.; Krouglova, T.; Engelborghs, Y.; Peumans, W.J.; Van Damme, E.J. Synergistic antifungal activity of two chitin-binding proteins from spindle tree (*Euonymus europaeus* L.). *Planta* **2004**, *219*, 221–232. [CrossRef] [PubMed]
146. Asensio, J.L.; Canada, F.J.; Bruix, M.; Gonzalez, C.; Khiar, N.; Rodriguez-Romero, A.; Jimenez-Barbero, J. Nmr investigations of protein-carbohydrate interactions: Refined three-dimensional structure of the complex between hevein and methyl beta-chitobioside. *Glycobiology* **1998**, *8*, 569–577. [CrossRef] [PubMed]
147. Harata, K.; Muraki, M. Crystal structures of urtica dioica agglutinin and its complex with tri-n-acetylchitotriose. *J. Mol. Biol.* **2000**, *297*, 673–681. [CrossRef] [PubMed]
148. Broekaert, W.F.; Marien, W.; Terras, F.R.; De Bolle, M.F.; Proost, P.; Van Damme, J.; Dillen, L.; Claeys, M.; Rees, S.B.; Vanderleyden, J.; *et al.* Antimicrobial peptides from amaranthus caudatus seeds with sequence homology to the cysteine/glycine-rich domain of chitin-binding proteins. *Biochemistry* **1992**, *31*, 4308–4314. [CrossRef] [PubMed]
149. Martins, J.C.; Maes, D.; Loris, R.; Pepermans, H.A.; Wyns, L.; Willem, R.; Verheyden, P. H nmr study of the solution structure of ac-amp2, a sugar binding antimicrobial protein isolated from amaranthus caudatus. *J. Mol. Biol.* **1996**, *258*, 322–333. [CrossRef] [PubMed]

150. Aboitiz, N.; Vila-Perello, M.; Groves, P.; Asensio, J.L.; Andreu, D.; Canada, F.J.; Jimenez-Barbero, J. Nmr and modeling studies of protein-carbohydrate interactions: Synthesis, three-dimensional structure, and recognition properties of a minimum hevein domain with binding affinity for chitooligosaccharides. *ChemBioChem* **2004**, *5*, 1245–1255. [CrossRef] [PubMed]
151. Koo, J.C.; Lee, S.Y.; Chun, H.J.; Cheong, Y.H.; Choi, J.S.; Kawabata, S.; Miyagi, M.; Tsunasawa, S.; Ha, K.S.; Bae, D.W.; *et al.* Two hevein homologs isolated from the seed of pharbitis nil l. Exhibit potent antifungal activity. *Biochim. Biophys. Acta* **1998**, *1382*, 80–90. [CrossRef]
152. Lee, O.S.; Lee, B.; Park, N.; Koo, J.C.; Kim, Y.H.; Prasad, D.T.; Karigar, C.; Chun, H.J.; Jeong, B.R.; Kim, D.H.; *et al.* Pn-amps, the hevein-like proteins from pharbitis nil confers disease resistance against phytopathogenic fungi in tomato, lycopersicum esculentum. *Phytochemistry* **2003**, *62*, 1073–1079. [CrossRef]
153. Koo, J.C.; Chun, H.J.; Park, H.C.; Kim, M.C.; Koo, Y.D.; Koo, S.C.; Ok, H.M.; Park, S.J.; Lee, S.H.; Yun, D.J.; *et al.* Over-expression of a seed specific hevein-like antimicrobial peptide from pharbitis nil enhances resistance to a fungal pathogen in transgenic tobacco plants. *Plant Mol. Biol.* **2002**, *50*, 441–452. [PubMed]
154. Li, S.S.; Claeson, P. Cys/gly-rich proteins with a putative single chitin-binding domain from oat (*Avena sativa*) seeds. *Phytochemistry* **2003**, *63*, 249–255. [CrossRef]
155. Huang, R.H.; Xiang, Y.; Liu, X.Z.; Zhang, Y.; Hu, Z.; Wang, D.C. Two novel antifungal peptides distinct with a five-disulfide motif from the bark of eucommia ulmoides oliv. *FEBS Lett.* **2002**, *521*, 87–90. [CrossRef]
156. Huang, R.H.; Xiang, Y.; Tu, G.Z.; Zhang, Y.; Wang, D.C. Solution structure of eucommia antifungal peptide: A novel structural model distinct with a five-disulfide motif. *Biochemistry* **2004**, *43*, 6005–6012. [CrossRef] [PubMed]
157. Xiang, Y.; Huang, R.H.; Liu, X.Z.; Zhang, Y.; Wang, D.C. Crystal structure of a novel antifungal protein distinct with five disulfide bridges from eucommia ulmoides oliver at an atomic resolution. *J. Struct. Biol* **2004**, *148*, 86–97. [CrossRef] [PubMed]
158. Odintsova, T.I.; Vassilevski, A.A.; Slavokhotova, A.A.; Musolyamov, A.K.; Finkina, E.I.; Khadeeva, N.V.; Rogozhin, E.A.; Korostyleva, T.V.; Pukhalsky, V.A.; Grishin, E.V.; *et al.* A novel antifungal hevein-type peptide from triticum kiharae seeds with a unique 10-cysteine motif. *FEBS J.* **2009**, *276*, 4266–4275. [CrossRef] [PubMed]
159. Dubovskii, P.V.; Vassilevski, A.A.; Slavokhotova, A.A.; Odintsova, T.I.; Grishin, E.V.; Egorov, T.A.; Arseniev, A.S. Solution structure of a defense peptide from wheat with a 10-cysteine motif. *Biochem. Biophys. Res. Commun.* **2011**, *411*, 14–18. [CrossRef] [PubMed]
160. Van den Bergh, K.P.; Proost, P.; Van Damme, J.; Coosemans, J.; Van Damme, E.J.; Peumans, W.J. Five disulfide bridges stabilize a hevein-type antimicrobial peptide from the bark of spindle tree (*Euonymus europaeus* L.). *FEBS Lett.* **2002**, *530*, 181–185. [CrossRef]
161. Chavez, M.I.; Vila-Perello, M.; Canada, F.J.; Andreu, D.; Jimenez-Barbero, J. Effect of a serine-to-aspartate replacement on the recognition of chitin oligosaccharides by truncated hevein. A 3d view by using nmr. *Carbohydr. Res.* **2010**, *345*, 1461–1468. [CrossRef] [PubMed]
162. Espinosa, J.F.; Asensio, J.L.; Garcia, J.L.; Laynez, J.; Bruix, M.; Wright, C.; Siebert, H.C.; Gabius, H.J.; Canada, F.J.; Jimenez-Barbero, J. Nmr investigations of protein-carbohydrate interactions binding studies and refined three-dimensional solution structure of the complex between the b domain of wheat germ agglutinin and n,n',n''-triacetylchitotriose. *Eur. J. Biochem.* **2000**, *267*, 3965–3978. [CrossRef] [PubMed]
163. Muraki, M. The importance of ch/pi interactions to the function of carbohydrate binding proteins. *Protein Pept. Lett.* **2002**, *9*, 195–209. [CrossRef] [PubMed]
164. Chavez, M.I.; Andreu, C.; Vidal, P.; Aboitiz, N.; Freire, F.; Groves, P.; Asensio, J.L.; Asensio, G.; Muraki, M.; Canada, F.J.; *et al.* On the importance of carbohydrate-aromatic interactions for the molecular recognition of oligosaccharides by proteins: Nmr studies of the structure and binding affinity of acamp2-like peptides with non-natural naphthyl and fluoroaromatic residues. *Chemistry* **2005**, *11*, 7060–7074. [CrossRef] [PubMed]
165. Slavokhotova, A.A.; Naumann, T.A.; Price, N.P.; Rogozhin, E.A.; Andreev, Y.A.; Vassilevski, A.A.; Odintsova, T.I. Novel mode of action of plant defense peptides - hevein-like antimicrobial peptides from wheat inhibit fungal metalloproteases. *FEBS J.* **2014**, *281*, 4754–4764. [CrossRef] [PubMed]
166. Pallaghy, P.K.; Nielsen, K.J.; Craik, D.J.; Norton, R.S. A common structural motif incorporating a cystine knot and a triple-stranded beta-sheet in toxic and inhibitory polypeptides. *Protein Sci.* **1994**, *3*, 1833–1839. [CrossRef] [PubMed]

167. Franco, O.L. Peptide promiscuity: An evolutionary concept for plant defense. *FEBS Lett.* **2011**, *585*, 995–1000. [CrossRef] [PubMed]
168. Rees, D.C.; Lipscomb, W.N. Refined crystal structure of the potato inhibitor complex of carboxypeptidase a at 2.5 a resolution. *J. Mol. Biol.* **1982**, *160*, 475–498. [CrossRef]
169. McDonald, N.Q.; Hendrickson, W.A. A structural superfamily of growth factors containing a cystine knot motif. *Cell* **1993**, *73*, 421–424. [CrossRef]
170. Craik, D.J.; Daly, N.L.; Bond, T.; Waine, C. Plant cyclotides: A unique family of cyclic and knotted proteins that defines the cyclic cystine knot structural motif. *J. Mol. Biol.* **1999**, *294*, 1327–1336. [CrossRef] [PubMed]
171. Gruber, C.W.; Elliott, A.G.; Ireland, D.C.; Delprete, P.G.; Dessein, S.; Goransson, U.; Trabi, M.; Wang, C.K.; Kinghorn, A.B.; Robbrecht, E.; *et al.* Distribution and evolution of circular miniproteins in flowering plants. *Plant Cell.* **2008**, *20*, 2471–2483. [CrossRef] [PubMed]
172. Poth, A.G.; Mylne, J.S.; Grassl, J.; Lyons, R.E.; Millar, A.H.; Colgrave, M.L.; Craik, D.J. Cyclotides associate with leaf vasculature and are the products of a novel precursor in petunia (solanaceae). *J. Biol. Chem.* **2012**, *287*, 27033–27046. [CrossRef] [PubMed]
173. Nguyen, G.K.; Zhang, S.; Nguyen, N.T.; Nguyen, P.Q.; Chiu, M.S.; Hardjojo, A.; Tam, J.P. Discovery and characterization of novel cyclotides originated from chimeric precursors consisting of albumin-1 chain a and cyclotide domains in the fabaceae family. *J. Biol. Chem.* **2011**, *286*, 24275–24287. [CrossRef] [PubMed]
174. Poth, A.G.; Colgrave, M.L.; Lyons, R.E.; Daly, N.L.; Craik, D.J. Discovery of an unusual biosynthetic origin for circular proteins in legumes. *Proc. Natl. Acad. Sci. USA* **2011**, *108*, 10127–10132. [CrossRef] [PubMed]
175. Mylne, J.S.; Chan, L.Y.; Chanson, A.H.; Daly, N.L.; Schaefer, H.; Bailey, T.L.; Nguyencong, P.; Cascales, L.; Craik, D.J. Cyclic peptides arising by evolutionary parallelism via asparaginyl-endopeptidase-mediated biosynthesis. *Plant Cell.* **2012**, *24*, 2765–2778. [CrossRef] [PubMed]
176. Nguyen, G.K.; Lian, Y.; Pang, E.W.; Nguyen, P.Q.; Tran, T.D.; Tam, J.P. Discovery of linear cyclotides in monocot plant panicum laxum of poaceae family provides new insights into evolution and distribution of cyclotides in plants. *J. Biol. Chem.* **2012**, *288*, 3370–3380. [CrossRef] [PubMed]
177. Ireland, D.C.; Colgrave, M.L.; Nguyencong, P.; Daly, N.L.; Craik, D.J. Discovery and characterization of a linear cyclotide from viola odorata: Implications for the processing of circular proteins. *J. Mol. Biol.* **2006**, *357*, 1522–1535. [CrossRef] [PubMed]
178. Gruber, C.W.; Cemazar, M.; Clark, R.J.; Horibe, T.; Renda, R.F.; Anderson, M.A.; Craik, D.J. A novel plant protein-disulfide isomerase involved in the oxidative folding of cystine knot defense proteins. *J. Biol. Chem.* **2007**, *282*, 20435–20446. [CrossRef] [PubMed]
179. Saska, I.; Gillon, A.D.; Hatsugai, N.; Dietzgen, R.G.; Hara-Nishimura, I.; Anderson, M.A.; Craik, D.J. An asparaginyl endopeptidase mediates *in vivo* protein backbone cyclization. *J. Biol. Chem.* **2007**, *282*, 29721–29728. [CrossRef] [PubMed]
180. Conlan, B.F.; Gillon, A.D.; Craik, D.J.; Anderson, M.A. Circular proteins and mechanisms of cyclization. *Biopolymers* **2010**, *94*, 573–583. [CrossRef] [PubMed]
181. Nguyen, G.K.T.; Wang, S.J.; Qiu, Y.B.; Hemu, X.; Lian, Y.L.; Tam, J.P. Butelase 1 is an asx-specific ligase enabling peptide macrocyclization and synthesis. *Nat. Chem. Biol.* **2014**, *10*, 732–738. [CrossRef] [PubMed]
182. Cao, Y.; Nguyen, G.K.; Tam, J.P.; Liu, C.F. Butelase-mediated synthesis of protein thioesters and its application for tandem chemoenzymatic ligation. *Chem. Commun. (Camb)* **2015**. [CrossRef] [PubMed]
183. Chagolla-Lopez, A.; Blanco-Labra, A.; Patthy, A.; Sanchez, R.; Pongor, S. A novel alpha-amylase inhibitor from amaranth (*Amaranthus hypocondriacus*) seeds. *J. Biol. Chem.* **1994**, *269*, 23675–23680. [PubMed]
184. Svensson, B.; Fukuda, K.; Nielsen, P.K.; Bonsager, B.C. Proteinaceous alpha-amylase inhibitors. *Biochim. Biophys. Acta* **2004**, *1696*, 145–156. [CrossRef] [PubMed]
185. Martins, J.C.; Enassar, M.; Willem, R.; Wieruzeski, J.M.; Lippens, G.; Wodak, S.J. Solution structure of the main alpha-amylase inhibitor from amaranth seeds. *Eur. J. Biochem.* **2001**, *268*, 2379–2389. [CrossRef] [PubMed]
186. Nguyen, P.Q.T.; Wang, S.J.; Kumar, A.; Yap, L.J.; Luu, T.T.; Lescar, J.; Tam, J.P. Discovery and characterization of pseudocyclic cystine-knot alpha-amylase inhibitors with high resistance to heat and proteolytic degradation. *FEBS J.* **2014**, *281*, 4351–4366. [CrossRef] [PubMed]
187. Nguyen, P.Q.; Luu, T.T.; Bai, Y.; Nguyen, G.K.; Pervushin, K.; Tam, J.P. Allotides: Proline-rich cystine knot alpha-amylase inhibitors from allamanda cathartica. *J. Nat. Prod.* **2015**, *78*, 695–704. [CrossRef] [PubMed]

188. Le-Nguyen, D.; Heitz, A.; Chiche, L.; el Hajji, M.; Castro, B. Characterization and 2d nmr study of the stable [9–21, 15–27] 2 disulfide intermediate in the folding of the 3 disulfide trypsin inhibitor eeti ii. *Protein Sci.* **1993**, *2*, 165–174. [CrossRef] [PubMed]
189. Heitz, A.; Le-Nguyen, D.; Chiche, L. Min-21 and min-23, the smallest peptides that fold like a cystine-stabilized beta-sheet motif: Design, solution structure, and thermal stability. *Biochemistry* **1999**, *38*, 10615–10625. [CrossRef] [PubMed]
190. Kolmar, H. Biological diversity and therapeutic potential of natural and engineered cystine knot miniproteins. *Curr. Opin. Pharmacol.* **2009**, *9*, 608–614. [CrossRef] [PubMed]
191. Colgrave, M.L.; Craik, D.J. Thermal, chemical, and enzymatic stability of the cyclotide kalata b1: The importance of the cyclic cystine knot. *Biochemistry* **2004**, *43*, 5965–5975. [CrossRef] [PubMed]
192. Heitz, A.; Avrutina, O.; Le-Nguyen, D.; Diederichsen, U.; Hernandez, J.F.; Gracy, J.; Kolmar, H.; Chiche, L. Knottin cyclization: Impact on structure and dynamics. *BMC Struct. Biol.* **2008**, *8*, 54. [CrossRef] [PubMed]
193. Ireland, D.C.; Colgrave, M.L.; Craik, D.J. A novel suite of cyclotides from viola odorata: Sequence variation and the implications for structure, function and stability. *Biochem. J.* **2006**, *400*, 1–12. [CrossRef] [PubMed]
194. Werle, M.; Kafedjiiski, K.; Kolmar, H.; Bernkop-Schnurch, A. Evaluation and improvement of the properties of the novel cystine-knot microprotein mcoeeti for oral administration. *Int. J. Pharm.* **2007**, *332*, 72–79. [CrossRef] [PubMed]
195. Werle, M.; Schmitz, T.; Huang, H.L.; Wentzel, A.; Kolmar, H.; Bernkop-Schnurch, A. The potential of cystine-knot microproteins as novel pharmacophoric scaffolds in oral peptide drug delivery. *J. Drug Target.* **2006**, *14*, 137–146. [CrossRef] [PubMed]
196. Gao, G.H.; Liu, W.; Dai, J.X.; Wang, J.F.; Hu, Z.; Zhang, Y.; Wang, D.C. Solution structure of pafp-s: A new knottin-type antifungal peptide from the seeds of phytolacca americana. *Biochemistry* **2001**, *40*, 10973–10978. [CrossRef] [PubMed]
197. Cammue, B.P.A.; Debolle, M.F.C.; Terras, F.R.G.; Proost, P.; Vandamme, J.; Rees, S.B.; Vanderleyden, J.; Broekaert, W.F. Isolation and characterization of a novel class of plant antimicrobial peptides from mirabilis-jalapa l seeds. *J. Biol. Chem.* **1992**, *267*, 2228–2233. [PubMed]
198. Hwang, J.S.; Lee, J.; Hwang, B.; Nam, S.H.; Yun, E.Y.; Kim, S.R.; Lee, D.G. Isolation and characterization of psacotheasin, a novel knottin-type antimicrobial peptide, from psacothea hilaris. *J. Microbiol. Biotechnol.* **2010**, *20*, 708–711. [CrossRef] [PubMed]
199. Konarev, A.V.; Anisimova, I.N.; Gavrilova, V.A.; Vachrusheva, T.E.; Konechnaya, G.Y.; Lewis, M.; Shewry, P.R. Serine proteinase inhibitors in the compositae: Distribution, polymorphism and properties. *Phytochemistry* **2002**, *59*, 279–291. [CrossRef]
200. Bode, W.; Greyling, H.J.; Huber, R.; Otlewski, J.; Wilusz, T. The refined 2.0 a x-ray crystal structure of the complex formed between bovine beta-trypsin and cmti-i, a trypsin inhibitor from squash seeds (*Cucurbita maxima*). Topological similarity of the squash seed inhibitors with the carboxypeptidase a inhibitor from potatoes. *FEBS Lett.* **1989**, *242*, 285–292. [PubMed]
201. Polanowski, A.; Wilusz, T.; Nienartowicz, B.; Cieslar, E.; Slominska, A.; Nowak, K. Isolation and partial amino acid sequence of the trypsin inhibitor from the seeds of cucurbita maxima. *Acta Biochim. Pol.* **1980**, *27*, 371–382. [PubMed]
202. Korsinczky, M.L.; Schirra, H.J.; Craik, D.J. Sunflower trypsin inhibitor-1. *Curr. Protein Pept. Sci.* **2004**, *5*, 351–364. [CrossRef] [PubMed]
203. Hass, G.M.; Ryan, C.A. Carboxypeptidase inhibitor from ripened tomatoes - purification and properties. *Phytochemistry* **1980**, *19*, 1329–1333. [CrossRef]
204. Arolas, J.L.; Lorenzo, J.; Rovira, A.; Vendrell, J.; Aviles, F.X.; Ventura, S. Secondary binding site of the potato carboxypeptidase inhibitor. Contribution to its structure, folding, and biological properties. *Biochemistry* **2004**, *43*, 7973–7982. [CrossRef] [PubMed]
205. Marino-Buslje, C.; Venhudova, G.; Molina, M.A.; Oliva, B.; Jorba, X.; Canals, F.; Aviles, F.X.; Querol, E. Contribution of c-tail residues of potato carboxypeptidase inhibitor to the binding to carboxypeptidase a a mutagenesis analysis. *Eur. J. Biochem.* **2000**, *267*, 1502–1509. [CrossRef] [PubMed]
206. Craik, D.J. Plant cyclotides: Circular, knotted peptide toxins. *Toxicon* **2001**, *39*, 1809–1813. [CrossRef]
207. Gould, A.; Ji, Y.; Aboye, T.L.; Camarero, J.A. Cyclotides, a novel ultrastable polypeptide scaffold for drug discovery. *Curr. Pharm. Des.* **2011**, *17*, 4294–4307. [CrossRef] [PubMed]

208. Daly, N.L.; Rosengren, K.J.; Craik, D.J. Discovery, structure and biological activities of cyclotides. *Adv. Drug Deliv. Rev.* **2009**, *61*, 918–930. [CrossRef] [PubMed]
209. Gran, L. On the effect of a polypeptide isolated from "kalata-kalata" (oldenlandia affinis dc) on the oestrogen dominated uterus. *Acta Pharmacol. Toxicol. (Copenh)* **1973**, *33*, 400–408. [CrossRef] [PubMed]
210. Rosengren, K.J.; Daly, N.L.; Plan, M.R.; Waine, C.; Craik, D.J. Twists, knots, and rings in proteins. Structural definition of the cyclotide framework. *J. Biol. Chem.* **2003**, *278*, 8606–8616. [CrossRef] [PubMed]
211. Tam, J.P.; Lu, Y.A.; Yang, J.L.; Chiu, K.W. An unusual structural motif of antimicrobial peptides containing end-to-end macrocycle and cystine-knot disulfides. *Proc. Natl. Acad. Sci. USA* **1999**, *96*, 8913–8918. [CrossRef] [PubMed]
212. Gran, L.; Sletten, K.; Skjeldal, L. Cyclic peptides from oldenlandia affinis dc. Molecular and biological properties. *Chem. Biodivers.* **2008**, *5*, 2014–2022. [CrossRef] [PubMed]
213. Pranting, M.; Loov, C.; Burman, R.; Goransson, U.; Andersson, D.I. The cyclotide cycloviolacin o2 from viola odorata has potent bactericidal activity against gram-negative bacteria. *J. Antimicrob. Chemother.* **2010**, *65*, 1964–1971. [CrossRef] [PubMed]
214. Wong, C.T.; Taichi, M.; Nishio, H.; Nishiuchi, Y.; Tam, J.P. Optimal oxidative folding of the novel antimicrobial cyclotide from hedyotis biflora requires high alcohol concentrations. *Biochemistry* **2011**, *50*, 7275–7283. [CrossRef] [PubMed]
215. Hernandez, J.F.; Gagnon, J.; Chiche, L.; Nguyen, T.M.; Andrieu, J.P.; Heitz, A.; Trinh Hong, T.; Pham, T.T.; Le Nguyen, D. Squash trypsin inhibitors from momordica cochinchinensis exhibit an atypical macrocyclic structure. *Biochemistry* **2000**, *39*, 5722–5730. [CrossRef] [PubMed]
216. Chiche, L.; Heitz, A.; Gelly, J.C.; Gracy, J.; Chau, P.T.; Ha, P.T.; Hernandez, J.F.; Le-Nguyen, D. Squash inhibitors: From structural motifs to macrocyclic knottins. *Curr. Protein Pept. Sci.* **2004**, *5*, 341–349. [CrossRef] [PubMed]
217. Heitz, A.; Hernandez, J.F.; Gagnon, J.; Hong, T.T.; Pham, T.T.; Nguyen, T.M.; Le-Nguyen, D.; Chiche, L. Solution structure of the squash trypsin inhibitor mcoti-ii. A new family for cyclic knottins. *Biochemistry* **2001**, *40*, 7973–7983. [CrossRef] [PubMed]
218. Henriques, S.T.; Craik, D.J. Cyclotides as templates in drug design. *Drug Discov. Today* **2010**, *15*, 57–64. [CrossRef] [PubMed]
219. Shenkarev, Z.O.; Nadezhdin, K.D.; Sobol, V.A.; Sobol, A.G.; Skjeldal, L.; Arseniev, A.S. Conformation and mode of membrane interaction in cyclotides. Spatial structure of kalata b1 bound to a dodecylphosphocholine micelle. *FEBS J.* **2006**, *273*, 2658–2672. [CrossRef] [PubMed]
220. Wang, C.K.; Colgrave, M.L.; Ireland, D.C.; Kaas, Q.; Craik, D.J. Despite a conserved cystine knot motif, different cyclotides have different membrane binding modes. *Biophys. J.* **2009**, *97*, 1471–1481. [CrossRef] [PubMed]
221. Wong, C.T.T.; Rowlands, D.K.; Wong, C.-H.; Lo, T.W.C.; Nguyen, G.K.T.; Li, H.-Y.; Tam, J.P. Orally active peptidic bradykinin b1 receptor antagonists engineered from a cyclotide scaffold for inflammatory pain treatment. *Angew. Chem. Int. Ed.* **2012**, *51*, 5620–5624. [CrossRef] [PubMed]
222. Hemu, X.; Taichi, M.; Qiu, Y.; Liu, D.-X.; Tam, J.P. Biomimetic synthesis of cyclic peptides using novel thioester surrogates. *Pept. Sci.* **2013**, *100*, 492–501. [CrossRef] [PubMed]
223. Qiu, Y.; Hemu, X.; Liu, D.X.; Tam, J.P. Selective bi-directional amide bond cleavage of *N*-methylcysteinyl peptide. *Eur. J. Org. Chem.* **2014**, *2014*, 4370–4380. [CrossRef]
224. Taichi, M.; Hemu, X.; Qiu, Y.; Tam, J.P. A thioethylalkylamido (tea) thioester surrogate in the synthesis of a cyclic peptide via a tandem acyl shift. *Org. Lett.* **2013**, *15*, 2620–2623. [CrossRef] [PubMed]
225. Tam, J.P.; Lu, Y.A. Synthesis of large cyclic cystine-knot peptide by orthogonal coupling strategy using unprotected peptide precursor. *Tetrahedron Lett.* **1997**, *38*, 5599–5602. [CrossRef]
226. Tam, J.P.; Lu, Y.A. A biomimetic strategy in the synthesis and fragmentation of cyclic protein. *Protein Sci.* **1998**, *7*, 1583–1592. [CrossRef] [PubMed]
227. Daly, N.L.; Love, S.; Alewood, P.F.; Craik, D.J. Chemical synthesis and folding pathways of large cyclic polypeptide: Studies of the cystine knot polypeptide kalata b1. *Biochemistry* **1999**, *38*, 10606–10614. [CrossRef] [PubMed]
228. Thongyoo, P.; Roque-Rosell, N.; Leatherbarrow, R.J.; Tate, E.W. Chemical and biomimetic total syntheses of natural and engineered mcoti cyclotides. *Org. Biomol. Chem.* **2008**, *6*, 1462–1470. [CrossRef] [PubMed]

229. Thongyoo, P.; Jaulent, A.M.; Tate, E.W.; Leatherbarrow, R.J. Immobilized protease-assisted synthesis of engineered cysteine-knot microproteins. *ChemBioChem* **2007**, *8*, 1107–1109. [CrossRef] [PubMed]
230. Kimura, R.H.; Tran, A.T.; Camarero, J.A. Biosynthesis of the cyclotide kalata b1 by using protein splicing. *Angew. Chem. Int. Ed.* **2006**, *45*, 973–976. [CrossRef] [PubMed]
231. Austin, J.; Wang, W.; Puttamadappa, S.; Shekhtman, A.; Camarero, J.A. Biosynthesis and biological screening of a genetically encoded library based on the cyclotide mcoti-i. *ChemBioChem* **2009**, *10*, 2663–2670. [CrossRef] [PubMed]
232. Tam, J.P.; Lu, Y.A.; Yu, Q.T. Thia zip reaction for synthesis of large cyclic peptides: Mechanisms and applications. *J. Am. Chem. Soc.* **1999**, *121*, 4316–4324. [CrossRef]
233. Duvick, J.P.; Rood, T.; Rao, A.G.; Marshak, D.R. Purification and characterization of a novel antimicrobial peptide from maize (*Zea mays* L.) kernels. *J. Biol. Chem.* **1992**, *267*, 18814–18820. [PubMed]
234. Marcus, J.P.; Green, J.L.; Goulter, K.C.; Manners, J.M. A family of antimicrobial peptides is produced by processing of a 7s globulin protein in macadamia integrifolia kernels. *Plant J.* **1999**, *19*, 699–710. [CrossRef] [PubMed]
235. Nolde, S.B.; Vassilevski, A.A.; Rogozhin, E.A.; Barinov, N.A.; Balashova, T.A.; Samsonova, O.V.; Baranov, Y.V.; Feofanov, A.V.; Egorov, T.A.; Arseniev, A.S.; *et al.* Disulfide-stabilized helical hairpin structure and activity of a novel antifungal peptide ecamp1 from seeds of barnyard grass (*Echinochloa crus-galli*). *J. Biol. Chem.* **2011**, *286*, 25145–25153. [CrossRef] [PubMed]
236. Utkina, L.L.; Andreev, Y.A.; Rogozhin, E.A.; Korostyleva, T.V.; Slavokhotova, A.A.; Oparin, P.B.; Vassilevski, A.A.; Grishin, E.V.; Egorov, T.A.; Odintsova, T.I. Genes encoding 4-cys antimicrobial peptides in wheat triticum kiharae dorof. Et migush.: Multimodular structural organization, instraspecific variability, distribution and role in defence. *FEBS J.* **2013**, *280*, 3594–3608. [CrossRef] [PubMed]
237. Slavokhotova, A.A.; Rogozhin, E.A.; Musolyamov, A.K.; Andreev, Y.A.; Oparin, P.B.; Berkut, A.A.; Vassilevski, A.A.; Egorov, T.A.; Grishin, E.V.; Odintsova, T.I. Novel antifungal alpha-hairpinin peptide from stellaria media seeds: Structure, biosynthesis, gene structure and evolution. *Plant. Mol. Biol.* **2014**. [CrossRef] [PubMed]
238. Conners, R.; Konarev, A.V.; Forsyth, J.; Lovegrove, A.; Marsh, J.; Joseph-Horne, T.; Shewry, P.; Brady, R.L. An unusual helix-turn-helix protease inhibitory motif in a novel trypsin inhibitor from seeds of veronica (veronica hederifolia l.). *J. Biol. Chem.* **2007**, *282*, 27760–27768. [CrossRef] [PubMed]
239. Oparin, P.B.; Mineev, K.S.; Dunaevsky, Y.E.; Arseniev, A.S.; Belozersky, M.A.; Grishin, E.V.; Egorov, T.A.; Vassilevski, A.A. Buckwheat trypsin inhibitor with helical hairpin structure belongs to a new family of plant defence peptides. *Biochem. J.* **2012**, *446*, 69–77. [CrossRef] [PubMed]
240. Ng, Y.M.; Yang, Y.; Sze, K.H.; Zhang, X.; Zheng, Y.T.; Shaw, P.C. Structural characterization and anti-hiv-1 activities of arginine/glutamate-rich polypeptide luffin p1 from the seeds of sponge gourd (*Luffa cylindrica*). *J. Struct. Biol.* **2011**, *174*, 164–172. [CrossRef] [PubMed]
241. Kader, J.C. Lipid-transfer proteins in plants. *Annu Rev. Plant. Physiol Plant. Mol. Biol* **1996**, *47*, 627–654. [CrossRef] [PubMed]
242. Carvalho Ade, O.; Gomes, V.M. Role of plant lipid transfer proteins in plant cell physiology-a concise review. *Peptides* **2007**, *28*, 1144–1153. [CrossRef] [PubMed]
243. Terras, F.R.G.; Goderis, I.J.; Vanleuven, F.; Vanderleyden, J.; Cammue, B.P.A.; Broekaert, W.F. Invitro antifungal activity of a radish (*Raphanus-sativus* L.) seed protein homologous to nonspecific lipid transfer proteins. *Plant. Physiol.* **1992**, *100*, 1055–1058. [CrossRef] [PubMed]
244. Molina, A.; Segura, A.; Garcia-Olmedo, F. Lipid transfer proteins (nsltps) from barley and maize leaves are potent inhibitors of bacterial and fungal plant pathogens. *FEBS Lett.* **1993**, *316*, 119–122. [CrossRef]
245. Segura, A.; Moreno, M.; Garcia-Olmedo, F. Purification and antipathogenic activity of lipid transfer proteins (ltps) from the leaves of arabidopsis and spinach. *FEBS Lett.* **1993**, *332*, 243–246. [CrossRef]
246. Cammue, B.P.; Thevissen, K.; Hendriks, M.; Eggermont, K.; Goderis, I.J.; Proost, P.; Van Damme, J.; Osborn, R.W.; Guerbette, F.; Kader, J.C.; *et al.* A potent antimicrobial protein from onion seeds showing sequence homology to plant lipid transfer proteins. *Plant Physiol.* **1995**, *109*, 445–455. [CrossRef] [PubMed]
247. Arondel, V.V.; Vergnolle, C.; Cantrel, C.; Kader, J. Lipid transfer proteins are encoded by a small multigene family in arabidopsis thaliana. *Plant Sci.* **2000**, *157*, 1–12. [CrossRef]

248. Douliez, J.P.; Pato, C.; Rabesona, H.; Molle, D.; Marion, D. Disulfide bond assignment, lipid transfer activity and secondary structure of a 7-kda plant lipid transfer protein, ltp2. *Eur. J. Biochem.* **2001**, *268*, 1400–1403. [CrossRef] [PubMed]
249. Pons, J.L.; de Lamotte, F.; Gautier, M.F.; Delsuc, M.A. Refined solution structure of a liganded type 2 wheat nonspecific lipid transfer protein. *J. Biol. Chem.* **2003**, *278*, 14249–14256. [CrossRef] [PubMed]
250. Samuel, D.; Liu, Y.J.; Cheng, C.S.; Lyu, P.C. Solution structure of plant nonspecific lipid transfer protein-2 from rice (*Oryza sativa*). *J. Biol. Chem.* **2002**, *277*, 35267–35273. [CrossRef] [PubMed]
251. Gomar, J.; Sodano, P.; Sy, D.; Shin, D.H.; Lee, J.Y.; Suh, S.W.; Marion, D.; Vovelle, F.; Ptak, M. Comparison of solution and crystal structures of maize nonspecific lipid transfer protein: A model for a potential *in vivo* lipid carrier protein. *Proteins* **1998**, *31*, 160–171. [CrossRef]
252. Tassin, S.; Broekaert, W.F.; Marion, D.; Acland, D.P.; Ptak, M.; Vovelle, F.; Sodano, P. Solution structure of ace-amp1, a potent antimicrobial protein extracted from onion seeds. Structural analogies with plant nonspecific lipid transfer proteins. *Biochemistry* **1998**, *37*, 3623–3637. [CrossRef] [PubMed]
253. Lee, J.Y.; Min, K.; Cha, H.; Shin, D.H.; Hwang, K.Y.; Suh, S.W. Rice non-specific lipid transfer protein: The 1.6 a crystal structure in the unliganded state reveals a small hydrophobic cavity. *J. Mol. Biol.* **1998**, *276*, 437–448. [CrossRef] [PubMed]
254. Han, G.W.; Lee, J.Y.; Song, H.K.; Chang, C.; Min, K.; Moon, J.; Shin, D.H.; Kopka, M.L.; Sawaya, M.R.; Yuan, H.S.; *et al.* Structural basis of non-specific lipid binding in maize lipid-transfer protein complexes revealed by high-resolution x-ray crystallography. *J. Mol. Biol.* **2001**, *308*, 263–278. [CrossRef] [PubMed]
255. Cheng, H.C.; Cheng, P.T.; Peng, P.; Lyu, P.C.; Sun, Y.J. Lipid binding in rice nonspecific lipid transfer protein-1 complexes from *Oryza sativa*. *Protein Sci.* **2004**, *13*, 2304–2315. [CrossRef] [PubMed]
256. Poznanski, J.; Sodano, P.; Suh, S.W.; Lee, J.Y.; Ptak, M.; Vovelle, F. Solution structure of a lipid transfer protein extracted from rice seeds. Comparison with homologous proteins. *Eur. J. Biochem.* **1999**, *259*, 692–708. [CrossRef] [PubMed]
257. Gincel, E.; Simorre, J.P.; Caille, A.; Marion, D.; Ptak, M.; Vovelle, F. Three-dimensional structure in solution of a wheat lipid-transfer protein from multidimensional 1h-nmr data. A new folding for lipid carriers. *Eur. J. Biochem.* **1994**, *226*, 413–422. [CrossRef] [PubMed]
258. Charvolin, D.; Douliez, J.P.; Marion, D.; Cohen-Addad, C.; Pebay-Peyroula, E. The crystal structure of a wheat nonspecific lipid transfer protein (ns-ltp1) complexed with two molecules of phospholipid at 2.1 a resolution. *Eur. J. Biochem.* **1999**, *264*, 562–568. [CrossRef] [PubMed]
259. Lerche, M.H.; Kragelund, B.B.; Bech, L.M.; Poulsen, F.M. Barley lipid-transfer protein complexed with palmitoyl coa: The structure reveals a hydrophobic binding site that can expand to fit both large and small lipid-like ligands. *Structure* **1997**, *5*, 291–306. [CrossRef]
260. Lerche, M.H.; Poulsen, F.M. Solution structure of barley lipid transfer protein complexed with palmitate. Two different binding modes of palmitate in the homologous maize and barley nonspecific lipid transfer proteins. *Protein Sci.* **1998**, *7*, 2490–2498. [CrossRef] [PubMed]
261. Gomar, J.; Petit, M.C.; Sodano, P.; Sy, D.; Marion, D.; Kader, J.C.; Vovelle, F.; Ptak, M. Solution structure and lipid binding of a nonspecific lipid transfer protein extracted from maize seeds. *Protein Sci.* **1996**, *5*, 565–577. [CrossRef] [PubMed]
262. Castro, M.S.; Gerhardt, I.R.; Orru, S.; Pucci, P.; Bloch, C., Jr. Purification and characterization of a small (7.3 kda) putative lipid transfer protein from maize seeds. *J. Chromatogr. B Analyt. Technol. Biomed. Life Sci.* **2003**, *794*, 109–114. [CrossRef]
263. Gizatullina, A.K.; Finkina, E.I.; Mineev, K.S.; Melnikova, D.N.; Bogdanov, I.V.; Telezhinskaya, I.N.; Balandin, S.V.; Shenkarev, Z.O.; Arseniev, A.S.; Ovchinnikova, T.V. Recombinant production and solution structure of lipid transfer protein from lentil lens culinaris. *Biochem. Biophys. Res. Commun.* **2013**, *439*, 427–432. [CrossRef] [PubMed]
264. Lin, K.F.; Liu, Y.N.; Hsu, S.T.; Samuel, D.; Cheng, C.S.; Bonvin, A.M.; Lyu, P.C. Characterization and structural analyses of nonspecific lipid transfer protein 1 from mung bean. *Biochemistry* **2005**, *44*, 5703–5712. [CrossRef] [PubMed]
265. Da Silva, P.; Landon, C.; Industri, B.; Marais, A.; Marion, D.; Ponchet, M.; Vovelle, F. Solution structure of a tobacco lipid transfer protein exhibiting new biophysical and biological features. *Proteins* **2005**, *59*, 356–367. [CrossRef] [PubMed]

266. Cheng, C.S.; Chen, M.N.; Lai, Y.T.; Chen, T.; Lin, K.F.; Liu, Y.J.; Lyu, P.C. Mutagenesis study of rice nonspecific lipid transfer protein 2 reveals residues that contribute to structure and ligand binding. *Proteins* **2008**, *70*, 695–706. [CrossRef] [PubMed]
267. Cheng, C.S.; Samuel, D.; Liu, Y.J.; Shyu, J.C.; Lai, S.M.; Lin, K.F.; Lyu, P.C. Binding mechanism of nonspecific lipid transfer proteins and their role in plant defense. *Biochemistry* **2004**, *43*, 13628–13636. [CrossRef] [PubMed]
268. Lin, P.; Xia, L.; Wong, J.H.; Ng, T.B.; Ye, X.; Wang, S.; Shi, X. Lipid transfer proteins from brassica campestris and mung bean surpass mung bean chitinase in exploitability. *J. Pept. Sci.* **2007**, *13*, 642–648. [CrossRef] [PubMed]
269. Molina, A.; Garcia-Olmedo, F. Enhanced tolerance to bacterial pathogens caused by the transgenic expression of barley lipid transfer protein ltp2. *Plant J.* **1997**, *12*, 669–675. [CrossRef] [PubMed]
270. Lascombe, M.B.; Bakan, B.; Buhot, N.; Marion, D.; Blein, J.P.; Larue, V.; Lamb, C.; Prange, T. The structure of "defective in induced resistance" protein of arabidopsis thaliana, dir1, reveals a new type of lipid transfer protein. *Protein Sci.* **2008**, *17*, 1522–1530. [CrossRef] [PubMed]
271. Yeats, T.H.; Rose, J.K. The biochemistry and biology of extracellular plant lipid-transfer proteins (ltps). *Protein Sci.* **2008**, *17*, 191–198. [CrossRef] [PubMed]
272. Kader, J.C. Proteins and intracellular exchange of lipids.1. Stimulation of phospholipid exchange between mitochondria and microsomal fractions by proteins isolated from potato-tuber. *Biochem. Biophys. Acta* **1975**, *380*, 31–44. [CrossRef]
273. Kader, J.C.; Julienne, M.; Vergnolle, C. Purification and characterization of a spinach-leaf protein capable of transferring phospholipids from liposomes to mitochondria or chloroplasts. *Eur. J. Biochem.* **1984**, *139*, 411–416. [CrossRef] [PubMed]
274. Thoma, S.; Kaneko, Y.; Somerville, C. A non-specific lipid transfer protein from arabidopsis is a cell wall protein. *Plant J.* **1993**, *3*, 427–436. [CrossRef] [PubMed]
275. Pyee, J.; Yu, H.S.; Kolattukudy, P.E. Identification of a lipid transfer protein as the major protein in the surface wax of broccoli (*Brassica oleracea*) leaves. *Archiv. Biochem. Biophys.* **1994**, *311*, 460–468. [CrossRef]
276. Regente, M.C.; Giudici, A.M.; Villalain, J.; de la Canal, L. The cytotoxic properties of a plant lipid transfer protein involve membrane permeabilization of target cells. *Lett. Appl. Microbiol.* **2005**, *40*, 183–189. [CrossRef] [PubMed]
277. Segura, A.; Moreno, M.; Madueno, F.; Molina, A.; Garcia-Olmedo, F. Snakin-1, a peptide from potato that is active against plant pathogens. *Mol. Plant Microbe Interact.* **1999**, *12*, 16–23. [CrossRef] [PubMed]
278. Berrocal-Lobo, M.; Segura, A.; Moreno, M.; Lopez, G.; Garcia-Olmedo, F.; Molina, A. Snakin-2, an antimicrobial peptide from potato whose gene is locally induced by wounding and responds to pathogen infection. *Plant Physiol.* **2002**, *128*, 951–961. [CrossRef] [PubMed]
279. Porto, W.F.; Franco, O.L. Theoretical structural insights into the snakin/gasa family. *Peptides* **2013**, *44*, 163–167. [CrossRef] [PubMed]
280. Bindschedler, L.V.; Whitelegge, J.P.; Millar, D.J.; Bolwell, G.P. A two component chitin-binding protein from french bean – association of a proline-rich protein with a cysteine-rich polypeptide. *FEBS Lett.* **2006**, *580*, 1541–1546. [CrossRef] [PubMed]
281. Daneshmand, F.; Zare-Zardini, H.; Ebrahimi, L. Investigation of the antimicrobial activities of snakin-z, a new cationic peptide derived from zizyphus jujuba fruits. *Nat. Prod. Res.* **2013**, *27*, 2292–2296. [CrossRef] [PubMed]
282. Mandal, S.M.; Porto, W.F.; Dey, P.; Maiti, M.K.; Ghosh, A.K.; Franco, O.L. The attack of the phytopathogens and the trumpet solo: Identification of a novel plant antifungal peptide with distinct fold and disulfide bond pattern. *Biochimie* **2013**, *2013*, 1939–1948. [CrossRef] [PubMed]
283. Tailor, R.H.; Acland, D.P.; Attenborough, S.; Cammue, B.P.; Evans, I.J.; Osborn, R.W.; Ray, J.A.; Rees, S.B.; Broekaert, W.F. A novel family of small cysteine-rich antimicrobial peptides from seed of impatiens balsamina is derived from a single precursor protein. *J. Biol. Chem.* **1997**, *272*, 24480–24487. [CrossRef] [PubMed]
284. Thevissen, K.; Francois, I.E.; Sijtsma, L.; van Amerongen, A.; Schaaper, W.M.; Meloen, R.; Posthuma-Trumpie, T.; Broekaert, W.F.; Cammue, B.P. Antifungal activity of synthetic peptides derived from impatiens balsamina antimicrobial peptides ib-amp1 and ib-amp4. *Peptides* **2005**, *26*, 1113–1119. [CrossRef] [PubMed]

285. Patel, S.U.; Osborn, R.; Rees, S.; Thornton, J.M. Structural studies of impatiens balsamina antimicrobial protein (ib-amp1). *Biochemistry* **1998**, *37*, 983–990. [CrossRef] [PubMed]
286. Wang, P.; Bang, J.K.; Kim, H.J.; Kim, J.K.; Kim, Y.; Shin, S.Y. Antimicrobial specificity and mechanism of action of disulfide-removed linear analogs of the plant-derived cys-rich antimicrobial peptide ib-amp1. *Peptides* **2009**, *30*, 2144–2149. [CrossRef] [PubMed]
287. Fujimura, M.; Ideguchi, M.; Minami, Y.; Watanabe, K.; Tadera, K. Amino acid sequence and antimicrobial activity of chitin-binding peptides, pp-amp 1 and pp-amp 2, from japanese bamboo shoots (phyllostachys pubescens). *Biosci. Biotechnol. Biochem.* **2005**, *69*, 642–645. [CrossRef] [PubMed]
288. Astafieva, A.A.; Rogozhin, E.A.; Odintsova, T.I.; Khadeeva, N.V.; Grishin, E.V.; Egorov Ts, A. Discovery of novel antimicrobial peptides with unusual cysteine motifs in dandelion taraxacum officinale wigg. Flowers. *Peptides* **2012**, *36*, 266–271. [CrossRef] [PubMed]
289. Astafieva, A.A.; Rogozhin, E.A.; Andreev, Y.A.; Odintsova, T.I.; Kozlov, S.A.; Grishin, E.V.; Egorov, T.A. A novel cysteine-rich antifungal peptide toamp4 from taraxacum officinale wigg. Flowers. *Plant Physiol. Biochem.* **2013**, *70*, 93–99. [CrossRef] [PubMed]
290. McManus, A.M.; Nielsen, K.J.; Marcus, J.P.; Harrison, S.J.; Green, J.L.; Manners, J.M.; Craik, D.J. Miamp1, a novel protein from macadamia integrifolia adopts a greek key beta-barrel fold unique amongst plant antimicrobial proteins. *J. Mol. Biol.* **1999**, *293*, 629–638. [CrossRef] [PubMed]
291. Silva, O.N.; Porto, W.F.; Migliolo, L.; Mandal, S.M.; Gomes, D.G.; Holanda, H.H.; Silva, R.S.; Dias, S.C.; Costa, M.P.; Costa, C.R.; *et al.* Cn-amp1: A new promiscuous peptide with potential for microbial infections treatment. *Biopolymers* **2012**, *98*, 322–331. [CrossRef] [PubMed]
292. Mandal, S.M.; Migliolo, L.; Das, S.; Mandal, M.; Franco, O.L.; Hazra, T.K. Identification and characterization of a bactericidal and proapoptotic peptide from cycas revoluta seeds with DNA binding properties. *J. Cell. Biochem.* **2012**, *113*, 184–193. [CrossRef] [PubMed]
293. Pelegrini, P.B.; Murad, A.M.; Silva, L.P.; Dos Santos, R.C.; Costa, F.T.; Tagliari, P.D.; Bloch, C., Jr.; Noronha, E.F.; Miller, R.N.; Franco, O.L. Identification of a novel storage glycine-rich peptide from guava (psidium guajava) seeds with activity against gram-negative bacteria. *Peptides* **2008**, *29*, 1271–1279. [CrossRef] [PubMed]
294. Tavares, L.S.; Rettore, J.V.; Freitas, R.M.; Porto, W.F.; Duque, A.P.; Singulani Jde, L.; Silva, O.N.; Detoni Mde, L.; Vasconcelos, E.G.; Dias, S.C.; *et al.* Antimicrobial activity of recombinant pg-amp1, a glycine-rich peptide from guava seeds. *Peptides* **2012**, *37*, 294–300. [CrossRef] [PubMed]
295. Park, C.J.; Park, C.B.; Hong, S.S.; Lee, H.S.; Lee, S.Y.; Kim, S.C. Characterization and cdna cloning of two glycine- and histidine-rich antimicrobial peptides from the roots of shepherd's purse, capsella bursa-pastoris. *Plant. Mol. Biol.* **2000**, *44*, 187–197. [CrossRef] [PubMed]
296. Rahnamaeian, M. Antimicrobial peptides: Modes of mechanism, modulation of defense responses. *Plant Signal. Behav.* **2011**, *6*, 1325–1332. [CrossRef] [PubMed]
297. Barbosa Pelegrini, P.; Del Sarto, R.P.; Silva, O.N.; Franco, O.L.; Grossi-de-Sa, M.F. Antibacterial peptides from plants: What they are and how they probably work. *Biochem. Res. Int.* **2011**, *2011*, 250349. [CrossRef] [PubMed]
298. Kagan, B.L.; Selsted, M.E.; Ganz, T.; Lehrer, R.I. Antimicrobial defensin peptides form voltage-dependent ion-permeable channels in planar lipid bilayer membranes. *Proc. Natl. Acad. Sci. USA* **1990**, *87*, 210–214. [CrossRef] [PubMed]
299. Miyazaki, Y.; Aoki, M.; Yano, Y.; Matsuzaki, K. Interaction of antimicrobial peptide magainin 2 with gangliosides as a target for human cell binding. *Biochemistry* **2012**, *51*, 10229–10235. [CrossRef] [PubMed]
300. Sarika; Iquebal, M.A.; Rai, A. Biotic stress resistance in agriculture through antimicrobial peptides. *Peptides* **2012**, *36*, 322–330. [CrossRef] [PubMed]
301. Montesinos, E. Antimicrobial peptides and plant disease control. *FEMS Microbiol. Lett.* **2007**, *270*, 1–11. [CrossRef] [PubMed]
302. Jagadish, K.; Camarero, J.A. Cyclotides, a promising molecular scaffold for peptide-based therapeutics. *Biopolymers* **2010**, *94*, 611–616. [CrossRef] [PubMed]
303. Yu, Q.; Lehrer, R.I.; Tam, J.P. Engineered salt-insensitive alpha-defensins with end-to-end circularized structures. *J. Biol. Chem.* **2000**, *275*, 3943–3949. [CrossRef] [PubMed]
304. Chan, L.Y.; Gunasekera, S.; Henriques, S.T.; Worth, N.F.; Le, S.J.; Clark, R.J.; Campbell, J.H.; Craik, D.J.; Daly, N.L. Engineering pro-angiogenic peptides using stable, disulfide-rich cyclic scaffolds. *Blood* **2011**, *118*, 6709–6717. [CrossRef] [PubMed]

305. Eliasen, R.; Daly, N.L.; Wulff, B.S.; Andresen, T.L.; Conde-Frieboes, K.W.; Craik, D.J. Design, synthesis, structural and functional characterization of novel melanocortin agonists based on the cyclotide kalata b1. *J. Biol. Chem.* **2012**, *287*, 40493–40501. [CrossRef] [PubMed]
306. Abdallah, N.A.; Shah, D.; Abbas, D.; Madkour, M. Stable integration and expression of a plant defensin in tomato confers resistance to fusarium wilt. *GM Crops* **2010**, *1*, 344–350. [CrossRef] [PubMed]

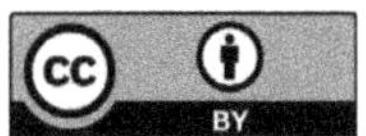

© 2015 by the authors. Licensee MDPI, Basel, Switzerland. This article is an open access article distributed under the terms and conditions of the Creative Commons Attribution (CC BY) license (http://creativecommons.org/licenses/by/4.0/).

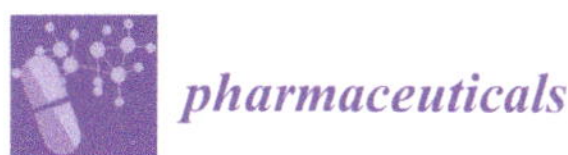

MDPI

Review

Chapter 4:

Lucifensins, the Insect Defensins of Biomedical Importance: The Story behind Maggot Therapy

Václav Čeřovský [1,*] and Robert Bém [2]

1 Institute of Organic Chemistry and Biochemistry, Academy of Sciences of the Czech Republic, Flemingovo nám. 2, Prague 6, 16610 Czech Republic

2 Diabetes Centre, Institute for Clinical and Experimental Medicine, Vídeňská 1958/9, Prague 4, 14021 Czech Republic; bemrob@yahoo.co.uk

* Author to whom correspondence should be addressed; cerovsky@uochb.cas.cz; Tel.: +420-220-183-378; Fax: +420-220-183-578.

Received: 10 December 2013; in revised form: 12 February 2014; Accepted: 20 February 2014; Published: 27 February 2014

Abstract: Defensins are the most widespread antimicrobial peptides characterised in insects. These cyclic peptides, 4–6 kDa in size, are folded into α-helical/β-sheet mixed structures and have a common conserved motif of three intramolecular disulfide bridges with a Cys1-Cys4, Cys2-Cys5 and Cys3-Cys6 connectivity. They have the ability to kill especially Gram-positive bacteria and some fungi, but Gram-negative bacteria are more resistant against them. Among them are the medicinally important compounds lucifensin and lucifensin II, which have recently been identified in the medicinal larvae of the blowflies *Lucilia sericata* and *Lucilia cuprina*, respectively. These defensins contribute to wound healing during a procedure known as maggot debridement therapy (MDT) which is routinely used at hospitals worldwide. Here we discuss the decades-long story of the effort to isolate and characterise these two defensins from the bodies of medicinal larvae or from their secretions/excretions. Furthermore, our previous studies showed that the free-range larvae of *L. sericata* acutely eliminated most of the Gram-positive strains of bacteria and some Gram-negative strains in patients with infected diabetic foot ulcers, but MDT was ineffective during the healing of wounds infected with *Pseudomonas* sp. and *Acinetobacter* sp. The bactericidal role of lucifensins secreted into the infected wound by larvae during MDT and its ability to enhance host immunity by functioning as immunomodulator is also discussed.

Keywords: antimicrobial peptide; insect defensin; lucifensin; maggot therapy; *Lucilia sericata*; *Lucilia cuprina*; peptide isolation; peptide identification

---

1. Introduction

Over the course of their evolution, insects have developed an amazing resistance to bacterial infection, resulting in exceptional adaptation to a variety of natural environments often considered rather unsanitary by human standards. Insects respond to bacterial challenge or injury by rapid production of antimicrobial peptides (AMPs) that have a broad spectrum of activity against Gram-positive and Gram-negative bacteria and fungi. These peptides are evolutionary conserved components of the host's innate immune system that form the first line of defence against infections and have been identified in almost all classes of life. Among the more than 2,000 AMPs listed in the Antimicrobial Peptide Database [1], peptides isolated from insects comprise the most abundant group. AMPs are synthesised in the fat body (the equivalent of the mammalian liver), epithelial cells, and in the certain cells of the haemolymph (the equivalent of mammalian blood) and then spread by the haemolymph over the entire body to fight infection [2]. The majority of these peptides belong to the class of cationic AMPs of molecular masses below 5 kDa [3]. Upon interacting with biological membrane or environments that mimic biological membranes, such as artificially made liposomes or sodium dodecyl sulfate, most are able to fold into highly amphipathic conformations with separated areas rich in positively charged and hydrophobic amino acid residues on the molecular surface [3–5]. The frequent occurrence of positively charged amino acid residues (Arg, Lys) in their molecules allows them to interact with the anionic phospholipids of bacterial membranes. This is followed by integration of the peptides into the lipid bilayer and disruption of the membrane structure via different modes that lead to leakage of cytoplasmic components and cell death [4–6]. Some studies have revealed that the killing process may proceed with relatively little membrane disruption but occurs rather by interfering with bacteria metabolism or interactions with putative key intracellular targets [7]. In contrast to conventional antibiotics, AMPs do not appear to induce microbial resistance and require only a short time to induce killing [6].

The AMPs isolated from insects may be classified on the basis of their sequence and structural features into three categories: (i) linear peptides which can form an α-helical structure and do not contain cysteine residues, such as cecropins; (ii) cyclic peptides containing disulfide bridges of which defensins are the most typical example and (iii) linear peptides with noticeable high content of one or two amino acid residues, mostly proline and/or glycine residues (pyrrhocoricins and diptericins) [2]. In this study, we will focus on the lucifensins [8,9]—two almost identical cyclic peptides of 40 amino acids residues and three intramolecular disulfide bridges belonging to the widely distributed family of insect defensins [10,11]. Lucifensin are the key antimicrobial peptides involved in the defence system of the blowfly larvae *Lucilia sericata* and *Lucilia cuprina*. These fly larvae are routinely used at hospitals worldwide during a procedure known as maggot debridement therapy (MDT) [12,13].

2. Insect Defensins

The first insect defensins were isolated from an embryonic cell line of *Sarcophaga peregrina* (flesh fly) [14] and from the haemolymph of immunised larvae of the black blowfly *Phormia terranovae* [15]. Since then, more than 70 defensins have been identified in various arthropods such as spiders, ticks, scorpions and in every insect species of the orders Diptera, Lepidoptera, Coleoptera, Hymenoptera, Hemiptera and Odonata investigated to date [10,11]. The defensins isolated from insects are 33 to 46 amino acid residues long with a few exceptions, such as the N-terminally extended defensin from the fly *Stomoxys calcitrans* [16] and C-terminally extended defensin found in the bee [17] and bumblebee [18]. They show sequence similarities ranging from 58 to 95% [2]. They may be further classified in two sub-families according to their *in vitro* activity against bacteria or filamentous fungi [11]: antimicrobial defensins that possesses activity against Gram-positive bacteria, including human pathogens, but are less effective against Gram-negative bacteria and fungi, and antifungal defensins that are mainly effective against filamentous fungi. Structurally, insect defensins possess an N-terminal flexible loop, a central α-helix and a C-terminal anti parallel β-sheet as has been determined by two-dimensional ^{1}H-NMR spectroscopy carried out on isolated *Sarcophaga peregrina* defensin [19] and on a recombinant *Phormia terranovae* defensin [20]. The antimicrobial defensins contain six cysteine residues engaged in a characteristic conserved motif of three intramolecular disulfide bridges connected in a Cys1-Cys4, Cys2-Cys5 and Cys3-Cys6 pattern. On the other hand, the antifungal defensin drosomycin from *Drosophila* encompasses an additional short terminal β-strand and four disulfide bridges [21]. With the exception of royalisin, the defensin of the royal jelly of the honeybee [17] and bumblebee defensin [18], the C-terminal residue of insect defensins is not amidated. Although insect defensins were originally thought to be structurally similar to mammalian defensins, their three-dimensional structure and disulfide bridges pattern are different.

3. Maggot Therapy

Maggot debridement therapy is a controlled application of cultured sterile larvae of the flies *L. sericata* or *L. cuprina* to an infected chronic non-healing wound, especially in patients with impaired healing due to underlying disorders (e.g., diabetes and cardiovascular disease). The maggots gently and completely remove necrotic tissue by mechanical action (debridement) and by proteolytic digestion over 3–5 days of application. They rapidly eliminate infecting microorganisms which pass through their digestive tract [22], stimulate wound granulation and repair and thus enhance the healing process [12,13]. In addition, the larvae both secrete (by salivary glands) and excrete into the wound numerous substances including antimicrobial compounds, and alkalise the wound environment [23].

Since the introduction of maggot therapy into clinical practice by Baer [24], many researchers, influenced by successful therapeutic experience, have been focusing on the identification of antimicrobial agents secreted/excreted by maggots in the infected wound. It is quite surprising that up to now only a few active compounds have been identified in maggot excretions/secretions (ES) with explicitly determined chemical structures. These compounds include low molecular mass organic compounds and recently discovered insect defensins—lucifensins [8,9].

4. The Brief History of the Search for Antimicrobial Agents in Medicinal Larvae

Starting in the 1930s, researchers began to investigate the underlying mechanisms which may be responsible for some of the beneficial effects of maggot therapy. The main focus of interest has been examining the antimicrobial activity of the components of larval secretions and faecal waste products. In one of the initial studies of Simmons [25], published in 1935, it was found that the excretions obtained from the washings of the non-sterile *L. sericata* maggots exhibited considerable antimicrobial activity against several species of pyogenic bacteria which were killed during five- to ten-minutes of exposure. The activity of the excretion was not destroyed by autoclaving. In the research carried out two decades later by Pavillard and Wright [26], the washings of maggots combined with a suspension of their excretions were fractionated using paper chromatography. The active fraction was active against *S. aureus*. By means of a cellulose column and a modification of the chromatography technique, it was possible to obtain relatively pure samples of the antibiotic fraction. A series of injections of this preparation protected mice from the lethal effects of intraperitoneal inoculation with pneumococci. The final purification of this active compound was never implemented. Subsequent research done at several laboratories has demonstrated that larval excretions/secretions (ES) of *L. sericata* contain a variety of alkaline components inhibiting bacterial growth and that the pH increase provides optimal conditions for the activity of larvae-secreted proteolytic enzymes that liquidise necrotic tissues [23]. It also has been proposed that larvae release antimicrobial ingredients into the wound in response to infection. Some of these ingredients are bacteriostatic low molecular weight compounds such as *p*-hydroxybenzoic acid, *p*-hydroxyphenylacetic acid, proline dioxopiperazine [27] or an "enigmatic compound" of the empirical formula $C_{10}H_{16}N_6O_9$ known as the antibiotic seraticin [13]. The other compounds may possibly be antimicrobial peptides originating from the larval immune system which are released into the wound and thus contribute to wound healing [28,29]. These peptides belong to the groups of insect defensins, cecropins and diptericins [10,11].

Since 2000, several research groups have been aiming to isolate and characterise such antimicrobial peptides from the ES by utilising current methods of protein purification. In the laboratory of Bexfield [29], the ES of maggots was fractionated using an ultrafiltration device with a 10 kDa and 500 Da molecular weight cut-off membrane generating three fractions of molecular weights: >10 kDa, 500 Da–10 kDa and <500 Da. The activity against *S. aureus* was detected in <500 Da fraction and 500 Da–10 kDa fraction, but not in the fraction above 10 kDa. Even though these fractions were investigated in further detail regarding their physicochemical properties and antimicrobial activities [30], their constituents were not identified. The antimicrobial properties of *L. sericata* larval ES and the attempts to characterise its components were independently studied in several other laboratories [31,32]. For example, the study of Kerridge *et al.* [32] revealed in the secretions the presence of small (<1 kDa) antimicrobial factors active against Gram-positive bacteria such as *S. aureus*, including both methicillin-resistant *S. aureus* (MRSA) and methicillin-sensitive *S. aureus* (MSSA), and *Streptococcus pyogenes*. However, Gram-negative *Pseudomonas aeruginosa* was less sensitive. This active factor passed through the filter of the 3 kDa cut-off when the secretion was fractionated by ultrafiltration procedure. In this case, anti-MRSA activity was also detected in the retenates of the 10 kDa and 5 kDa filters indicating the presence of at least one additional larger antimicrobial agent. The authors concluded that the activities in the secretions possess characteristics consistent with insect antimicrobial peptides and are considered to be of low molecular weight, highly stable and a systemic part of the larva [32].

In 2013, Chinese researchers described the isolation of antimicrobial protein from an extract of the homogenate of *L. sericata* larvae using an ultrafiltration procedure [33]. The crude material obtained was named "antibacterial protein from maggots" (MAMP). MAMP demonstrated inhibitory activity against both standard strains and clinically isolated antibiotic-resistant strains of *S. aureus in vitro*. The topical use of MAMP effectively decreased the viability of *S. aureus* and promoted wound healing in an *S. aureus* mouse skin infection model. Although the authors claim the molecular weight of MAMP to be lower than 10 kDa, neither the chemical structure nor other specific identification of this "protein" was published.

Russian researchers [34] detected several inducible antimicrobial compounds by the "chromato-mass-spectrometry" method in the *L. sericata* larvae haemolymph and in the exosecretion released by the larvae. According to the authors, some of these compounds correspond to insect defensins and diptericins. Particularly, the molecular mass 4,117 Da of the peptide detected in the haemolymph matches well the molecular mass of lucifensin [8]. All the other compounds were identified solely based on their molecular masses, but their primary structures were not determined.

5. Lucifensin—The Defensin from *L. sericata*

5.1. Purification and Sequence Determination

Since 2007, we have been engaged in the identification of *L. sericata* AMPs by focusing on insect defensins. We have aimed to detect defensins in larval ES as well as different parts of the larval bodies, purify them and determine their primary structure. In our experience, it is evident that only the use of modern separation techniques such as high performance liquid chromatography (HPLC) as a part of the purification procedure may result in the discovery of the sought peptides.

The physicochemical properties of insect defensins (medium size, cationic molecule, contains disulfide bridges) influenced us in the selection of the purification procedure. Starting with the extractions of *L. sericata* larval guts, a strongly acidic acetonitrile/water/0.5% trifluoroacetic acid mixture, which provides good solubility for cationic peptides while protecting its stability against enzymatic digestion and disulfide bridges reshuffling, was the extraction solvent of choice. Successive ultrafiltration of crude extract, the size exclusion HPLC and following reversed phase HPLC (RP-HPLC) applied as the final steps of the purification procedure resulted in the peptide of the purity satisfactory for sequencing by Edman degradation [8].

The Edman degradation using 40 cycles yielded the following N-terminal sequence: Ala-Thr-X-Asp-Leu-Leu-Ser-Gly-Thr-Gly-Val-Lys-His-Ser-Ala-X-Ala-Ala-His-X-Leu-Leu-Arg-Gly-Asn-Arg-Gly-Gly-Tyr-X-Asn-Gly-Arg-Ala-Ile-X-Val-X-Arg-Asn, assuming that all six undetermined amino acid residues (X) were cysteines. The molecular mass of this defensin measured by ESI-QTOF MS was determined to be 4113.6. This was in good agreement with the calculated value of 4113.89, based on the sequence determined by Edman degradation and assuming that the six cysteine residues form three disulfide bridges [8]. Our results showed that *L. sericata* defensin, which we term lucifensin, differs from *Phormia terranovae* defensins A and B and from *Sarcophaga peregrina* sapecin by five amino acid residues (Val11, Lys12, Arg33, Ala34, and ILe35).

Knowing the properties of lucifensin, we were able to detect its presence in the extracts of other larval tissues such as the salivary glands, fat body, haemolymph as well as in the larval ES [8]. However, no antimicrobial peptide from other families such as cecropins, diptericins or Pro-rich peptides was detected in the frame of our study.

5.2. Synthetic Lucifensin

In 2011, we reported a total chemical synthesis of lucifensin using the methodology of solid phase peptide synthesis [35]. In the first step of the synthesis, we prepared the linear peptide of 40 amino acid residues containing six cysteines in the sequence. Oxidative folding of this linear peptide yielded a cyclic peptide with the disulfide bridges formed between Cys3-Cys30, Cys16-Cys36 and Cys20-Cys38; this disulfide bridges pattern corresponds to that of natural lucifensin.

Synthetic lucifensin was highly active against *M. luteus* and *Bacillus subtilis* with MIC values of 0.6 and 1.2 μM, respectively, while lower but significant activity was observed against *S. aureus* with MIC value of 41 μM. No activity was detected against *E. coli*, thus confirming the generally recognised fact that insect defensins are more active against Gram-positive than Gram-negative bacteria. The peptide showed slight antifungal activity against *C. albicans* (MIC = 86 μM) and was not haemolytic against human red blood cells [35]. These findings corresponded to the clinical effect of maggot therapy and supported our hypothesis that lucifensin is the long-sought antimicrobial factor of medicinal maggots.

To confirm the importance of disulfide bridges for its activity and structure, we synthesised three lucifensin analogs, each of which was cyclised through only one native disulfide bridge in different positions and having the remaining four cysteines substituted by alanine [35]. The analog cyclised through a Cys16-Cys36 disulfide bridge showed weak antimicrobial activity, while the other two analogs containing one disulfide bridge were inactive. These results indicate that the presence of disulfide bridges in lucifensin is essential for its antimicrobial activity as it is necessary for preserving its three-dimensional structure. The synthesis of truncated lucifensin at the N-terminal by 10 amino acid residues resulted in an almost inactive analog [35].

5.3. Three Dimensional Structure and Mode of Action

The tertiary structure of lucifensin determined using NMR [36] showed a high degree of similarity to the structure of other insect defensins: sapecin [19] and insect defensin A [20]. Lucifensin adopts a characteristic insect defensin structure that includes an N-terminal loop (residues 1–12), followed by an α-helix (residues 13–23), which is linked by a turn to a pair of β-strands (residues 28–31 and 34–38) folded into an antiparallel β-sheet (Figure 1). The Cys3-Cys30 disulfide bridge connects the N-terminal loop with the first β-strand and the other two bridges (Cys16-Cys36, Cys20-Cys38) link the α-helix and second β-strand [36]. The α-helix and β-structure connected by two disulfide bridges form a common structural element typical for insect defensins, known as the cysteine-stabilised αβ (CS αβ) motif, which is essential for their antimicrobial activity [19,20].

The action mechanism of lucifensin relates to the study on homologous sapecin—the defensin of *Sarcophaga peregrina* for which a putative mechanistic model for membrane permeabilisation has been already proposed [37]. According to this model obtained on the basis of NMR experiments, sapecin oligomerises in the bacterial membrane and thus forms the channels therein which results in consequent leakage of cytoplasmic components and bacterial cell death. This putative model of sapecin oligomerisation is based on an electrostatic interaction between Asp4 of one sapecin molecule and Arg23 of another sapecin molecule, as these two residues are situated at opposite ends of the oligomerisation site. Since the sequences of the lucifensin differs from that of sapecin by only four amino acid residues (positions 11, 12, 33 and 35) and residues Asp4 and Arg23 are conserved in lucifensin, we may speculate that the mechanism of the lucifensins antimicrobial action is the same as that proposed for sapecin [37]. We may then suppose that the absence of Asp4 in the truncated analog of lucifensin might be the reason that its antimicrobial activity significantly decreased.

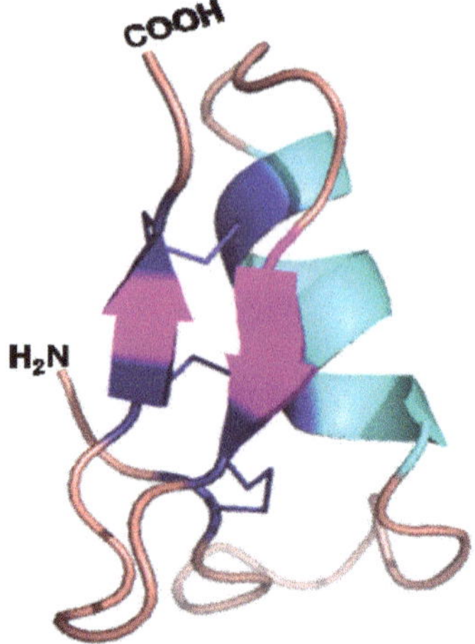

Figure 1. An illustrated representation of the three-dimensional structure of lucifensin (*L. sericata* defensin) which was generated in Pymol [38] by using the solution structure of lucifensin (PDB code 2LLD).

As illustrated in Figure 2, the treatment of *B. subtilis* by lucifensin followed by transmission electron microscopy revealed significant changes in the bacterial envelope leading to final breakup of bacterial cells [35], just demonstrating the generally accepted mechanism of the action for cationic antimicrobial peptides, such as insect defensins.

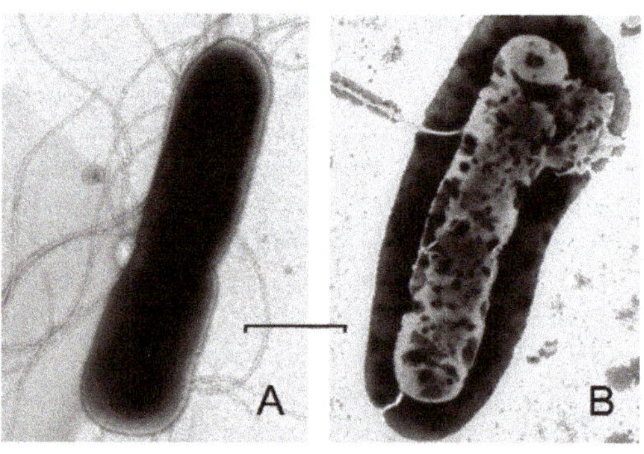

1 µm

Figure 2. Electron micrographs of negatively stained *Bacillus subtilis* either untreated (**A**) or treated by lucifensin for 60 min (**B**). Scale bars represent 1 µm.

6. Lucifensin II—The Defensin from *L. cuprina*

The homolog of insect defensin designated lucifensin II was recently isolated from an extract of the haemolymph of the fly larva *Lucilia cuprina* in our laboratory [9]. We applied an improved purification procedure comprising of two ultrafiltration steps, RP-HPLC, modified size exclusion HPLC and a final RP-HPLC purification leading to the successful determination of its full-length primary sequence. This sequence determined by ESI-orbitrap mass spectrometry and Edman degradation shows almost the same identity to the sequence of lucifensin (*Lucilia sericata* defensin). The lucifensin II sequence differs from that of lucifensin by only one amino acid residue; that is by isoleucine instead of valine at position 11. The presence of lucifensin II was also detected in the extracts of other larval tissues such as gut, salivary glands, fat body and whole body extract [9].

We isolated lucifensin II from the haemolymph of non-sterile maggots which has led to the question of whether lucifensin II is produced in response to poly-microbial challenge or is it constitutively expressed by the larval immune system. Accordingly, we analysed the anti-*M. luteus* active RP-HPLC fractions of 50 kDa filtrate obtained either from the haemolymph of non-sterile maggots or haemolymph of maggots treated individually with the *S. aureus*, *P. aeruginosa* and *Proteus mirabilis*, by mass spectrometry. The presence of lucifensin II was detected in all corresponding fractions independently of whether the maggots were challenged by infection or were kept sterile [9]. This observation is not in agreement with a hypothesis predicting no antibacterial activity in larvae without bacterial challenge [39]. In addition, we were not able to detect any other cationic antimicrobial peptides in the haemolymph of *L. cuprina* in the course of lucifensin II purification.

7. Molecular Biology Approaches for the Identification of Lucifensin in Medicinal Larvae

Using suppression subtractive hybridisation methodology, Altincicek *et al.* [40] identified numerous genes that are up-regulated in larvae of *L. sericata* upon septic injury. These genes encode signalling proteins, proteinases and homeostasis proteins and also potential antimicrobial peptides. The deduced peptides share sequence similarities with insect defensins, diptericins and proline-rich peptides which are conserved within Diptera. However, none of these deduced sequences match to that of lucifensin.

Danish researchers used for the identification of lucifensin in *L. sericata* maggots a transposon-assisted signal trapping, a methodology specially developed for identification of secreted proteins and peptides. They applied this method to *L. sericata* maggots induced with external stimuli mimicking those encountered by the maggots during MDT [41]. The lucifensin sequence determined in that laboratory [41] was identical to that published by us [8]. They also produced a few milligrams of recombinant peptide and estimated its antimicrobial activity against both Gram-positive and Gram-negative bacteria. Lucifensin was active against *S. carnosus*, *Streptococcus pyogenes* and *Streptococcus pneumoniae* with MIC values of 2 mg/L, and against *Enterococcus faecalis* and *S. aureus* with MIC values of 32 and 16 mg/L, respectively, but did not show any antimicrobial activity towards the Gram-negative bacteria tested at concentrations <128 mg/L. The MIC of lucifensin for a selection of 15 MRSA and glycopeptide-intermediate *S. aureus* isolates tested ranged from 8 to 128 mg/L [41].

The expression of lucifensin in various larval tissues during *L. sericata* development and in maggots exposed to infections was recently examined by Slovak researchers [42]. Using an *in situ* hybridisation method, they revealed lucifensin expression in the salivary glands of all larval stages. No differences were detected in the salivary glands after stimulation by bacteria. However, lucifensin expression was strongly stimulated in the fat body in response to the infectious environment and it was found that it is secreted solely from this tissue into the haemolymph [42].

8. Lucifensin Released by Maggots to the Wound

We analysed the extract of the swabs taken from the infected diabetic foot ulcers (DFU) during maggot treatment or immediately after removal of the maggots from the wound (Figure 3). The extracts of these samples were pre-purified by ultrafiltration through 10 kDa molecular weight cut-off membrane to remove high molecular mass components and then the filtrates were lyophilised. The HPLC profile of obtained material (Figure 3) indicates the presence of a tiny amount of lucifensin together with two human α-defensins (HNP1 and HNP2). In a drop diffusion test against *M. luteus*, the fraction of lucifensin exhibited almost equal antimicrobial activity against Gram-positive bacteria as the fraction corresponding to the mixtures of these two HNPs (Figure 3). These two host defence peptides were apparently produced and released into the wound by the components of the human immune system, including some blood cells (neutrophils) as the innate immune response against infection.

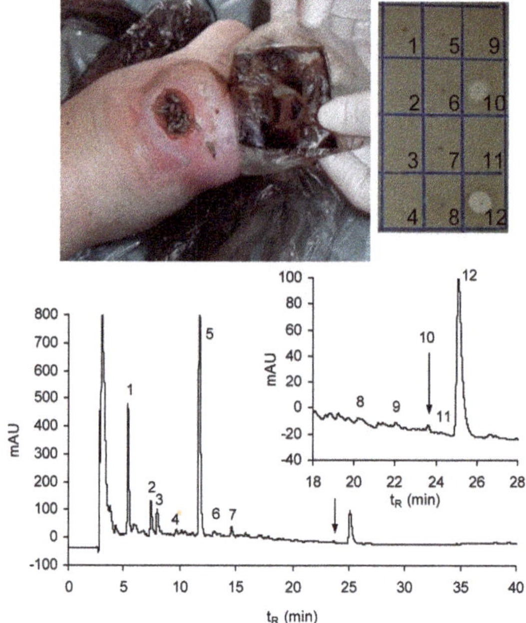

Figure 3. RP-HPLC profile (at 220 nm) of the lyophilised filtrate obtained by ultrafiltration through 10 kDa cut-off membrane of the swab extract taken from the wound (photo) immediately after removal of the larvae. An elution gradient of solvents from 5% to 70% acetonitrile/water/0.1% TFA was applied for 60 min at a flow rate 1 mL/min. Arrows indicate the anti-*M. luteus* active peak (10) containing lucifensin. The larger peak at t_R = 25 min (12) represents a mixture of two human α-defensins: HNP1 and HNP2. Inset: Anti-*M. luteus* activity (clear zones in the drop diffusion test) of selected peaks delineated in the profile.

The antimicrobial effect of maggots was investigated in several *in vivo* studies by comparing bacterial diversity in the wounds before and after their application. Our study in 91 patients with DFU demonstrated that maggot therapy by free-range larvae applied to the wound for an average 3 days acutely eliminated most of the Gram-positive and Gram-negative strains including methicillin-resistant *Staphylococcus aureus* (MRSA), but maggots were ineffective against *Pseudomonas* sp. and *Acinetobacter* sp. [43]. The antimicrobial effect persisted 7–13 days after removal of the larvae. These results are in accordance with the observations of other researchers [31,44] and signify that lucifensin, as an external antimicrobial peptide presented in DFU, may play a key role as a microbicide and as a healing factor in the majority of maggot-treated DFU. In cases of ulcers infected by *P. aeruginosa* or some other Gram-negative bacteria, we hypothesize that maggot therapy fails due to the specific activity of lucifensin against Gram-positive bacteria.

In addition to killing bacteria directly, lucifensin and other antimicrobial compounds from maggots have a number of immunomodulatory functions that may be involved in the clearance of infection and support of wound healing, including the ability to influence host innate and adaptive immune response. Regarding the innate immune system, a wide variety of human antimicrobial peptides is expressed by the epidermal cells and neutrophils, such as human β-defensins and HNPs [45]. Besides their antimicrobial effect, AMPs also support processes of wound healing, such as proliferation and angiogenesis or keratinocyte migration [46]. In contrast to acute wound healing, chronic wounds are marked by a prolonged and dysregulated inflammatory phase. Inflammatory cells like neutrophils, monocytes and macrophages are not only present in excess numbers, they also have enhanced production and release of pro-inflammatory cytokines, proteases and reactive oxygen species, leading to growth factor inactivation and tissue destruction [47]. Moreover, chronic ulcers from diabetic patients showed β-defensins up-regulation; the production of these antimicrobial peptides might be insufficient to mount proper antimicrobial control and wound healing [48]. Lucifensin and other antimicrobial compounds from maggots may turn this unfavourable situation and transfer the wound to satisfactory healing. Maggot secretions potently inhibit the pro-inflammatory responses of human neutrophils without affecting their antimicrobial activities [49]. In addition to reducing the production of proinflammatory cytokines and host antimicrobial peptides, maggot secretions also increased the production of pro-angiogenic growth factors bFGF and VEGF in anti-inflammatory macrophages [50]. Simultaneously, the increased pro-angiogenic activity of anti-inflammatory macrophages may induce neovascularisation and the concurrent formation of granulation tissue. In addition, maggots increase the expression of bFGF in ulcer tissue and induce the formation of granulation tissue.

9. Perspectives on the Future of Lucifensins

Bacterial resistance to conventional antibiotics is a major concern and the main reason for extensive, ongoing research to develop new therapeutics. Antimicrobial peptides could both affect the pathogens and simultaneously activate and modulate innate and adaptive immune systems of the host. Lucifensins have interesting features for topical application to treat wound infection and promote wound healing. These peptides that act simultaneously on the pathogens as well as on the host offer a unique opportunity to minimise the direct selective pressures for pathogen resistance. For lucifensin, there are several different potential strategies for its therapeutic application: (i) as single anti-infective agent, (ii) in combination with conventional antibiotics, (iii) in combination with other antimicrobial peptides. The reason for using lucifensin with conventional antibiotics is a formation of bacterial biofilm in the wound. Bacteria within chronic wounds often reside in biofilms that protect them from antibiotics and the immune system. A combination of lucifensin and antibiotics may ensure complete breakdown of the biofilms, thereby preventing bacterial re-growth from the remaining matrix, and prompt antibiotic action against the bacteria released from the biofilms. Preclinical studies with lucifensin for testing of safety, pharmacokinetics and toxicity are needed. After that, clinical studies may be initiated.

10. Conclusions

We propose that lucifensins are key antimicrobial factors involved in the defence system of medicinal larvae *L. sericata* and *L. cuprina* which protect maggots when they are exposed to the highly infectious environment of a wound during maggot therapy. They act as a microbicide and healing factor within the wound. Their discovery as a crucial disinfectant secreted/excreted by maggots to the wound broadened the understanding of the healing mechanism of maggot therapy. As the deliberate treatment of non-healing wounds by maggots has been in practice since the 1930s, can we possibly consider lucifensin as a prime example of the practical application of antimicrobial peptide in medicine?

Acknowledgments: This study was supported by Czech Science Foundation, Grant no. 203/08/0536, by research project RVO 61388963 of the Institute of Organic Chemistry and Biochemistry, Academy of Sciences of the Czech Republic and by project MH CZ – DRO, IN 00023001 of the Institute for Clinical and Experimental Medicine.

Conflicts of Interest: The authors declare that they have no conflicts of interest

References

1. Wang, G.; Li, X.; Wang, Z. APD2: The updated antimicrobial peptide database and its application in peptide design. *Nucleic Acids Res.* **2009**, *37*, D933–D937. [CrossRef]
2. Bulet, P.; Hetru, C.; Dimarcq, J.-L.; Hoffmann, D. Antimicrobial peptides in insects; structure and function. *Dev. Comp. Immunol.* **1999**, *23*, 329–344. [CrossRef]

3. Brown, K.L.; Hancock, R.E.W. Cationic host defense (antimicrobial) peptides. *Curr. Opin. Immunol.* **2006**, *18*, 24–30. [CrossRef]
4. Tossi, A.; Sandri, L.; Giangaspero, A. Amphipathic, α-helical antimicrobial peptides. *Biopolymers* **2000**, *55*, 4–30. [CrossRef]
5. Toke, O. Antimicrobial peptides: New candidates in the fight against bacterial infections. *Biopolymers* **2005**, *80*, 717–735. [CrossRef]
6. Yeaman, M.R.; Yount, N.Y. Mechanisms of antimicrobial peptide action and resistance. *Pharmacol. Rev.* **2003**, *55*, 27–55. [CrossRef]
7. Giuliani, A.; Pirri, G.; Nicoletto, S.F. Antimicrobial peptides: An overview of a promising class of therapeutics. *Centr. Eur. J. Biol.* **2007**, *2*, 1–33. [CrossRef]
8. Čeřovský, V.; Ždárek, J.; Fučík, V.; Monincová, L.; Voburka, Z.; Bém, R. Lucifensin, the long-sought antimicrobial factor of medicinal maggots of the blowfly *Lucilia sericata*. *Cell. Mol. Life Sci.* **2010**, *67*, 455–466. [CrossRef]
9. El Shazely, B.; Veverka, V.; Fučík, V.; Voburka, Z.; Žd'árek, J.; Čeřovský, V. Lucifensin II, a defensin of medicinal maggots of the blowfly *Lucilia cuprina* (Diptera: Calliphoridae). *J. Med. Entomol.* **2013**, *50*, 571–578. [CrossRef]
10. Hoffmann, J.A.; Hetru, C. Insect defensins: inducible antimicrobial peptides. *Immunol. Today* **1992**, *13*, 411–415. [CrossRef]
11. Bulet, P.; Stöcklin, R. Insect antimicrobial peptides: Structures, properties and gene regulation. *Protein Peptide Lett.* **2005**, *12*, 3–11. [CrossRef]
12. Sherman, R.A.; Hall, M.J.R.; Thomas, S. Medicinal maggots: An ancient remedy for some contemporary afflictions. *Annu. Rev. Entomol.* **2000**, *45*, 55–81. [CrossRef]
13. Nigam, Y.; Dudley, E.; Bexfield, A.; Bond, A.E.; Evans, J.; James, J. The physiology of wound healing by the medicinal maggot, *Lucilia sericata*. *Adv. Insect Physiol.* **2010**, *39*, 39–81. [CrossRef]
14. Matsuyama, K.; Natori, S. Purification of three antibacterial proteins from the culture medium of NIH-Sape-4, an embryonic cell line of *Sarcophaga peregrina*. *J. Biol. Chem.* **1988**, *263*, 17112–17116.
15. Lambert, J.; Keppi, E.; Dimarcq, J.-L.; Wicker, C.; Reichhart, J.-M.; Dunbar, B.; Lepage, P.; Van Dorsselaer, A.; Hoffmann, J.; Forthergill, J.; Hoffmann, D. Insect immunity: isolation from immune blood of the dipteran *Phormia terranovae* of two insect antibacterial peptides with sequence homology to rabbit lung macrophage bactericidal peptides. *Proc. Natl. Acad. Sci. USA* **1989**, *86*, 262–266. [CrossRef]
16. Lehane, M.J.; Wu, D.; Lehane, S.M. Midgut-specific immune molecules are produced by the blood-sucking insect *Stomoxys calcitrans*. *Proc. Natl. Acad. Sci.USA* **1997**, *94*, 11502–11507. [CrossRef]
17. Fujiwara, S.; Imai, J.; Fujiwara, M.; Yaeshima, T.; Kawashima, T.; Kobayashi, K. A potent antimicrobial protein in royal jelly. Purification and determination of the primary structure of royalisin. *J. Biol. Chem.* **1990**, *265*, 11333–11337.
18. Rees, J.A.; Moniatte, M.; Bulet, P. Novel antimicrobial peptides isolated from a European bumblebee, *Bombus pascuorum* (Hymenoptera, Apoidea). *Insect. Biochem. Molec. Biol.* **1997**, *27*, 413–422. [CrossRef]
19. Hanzawa, H.; Shimada, I.; Kuzuhara, T.; Komano, H.; Kohda, D.; Inagaki, F.; Natori, S.; Arata, Y. ^{1}H nuclear magnetic resonance study of the solution conformation of an antibacterial protein, sapecin. *FEBS Lett.* **1990**, *269*, 413–420. [CrossRef]
20. Cornet, B.; Bonmatin, J.-M.; Hetru, C.; Hoffmann, J.A.; Ptak, M.; Vovelle, F. Refined three-dimensional solution structure of insect defensin A. *Structure* **1995**, *3*, 435–448. [CrossRef]
21. Landon, C.; Sodano, P.; Hetru, C.; Hoffmann, J.; Ptak, M. Solution structure of drosomycin, the first inducible antifungal protein from insects. *Protein Sci.* **1997**, *6*, 1878–1884. [CrossRef]
22. Mumcuoglu, K. Y.; Miller, J.; Mumcuoglu, M.; Friger, M.; Tarshis, M. Destruction of bacteria in the digestive tract of the maggot of *Lucilia sericata* (Diptera: Calliphoridae). *J. Med. Entomol.* **2001**, *38*, 161–166. [CrossRef]
23. Parnés, A.; Lagan, K. M. Larval therapy in wound management: A review. *Int. J. Clin. Pract.* **2007**, *61*, 488–493. [CrossRef]
24. Baer, W.S. The treatment of chronic osteomyelitis with the maggots (larva of the blowfly). *J. Bone Joint. Surg.* **1931**, *13*, 438.
25. Simons, S.W. A bactericidal principle in excretions of surgical maggots which destroys important etiological agents of pyogenic infections. *J. Bacteriol.* **1935**, *30*, 253–267.
26. Pavillard, E.R.; Wright, E.A. An antibiotic from maggots. *Nature* **1957**, *180*, 916–917. [CrossRef]

27. Huberman, L.; Gollop, N.; Mumcuoglu, K.Y.; Breuer, E.; Bhusare, S.R.; Shai, Y.; Galun, R. Antibacterial substances of low molecular weight isolated from the blowfly, *Lucilia sericata*. *Med. Vet. Entomol.* **2007**, *21*, 127–131. [CrossRef]
28. Thomas, S.; Andrews, A.M.; Hay, N.P.; Bourgoise, S. The anti-microbial activity of maggot secretions: results of a preliminary study. *J. Tissue Viability* **1999**, *9*, 127–132.
29. Bexfield, A.; Nigam, Y.; Thomas, S.; Ratcliffe, N.A. Detection and partial characterisation of two antibacterial factors from the excretions/secretions of the medicinal maggot *Lucilia sericata* and their activity against methicillin-resistant *Staphylococcus aureus* (MRSA). *Microbes Infect.* **2004**, *6*, 1297–1304. [CrossRef]
30. Bexfield, A.; Bond, A.E.; Roberts, E.C.; Dudley, E.; Nigam, Y.; Thomas, S.; Newton, R.P.; Ratcliffe, N.A. The antibacterial activity against MRSA strains and other bacteria of a <500 Da fraction from maggot excretions/secretions of *Lucilia sericata* (Diptera: Calliphoridae). *Microbes Infect.* **2008**, *10*, 325–333. [CrossRef]
31. Jaklič, D.; Lapanje, A.; Zupančič, K.; Smrke, D.; Gunde-Cimerman, N. Selective antimicrobial activity of maggots against pathogenic bacteria. *J. Med. Microbiol.* **2008**, *57*, 617–625. [CrossRef]
32. Kerridge, A.; Lappin-Scott, H.; Stevens, J.R. Antibacterial properties of larval secretions of the blowfly, *Lucilia sericata*. *Med. Vet. Entomol.* **2005**, *19*, 333–337. [CrossRef]
33. Zhang, Z.; Wang, J.; Zhang, B.; Liu, H.; Song, W.; He, J.; Lv, D.; Wang, S.; Xu, X. Activity of antimicrobial protein from maggots against *Staphylococcus aureus in vitro* and *in vivo*. *Int. J. Mol. Med.* **2013**, *31*, 1159–1165.
34. Kruglikova, A.A.; Chernysh, S.I. Antimicrobial compounds from the excretions of surgical maggots, *Lucilia sericata* (Meigen) (Diptera, Calliphoridae). *Entomol. Rev.* **2011**, *91*, 813–819. [CrossRef]
35. Čeřovský, V.; Slaninová, J.; Fučík, V.; Monincová, L.; Bednárová, L.; Maloň, P.; Štokrová, J. Lucifensin, a novel insect defensin of medicinal maggots: Synthesis and structural study. *ChemBioChem* **2011**, *12*, 1352–1361. [CrossRef]
36. Nygaard, M.K.E.; Andersen, A.S.; Kristensen, H-H.; Krogfelt, K.A.; Fojan, P.; Wimmer, R. The insect defensin lucifensin from *Lucilia sericata*. *J. Biomol. NMR* **2012**, *52*, 277–282. [CrossRef]
37. Takeuchi, K.; Takahashi, H.; Sugai, M.; Iwai, H.; Kohno, T.; Sekimizu, K.; Natori, S.; Shimada, I. Channel-forming membrane permeabilization by an antimicrobial protein, sapecin. *J. Biol. Chem.* **2004**, *279*, 4981–4987.
38. Pymol. Available online: http://www.pymol.org/ (accessed on 12 February 2014).
39. Cociancich, S.; Bulet, P.; Hetru, C.; Hoffmann, J.A. The inducible antimicrobial peptides of insects. *Parasitol. Today* **1994**, *10*, 132–138. [CrossRef]
40. Altincicek, B.; Vilcinskas, A. Septic injury-inducible genes in medicinal maggots of the green blow fly *Lucilia sericata*. *Insect Mol. Biol.* **2009**, *18*, 119–125. [CrossRef]
41. Andersen, A.S.; Sandvang, D.; Schnorr, K.M.; Kruse, T.; Neve, S.; Joergensen, B.; Karlsmark, T.; Krogfelt, K.A. A novel approach to the antimicrobial activity of maggot debridement therapy. *J. Antimicrob. Chemother.* **2010**, *65*, 1646–1654. [CrossRef]
42. Valachová, I.; Bohová, J.; Pálošová, Z.; Takáč, P.; Kozánek, M.; Majtán, J. Expression of lucifensin in *Lucilia sericata* medicinal maggots in infected environments. *Cell Tissue Res.* **2013**, *353*, 165–171. [CrossRef]
43. Bém, R.; Jirkovská, A.; Fejfarová, V.; Dubský, M.; Skibová, J.; Čeřovský, V. Acute antimicrobial effect of maggot therapy on diabetic foot ulcer infection as a basis for identification of antimicrobial peptides from maggots (Abstract). *Diabetologia* **2010**, *53*, 56.
44. Bowling, F.L.; Salgami, E.V.; Boulton, A.J. Larval therapy: a novel treatment in eliminating methicillin-resistant *Staphylococcus aureus* from diabetic foot ulcers. *Diabetes Care* **2007**, *30*, 370–371. [CrossRef]
45. Harder, J.; Meyer-Hoffert, U.; Wehkamp, K.; Schwichtenberg, L.; Schroder, J.M. Differential gene induction of human beta-defensins (hBD-1, -2, -3, and -4) in keratinocytes is inhibited by retinoic acid. *J. Invest. Dermatol.* **2004**, *123*, 522–529. [CrossRef]
46. Khanolkar, M.P.; Bain, S.C.; Stephens, J.W. The diabetic foot. *QJM* **2008**, *101*, 685–695. [CrossRef]
47. Lobmann, R.; Schultz, G.; Lehnert, H. Proteases and the diabetic foot syndrome: mechanisms and therapeutic implications. *Diabetes Care* **2005**, *28*, 461–471. [CrossRef]
48. Rivas-Santiago, B.; Trujillo, V.; Montoya, A.; Gonzalez-Curiel, I.; Castaneda-Delgado, J.; Cardenas, A.; Rincon, K.; Hernandez, M.L.; Hernandez-Pando, R. Expression of antimicrobial peptides in diabetic foot ulcer. *J. Dermatol. Sci.* **2012**, *65*, 19–26. [CrossRef]

49. Van der Plas, M.J.A; van der Does, A.M; Baldry, M.; Dogterom-Ballering, H.C.M; van Gulpen, C; van Dissel, J.T.; Nibbering, P.H; Jukema, G.N. Maggot excretions/secretions inhibit multiple neutrophil pro-inflammatory responses. *Microbes Infect.* **2007**, *9*, 507–514. [CrossRef]
50. Horobin, A.J.; Shakesheff, K.M.; Pritchard, D.I. Promotion of human dermal fibroblast migration, matrix remodeling and modification of fibroblast morphology within a novel 3D model by *Lucilia sericata* larval secretions. *J. Invest. Dermatol.* **2006**, *126*, 1410–1418. [CrossRef]

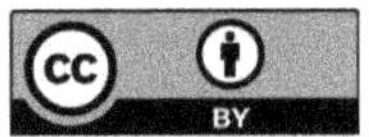

© 2014 by the authors. Licensee MDPI, Basel, Switzerland. This article is an open access article distributed under the terms and conditions of the Creative Commons Attribution (CC BY) license (http://creativecommons.org/licenses/by/4.0/).

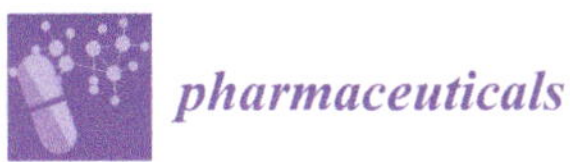

MDPI

Review

Chapter 5:
Antimicrobial Peptides from Fish

Jorge A. Masso-Silva [1] and Gill Diamond [2,*]

[1] Department of Pediatrics and Graduate School of Biomedical Sciences, Rutgers New Jersey Medical School, Newark, NJ 07101, USA; massoja@gsbs.rutgers.edu

[2] Department of Oral Biology, University of Florida, Box 100424, Gainesville, FL 32610, USA

* Author to whom correspondence should be addressed; gdiamond@dental.ufl.edu; Tel.: +1-352-273-8861; Fax: +1-352-273-8829.

Received: 15 January 2014; in revised form: 6 February 2014; Accepted: 18 February 2014; Published: 3 March 2014

Abstract: Antimicrobial peptides (AMPs) are found widely distributed through Nature, and participate in the innate host defense of each species. Fish are a great source of these peptides, as they express all of the major classes of AMPs, including defensins, cathelicidins, hepcidins, histone-derived peptides, and a fish-specific class of the cecropin family, called piscidins. As with other species, the fish peptides exhibit broad-spectrum antimicrobial activity, killing both fish and human pathogens. They are also immunomodulatory, and their genes are highly responsive to microbes and innate immuno-stimulatory molecules. Recent research has demonstrated that some of the unique properties of fish peptides, including their ability to act even in very high salt concentrations, make them good potential targets for development as therapeutic antimicrobials. Further, the stimulation of their gene expression by exogenous factors could be useful in preventing pathogenic microbes in aquaculture.

Keywords: defensin; pleurocidin; cathelicidin; hepcidin; piscidin

---

1. Introduction

Antimicrobial peptides (AMPs) represent a broad category of different families of highly conserved peptides widely found throughout Nature, which exhibit broad-spectrum antimicrobial activity *in vitro* and *in vivo*. While vertebrate antimicrobial peptides were initially discovered in amphibians, humans and rabbits in the mid-1980s [1–3], The antimicrobial activity of fish peptides was not described for another decade. Initially, a toxic peptide from the Moses sole fish *Pardachirus marmoratus*, called pardaxin, was characterized in 1980 [4], but its antimicrobial activity wasn't observed until 1996 [5]. Shortly thereafter, Cole *et al*. described a peptide isolated from the skin secretions of the winter flounder (*Pleuronectes americanus*) [6] using antimicrobial activity as a screening method. Since then, the field has progressed as with other vertebrate species, with the identification of homologous peptides in the piscidin family (unique to fish, but homologous to cecropins), as well as the defensin, cathelicidin, and hepcidin families, which are found in many other species. Many of the peptides were identified by purification of the peptides with antibiotic activity, although as with other species, the increased use of bioinformatics techniques has allowed the identification of even more peptides [7]. The results of the research described here demonstrate that AMPs from fish exhibit many if not all of the same characteristics as other vertebrate AMPs, like broad-spectrum (but often species-specific) antimicrobial activities, as well as immunomodulatory functions. In addition, there appear to be interesting differences, specific to fish, that have evolved to address the unique aquatic environments and microbes encountered by these species. There has also been a recent effort to study the potential for using these peptides as therapeutic agents, both in human medicine and in aquaculture. Below we will examine the various peptide families (whose members are shown in Table 1), and discuss their role in host defense and potential for future use.

Table 1. Characterized antimicrobial peptides from fish, by species. Listed is the number of peptides of each family [reference].

Species			Piscidins	Defensins	Hepcidins	Cathelicidins	Histone-derived
Common name	Scientific name	Habitat					
American plaice	*Hippoglossoides platessoides*	Marine	2 [8]				
Antarctic toothfish	*Dissostichus mawsoni*	Marine			3 [9]		
Atlantic cod	*Gadus morhua*	Marine and brackish	2 [10]	1 [11]	1 [12]	1 [13]	1 [14]
Antarctic eelpout	*Lycodichthys dearborni*	Marine			2 [9]		
Atlantic hagfish	*Myxine glutinosa*	Marine				3 [15]	
Atlantic salmon	*Salmo salar*	Marine, brackish and freshwater			2 [16]	2 [17]	1 [18]
Ayu	*Plecoglossus altivelis*	Marine, brackish and freshwater			1 [19]	1 [20]	
Barramundi	*Lates calcarifer*	Marine, brackish and freshwater			2 [21]		
Black porgy	*Acanthopagrus schlegelii*	Marine and brackish			7 [22,23]		
Black rockfish	*Sebastes schlegelii*	Marine			2 [24]		
Blotched snakehead	*Channa maculata*	Freshwater			1 [25]		
Blue catfish	*Ictalurus furcatus*	Freshwater and brackish			1 [26]		
Blunt snout bream	*Megalobrama amblycephala*	Freshwater			1 [27]		
Brook trout	*Salvelinus fontinalis*	Marine, brackish and freshwater				2 [28]	
Brown trout	*Salmo trutta fario*	Marine, brackish and freshwater				1 [28]	
Channel catfish	*Ictalurus punctatus*	Freshwater			1 [26]		1 [29]
Chinese loach	*Paramisgurnus dabryanus*	Freshwater		1 [30]			
Common carp	*Cyprinus carpio* L.	Freshwater and brackish		2 [31]	1 [32]		
European seabass	*Dicentrarchus labrax*	Marine, brackish and freshwater	1 [33]		1 [34]		
Gilthead seabream	*Sparus aurata*	Marine and brackish		1 [35]	1 [36]		
Grayling	*Thymallus thymallus*	Freshwater and brackish				1 [28]	
Half-smooth tongue sole	*Cynoglossus semilaevis*	Marine, brackish and freshwater			1 [37]		
Atlantic halibut	*Hippoglossus hippoglossus*	Marine	1 [8]				1 [38]
Hybrid striped bass	*Morone saxatilis x M. chrysops*	Marine, brackish and freshwater	4 [39–41]		1 [42]		
Icefish	*Chionodraco hamatus*	Marine	1 [43]				
Olive flounder	*Paralichthys olivaceus*	Marine			2 [16]		
Japanese rice fish	*Oryzias latipes*	Freshwater and brackish			1 [16]		
Japanese pufferfish	*Takifugu rubripes*	Marine, brackish and freshwater		1 [44]			
Japanese seabass	*Lateolabrax japonicus*	Marine, brackish and freshwater			1 [45]		
Largemouth bass	*Micropterus salmoides*	Freshwater			2 [46]		
Large yellow croaker	*Pseudosciaena crocea*	Marine and brackish	1 [47]		1 [48,49]		
Mandarin fish	*Siniperca chuatsi*	Freshwater	1 [50]	1 [51]			
Maori chief	*Notothenia angustata*	Marine			5 [9]		
Medaka	*Oryzias melastigma*	Freshwater and brackish		1 [52]	2 [53]		
Miiuy croaker	*Miichthys miiuy*	Marine and brackish			1 [54]		

Table 1. *Cont.*

Species			Piscidins	Defensins	Hepcidins	Cathelicidins	Histone-derived
Common name	Scientific name	Habitat					
Mud dab	*Limanda limanda*	Marine	1 [55]				
Mud loach	*Misgurnus mizolepis*	Freshwater			[56]		
Olive flounder	*Paralichthys olivaceus*	Marine		5 [57]			
Orange-spotted grouper	*Epinephelus coioides*	Marine and brackish	1 [58]	2 [59,60]	3 [61,62]		
Pacific mutton hamlet	*Alphestes immaculatus*	Marine			1 [63]		
Rainbow trout	*Oncorhynchus mykiss*	Marine, brackish and freshwater		4 [64,65]		2 [17]	3 [66–69]
Redbanded seabream	*Pagrus auriga*	Marine			4 [70]		
Red sea bream	*Chrysophrys major*	Marine	1 [71]		1 [72]		
Rockbream	*Oplegnathus fasciatus*	Marine			4 [73]		
Sea bass	*Dicentrarchus labrax*	Marine, brackish and freshwater					1 [74]
Seahorse	*Hippocampus kuda*	Marine and brackish	1 [75]				
Smallmouth bass	*Micropterus dolomieu*	Freshwater			2 [46]		
Snowtrout	*Schizothorax richardsonii*	Freshwater			1 [76]		
Spotted-green pufferfish	*Tetraodon nigroviridis*	Freshwater and brackish		2 [44]			
Sunshine bass	Marine, brackish and freshwater						1 [69]
Thick-lipped lenok	*Brachymystax lenok*	Freshwater				1 [77]	
Tilapia	Oreochromis mossambicus	Freshwater and brackish	5 [78]		3 [79]		
Turbot	*Scophthalmus maximus*	Marine and brackish			2 [80,81]		
Winter flounder	*Pleuronectesamericanus*	Marine	6 [6,82,83]		5 [16]		
Witch flounder	*Glyptocephalus cynoglossus*	Marine	5 [8]				
Yellowtail flounder	*Pleuronectes ferruginea*	Marine	1 [8]				
Zebrafish	*Danio rerio*	Freshwater		3 [44]	2 [84]		

2. Piscidins

Piscidins and pleurocidins comprise a family of linear, amphipathic AMPs, evolutionarily related to similarly structured peptides found in amphibian skin and insects [85]. The first member of the family identified was a 25-residue peptide isolated and characterized from skin mucous secretions of the winter flounder, *Pleuronectes americanus*, called pleurocidin [6]. Further research identified other homologous pleurocidins in related species [8,83]. These were shown to exhibit an amphipathic, α-helical structure, similar to magainins and cecropins. A similarly structured peptide was identified in the loach, *Misgurunus anguillicaudatus*, called misgurin [86], and a family of peptides, termed piscidins, were identified in the mast cells of the hybrid striped bass [87], as well as numerous other fish taxa [88]. Other similar peptides, including moronecidin, epinecidin, dicentracin, have been identified [33,41,89]. An alignment of primary amino acid sequences of some members of this class are shown in Figure 1. The similarities of the mature peptide predicted secondary structure [6,41,78,90] as well as an analysis of their gene structures [33,50] suggested that they all belong to the same evolutionarily related family, which we will refer to as the piscidins. In addition, positive selection has been found influencing evolution of these peptides, where the highest diversity is found in the mature peptide that suggest adaptation for attacking new pathogens or strains that are coevolving with the host [91,92].

```
                             10        20        30        40        50        60        70        80
pleurocidin          MKFTATFLMIAIFVLMVEPGECGWGS-FFKKAAHVGKHVGKAALTHY------------LGDKQELNKRAVDEDPNVIVFE-
cod piscidin-1       MRYIVLLVVVLLLAMMVQPADCFIHH------IIGWISHGVRAIHR-----------AIHGEKAEEYIMVD---------
Rock bream pisc      MKCIVIFLVLSMVVLMAEPGEGFLGM-LLHGVGHA---IHGLIHGKQN-------VEEQQQQQEQLDKRSVDYNPGQPNLD-
Red drum_piscid      MKCTAVFLVLFMVVLMAEPGECIWGL-IAHGVAHVGSLIHGLVNGNHG-------GNQAEEQQEQLNKRSLSYD--HP----
Malabar grouper p1   MRCIALFLVLSLVVLMAEPGEGFFFH-IIKGLFHAGRMIHGLVNRRR--------HRHGMEEL-DLDQRAFEREK-AFA---
Malabar grouper p2   MRCIALFLVLSLVVLMAEPGEGFIFH-IIKGLFHAGKMIHGLVTRR----------RHGVEELQDLDQRAFEREK-AFA---
moronecidin          MKCITLFLVLSLVVLMAEPGECFFHHHIYHGYIKLHQAIRCLVRAA-------------MTEQQEMEQRAFDRER-AFA---
cod piscidin-2       MRCIFLLFVVLLLAMMVLPAEGFLHH------IVGLIHHGLSLFG-------------DRADKAEEYIAVD---------
striped bass p5      MKCVMIFLVLTLVVLMAEPGEGLIGS-LFRGAKAIFRGARQGWRSHK---------AVSRYRARYVRRPVIYYHRVYPNEER
striped bass p4      MKCVMIFLVLTLVVLMAEPGEGFFRH-LFRGAKAIFRGARQGWRAHK---------VVSRYRNRDV--PETDNNQEEPYNQR
Striped bass p1      MKCATLFLVLSMVVLMAEPGDAFFHH-IFRGIVHVGKTIHRLVTGGKAEQDQQDQQYQQEQQEQQAQQYQRFNRERAAFD---
Drosophila cecropin  MNFYNIFVFVAL-ILAITIGQSEAGW-----LKKIGKKIERVGQHTR----------DATIQGLGIAQQAANVAATARG---
```

Figure 1. Alignment of piscidins. Mature peptide sequences were obtained from published data and from the PubMed protein database, and were aligned using MacVector software. The Drosophila cecropin A1 sequences is provided for comparison as a representative member of the cecropin family.

Alignment of primary amino acid sequences shows that piscidins as a group have little direct sequence identity (Figure 1), but are as a group predicted to possess an amphipatic α-helical structure [6,41,78,90]. However, CD spectroscopy of the piscidin from brooding pouch suggests that it might have a β-sheet or β-strand motif instead of α-helix [75]. Their gene structure is composed of four exons and three introns, encoding a peptide precursor containing a signal peptide, a mature piscidin and a carboxy-terminal prodomain [41,50,82]. However, in tilapia and grouper a three-exon/two-intron and five-exon/four-intron structure, respectively was found [78,89]. Moreover, multiple piscidin isoforms have been found in the same species [78,83].

Piscidins exhibit potent antimicrobial activity against a variety of microorganisms. They are widely active against bacteria Gram-positive and -negative species, with the best antibacterial values obtained against several *Streptococcus*, *Pseudomonas*, *Bacillus* and *Vibrio* species (for a full listing of fish antimicrobial peptides and their activities, see Supplementary Table S1). Interestingly, chrysophsin-3 was observed to kill the three stages of *Bacillus anthracis* (sporulated, germinated and vegetative), being able to penetrate and kill the spores without full germination [93]. Piscidins have also been shown to possess anti-fungal activity [47,94,95], anti-parasitic activity [47,96–98], and anti-viral activity [99,100]. An interesting study showed that piscidin-2 was highly potent against the water mold *Saprolegnia* sp. (Oomycetes) with a MIC within the physiological piscidin-2 levels [98].

Piscidins are mainly expressed in gill, skin and intestine, although can be also found in head-kidney and spleen [10,43,47,50,58,101,102]. However, in Atlantic cod piscidin was found to be ubiquitous, being detected in chondrocytes, heart, oocytes, exocrine and endocrine glands, swim bladder, and other tissues [103]. Nevertheless, the expression profiles vary depending on the isoform [39,78,83]. Moreover, specifically among the cell types where piscidin has shown to be expressed are mast cells, rodlet cells, phagocytic granulocytes and eosinophilic granular cells [43,88,102,104,105]. Interestingly, there is evidence that granulocytes can destroy bacteria in phagosome by intracellular release of piscidin, meaning that piscidin can act against extra and intracellular bacteria [102]. In addition, pleurocidin expression is expressed at 13 days post-hatch in the winter flounder, which is suggested to play an important role in defense during development [101].

Like AMP genes from mammals, piscidin genes can be induced by a variety of stimuli, including Gram-positive and -negative bacteria [78], bacteria cell components like LPS [43,50,58] or the bacterial antigen ASAL [10]. The LPS-mediated induction of epinecidin-1 in zebrafish was shown to require hepatocyte nuclear factor 1 [89]. Furthermore, piscidin genes are induced by parasites [47,104,106], viruses [107], and poly I:C [43,58]. Another study demonstrated that high biomass density (*i.e.*, a higher concentration of fish per volume water in an experimental tank) used as an acute stressor component, led to an to up-regulation of dicentracin in gills and skin as well [74].

Besides microorganisms, piscidin-mediated anti-tumor activity has been shown by the growth inhibition and/or killing of a variety of different cancer-derived cell lines like A549 [108], HT1080 [108–110], U937 [111], HL60 [112], U937 [110], HeLa [110] and different breast cancer-derived cell lines including MDA-MB-468, T47-D, SKBR3, MCF7, MCF7-TX400 (paclitaxel-resistant MCF7), MDA-MB-231 and 4T1 [113]. Furthermore, pleurocidin is able to kill breast cancer xenografts in NOD SCID mice, where cell death was caused by mitochondrial membrane damage and ROS production [113]. In addition, disruption of cancer cell membrane has been also shown to occur [110]. Moreover, *in vitro* inhibition of proliferation of U937 and HT1080 was suggested to occur by inducing apoptosis in response to cytokine production like TNF-α, IL-10, IL-15, IL-6, the tumor suppressor p53 [111], and caspases [110]. Also, pleurocidin showed the ability to inhibit HT1080 migration in a dose-dependent manner [109] as well as the rapid killing of a human leukemia cell line [112]. In contrast, pleurocidin showed no lysis of human dermal fibroblasts, umbilical vein endothelial cells and erythrocytes [113].

Several studies have shown that piscidin can disrupt the plasma membranes and cause cellular material efflux by pore formation [114,115]. However, use of membrane models has suggested that membrane composition is an important factor in the lytic capacity of piscidin to disrupt cell membranes [116]. In addition, using site-specific high-resolution solid-state NMR orientational restraints and circular dichroism it was shown that piscidin-1 and -3 induce a membrane-AMP interaction by parallel orientation of the α-helical in membrane model surfaces where fast and large amplitude backbone motions occur [117,118]. Moreover, at very low inhibitory concentrations piscidin does not cause significant cell membrane damage but is capable to inhibit macromolecular synthesis in bacteria [119]. Against fungi, pleurocidin was active against *C. albicans* by causing protoplast regeneration and membrane disruption [95,112] and it has been suggested to cause oxidative stress, triggering apoptosis in *C. albicans* by inducing intracellular reactive oxygen species (ROS) and activation of metacaspases, leading to externalization of phosphatidylserine [94].

Among other attractive features of piscidin includes their ability to retain antibacterial activity at high salt concentrations [41], thermostability (piscidin from seahorse brooding pouch retained full activity after exposing from 20–80 °C for 30 min, and only 20% loss of activity when boiling at 100 °C for 30 min) [75], and relatively low cytotoxicity against mammalian cells [120]. However, in tilapia some piscidin isoforms were hemolytic for tilapia red blood cells. The peptide with the greatest hemolysis activity was also the one with the best antibacterial activity, which is associated with the amphiphilic α-helical cationic structure [78].

The immunomodulatory capacity of piscidins is another feature that has been widely assessed. In fish, they are able to modulate the expression of pro-inflammatory and other immune-related genes like IL-1β, IL-10, IL-22, IL-26, TNF-α, IFN-γ, NF-κB, lysozyme, NOS2, MyD88, TLR4a, TLR1, TLR3, [121–125]. Moreover, in mice this immunomodulatory effect also has been observed, with the modulation of the genes encoding IL-6, IL-10, IL-12, MCP-1, TNF-α, IFN-γ and IgG1 [126–128].

Recently, some pleurocidins have shown to be able stimulate human mast cell chemotaxis increasing Ca2+ mobilization, and inducing the production of pro-inflammatory cytokines (like CCL2, 1β/CCL4) in mast cells, which was suggested to occur through G-proteins. In addition, it is able to cause mast cells to adhere, migrate, degranulate, and release cysteinyl leukotrienes and prostaglandin D2 [129].

Overall, it appears that piscidins represent an evolutionarily conserved family of peptides, which, while unique to fish, exhibit broad homology to the linear, amphipathic classes of antimicrobial peptides found in many other species.

3. β-Defensins

A general term for cysteine-rich, cationic antimicrobial peptides found in plants, fungi, invertebrates and vertebrates [130–132], defensins exhibit a general conformation made by cysteine-stabilized α-helical and β–sheet folds (reviewed in [131,133]). In mammals three types of defensins have been identified based on their structure, α-, β-, and θ-defensins (last one found only in certain nonhuman primates, including the rhesus macacque) [130,134,135]. However in fish, sequence and structural analysis have revealed that fish defensins are solely β-defensin-like proteins [35,44,51,64] including the conserved 6-cyteine motif (Figure 2). To date, up to four genes and five isoforms of defensins have been found in a single species [57,65], apparently as result of gene duplication events that had occurred in vertebrate β-defensins [133]. Fish defensins were first identified in zebrafish, Fugu and tetraodon by a database mining approach [44], but currently defensins have been identified in many other marine and freshwater fish species (see Table 1). Interestingly, a phylogenetic analysis using defensins from human and fish revealed that hBD-4 is the only human defensin that clustered with fish defensins, suggesting possible similar biological properties [35].

The human β-defensin gene has two exons and one intron, fairly typical of most β-defensin genes. Furthermore, mammalian β-defensins are translated as prepeptides, with the mature peptide sequence immediately downstream from the signal sequence [136]. However, in fish three exons and two introns are found [65], encoding a prepropeptide (including signal peptide, propeptide and mature peptide) comprised of 60 to 77 amino acids, and a mature peptide from 38 to 45 amino acids with cationic nature with a *pI* around 8 (except for those in olive flounder, which are around 4, indicating anionic nature [57]). Due its cationic nature they present a net positive charge that can go from +1 to +5. As with all vertebrate β-defensins, there are six conserved cysteines, although in human and birds these are located in a single exon, while in fish they span two exons [57].

```
                                   10        20      * 30        40        50        60        70
Orange_spotted_grouper_BD  MKGLSLVLLVLLLMLTVGEGNDPEMQY---WTCG-YRGLCR--RFCHAQ-EYIVGHHG-CP-RRYRCCAVRS-
Rainbow_trout_BD4          .KYHCTML....AF..IACDVNEAAAFPIPWG.SNYS.V..--AV.LSA-.LPF.PF.-.A-KGFV..VAHVF
Rainbow_trout_BD3          .NCLMIFM..A..VI.CGIQESSASLH----L.FISG.G..NLRL.LAP.GTNI.KM.-.T-WPNV..K----
Rainbow_trout_BD2          .GRLGLVM.....LT.V-QADDTKVQG---.T.G-YR.A..--KY.YAQ-.YMV.YH.-.P-RRLR..ALRF-
Rainbow_trout_BD1          .SCQRMVT....VF.LLNVVEDEAASF--.FS.PTLS.V..--KL.LPT-.MFF.PL.-.G-KGFL..VSHF-
Mandarin_fish_BD           .KGLSLVL.....M..VGEGNDPEMQY---.T.G-YR.L..--RF.YAQ-.YIV.HH.-.P-RRYR..AMRS-
Cod_BD                     .SCHRVWV....AV..LNFVENEAAAF--..S.PTLS.V..--KV.LPT-.MFF.PL.-.G-KEFQ..VSHFF
TAP                        MRLHHLLLALLFLVLSAWSGFTQGVGN--PVSCVRNK.I.VP-IR.PGS---MKQI.T.VGRAVK..RKK---
Consensus                  M                                    G C     C           C C      CC
```

Figure 2. Alignment of β-defensins. Precursor peptide sequences were obtained from published data and from the PubMed protein database, and were aligned using MacVector software. The bovine β-defensin, Tracheal Antimicrobial Peptide (TAP) is shown for comparison. The conserved β-defensin cysteine spacing is shown in the consensus line. The first residue of the mature peptide region (based on the isolated TAP sequence) is denoted with an asterisk.

Fish β-defensins have proven to be active against both Gram-negative and -positive bacteria (for specific inhibitory values see Supplementary Table S1), although with rather moderate activity. Exceptions to those reports of MICs in the high μM range are *Planococcus citreus* (Gram-positive) [11] and *Aeromonas hydrophila* (Gram-negative) [52], with low MIC values. Other studies using supernatant of lysates HEK293T cells transfected with β-defensins from the Chinese loach or the gilthead seabream showed significant growth inhibition of the Gram-negative *A. hydrophila* and the Gram-positive *B. subtilis* [30,35]. Moreover, β-defensins are also active against fish-specific viruses such as *Singapore grouper iridovirus* (SGIV), *viral nervous necrosis virus* (VNNV), *haemorrhagic septicaemia virus* (VHSV), and the frog-specific *Rana grylio virus* (RGV) [59,60,64]. In addition it has been shown that the α-defensin human defensin-1 (HD-1) is highly active against VHSV, a salmonid rhabdovirus, causing its inactivation and inhibition [137]. However, no assessment has been carried out testing fish-derived defensins against human viruses so far, nor about their potential mechanism of action. Similarly, there are no published studies examining the activity of fish defensins against parasites. A small number of studies demonstrate the activity of human defensins against parasites, showing, for example, that HD-1 is capable to destroy the parasite *Trypanosoma cruzi* by pore formation and induction of nuclear and mitochondrial DNA fragmentation [138], and that hd-5 is able to reduce *Toxoplasma gondii* viability by aggregation [139]. This is an area with great potential both for fish and human biology. As with parasites, there are no studies related to the antifungal activity of fish defensins, in spite of the many studies showing such activity of β-defensins from other species (e.g., those described in [140–142].

In addition to their antimicrobial activities, β-defensins have been shown to exhibit multiple immunomodulatory activities (reviewed in [143]). For example, recombinant mBD4 and hBD2 (both β-defensins in mice and human, respectively) have shown to possess chemotactic activity for CCR6-expressing cells (which include monocytes, dendritic cells and T-lymphocytes), which was confirmed using its chemokine ligand CCL20 that competed with these β-defensins [144]. Similar activity has been observed in a fish homologue. β-defensins from the gilthead seabream exhibited chemotactic activity, showing the capacity to attract head-kidney leukocytes [35]. There is evidence of CCR6 mammalian orthologs in zebrafish [145] and rainbow trout [146] that may help address the mechanism. In addition, chemotactic capacity of HNP1 (human α-defensin) towards trout leucocytes has been shown [147]. Furthermore, a β-defensin from Atlantic cod is capable of stimulating antimicrobial activity in phagocytes [11]. Together, the studies suggest that fish β-defensins function similarly to their mammalian counterparts, contributing to the innate host defense in multiple ways.

In mammals, β-defensin expression was initially identified and studied predominantly in skin and mucosal membranes from respiratory, gastrointestinal and genitourinary tracts (reviewed in [148]. More recently, however, numerous β-defensin isoforms have been identified in sperm, with associations to reproduction being demonstrated [149]. While some β-defensins (mostly hBD-1 and its homologue) are constitutively expressed, the expression of most β-defensins can be induced by a variety of factors, including many innate immune mediators and microbe-associated molecular patterns (reviewed in [150]). Furthermore, their expression is observed not only in adult tissues, but during embryonic development as well [151,152]. In fish, constitutive expression seems to start early in the development probably as part of the need of defense in vulnerable stages that rely significantly in the innate immune response [11,57]. However, it is hard to establish specific expression patterns, because this appears to vary between species and isoform [31,44,59,60,65], although in most of the characterized fish β-defensins, skin is one of the tissues with the highest basal expression [31,35,44,65], a widely distributed feature among vertebrate defensins [148,153]. After skin, head-kidney and spleen are the tissues with also high expression, which are the main immune organs in fish [51,52,65]. Nevertheless, in some studies some isoforms of fish β-defensins have shown to possess a widespread constitutive expression [30,52,65]. Furthermore, high expression in eye has been found, suggesting a relevant role in ocular infections [30,52]. In addition, a study in the orange-spotted grouper suggest a relationship of fish β-defensin and reproduction endocrine regulation, finding an isoform that is exclusively expressed in pituitary and testis, where such expression is up-regulated from intersexual gonad to testis in sex reversal, and a deeper analysis proved that the pituitary-specific POU1F1 transcription binding site and the testis-specific SRY site are responsible for this phenomenon [60]. Fish β-defensin genes are induced by a variety of stimuli including cell wall components like LPS [52,59], β-glucans [31] and peptidoglycan [154]. They are stimulated by bacterial challenges from *A. hydrophila* [30], *Y. ruckeri* [65], *V. anguillarum* [11] and *E. tarda* [57]; and by viral challenges, including SGIV [59] or the TLR-3 agonist poly(I:C), to emulate a viral infection [59,65]. In addition, supplemented diets with the diatom *Naviluca* sp. and the lactobacillus *Lactobacillus sakei* have shown to induced β-defensin in gilthead seabream [155]. Thus, β-defensins in fish are true orthologues, exhibiting both structural and functional similarities to mammalian peptides, as well as their patterns of expression. This further supports the hypothesis that β-defensins are an ancient and highly conserved mechanism of host defense in animal species [133].

4. Hepcidins

Hepcidins are cysteine-rich peptides with antimicrobial activity that were first discovered in humans [156,157]. Since then, hepcidins have been identified in many other vertebrates including reptiles, amphibians and fish. Although, in birds the existence of a hepcidin needs to be better confirmed [158]. Fish hepcidin was first identified and isolated from the hybrid striped bass [42] and since then hepcidins have been identified in at least 37 fish species. The general structure of human hepcidin is a β-sheet-composed harpin-shaped with four disulfide bridges (formed by eight cysteines) with an unusual vicinal bridge at the hairpin turn [159], which is also the general structure in fish hepcidin [76,79]. However, sequence analysis of fish hepcidins has shown the presence of hepcidins containing 7, 6 or 4 cysteines [9,48].

Fish hepcidin genes have undergone duplication and diversification processes that have produced multiple gene copies [9], and up to eight copies have been identified [22,34,73]. Hepcidin genes are composed of three exons and two introns encoding a signal peptide, a prodomain and a mature peptide [22,34,72]. The pre-prohepcidin size can range from 81 to 96 amino acids, and the mature hepcidin from 19 to 31, with a molecular weight around 2–3 kDa. Representative sequences are shown in Figure 3. An average *pI* generally above 8 demonstrates their cationic nature. However, a predicted low *pI* of 5.4 of the orange-spotted grouper, indicates the existence of anionic hepcidin [61].

```
                              10        20        30        40        50        60        70 *      80        90
Pacific_mutton_hamlet         --MKAFSIAVAVTLVLAFICILESSAVP----FTGVQELEEAASNDTPVAAYQEMSMESRMMPDH---VRQKRQSHLSLCRWCCNCCRGNKGCGFCCKF
Red_spotted_grouper_hepcidin  --..TF.V....AV...FI.TQ....L.----V.GVEE.V.LV.S.D..ADH.ELPV.LGERLFN---I.K..--AP-K.TPY.YPTRDGSK..M...T
Mud_loach_hepcidin            --..LTRFFLVAVFIV.CF.F.QTA.S.----F.QEVQH.DEMNS-GAPQVNYHSTETTPEQSNPLALF.S.......M..Y..K..R.-VF..V.D-.
Carp_hepcidin                 --.RAM.I.C..AVII.CV.A.Q.A.L.SEVRLDPEVR...PEDSEAARSID.GVAAALAKETSPEVRF.T.......L..Y.....K.-K........
Atlantic_salmon_hepcidin      ----MKAFS...VL.I.CMFI...T.V.-----FSEVRT..VG.F.S..GEH.QPGG.SMHLPEP---F.F...I...L.GL.....H.-K......R.
Bass_hepcidin                 --..TF.V....AV...FI.LQ....V.----V.EVQE...PM.N-----EY.EMPV.SWKMPYN---N.H..H.SPGG..F.....P.MI........
Human_hepcidin                MALSSQIW.ACLLLL.LLASLTSG.VF.-----QQTGQ.A.LQPQ-----DRAGARASWMPMFQR----.RR.DT.FPI.IF..G..HR-S...V..R.
Consensus                                                P                                       R  R      C   C        CG C
```

Figure 3. Alignment of hepcidins. Representative precursor peptide sequences were obtained from published data and from the PubMed protein database, and were aligned using MacVector software. Human hepcidin is shown for comparison. The first residue of the mature peptide region is denoted with an asterisk.

Fish have two types of hepcidins, HAMP1 and HAMP2. However, although HAMP1 is present in actinopterygian and non-actinopterygian fish, HAMP2 has been only found in actinopterygian fish [54,63,158]. Moreover, a phylogenetic study has shown positive Darwinian selection in HAMP2 (but not HAMP1 and its mammalian orthologue) that suggest adaptive evolution probably associated with the host-pathogen interaction in different environments [9,54,160].

Hepcidin expression can be detected as early as in the fertilized egg in blunt snout bream [27] or at 8 h after fertilization in channel catfish [26]. However, in winter flounder and tongue sole it was not detected until day 5 and 6, respectively (larvae stage) [16,37]. Nevertheless, it has been shown that hepcidin isoforms have different expression pattern and kinetics in larval development [70]. In addition, different hepcidin types in a single species can have different rates of expression within the same tissue [80] that can be affected by different stimuli [24,70,73,79]. Interestingly, some isoforms have high basal hepcidin expression in liver, but some have not, where the highest expression often occurs in spleen, kidney and intestine [9,70,73,79].

Similar to other AMP genes, fish hepcidins can be induced by exposure to both Gram-positive and Gram-negative bacteria [12,19,25–27,34,36,37,42,48,53,56,61,63,72,73,161–166]. Moreover, fungi like *Saccharomyces cerevisiae* [36,61], and tumor cell lines like L-1210 and SAF-1 have shown to induce hepcidin expression as well [36]. Hepcidin genes in fish are also induced by viruses [36,61,73,165], and poly I:C [12,36,164], as well as mitogens [36]. Moreover, environmental estrogenic endocrine disrupting chemicals like 17β-estradiol down-regulates one of the hepcidin isoforms expression in liver in largemouth bass [46].

In humans, hepcidin acts as a type II actue-phase protein [167]. Related to this, time-course experiments under bacterial challenge of fish have shown that the highest expression of hepcidin occurs at 3–6 h and decay after that [23,32,163]. Also, the expression of hepcidin occurs along with other acute phase response proteins like IL-1β, serum amyloid A and precerebellin after infection with *Yersinia ruckeri* in rainbow trout [168]. Related to this, mud loach infected with Gram-negative bacteria showed a high IL-1β-like gene expression-mediated response [56]. Together, these results suggest that hepcidins can also act as a type II acute phase protein, and function as part of a broad innate immune response in fish.

Fish hepcidins are active against a wide variety of bacteria, both Gram-positive and -negative at the low μM range, including potent activity against a large number of fish pathogens (see Supplementary Table S1 for a complete listing). This includes rapid killing kinetics against *S. aureus* and *Pseudomonas stutzeri* [23,62]. Furthermore, synergy between bass hepcidin and moronecidin against *S. iniae* and *Y. enterocolitica* has been demonstrated [161]. In addition, they are active against a number of viruses [80, 99,169–171], and a recent study indicates that human Hepc25 is able to affect HCV replication in cell culture by inducing STAT3 activation leading to an antiviral state of the cell [172]. In contrast, their quantified activity against fungi appears to be rather low [23,48,161].

A few studies have tried to elucidate the mechanism of action of hepcidin against bacteria. With human Hepc25, the lack of SYTOX uptake showed that membrane permeabilization does not occur [173] in contrast to most antimicrobial peptides [150]. Similar results have been observed with fish peptides, using light emission kinetics, which showed that Medaka recombinant pro-hepcidin and synthetic hepcidin also do not cause membrane permeabilization in *E. coli* [171]. However, human Hepc25 has shown binding to DNA with high efficiency in a retardation assay [173].

Fish hepcidins have also shown the capacity of affect cancer cells viability. For example, tilapia hepcidin TH2-3, have shown inhibition of proliferation and migration of human fibrosarcoma cell line HT1080a in a concentration-dependent manner. Furthermore, TH2-3 was able to cause cell membrane disruption in HT1080 and results also suggest that TH2-3 down-regulates c-Jun leading to apoptosis [174]. TH1-5 inhibit the proliferation of tumor cells (HeLa, HT1080 and HepG2) altering membrane structure and inducing apoptosis at low dose. Also, TH1-5 showed modulation of immune-related genes [175]. A study with medaka hepcidin showed 40% decrease in HepG2 cell viability by addition of 25 and 5 μM of synthetic mature Om-hep1 and recombinant pro-Om-hep1 (prohepcidin), respectively [171]. Interestingly, Pro-Omhep1 has better anti-tumor activity compared with Om-hep1, using HepG2 cells [171].

Fish hepcidins have also shown the ability to modulate the expression of different immune-related genes not only in fish but also in mice. Transgenic zebrafish expressing TH1-5 showed upregulation of IL-10, IL-21, IL-22, lysozyme, TLR-1, TLR-3, TNF-α and NF-κB [176]. However, TH2-3 showed to downregulate some of those upregulated by TH1-5 [177]. In the same context, TH2-3 reduced the amount of TNF-α, IL-1α, IL-1β, IL-6 and COX-2 in mouse macrophages challenged with LPS [178]. Related to this, in turbot it has been shown that hepcidin is able to increase the activation of NF-κB (which control a variety of inflammatory cytokines) through an undetermined yet signaling pathway [165]. TH2-3 have also shown to be able to modulate protein kinase C isoforms in the mouse macrophage RAW264.7 cell line [179], and was also capable to induce morphology changes in these cells similar to PMA-induced changes [179]. Moreover, TH1-5 modulates the expression of certain interferons and annexin (viral-responsive genes) in pancreatic necrosis virus-infected fish [170].

However, despite the potential antimicrobial and immunomodulatory effect, hepcidin is better known for being a key iron regulator controlling ferroportin, which is able to degrade by its internalization, which decrease iron transfer into blood [180]. In fish, although ferroportin internalization by hepcidin has not been proven yet, there is evidence suggesting that fish hepcidin also controls iron [34,56,73,80,162,165,166,181]. It may also serve as a pleiotropic sensor for other divalent metals, because it is up-regulated by exposure to other metals like copper [56] and cadmium [182], which can be considered waterborne or toxic.

5. Cathelicidins

Unusual among the AMPs, cathelicidins share little sequence homology between the mature peptides. Rather, they are defined by a homologous *N*-terminal region of the precursor peptide, called a cathelin domain, found just after a conserved signal domain (reviewed in [183]). The active, mature peptide is released upon protolytic cleavage by elastase and possibly other enzymes [184]. In mammals, the mature AMP sequence varies greatly, not only between species but also among the often multiple cathelicidin peptides within a single species. In general, however, all mammalian cathelicidin mature peptides are cationic and exhibit an amphipathic characteristic, as well as broad-spectrum antimicrobial activity *in vitro*. As can be seen by the alignment of primary amino acid sequences in Figure 4, there are significant sequence similarities in the C-terminal region, and in several short domains, which are highly cationic and glycine-rich.

The first cathelicidins identified in fish were initially isolated as antimicrobial peptides from the Atlantic hagfish, *Myxine glutinosa* [15]. Upon sequence analysis of the cDNA that encoded these peptides, it was discovered that they exhibited homology to cathelicidins, previously only found in mammals to this point. As cathelicidins were discovered in other more conventional fish species, primarily by sequence homology from the cathelin region (e.g., [17,28,77,185]), or more recently by peptide isolation [186], new patterns emerged. In some of the more recently studied fish cathelicidins, while a high degree of homology is maintained in the cathelin domain (see [185] for a comprehensive alignment), there appears to be a higher degree of sequence similarity of the mature peptide than seen in mammals. Thus, fish cathelicidins can now be subdivided into two classes—the linear peptides, and those that exhibit a characteristic disulphide bond. In contrast to mammalian cathelicidins, there is significant sequence homology among members of the classes (up to 90%), and little homology between the classes. In addition, the recently identified cathelicidins found in cod appear to comprise a third class, based on sequence homology between themselves, and a lack of homology with either of the other two classes [185]. An alignment of representative fish cathelicidins is shown in Figure 4.

```
                   10        20        30        40        50        60        70        80        90        100
AsCath1   RRSQARKCSRGN------GGKIGSIRCRGGG-------------TRLGGGSLIG---------RLRVALLLGVAPFLLDLSQINVMEIAFA-----------
AsCath2   RRGKPSGGSRGS------KMG--SKDSKGGWRG------------RPGSGS------------RPGFGSSIAGASG-RDQGGTRNA----------------
RtCath1   RRSKVRICSRGKNCVSRPGVGS-IIGRPGGGSL----------IGRPGGGSVIG---------RPGGGSPPGGGSFNDEFIRDHSDGNRFA-----------
RtCath2   RRGKDSGGPK---------MG--RKDSKGGWRG------------RPGSGS------------RPLGGSGIAGASG-GNHVGTLTASNSTTHPLDNCKISPQ
CsCath    RRGKDSGGS--------------RGSKMWGWRG------------RPGLRS------------RPLGGSGIAGASG-GNHVGTLTA----------------
BtrCath   RRSQARKCSRGN------GGG---IRCPGGG------------I-RLGGGSLIG---------RPKGGSPPGGGSFTAGFIRDQRDGNRFA-----------
AcCath    RRGKASGGSSDS------NMG--RRDSKGGRRG------------RPGSGS------------RPGFGSSIAGASG-VNHGGTRTA----------------
BtCath    RRGKASGGSSDS------NMG--RKDSKGGRRG------------RPGSGS------------RPGFGSSIAGASG-VNHGGTRTA----------------
CodCath2  RRSRSGRGSGKG------GRG-GSRESSGSRGS------------RGSKGS------------RGGLGSTIGRNLKKRRTCPVRPL----------------
CodCath1  RRSRSGRGSGKG------GRG-GSRGSSGSRGSKGPSGSRGSSGSRGSKGS---------RGGRSGRGSTIAGNGN-RNNGGTRTA----------------
CodCath3  RRSRSGRGSGKG------GRG-GSRGSSGSRGSKGPSGSRGSSGSRGSKGSSGSRGSKGSRGGRSGRGSTIAGNGN-RNNGGTR------------------
AyuCath   RRSKSGKGSG-G------SKGSGSKGSKGSKGS--------GSKGSGSKGG-----------SRPGGGSSIAGGGS-KGKGGTQTA----------------
JeCath    RRSKAGKGSG------------GNKGNKGSGGN------------KGNKGS------------RPGGGSSIAGRDK--GDSGTRTA----------------
```

Figure 4. Alignment of fish cathelicidins. Mature peptide sequences were obtained from published data and from the PubMed protein database, and were aligned using MacVector software. Characteristic cysteine residues found in certain classes of fish cathelicidins are underlined. As, Atlantic salmon; Rt, Rainbow trout; Cs, Chinook salmon; Btr, Brown trout; Ac, Arctic char; Bt, Brook trout; Je, Japanese eel.

As cathelicidin peptides are purified from more species, their *in vitro* antibacterial activities appear to exhibit significant variability with respect to selectivity, depending on the species. For example, cod cathelicidin (codCATH) is highly active against those Gram-negative bacterial species examined, but almost inactive against the Gram-positive species. It also exhibits potent antifungal activity against *C. albicans* [13]. In contrast, the hagfish cathelicidins are active against both Gram-positive and -negative bacteria, but inactive against Candida [15]. Even more specifically, rainbow trout cathelicidins are active against *Y. ruckeri*, while Atlantic salmon cathelicidins are not [187]. Thus, the variability in the mature peptide sequence of these molecules appears to direct the antimicrobial activities, and is probably a result of an evolutionary divergence to address specific pathogens.

Based on their antimicrobial activity, most of the work to elucidate their role *in vivo* has examined the expression of the cathelicidin genes in the various fish species with respect to induction by innate immune regulators, such as bacteria and to different pathogen-associated molecular patterns (PAMPs). Importantly, cathelicidin expression is observed early in embryonic development, suggesting that its role in immunity is present early on [186]. *In vitro*, both bacteria and bacterial DNA were sufficient to induce cathelicidin expression in a cultured embryonic salmon cell line [188], suggesting that like mammalian cathelicidins, the fish homologs play a similar role in antibacterial host defense. Surprisingly, purified LPS (that is, treated with DNase I) could not induce the gene. This regulation has been further elucidated by the demonstration of a wide variability of the Chinook salmon embryonic cell line's response to different bacteria and to poly I:C, LPS and flagellin [189]. Further *in vitro* evidence of this role was demonstrated by the induction of rainbow trout cathelicidin in a macrophage cell line from that species by IL-6, an important mediator of the innate immune response [190], and by a novel TNF-α isoform [191]. Similarly, stimulation of a cell line from Atlantic cod with poly I:C induced expression of the gmCath1 (from cod) gene promoter [192]. In addition to bacteria and their products, trout cell lines were shown to induce cathelicidin gene expression upon incubation with the oomycete *Saprolegnia parasitica* [193].

In vivo studies further support this hypothesis. When ayu were injected with live pathogenic bacteria, there was a time-dependent induction of cathelicidin expression in numerous tissues, including gill, liver, spleen and intestine [20]. Further, Atlantic salmon and rainbow trout infected with *Y. ruckeri* led to an induction in cathelicidin expression [187,194]. In the Atlantic cod, a difference in inducibility was observed. Cathelicidin experession in the gills was induced by a 3-h incubation with *Aeromonas salmonicida*, but not *V. anguillarum*, suggesting a more complex role is played by these peptides in host defense.

In mammals, cathelicidins have been demonstrated to exhibit multiple activities, both immune and non-immune, well in excess of their *in vitro* antimicrobial activities (reviewed in [195]). While research in fish has not approached this level, a recent study demonstrated that two Atlantic salmon cathelicidins induced the rapid and transient expression of IL-8 in peripheral blood leukocytes [187]. This suggests that the immunomodulatory activities seen by mammalian cathelicidins may be shared by their fish counterparts, and may thus be an evolutionarily conserved mechanism of innate immune regulation.

6. Histone-Derived Peptides

While examining an amphibian species for novel antimicrobial peptides, Park *et al.* [196] described a new peptide from the Asian toad, *Bufo bufo gargarizans*, which they called Buforin I. This turned out to be identical to the *N*-terminal portion of histone 2A. This led to the demonstration of antimicrobial activity of histone fragments from numerous species (reviewed in [197]), suggesting that these proteolytic fragments are part of an ancient innate immune mechanism. Histone-derived AMPs have been identified in a number of fish species, with broad-spectrum activity against both human and fish pathogens (reviewed in [198]), including water molds [199] and a parasitic dinoflagellate [69]. They are expressed and secreted in fish skin, and found in other tissues, including gill, speen and the gut. They are not limited to the *N*-terminus of the histones, as was found for the Buforin peptide, but can be found as fragments of both termini, from histones H1, H2A, H2B and H6 (see Figure 5). Further evidence that they play a role in host defense of the fish comes from studies showing that expression of histone-derived AMP genes are induced under conditions of stress in specific tissues of different fish species [74,200].

```
                                         10        20        30        40        50        60        70
Rainbow trout oncorhyncin III (H6)   MPKRKSATKGDEPARRSARLSARPVPKPAAKPKKAAAPKKAVKGKKAAENGDAKAEAKVQAAGDGAGNAK
Halibut hipposin {H2A}               .SG-----R.KTGG.--------ARA.AKTRSSR.GLQFP--V.RVHRLLRKGNYAHR---V.A..PVYL
Atlantic salmon H1                   .AEVAP.PAAAA..K-------A.KK.A......G-.S---V.ELIVKAVS.SK.R----S.VSLAAL.
```

Figure 5. Alignment of histone-derived peptides. Representative peptide sequences were obtained from published data and from the PubMed protein database, and were aligned using MacVector software. Since the sequences are homolgous to different histone peptide fragments, there is no shared sequence homology.

7. Therapeutics

All AMPs have common characteristics that support their development as therapeutic antimicrobials. These include broad-spectrum activity against a wide variety of pathogens; potent activity under a wide range of conditions, including temperature and in secretions such as saliva; and a reduced capacity to the development of resistance by bacteria. The identification and characterization of peptides from fish has provided a unique contribution in this arena. While the structural characteristics of fish peptides do not appear particularly different from their mammalian, insect or amphibian homologues, there may be specific differences with respect to activity. It appears that overall their antimicrobial activities against human pathogens is in the same range as AMPs from other species. However, it is possible that they are more active against fish pathogens, as they most likely have evolved together with those pathogens. It is difficult to know this, however, as few studies have compared non-fish peptides with fish peptides against fish pathogens. One area where fish peptides may provide an advantage is in food preservation [201], as they are derived from a natural food source, and thus may be more amenable to being consumed.

Since many AMPs are sensitive to high salt concentrations [202–204], the ability of some fish AMPs to kill microbes even at extremely high salt concentrations, such as those found in the marine environment, make them important targets for investigation. Pleurocidin, for example, maintains its antibacterial activity even up to 300 mM NaCl [6], similar to other piscidins [41,205]. Understanding the structural foundation that supports this salt-independent activity could aid in the design of novel peptides [206] or mimetics that could address infections under a wide range of normal and abnormal salt concentrations, whether in serum, tear film hyperosmolarity, or in saliva to address dental caries [207]. In addition to their potential uses as antimicrobials, some fish AMPs have been observed to exhibit *in vitro* cytotoxic activity against a variety of cancer cells [113,208].

Different applications of piscidin have been promising. For example, epinecidin-1, when administrated orally or injected (in pre-, co- and post-infection) can significantly enhance survival in zebrafish and grouper that were challenged with *Vibrio vulnificus* [58,123,124]. Related to this, electrotransfer of epinecidin-1 in zebrafish and grouper muscle showed significant reduction in *V. vulnificus* and *Streptococcus agalactiae* bacterial counts [121,122,125]. Moreover, treatment of lethally-challenged methicillin-resistant *S. aureus* (MRSA) mice with epinecidin-1 allowed mice to survive by decreasing considerably the bacterial counts, where also there was evidence of wound closure and angiogenesis enhancement [128].

In oral disease treatment piscidins are also promising due to the potent effect of chrysophsin-1 in killing the cariogenic pathogen *Streptococcus mutans* [209]. Furthermore, pleurocidin also demonstrated anti-cariogenic activity by being able to kill both *S. mutans* and *S. sobrinus*, where killing of biofilms occurred in a dose-dependent manner. In addition, it showed to retained its activity in physiological or higher salt concentration, and was relatively stable in presence of human saliva and no hemolysis was found [207,210].

Epinecidin-1 showed to be a potential candidate for topical application that can prevent vaginal or skin infections due to the synergistic effect that possess with commercial cleaning solutions, where such effect was not affected by low pH or after being stored at room temperature and at 4 °C for up to 14 days [211]. The synergistic effect of pleurocidin and several antibiotics [212], bacteroricin [213] and histone-derived [214] has also been shown [212,213]. Furthermore, the creation of antimicrobial surfaces has been made by the immobilization of chrysophsin-1 resulting in a surface with antibacterial activity capable to killed around 82% of *E. coli* bacteria [215].

A recent interest finding is the ability of epinecidin-1 to create inactivated virus for vaccination purposes. Huang *et al.* found that mice injected with Epi-1-based inactivated Japanese encephalitis virus (JEV) reached 100% survival (in a dose-dependent manner), and the performance was better than the formalin-based JEV-inactivated vaccine. This was caused by the modulation of immune-related genes, including the increase of anti-JEV-neutralizing antibodies in serum, which suppressed the multiplication of JEV in brain sections [126].

Fish hepcidins are also under examination for development as therapeutics. One example of this is the study carried out by Pan *et al.* [216], where injections with pre-incubated tilapia hepcidin TH2-3 and 10^8 cfu of *Vibrio vulnificus* for 30 min enhanced the survival of infected and re-infected mice, obtaining up to 60% of survival with a dose of 40 μg/mice. In addition, TH2-3 also showed significant prophylactic effect by administration prior infection, where survival rates of 100% were obtained after 7 days of infection. Also, curative effects were shown when fish were first infected and later injected with 40 μg/mice of TH2-3, obtaining survival rates up to 50%. But more interesting, was the fact that TH2-3 had better bacteriostatic effect than tetracycline in controlling the bacterial burden in blood, although in liver there was no significant difference, demonstrating the capacity of TH2-3 to control multiplication of *V. vulnificus* in mice. Although the direct *in vivo* TH2-3-mediated killing was not confirmed, a microarray analysis showed that TH2-3 clearly altered the gene expression profiles improving the host response in mice [216]. In addition, a transgenic zebrafish expressing TH2-3 showed to be able to decrease *V. vulnificus* burden significantly, but not *S. agalactiae* [177]. Zebrafish expressing TH1-5 exhibited enhanced bacterial resistance by decreasing the bacterial burden of both same pathogens [176]. In addition, TH1-5 has showed to be effective at increasing survival and decreasing the number of infectious bacteria in ducks challenged with *Riemerella anatipestifer*, which also showed to be able to modulate the expression of immune-related genes [114].

However, as with other AMPs, they share the similar problems that hinder their further development, especially for use in human medicine. These include a tendency to be inactivated in the body, increased expense of peptide synthesis, and sensitivity to protease digestion. Attempts to address these issues with fish peptides, include the identification of smaller peptide fragments that might exhibit better activity with smaller molecules [217], and the observation of high levels of synergy with bacterial AMPs [213,214], as well as conventional antibiotics [218] allowing for reduced concentrations. One strategy that may have some success is the design of small molecule peptide mimetics that incorporate the structural characteristics of the peptides necessary for their activity (reviewed in [219]). Initial *in vitro* and *in vivo* results with molecules designed from magainins and defensins have been encouraging, demonstrating antibacterial [220] and antifungal [221] activities, as well as immunomodulatory activity [222]. Another strategy that has been examined extensively in other species (reviewed in [223]) is the use of exogenous agents to modulate the expression of endogenous AMPs in the fish. Terova *et al.* have demonstrated the induction of an AMP initially isolated from sea bass [33] by feeding them a cell wall extract from *S. cerevisiae* [224], suggesting a novel method for enhancing the natural defense mechanism of the fish. Incorporation of an enhancer of AMP expression in the diet could be a cost-effective part of an overall strategy of modulating the innate immune system of the fish to control infection in aquaculture (reviewed in [198]).

8. Conclusions

The comprehensive characterization of AMPs from fish, on the structural, genetic and functional levels, has provided a wealth of information. Examination of AMPs in a single species, such as the Atlantic cod, where members of all five groups of AMPs have been identified can help understand the role of these peptides in innate host defense of the fish. Studies on the similarities and differences with peptides from non-fish species contribute to our understanding of the evolutionary relationships of innate host defense mechanisms among vertebrates. Furthermore, they can provide important information for the better design of novel therapeutic agents, both for microbial infections as well as cancer and other conditions. Unique for the field of fish AMPs is the potential application to aquaculture. The constant risk of large-scale microbial infection that can lead to significant economic losses demands new strategies to prevent or treat these pathogens. Many of the studies described above have demonstrated that specific fish AMPs have potent activity against fish pathogens. Furthermore, other studies have shown that some pathogens induce potent innate immune responses in the fish. Complicating this is the evolutionary battle with the pathogens. For example, challenge of Atlantic cod with the pathogen *V. anguillarum* induces the expression of a β-defensin, which is antibacterial against other species, but not the inducing *V. anguillarum* [11]. Thus, the large body of work described above provides a solid foundation for strong future work to better understand both the role of these peptides in host defense of the fish, as well as the development of these peptides and their derivatives as potential therapeutics.

Acknowledgments: GD is funded by US Public Health Service Grants R01 DE22723 and R21 AI100379.

Author Contributions: Both authors contributed to the writing and editing of this review

Conflicts of Interest: The authors declare no conflict of interest.

References

1. Ganz, T.; Selsted, M.E.; Szklarek, D.; Harwig, S.S.; Daher, K.; Bainton, D.F.; Lehrer, R.I. Defensins. Natural peptide antibiotics of human neutrophils. *J. Clin. Investig.* **1985**, *76*, 1427–1435. [CrossRef]
2. Lehrer, R.I.; Selsted, M.E.; Szklarek, D.; Fleischmann, J. Antibacterial activity of microbicidal cationic proteins 1 and 2, natural peptide antibiotics of rabbit lung macrophages. *Infect. Immun.* **1983**, *42*, 10–14.
3. Zasloff, M. Magainins, a class of antimicrobial peptides from Xenopus skin: Isolation, characterization of two active forms, and partial cDNA sequence of a precursor. *Proc. Natl. Acad. Sci. USA* **1987**, *84*, 5449–5453. [CrossRef]
4. Primor, N.; Tu, A.T. Conformation of pardaxin, the toxin of the flatfish Pardachirus marmoratus. *Biochim. Biophys. Acta* **1980**, *626*, 299–306. [CrossRef]
5. Oren, Z.; Shai, Y. A class of highly potent antibacterial peptides derived from pardaxin, a pore-forming peptide isolated from Moses sole fish Pardachirus marmoratus. *Eur. J. Biochem.* **1996**, *237*, 303–310.
6. Cole, A.M.; Weis, P.; Diamond, G. Isolation and characterization of pleurocidin, an antimicrobial peptide in the skin secretions of winter flounder. *J. Biol. Chem.* **1997**, *272*, 12008–12013. [CrossRef]
7. Tessera, V.; Guida, F.; Juretic, D.; Tossi, A. Identification of antimicrobial peptides from teleosts and anurans in expressed sequence tag databases using conserved signal sequences. *FEBS J.* **2012**, *279*, 724–736. [CrossRef]
8. Patrzykat, A.; Gallant, J.W.; Seo, J.K.; Pytyck, J.; Douglas, S.E. Novel antimicrobial peptides derived from flatfish genes. *Antimicrob. Agents Chemother.* **2003**, *47*, 2464–2470. [CrossRef]
9. Xu, Q.; Cheng, C.H.; Hu, P.; Ye, H.; Chen, Z.; Cao, L.; Chen, L.; Shen, Y.; Chen, L. Adaptive evolution of hepcidin genes in antarctic notothenioid fishes. *Mol. Biol. Evol.* **2008**, *25*, 1099–1112. [CrossRef]
10. Browne, M.J.; Feng, C.Y.; Booth, V.; Rise, M.L. Characterization and expression studies of Gaduscidin-1 and Gaduscidin-2; paralogous antimicrobial peptide-like transcripts from Atlantic cod (Gadus morhua). *Dev. Comp. Immunol.* **2011**, *35*, 399–408. [CrossRef]
11. Ruangsri, J.; Kitani, Y.; Kiron, V.; Lokesh, J.; Brinchmann, M.F.; Karlsen, B.O.; Fernandes, J.M. A novel beta-defensin antimicrobial peptide in Atlantic cod with stimulatory effect on phagocytic activity. *PLoS One* **2013**, *8*, e62302.
12. Solstad, T.; Larsen, A.N.; Seppola, M.; Jorgensen, T.O. Identification, cloning and expression analysis of a hepcidin cDNA of the Atlantic cod (*Gadus morhua* L.). *Fish Shellfish Immunol.* **2008**, *25*, 298–310. [CrossRef]
13. Broekman, D.C.; Zenz, A.; Gudmundsdottir, B.K.; Lohner, K.; Maier, V.H.; Gudmundsson, G.H. Functional characterization of codCath, the mature cathelicidin antimicrobial peptide from Atlantic cod (Gadus morhua). *Peptides* **2011**, *32*, 2044–2051. [CrossRef]

14. Bergsson, G.; Agerberth, B.; Jornvall, H.; Gudmundsson, G.H. Isolation and identification of antimicrobial components from the epidermal mucus of Atlantic cod (Gadus morhua). *FEBS J.* **2005**, *272*, 4960–4969. [CrossRef]
15. Uzzell, T.; Stolzenberg, E.D.; Shinnar, A.E.; Zasloff, M. Hagfish intestinal antimicrobial peptides are ancient cathelicidins. *Peptides* **2003**, *24*, 1655–1667. [CrossRef]
16. Douglas, S.E.; Gallant, J.W.; Liebscher, R.S.; Dacanay, A.; Tsoi, S.C. Identification and expression analysis of hepcidin-like antimicrobial peptides in bony fish. *Dev. Comp. Immunol.* **2003**, *27*, 589–601. [CrossRef]
17. Chang, C.I.; Zhang, Y.A.; Zou, J.; Nie, P.; Secombes, C.J. Two cathelicidin genes are present in both rainbow trout (Oncorhynchus mykiss) and atlantic salmon (Salmo salar). *Antimicrob. Agents Chemother.* **2006**, *50*, 185–195. [CrossRef]
18. Richards, R.C.; O'Neil, D.B.; Thibault, P.; Ewart, K.V. Histone H1: An antimicrobial protein of Atlantic salmon (Salmo salar). *Biochem. Biophys. Res. Commun.* **2001**, *284*, 549–555. [CrossRef]
19. Chen, M.Z.; Chen, J.; Lu, X.J.; Shi, Y.H. Molecular cloning, sequence analysis and expression pattern of hepcidin gene in ayu (Plecoglossus altivelis). *Dongwuxue Yanjiu* **2010**, *31*, 595–600.
20. Lu, X.J.; Chen, J.; Huang, Z.A.; Shi, Y.H.; Lv, J.N. Identification and characterization of a novel cathelicidin from ayu, Plecoglossus altivelis. *Fish Shellfish Immunol.* **2011**, *31*, 52–57. [CrossRef]
21. Barnes, A.C.; Trewin, B.; Snape, N.; Kvennefors, E.C.; Baiano, J.C. Two hepcidin-like antimicrobial peptides in Barramundi Lates calcarifer exhibit differing tissue tropism and are induced in response to lipopolysaccharide. *Fish Shellfish Immunol.* **2011**, *31*, 350–357. [CrossRef]
22. Yang, M.; Wang, K.J.; Chen, J.H.; Qu, H.D.; Li, S.J. Genomic organization and tissue-specific expression analysis of hepcidin-like genes from black porgy (Acanthopagrus schlegelii B). *Fish Shellfish Immunol.* **2007**, *23*, 1060–1071. [CrossRef]
23. Yang, M.; Chen, B.; Cai, J.J.; Peng, H.; Ling, C.; Yuan, J.J.; Wang, K.J. Molecular characterization of hepcidin AS-hepc2 and AS-hepc6 in black porgy (Acanthopagrus schlegelii): Expression pattern responded to bacterial challenge and *in vitro* antimicrobial activity. *Comp. Biochem. Physiol. B Biochem. Mol. Biol.* **2011**, *158*, 155–163. [CrossRef]
24. Kim, Y.O.; Park, E.M.; Nam, B.H.; Kong, H.J.; Kim, W.J.; Lee, S.J. Identification and molecular characterization of two hepcidin genes from black rockfish (*Sebastes schlegelii*). *Mol. Cell. Biochem.* **2008**, *315*, 131–136. [CrossRef]
25. Gong, L.C.; Wang, H.; Deng, L. Molecular characterization, phylogeny and expression of a hepcidin gene in the blotched snakehead *Channa maculata*. *Dev. Comp. Immunol.* **2014**, *44*, 1–11. [CrossRef]
26. Bao, B.; Peatman, E.; Li, P.; He, C.; Liu, Z. Catfish hepcidin gene is expressed in a wide range of tissues and exhibits tissue-specific upregulation after bacterial infection. *Dev. Comp. Immunol.* **2005**, *29*, 939–950. [CrossRef]
27. Liang, T.; Ji, W.; Zhang, G.R.; Wei, K.J.; Feng, K.; Wang, W.M.; Zou, G.W. Molecular cloning and expression analysis of liver-expressed antimicrobial peptide 1 (LEAP-1) and LEAP-2 genes in the blunt snout bream (*Megalobrama amblycephala*). *Fish Shellfish Immunol.* **2013**, *35*, 553–563. [CrossRef]
28. Scocchi, M.; Pallavicini, A.; Salgaro, R.; Bociek, K.; Gennaro, R. The salmonid cathelicidins: A gene family with highly varied C-terminal antimicrobial domains. *Comp. Biochem. Physiol. B Biochem. Mol. Biol.* **2009**, *152*, 376–381. [CrossRef]
29. Park, I.Y.; Park, C.B.; Kim, M.S.; Kim, S.C. Parasin I, an antimicrobial peptide derived from histone H2A in the catfish, Parasilurus asotus. *FEBS Lett.* **1998**, *437*, 258–262. [CrossRef]
30. Chen, Y.; Zhao, H.; Zhang, X.; Luo, H.; Xue, X.; Li, Z.; Yao, B. Identification, expression and bioactivity of Paramisgurnus dabryanus beta-defensin that might be involved in immune defense against bacterial infection. *Fish Shellfish Immunol.* **2013**, *35*, 399–406. [CrossRef]
31. Marel, M.; Adamek, M.; Gonzalez, S.F.; Frost, P.; Rombout, J.H.; Wiegertjes, G.F.; Savelkoul, H.F.; Steinhagen, D. Molecular cloning and expression of two beta-defensin and two mucin genes in common carp (*Cyprinus carpio* L.) and their up-regulation after beta-glucan feeding. *Fish Shellfish Immunol.* **2012**, *32*, 494–501. [CrossRef]
32. Li, H.; Zhang, F.; Guo, H.; Zhu, Y.; Yuan, J.; Yang, G.; An, L. Molecular characterization of hepcidin gene in common carp (*Cyprinus carpio* L.) and its expression pattern responding to bacterial challenge. *Fish Shellfish Immunol.* **2013**, *35*, 1030–1038. [CrossRef]

33. Salerno, G.; Parrinello, N.; Roch, P.; Cammarata, M. cDNA sequence and tissue expression of an antimicrobial peptide, dicentracin; a new component of the moronecidin family isolated from head kidney leukocytes of sea bass, Dicentrarchus labrax. *Comp. Biochem. Physiol. B Biochem. Mol. Biol.* **2007**, *146*, 521–529. [CrossRef]
34. Rodrigues, P.N.; Vazquez-Dorado, S.; Neves, J.V.; Wilson, J.M. Dual function of fish hepcidin: Response to experimental iron overload and bacterial infection in sea bass (Dicentrarchus labrax). *Dev. Comp. Immunol.* **2006**, *30*, 1156–1167. [CrossRef]
35. Cuesta, A.; Meseguer, J.; Esteban, M.A. Molecular and functional characterization of the gilthead seabream beta-defensin demonstrate its chemotactic and antimicrobial activity. *Mol. Immunol.* **2011**, *48*, 1432–1438. [CrossRef]
36. Cuesta, A.; Meseguer, J.; Esteban, M.A. The antimicrobial peptide hepcidin exerts an important role in the innate immunity against bacteria in the bony fish gilthead seabream. *Mol. Immunol.* **2008**, *45*, 2333–2342. [CrossRef]
37. Wang, Y.; Liu, X.; Ma, L.; Yu, Y.; Yu, H.; Mohammed, S.; Chu, G.; Mu, L.; Zhang, Q. Identification and characterization of a hepcidin from half-smooth tongue sole Cynoglossus semilaevis. *Fish Shellfish Immunol.* **2012**, *33*, 213–219. [CrossRef]
38. Birkemo, G.A.; Luders, T.; Andersen, O.; Nes, I.F.; Nissen-Meyer, J. Hipposin, a histone-derived antimicrobial peptide in Atlantic halibut (*Hippoglossus hippoglossus* L.). *Biochim. Biophys. Acta* **2003**, *1646*, 207–215. [CrossRef]
39. Salger, S.A.; Reading, B.J.; Baltzegar, D.A.; Sullivan, C.V.; Noga, E.J. Molecular characterization of two isoforms of piscidin 4 from the hybrid striped bass (Morone chrysops x *Morone saxatilis*). *Fish Shellfish Immunol.* **2011**, *30*, 420–424. [CrossRef]
40. Noga, E.J.; Silphaduang, U.; Park, N.G.; Seo, J.K.; Stephenson, J.; Kozlowicz, S. Piscidin 4, a novel member of the piscidin family of antimicrobial peptides. *Comp. Biochem. Physiol. B Biochem. Mol. Biol.* **2009**, *152*, 299–305. [CrossRef]
41. Lauth, X.; Shike, H.; Burns, J.C.; Westerman, M.E.; Ostland, V.E.; Carlberg, J.M.; van Olst, J.C.; Nizet, V.; Taylor, S.W.; Shimizu, C.; *et al.* Discovery and characterization of two isoforms of moronecidin, a novel antimicrobial peptide from hybrid striped bass. *J. Biol. Chem.* **2002**, *277*, 5030–5039. [CrossRef]
42. Shike, H.; Lauth, X.; Westerman, M.E.; Ostland, V.E.; Carlberg, J.M.; van Olst, J.C.; Shimizu, C.; Bulet, P.; Burns, J.C. Bass hepcidin is a novel antimicrobial peptide induced by bacterial challenge. *Eur. J. Biochem.* **2002**, *269*, 2232–2237. [CrossRef]
43. Buonocore, F.; Randelli, E.; Casani, D.; Picchietti, S.; Belardinelli, M.C.; de Pascale, D.; de Santi, C.; Scapigliati, G. A piscidin-like antimicrobial peptide from the icefish Chionodraco hamatus (Perciformes: Channichthyidae): Molecular characterization, localization and bactericidal activity. *Fish Shellfish Immunol.* **2012**, *33*, 1183–1191. [CrossRef]
44. Zou, J.; Mercier, C.; Koussounadis, A.; Secombes, C. Discovery of multiple beta-defensin like homologues in teleost fish. *Mol. Immunol.* **2007**, *44*, 638–647. [CrossRef]
45. Ren, H.L.; Wang, K.J.; Zhou, H.L.; Yang, M. Cloning and organisation analysis of a hepcidin-like gene and cDNA from Japan sea bass, Lateolabrax japonicus. *Fish Shellfish Immunol.* **2006**, *21*, 221–227. [CrossRef]
46. Robertson, L.S.; Iwanowicz, L.R.; Marranca, J.M. Identification of centrarchid hepcidins and evidence that 17beta-estradiol disrupts constitutive expression of hepcidin-1 and inducible expression of hepcidin-2 in largemouth bass (*Micropterus salmoides*). *Fish Shellfish Immunol.* **2009**, *26*, 898–907. [CrossRef]
47. Niu, S.F.; Jin, Y.; Xu, X.; Qiao, Y.; Wu, Y.; Mao, Y.; Su, Y.Q.; Wang, J. Characterization of a novel piscidin-like antimicrobial peptide from Pseudosciaena crocea and its immune response to *Cryptocaryon irritans*. *Fish Shellfish Immunol.* **2013**, *35*, 513–524. [CrossRef]
48. Wang, K.J.; Cai, J.J.; Cai, L.; Qu, H.D.; Yang, M.; Zhang, M. Cloning and expression of a hepcidin gene from a marine fish (*Pseudosciaena crocea*) and the antimicrobial activity of its synthetic peptide. *Peptides* **2009**, *30*, 638–646. [CrossRef]
49. Zhang, J.; Yan, Q.; Ji, R.; Zou, W.; Guo, G. Isolation and characterization of a hepcidin peptide from the head kidney of large yellow croaker, *Pseudosciaena crocea. Fish Shellfish Immunol.* **2009**, *26*, 864–870. [CrossRef]
50. Sun, B.J.; Xie, H.X.; Song, Y.; Nie, P. Gene structure of an antimicrobial peptide from mandarin fish, *Siniperca chuatsi* (Basilewsky), suggests that moronecidins and pleurocidins belong in one family: The piscidins. *J. Fish Dis.* **2007**, *30*, 335–343. [CrossRef]

51. Wang, G.; Li, J.; Zou, P.; Xie, H.; Huang, B.; Nie, P.; Chang, M. Expression pattern, promoter activity and bactericidal property of beta-defensin from the mandarin fish Siniperca chuatsi. *Fish Shellfish Immunol.* **2012**, *33*, 522–531. [CrossRef]
52. Zhao, J.G.; Zhou, L.; Jin, J.Y.; Zhao, Z.; Lan, J.; Zhang, Y.B.; Zhang, Q.Y.; Gui, J.F. Antimicrobial activity-specific to Gram-negative bacteria and immune modulation-mediated NF-kappaB and Sp1 of a medaka beta-defensin. *Dev. Comp. Immunol.* **2009**, *33*, 624–637.
53. Bo, J.; Cai, L.; Xu, J.H.; Wang, K.J.; Au, D.W. The marine medaka Oryzias melastigma—A potential marine fish model for innate immune study. *Mar. Pollut. Bull.* **2011**, *63*, 267–276. [CrossRef]
54. Xu, T.; Sun, Y.; Shi, G.; Wang, R. Miiuy croaker hepcidin gene and comparative analyses reveal evidence for positive selection. *PLoS One* **2012**, *7*, e35449.
55. Brocal, I.; Falco, A.; Mas, V.; Rocha, A.; Perez, L.; Coll, J.M.; Estepa, A. Stable expression of bioactive recombinant pleurocidin in a fish cell line. *Appl. Microbiol. Biotechnol.* **2006**, *72*, 1217–1228. [CrossRef]
56. Nam, Y.K.; Cho, Y.S.; Lee, S.Y.; Kim, B.S.; Kim, D.S. Molecular characterization of hepcidin gene from mud loach (*Misgurnus mizolepis*; Cypriniformes). *Fish Shellfish Immunol.* **2011**, *31*, 1251–1258. [CrossRef]
57. Nam, B.H.; Moon, J.Y.; Kim, Y.O.; Kong, H.J.; Kim, W.J.; Lee, S.J.; Kim, K.K. Multiple beta-defensin isoforms identified in early developmental stages of the teleost Paralichthys olivaceus. *Fish Shellfish Immunol.* **2010**, *28*, 267–274. [CrossRef]
58. Pan, C.Y.; Chen, J.Y.; Cheng, Y.S.; Chen, C.Y.; Ni, I.H.; Sheen, J.F.; Pan, Y.L.; Kuo, C.M. Gene expression and localization of the epinecidin-1 antimicrobial peptide in the grouper (*Epinephelus coioides*), and its role in protecting fish against pathogenic infection. *DNA Cell Biol.* **2007**, *26*, 403–413. [CrossRef]
59. Guo, M.; Wei, J.; Huang, X.; Huang, Y.; Qin, Q. Antiviral effects of beta-defensin derived from orange-spotted grouper (*Epinephelus coioides*). *Fish Shellfish Immunol.* **2012**, *32*, 828–838. [CrossRef]
60. Jin, J.Y.; Zhou, L.; Wang, Y.; Li, Z.; Zhao, J.G.; Zhang, Q.Y.; Gui, J.F. Antibacterial and antiviral roles of a fish beta-defensin expressed both in pituitary and testis. *PLoS One* **2010**, *5*, e12883.
61. Zhou, J.G.; Wei, J.G.; Xu, D.; Cui, H.C.; Yan, Y.; Ou-Yang, Z.L.; Huang, X.H.; Huang, Y.H.; Qin, Q.W. Molecular cloning and characterization of two novel hepcidins from orange-spotted grouper, *Epinephelus coioides*. *Fish Shellfish Immunol.* **2011**, *30*, 559–568. [CrossRef]
62. Qu, H.; Chen, B.; Peng, H.; Wang, K. Molecular cloning, recombinant expression, and antimicrobial activity of EC-hepcidin3, a new four-cysteine hepcidin isoform from *Epinephelus coioides*. *Biosci. Biotechnol. Biochem.* **2013**, *77*, 103–110. [CrossRef]
63. Masso-Silva, J.; Diamond, G.; Macias-Rodriguez, M.; Ascencio, F. Genomic organization and tissue-specific expression of hepcidin in the pacific mutton hamlet, Alphestes immaculatus (Breder, 1936). *Fish Shellfish Immunol.* **2011**, *31*, 1297–1302. [CrossRef]
64. Falco, A.; Chico, V.; Marroqui, L.; Perez, L.; Coll, J.M.; Estepa, A. Expression and antiviral activity of a beta-defensin-like peptide identified in the rainbow trout (*Oncorhynchus mykiss*) EST sequences. *Mol. Immunol.* **2008**, *45*, 757–765.
65. Casadei, E.; Wang, T.; Zou, J.; Gonzalez Vecino, J.L.; Wadsworth, S.; Secombes, C.J. Characterization of three novel beta-defensin antimicrobial peptides in rainbow trout (*Oncorhynchus mykiss*). *Mol. Immunol.* **2009**, *46*, 3358–3366. [CrossRef]
66. Fernandes, J.M.; Kemp, G.D.; Molle, M.G.; Smith, V.J. Anti-microbial properties of histone H2A from skin secretions of rainbow trout, *Oncorhynchus mykiss*. *Biochem. J.* **2002**, *368*, 611–620. [CrossRef]
67. Fernandes, J.M.; Molle, G.; Kemp, G.D.; Smith, V.J. Isolation and characterisation of oncorhyncin II, a histone H1-derived antimicrobial peptide from skin secretions of rainbow trout, *Oncorhynchus mykiss*. *Dev. Comp. Immunol.* **2004**, *28*, 127–138. [CrossRef]
68. Fernandes, J.M.; Saint, N.; Kemp, G.D.; Smith, V.J. Oncorhyncin III: A potent antimicrobial peptide derived from the non-histone chromosomal protein H6 of rainbow trout, *Oncorhynchus mykiss*. *Biochem. J.* **2003**, *373*, 621–628. [CrossRef]
69. Noga, E.J.; Fan, Z.; Silphaduang, U. Histone-like proteins from fish are lethal to the parasitic dinoflagellate *Amyloodinium ocellatum*. *Parasitology* **2001**, *123*, 57–65.
70. Martin-Antonio, B.; Jimenez-Cantizano, R.M.; Salas-Leiton, E.; Infante, C.; Manchado, M. Genomic characterization and gene expression analysis of four hepcidin genes in the redbanded seabream (*Pagrus auriga*). *Fish Shellfish Immunol.* **2009**, *26*, 483–491. [CrossRef]

71. Iijima, N.; Tanimoto, N.; Emoto, Y.; Morita, Y.; Uematsu, K.; Murakami, T.; Nakai, T. Purification and characterization of three isoforms of chrysophsin, a novel antimicrobial peptide in the gills of the red sea bream, *Chrysophrys major*. *Eur. J. Biochem.* **2003**, *270*, 675–686. [CrossRef]
72. Chen, S.L.; Xu, M.Y.; Ji, X.S.; Yu, G.C.; Liu, Y. Cloning, characterization, and expression analysis of hepcidin gene from red sea bream (*Chrysophrys major*). *Antimicrob. Agents Chemother.* **2005**, *49*, 1608–1612. [CrossRef]
73. Cho, Y.S.; Lee, S.Y.; Kim, K.H.; Kim, S.K.; Kim, D.S.; Nam, Y.K. Gene structure and differential modulation of multiple rockbream (*Oplegnathus fasciatus*) hepcidin isoforms resulting from different biological stimulations. *Dev. Comp. Immunol.* **2009**, *33*, 46–58. [CrossRef]
74. Terova, G.; Cattaneo, A.G.; Preziosa, E.; Bernardini, G.; Saroglia, M. Impact of acute stress on antimicrobial polypeptides mRNA copy number in several tissues of marine sea bass (*Dicentrarchus labrax*). *BMC Immunol.* **2011**, *12*, 69. [CrossRef]
75. Sun, D.; Wu, S.; Jing, C.; Zhang, N.; Liang, D.; Xu, A. Identification, synthesis and characterization of a novel antimicrobial peptide HKPLP derived from *Hippocampus kuda* Bleeker. *J. Antibiot. (Tokyo)* **2012**, *65*, 117–121. [CrossRef]
76. Chaturvedi, P.; Dhanik, M.; Pande, A. Characterization and structural analysis of hepcidin like antimicrobial peptide from schizothorax richardsonii (Gray). *Protein J.* **2014**, *33*, 1–10. [CrossRef]
77. Li, Z.; Zhang, S.; Gao, J.; Guang, H.; Tian, Y.; Zhao, Z.; Wang, Y.; Yu, H. Structural and functional characterization of CATH_BRALE, the defense molecule in the ancient salmonoid, *Brachymystax lenok*. *Fish Shellfish Immunol.* **2013**, *34*, 1–7. [CrossRef]
78. Peng, K.C.; Lee, S.H.; Hour, A.-L.; Pan, C.Y.; Lee, L.H.; Chen, J. Five different piscidins from nile tilapia, oreochromis niloticus: Analysis of their expressions and biological functions. *PLoS One* **2012**, *7*, e50263.
79. Huang, P.H.; Chen, J.Y.; Kuo, C.M. Three different hepcidins from tilapia, Oreochromis mossambicus: Analysis of their expressions and biological functions. *Mol. Immunol.* **2007**, *44*, 1922–1934. [CrossRef]
80. Pereiro, P.; Figueras, A.; Novoa, B. A novel hepcidin-like in turbot (*Scophthalmus maximus* L.) highly expressed after pathogen challenge but not after iron overload. *Fish Shellfish Immunol.* **2012**, *32*, 879–889. [CrossRef]
81. Chen, S.L.; Li, W.; Meng, L.; Sha, Z.X.; Wang, Z.J.; Ren, G.C. Molecular cloning and expression analysis of a hepcidin antimicrobial peptide gene from turbot (*Scophthalmus maximus*). *Fish Shellfish Immunol.* **2007**, *22*, 172–181. [CrossRef]
82. Cole, A.M.; Darouiche, R.O.; Legarda, D.; Connell, N.; Diamond, G. Characterization of a fish antimicrobial peptide: Gene expression, subcellular localization, and spectrum of activity. *Antimicrob. Agents Chemother.* **2000**, *44*, 2039–2045. [CrossRef]
83. Douglas, S.E.; Patrzykat, A.; Pytyck, J.; Gallant, J.W. Identification, structure and differential expression of novel pleurocidins clustered on the genome of the winter flounder, *Pseudopleuronectes americanus* (Walbaum). *Eur. J. Biochem.* **2003**, *270*, 3720–3730. [CrossRef]
84. Shike, H.; Shimizu, C.; Lauth, X.; Burns, J.C. Organization and expression analysis of the zebrafish hepcidin gene, an antimicrobial peptide gene conserved among vertebrates. *Dev. Comp. Immunol.* **2004**, *28*, 747–754. [CrossRef]
85. Tamang, D.G.; Saier, M.H., Jr. The cecropin superfamily of toxic peptides. *J. Mol. Microbiol. Biotechnol.* **2006**, *11*, 94–103. [CrossRef]
86. Park, C.B.; Lee, J.H.; Park, I.Y.; Kim, M.S.; Kim, S.C. A novel antimicrobial peptide from the loach, *Misgurnus anguillicaudatus*. *FEBS Lett.* **1997**, *411*, 173–178. [CrossRef]
87. Silphaduang, U.; Noga, E.J. Peptide antibiotics in mast cells of fish. *Nature* **2001**, *414*, 268–269. [CrossRef]
88. Silphaduang, U.; Colorni, A.; Noga, E.J. Evidence for widespread distribution of piscidin antimicrobial peptides in teleost fish. *Dis. Aquat. Org.* **2006**, *72*, 241–252. [CrossRef]
89. Pan, C.Y.; Chen, J.Y.; Ni, I.H.; Wu, J.L.; Kuo, C.M. Organization and promoter analysis of the grouper (*Epinephelus coioides*) epinecidin-1 gene. *Comp. Biochem. Physiol. B Biochem. Mol. Biol.* **2008**, *150*, 358–367. [CrossRef]
90. Syvitski, R.T.; Burton, I.; Mattatall, N.R.; Douglas, S.E.; Jakeman, D.L. Structural characterization of the antimicrobial peptide pleurocidin from winter flounder. *Biochemistry* **2005**, *44*, 7282–7293. [CrossRef]
91. Fernandes, J.M.O.; Ruangsri, J.; Kiron, V. Atlantic cod piscidin and its diversification through positive selection. *PLoS One* **2010**, *5*, e9501. [CrossRef]
92. Tennessen, J.A. Enhanced synonymous site divergence in positively selected vertebrate antimicrobial peptide genes. *J. Mol. Evol.* **2005**, *61*, 445–455. [CrossRef]

93. Pinzon-Arango, P.A.; Nagarajan, R.; Camesano, T.A. Interactions of antimicrobial peptide chrysophsin-3 with Bacillus anthracis in sporulated, germinated, and vegetative states. *J. Phys. Chem. B* **2013**, *117*, 6364–6372. [CrossRef]
94. Cho, J.; Lee, D.G. Oxidative stress by antimicrobial peptide pleurocidin triggers apoptosis in *Candida albicans*. *Biochimie* **2011**, *93*, 1873–1879. [CrossRef]
95. Jung, H.J.; Park, Y.; Sung, W.S.; Suh, B.K.; Lee, J.; Hahm, K.S.; Lee, D.G. Fungicidal effect of pleurocidin by membrane-active mechanism and design of enantiomeric analogue for proteolytic resistance. *Biochim. Biophys. Acta* **2007**, *1768*, 1400–1405. [CrossRef]
96. Pan, C.Y.; Chen, J.Y.; Lin, T.L.; Lin, C.H. *In vitro* activities of three synthetic peptides derived from epinecidin-1 and an anti-lipopolysaccharide factor against *Propionibacterium acnes*, *Candida albicans*, and *Trichomonas vaginalis*. *Peptides* **2009**, *30*, 1058–1068. [CrossRef]
97. Colorni, A.; Ullal, A.; Heinisch, G.; Noga, E.J. Activity of the antimicrobial polypeptide piscidin 2 against fish ectoparasites. *J. Fish Dis.* **2008**, *31*, 423–432. [CrossRef]
98. Zahran, E.; Noga, E.J. Evidence for synergism of the antimicrobial peptide piscidin 2 with antiparasitic and antioomycete drugs. *J. Fish Dis.* **2010**, *33*, 995–1003. [CrossRef]
99. Wang, Y.D.; Kung, C.W.; Chen, J.Y. Antiviral activity by fish antimicrobial peptides of epinecidin-1 and hepcidin 1–5 against nervous necrosis virus in medaka. *Peptides* **2010**, *31*, 1026–1033. [CrossRef]
100. Chinchar, V.G.; Bryan, L.; Silphadaung, U.; Noga, E.; Wade, D.; Rollins-Smith, L. Inactivation of viruses infecting ectothermic animals by amphibian and piscine antimicrobial peptides. *Virology* **2004**, *323*, 268–275. [CrossRef]
101. Douglas, S.E.; Gallant, J.W.; Gong, Z.; Hew, C. Cloning and developmental expression of a family of pleurocidin-like antimicrobial peptides from winter flounder, *Pleuronectes americanus* (Walbaum). *Dev. Comp. Immunol.* **2001**, *25*, 137–147. [CrossRef]
102. Mulero, I.; Noga, E.J.; Meseguer, J.; Garcia-Ayala, A.; Mulero, V. The antimicrobial peptides piscidins are stored in the granules of professional phagocytic granulocytes of fish and are delivered to the bacteria-containing phagosome upon phagocytosis. *Dev. Comp. Immunol.* **2008**, *32*, 1531–1538. [CrossRef]
103. Ruangsri, J.; Fernandes, J.M.; Rombout, J.H.; Brinchmann, M.F.; Kiron, V. Ubiquitous presence of piscidin-1 in Atlantic cod as evidenced by immunolocalisation. *BMC Vet. Res.* **2012**, *8*, 46. [CrossRef]
104. Dezfuli, B.S.; Pironi, F.; Giari, L.; Noga, E.J. Immunocytochemical localization of piscidin in mast cells of infected seabass gill. *Fish Shellfish Immunol.* **2010**, *28*, 476–482. [CrossRef]
105. Murray, H.M.; Gallant, J.W.; Douglas, S.E. Cellular localization of pleurocidin gene expression and synthesis in winter flounder gill using immunohistochemistry and *in situ* hybridization. *Cell Tissue Res.* **2003**, *312*, 197–202.
106. Dezfuli, B.S.; Castaldelli, G.; Bo, T.; Lorenzoni, M.; Giari, L. Intestinal immune response of Silurus glanis and Barbus barbus naturally infected with *Pomphorhynchus laevis* (Acanthocephala). *Parasite Immunol.* **2011**, *33*, 116–23. [CrossRef]
107. Dezfuli, B.S.; Lui, A.; Giari, L.; Castaldelli, G.; Mulero, V.; Noga, E.J. Infiltration and activation of acidophilic granulocytes in skin lesions of gilthead seabream, *Sparus aurata*, naturally infected with lymphocystis disease virus. *Dev. Comp. Immunol.* **2012**, *36*, 174–182. [CrossRef]
108. Lin, W.J.; Chien, Y.L.; Pan, C.Y.; Lin, T.L.; Chen, J.Y.; Chiu, S.J.; Hui, C.F. Epinecidin-1, an antimicrobial peptide from fish (*Epinephelus coioides*) which has an antitumor effect like lytic peptides in human fibrosarcoma cells. *Peptides* **2009**, *30*, 283–290. [CrossRef]
109. Lin, H.J.; Huang, T.C.; Muthusamy, S.; Lee, J.F.; Duann, Y.F.; Lin, C.H. Piscidin-1, an antimicrobial peptide from fish (hybrid striped bass morone saxatilis x M. chrysops), induces apoptotic and necrotic activity in HT1080 cells. *Zool. Sci.* **2012**, *29*, 327–332. [CrossRef]
110. Hsu, J.C.; Lin, L.C.; Tzen, J.T.; Chen, J.Y. Characteristics of the antitumor activities in tumor cells and modulation of the inflammatory response in RAW264.7 cells of a novel antimicrobial peptide, chrysophsin-1, from the red sea bream (*Chrysophrys major*). *Peptides* **2011**, *32*, 900–910. [CrossRef]
111. Chen, J.Y.; Lin, W.J.; Wu, J.L.; Her, G.M.; Hui, C.F. Epinecidin-1 peptide induces apoptosis which enhances antitumor effects in human leukemia U937 cells. *Peptides* **2009**, *30*, 2365–2373. [CrossRef]
112. Morash, M.G.; Douglas, S.E.; Robotham, A.; Ridley, C.M.; Gallant, J.W.; Soanes, K.H. The zebrafish embryo as a tool for screening and characterizing pleurocidin host-defense peptides as anti-cancer agents. *Dis. Model. Mech.* **2011**, *4*, 622–633. [CrossRef]

113. Hilchie, A.L.; Doucette, C.D.; Pinto, D.M.; Patrzykat, A.; Douglas, S.; Hoskin, D.W. Pleurocidin-family cationic antimicrobial peptides are cytolytic for breast carcinoma cells and prevent growth of tumor xenografts. *Breast Cancer Res.* **2011**, *13*, R102. [CrossRef]
114. Pan, C.Y.; Chow, T.Y.; Yu, C.Y.; Yu, C.Y.; Chen, J.C.; Chen, J.Y. Antimicrobial peptides of an anti-lipopolysaccharide factor, epinecidin-1, and hepcidin reduce the lethality of Riemerella anatipestifer sepsis in ducks. *Peptides* **2010**, *31*, 806–815. [CrossRef]
115. Sung, W.S.; Lee, D.G. Pleurocidin-derived antifungal peptides with selective membrane-disruption effect. *Biochem. Biophys. Res. Commun.* **2008**, *369*, 858–861. [CrossRef]
116. Rahmanpour, A.; Ghahremanpour, M.M.; Mehrnejad, F.; Moghaddam, M.E. Interaction of Piscidin-1 with zwitterionic *versus* anionic membranes: A comparative molecular dynamics study. *J. Biomol. Struct. Dyn.* **2013**, *31*, 1393–1403. [CrossRef]
117. Chekmenev, E.Y.; Jones, S.M.; Nikolayeva, Y.N.; Vollmar, B.S.; Wagner, T.J.; Gor'kov, P.L.; Brey, W.W.; Manion, M.N.; Daugherty, K.C.; Cotten, M. High-field NMR studies of molecular recognition and structure-function relationships in antimicrobial piscidins at the water-lipid bilayer interface. *J. Am. Chem. Soc.* **2006**, *128*, 5308–5309. [CrossRef]
118. Mason, A.J.; Bertani, P.; Moulay, G.; Marquette, A.; Perrone, B.; Drake, A.F.; Kichler, A.; Bechinger, B. Membrane interaction of chrysophsin-1, a histidine-rich antimicrobial peptide from red sea bream. *Biochemistry* **2007**, *46*, 15175–15187. [CrossRef]
119. Patrzykat, A.; Friedrich, C.L.; Zhang, L.; Mendoza, V.; Hancock, R.E. Sublethal concentrations of pleurocidin-derived antimicrobial peptides inhibit macromolecular synthesis in *Escherichia coli*. *Antimicrob. Agents Chemother.* **2002**, *46*, 605–614. [CrossRef]
120. Kim, J.K.; Lee, S.A.; Shin, S.; Lee, J.Y.; Jeong, K.W.; Nan, Y.H.; Park, Y.S.; Shin, S.Y.; Kim, Y. Structural flexibility and the positive charges are the key factors in bacterial cell selectivity and membrane penetration of peptoid-substituted analog of Piscidin 1. *Biochim. Biophys. Acta* **2010**, *1798*, 1913–1925.
121. Lin, S.B.; Fan, T.W.; Wu, J.L.; Hui, C.F.; Chen, J.Y. Immune response and inhibition of bacterial growth by electrotransfer of plasmid DNA containing the antimicrobial peptide, epinecidin-1, into zebrafish muscle. *Fish Shellfish Immunol.* **2009**, *26*, 451–458. [CrossRef]
122. Lee, L.H.; Hui, C.F.; Chuang, C.M.; Chen, J.Y. Electrotransfer of the epinecidin-1 gene into skeletal muscle enhances the antibacterial and immunomodulatory functions of a marine fish, grouper (*Epinephelus coioides*). *Fish Shellfish Immunol.* **2013**, *35*, 1359–1368. [CrossRef]
123. Pan, C.Y.; Wu, J.L.; Hui, C.F.; Lin, C.H.; Chen, J.Y. Insights into the antibacterial and immunomodulatory functions of the antimicrobial peptide, epinecidin-1, against Vibrio vulnificus infection in zebrafish. *Fish Shellfish Immunol.* **2011**, *31*, 1019–1025. [CrossRef]
124. Pan, C.Y.; Huang, T.C.; Wang, Y.D.; Yeh, Y.C.; Hui, C.F.; Chen, J.Y. Oral administration of recombinant epinecidin-1 protected grouper (*Epinephelus coioides*) and zebrafish (*Danio rerio*) from Vibrio vulnificus infection and enhanced immune-related gene expressions. *Fish Shellfish Immunol.* **2012**, *32*, 947–957. [CrossRef]
125. Peng, K.C.; Pan, C.Y.; Chou, H.N.; Chen, J.Y. Using an improved Tol2 transposon system to produce transgenic zebrafish with epinecidin-1 which enhanced resistance to bacterial infection. *Fish Shellfish Immunol.* **2010**, *28*, 905–917. [CrossRef]
126. Huang, H.N.; Pan, C.Y.; Rajanbabu, V.; Chan, Y.L.; Wu, C.J.; Chen, J.Y. Modulation of immune responses by the antimicrobial peptide, epinecidin (Epi)-1, and establishment of an Epi-1-based inactivated vaccine. *Biomaterials* **2011**, *32*, 3627–3636. [CrossRef]
127. Lee, S.C.; Pan, C.Y.; Chen, J.Y. The antimicrobial peptide, epinecidin-1, mediates secretion of cytokines in the immune response to bacterial infection in mice. *Peptides* **2012**, *36*, 100–108. [CrossRef]
128. Huang, H.N.; Rajanbabu, V.; Pan, C.Y.; Chan, Y.L.; Wu, C.J.; Chen, J.Y. Use of the antimicrobial peptide Epinecidin-1 to protect against MRSA infection in mice with skin injuries. *Biomaterials* **2013**, *34*, 10319–10327. [CrossRef]
129. Pundir, P.; Catalli, A.; Leggiadro, C.; Douglas, S.E.; Kulka, M. Pleurocidin, a novel antimicrobial peptide, induces human mast cell activation through the FPRL1 receptor. *Mucosal Immunol.* **2014**, *7*, 177–187. [CrossRef]
130. Bulet, P.; Stocklin, R.; Menin, L. Anti-microbial peptides: From invertebrates to vertebrates. *Immunol. Rev.* **2004**, *198*, 169–184. [CrossRef]

131. Aerts, A.M.; Francois, I.E.; Cammue, B.P.; Thevissen, K. The mode of antifungal action of plant, insect and human defensins. *Cell. Mol. Life Sci.* **2008**, *65*, 2069–2079. [CrossRef]
132. Zhu, S. Discovery of six families of fungal defensin-like peptides provides insights into origin and evolution of the CSalphabeta defensins. *Mol. Immunol.* **2008**, *45*, 828–838. [CrossRef]
133. Zhu, S.; Gao, B. Evolutionary origin of beta-defensins. *Dev. Comp. Immunol.* **2013**, *39*, 79–84. [CrossRef]
134. Liu, L.; Zhao, C.; Heng, H.H.; Ganz, T. The human beta-defensin-1 and alpha-defensins are encoded by adjacent genes: Two peptide families with differing disulfide topology share a common ancestry. *Genomics* **1997**, *43*, 316–320. [CrossRef]
135. Tang, Y.Q.; Yuan, J.; Osapay, G.; Osapay, K.; Tran, D.; Miller, C.J.; Ouellette, A.J.; Selsted, M.E. A cyclic antimicrobial peptide produced in primate leukocytes by the ligation of two truncated alpha-defensins. *Science* **1999**, *286*, 498–502. [CrossRef]
136. Beckloff, N.; Diamond, G. Computational analysis suggests beta-defensins are processed to mature peptides by signal peptidase. *Protein Pept. Lett.* **2008**, *15*, 536–540. [CrossRef]
137. Falco, A.; Mas, V.; Tafalla, C.; Perez, L.; Coll, J.M.; Estepa, A. Dual antiviral activity of human alpha-defensin-1 against viral haemorrhagic septicaemia rhabdovirus (VHSV): Inactivation of virus particles and induction of a type I interferon-related response. *Antivir. Res.* **2007**, *76*, 111–123. [CrossRef]
138. Madison, M.N.; Kleshchenko, Y.Y.; Nde, P.N.; Simmons, K.J.; Lima, M.F.; Villalta, F. Human defensin alpha-1 causes Trypanosoma cruzi membrane pore formation and induces DNA fragmentation, which leads to trypanosome destruction. *Infect. Immun.* **2007**, *75*, 4780–4791. [CrossRef]
139. Tanaka, T.; Rahman, M.M.; Battur, B.; Boldbaatar, D.; Liao, M.; Umemiya-Shirafuji, R.; Xuan, X.; Fujisaki, K. Parasiticidal activity of human alpha-defensin-5 against *Toxoplasma gondii*. *In Vitro Cell. Dev. Biol. Anim.* **2010**, *46*, 560–565. [CrossRef]
140. Krishnakumari, V.; Rangaraj, N.; Nagaraj, R. Antifungal activities of human beta-defensins HBD-1 to HBD-3 and their C-terminal analogs Phd1 to Phd3. *Antimicrob. Agents Chemother.* **2009**, *53*, 256–260. [CrossRef]
141. Jiang, Y.; Wang, Y.; Wang, B.; Yang, D.; Yu, K.; Yang, X.; Liu, F.; Jiang, Z.; Li, M. Antifungal activity of recombinant mouse beta-defensin 3. *Lett. Appl. Microbiol.* **2010**, *50*, 468–473. [CrossRef]
142. Aerts, A.M.; Thevissen, K.; Bresseleers, S.M.; Sels, J.; Wouters, P.; Cammue, B.P.; Francois, I.E. Arabidopsis thaliana plants expressing human beta-defensin-2 are more resistant to fungal attack: Functional homology between plant and human defensins. *Plant Cell Rep.* **2007**, *26*, 1391–1398. [CrossRef]
143. Semple, F.; Dorin, J.R. Beta-Defensins: Multifunctional modulators of infection, inflammation and more? *J. Innate Immun.* **2012**, *4*, 337–348. [CrossRef]
144. Rohrl, J.; Yang, D.; Oppenheim, J.J.; Hehlgans, T. Specific binding and chemotactic activity of mBD4 and its functional orthologue hBD2 to CCR6-expressing cells. *J. Biol. Chem.* **2010**, *285*, 7028–7034.
145. Liu, Y.; Chang, M.X.; Wu, S.G.; Nie, P. Characterization of C-C chemokine receptor subfamily in teleost fish. *Mol. Immunol.* **2009**, *46*, 498–504.
146. Dixon, B.; Luque, A.; Abos, B.; Castro, R.; Gonzalez-Torres, L.; Tafalla, C. Molecular characterization of three novel chemokine receptors in rainbow trout (*Oncorhynchus mykiss*). *Fish Shellfish Immunol.* **2013**, *34*, 641–651.
147. Falco, A.; Brocal, I.; Perez, L.; Coll, J.M.; Estepa, A.; Tafalla, C. *In vivo* modulation of the rainbow trout (*Oncorhynchus mykiss*) immune response by the human alpha defensin 1, HNP1. *Fish Shellfish Immunol.* **2008**, *24*, 102–112. [CrossRef]
148. Lehrer, R.I.; Ganz, T. Defensins of vertebrate animals. *Curr. Opin. Immunol.* **2002**, *14*, 96–102. [CrossRef]
149. Tollner, T.L.; Venners, S.A.; Hollox, E.J.; Yudin, A.I.; Liu, X.; Tang, G.; Xing, H.; Kays, R.J.; Lau, T.; Overstreet, J.W.; *et al.* A common mutation in the defensin DEFB126 causes impaired sperm function and subfertility. *Sci. Transl. Med.* **2011**, *3*, 92–ra65.
150. Diamond, G.; Beckloff, N.; Weinberg, A.; Kisich, K.O. The roles of antimicrobial peptides in innate host defense. *Curr. Pharm. Des.* **2009**, *15*, 2377–2392. [CrossRef]
151. Dorschner, R.A.; Lin, K.H.; Murakami, M.; Gallo, R.L. Neonatal skin in mice and humans expresses increased levels of antimicrobial peptides: Innate immunity during development of the adaptive response. *Pediatr. Res.* **2003**, *53*, 566–572. [CrossRef]
152. Huttner, K.M.; Brezinski-Caliguri, D.J.; Mahoney, M.M.; Diamond, G. Antimicrobial peptide expression is developmentally-regulated in the ovine gastrointestinal tract. *J. Nutr.* **1998**, *128*, 297S–299S.
153. Ganz, T. Defensins: Antimicrobial peptides of innate immunity. *Nat. Rev. Immunol.* **2003**, *3*, 710–720. [CrossRef]

154. Casadei, E.; Bird, S.; Vecino, J.L.; Wadsworth, S.; Secombes, C.J. The effect of peptidoglycan enriched diets on antimicrobial peptide gene expression in rainbow trout (*Oncorhynchus mykiss*). *Fish Shellfish Immunol.* **2013**, *34*, 529–537. [CrossRef]
155. Reyes-Becerril, M.; Guardiola, F.; Rojas, M.; Ascencio-Valle, F.; Esteban, M.A. Dietary administration of microalgae Navicula sp. affects immune status and gene expression of gilthead seabream (*Sparus aurata*). *Fish Shellfish Immunol.* **2013**, *35*, 883–889. [CrossRef]
156. Krause, A.; Neitz, S.; Magert, H.J.; Schulz, A.; Forssmann, W.G.; Schulz-Knappe, P.; Adermann, K. LEAP-1, a novel highly disulfide-bonded human peptide, exhibits antimicrobial activity. *FEBS Lett.* **2000**, *480*, 147–150. [CrossRef]
157. Park, C.H.; Valore, E.V.; Waring, A.J.; Ganz, T. Hepcidin, a urinary antimicrobial peptide synthesized in the liver. *J. Biol. Chem.* **2001**, *276*, 7806–7810. [CrossRef]
158. Hilton, K.B.; Lambert, L.A. Molecular evolution and characterization of hepcidin gene products in vertebrates. *Gene* **2008**, *415*, 40–48. [CrossRef]
159. Hunter, H.N.; Fulton, D.B.; Ganz, T.; Vogel, H.J. The solution structure of human hepcidin, a peptide hormone with antimicrobial activity that is involved in iron uptake and hereditary hemochromatosis. *J. Biol. Chem.* **2002**, *277*, 37597–37603.
160. Padhi, A.; Verghese, B. Evidence for positive Darwinian selection on the hepcidin gene of Perciform and Pleuronectiform fishes. *Mol. Divers.* **2007**, *11*, 119–130. [CrossRef]
161. Lauth, X.; Babon, J.J.; Stannard, J.A.; Singh, S.; Nizet, V.; Carlberg, J.M.; Ostland, V.E.; Pennington, M.W.; Norton, R.S.; Westerman, M.E. Bass hepcidin synthesis, solution structure, antimicrobial activities and synergism, and *in vivo* hepatic response to bacterial infections. *J. Biol. Chem.* **2005**, *280*, 9272–9282.
162. Hu, X.; Camus, A.C.; Aono, S.; Morrison, E.E.; Dennis, J.; Nusbaum, K.E.; Judd, R.L.; Shi, J. Channel catfish hepcidin expression in infection and anemia. *Comp. Immunol. Microbiol. Infect. Dis.* **2007**, *30*, 55–69. [CrossRef]
163. Pridgeon, J.W.; Mu, X.; Klesius, P.H. Expression profiles of seven channel catfish antimicrobial peptides in response to *Edwardsiella ictaluri* infection. *J. Fish Dis.* **2012**, *35*, 227–237. [CrossRef]
164. Chiou, P.P.; Lin, C.M.; Bols, N.C.; Chen, T.T. Characterization of virus/double-stranded RNA-dependent induction of antimicrobial peptide hepcidin in trout macrophages. *Dev. Comp. Immunol.* **2007**, *31*, 1297–1309. [CrossRef]
165. Yang, C.G.; Liu, S.S.; Sun, B.; Wang, X.L.; Wang, N.; Chen, S.L. Iron-metabolic function and potential antibacterial role of Hepcidin and its correlated genes (Ferroportin 1 and Transferrin Receptor) in turbot (*Scophthalmus maximus*). *Fish Shellfish Immunol.* **2013**, *34*, 744–755. [CrossRef]
166. Alvarez, C.A.; Santana, P.A.; Guzman, F.; Marshall, S.; Mercado, L. Detection of the hepcidin prepropeptide and mature peptide in liver of rainbow trout. *Dev. Comp. Immunol.* **2013**, *41*, 77–81. [CrossRef]
167. Nemeth, E.; Valore, E.V.; Territo, M.; Schiller, G.; Lichtenstein, A.; Ganz, T. Hepcidin, a putative mediator of anemia of inflammation, is a type II acute-phase protein. *Blood* **2003**, *101*, 2461–2463. [CrossRef]
168. Skov, J.; Kania, P.W.; Holten-Andersen, L.; Fouz, B.; Buchmann, K. Immunomodulatory effects of dietary beta-1,3-glucan from Euglena gracilis in rainbow trout (*Oncorhynchus mykiss*) immersion vaccinated against *Yersinia ruckeri*. *Fish Shellfish Immunol.* **2012**, *33*, 111–120. [CrossRef]
169. Chia, T.J.; Wu, Y.C.; Chen, J.Y.; Chi, S.C. Antimicrobial peptides (AMP) with antiviral activity against fish nodavirus. *Fish Shellfish Immunol.* **2010**, *28*, 434–439. [CrossRef]
170. Rajanbabu, V.; Chen, J.Y. Antiviral function of tilapia hepcidin 1–5 and its modulation of immune-related gene expressions against infectious pancreatic necrosis virus (IPNV) in Chinook salmon embryo (CHSE)-214 cells. *Fish Shellfish Immunol.* **2011**, *30*, 39–44. [CrossRef]
171. Cai, L.; Cai, J.J.; Liu, H.P.; Fan, D.Q.; Peng, H.; Wang, K.J. Recombinant medaka (Oryzias melastigmus) pro-hepcidin: Multifunctional characterization. *Comp. Biochem. Physiol. B Biochem. Mol. Biol.* **2012**, *161*, 140–147. [CrossRef]
172. Liu, H.; Trinh, T.L.; Dong, H.; Keith, R.; Nelson, D.; Liu, C. Iron regulator hepcidin exhibits antiviral activity against hepatitis C virus. *PLoS One* **2012**, *7*, e46631.
173. Hocquellet, A.; le Senechal, C.; Garbay, B. Importance of the disulfide bridges in the antibacterial activity of human hepcidin. *Peptides* **2012**, *36*, 303–307. [CrossRef]
174. Chen, J.Y.; Lin, W.J.; Lin, T.L. A fish antimicrobial peptide, tilapia hepcidin TH2–3, shows potent antitumor activity against human fibrosarcoma cells. *Peptides* **2009**, *30*, 1636–1642. [CrossRef]

175. Chang, W.T.; Pan, C.Y.; Rajanbabu, V.; Cheng, C.W.; Chen, J.Y. Tilapia (Oreochromis mossambicus) antimicrobial peptide, hepcidin 1–5, shows antitumor activity in cancer cells. *Peptides* **2011**, *32*, 342–352. [CrossRef]
176. Pan, C.Y.; Peng, K.C.; Lin, C.H.; Chen, J.Y. Transgenic expression of tilapia hepcidin 1–5 and shrimp chelonianin in zebrafish and their resistance to bacterial pathogens. *Fish Shellfish Immunol.* **2011**, *31*, 275–285. [CrossRef]
177. Hsieh, J.C.; Pan, C.Y.; Chen, J.Y. Tilapia hepcidin (TH)2-3 as a transgene in transgenic fish enhances resistance to Vibrio vulnificus infection and causes variations in immune-related genes after infection by different bacterial species. *Fish Shellfish Immunol.* **2010**, *29*, 430–439. [CrossRef]
178. Rajanbabu, V.; Pan, C.Y.; Lee, S.C.; Lin, W.J.; Lin, C.C.; Li, C.L.; Chen, J.Y. Tilapia hepcidin 2-3 peptide modulates lipopolysaccharide-induced cytokines and inhibits tumor necrosis factor-alpha through cyclooxygenase-2 and phosphodiesterase 4D. *J. Biol. Chem.* **2010**, *285*, 30577–30586.
179. Rajanbabu, V.; Chen, J.Y. The antimicrobial peptide, tilapia hepcidin 2-3, and PMA differentially regulate the protein kinase C isoforms, TNF-alpha and COX-2, in mouse RAW264.7 macrophages. *Peptides* **2011**, *32*, 333–341. [CrossRef]
180. Ganz, T.; Nemeth, E. The hepcidin-ferroportin system as a therapeutic target in anemias and iron overload disorders. *Hematol. Am. Soc. Hematol. Educ. Program.* **2011**, *2011*, 538–542. [CrossRef]
181. Fraenkel, P.G.; Gibert, Y.; Holzheimer, J.L.; Lattanzi, V.J.; Burnett, S.F.; Dooley, K.A.; Wingert, R.A.; Zon, L.I. Transferrin-a modulates hepcidin expression in zebrafish embryos. *Blood* **2009**, *113*, 2843–2850. [CrossRef]
182. Chen, J.; Shi, Y.H.; Li, M.Y. Changes in transferrin and hepcidin genes expression in the liver of the fish Pseudosciaena crocea following exposure to cadmium. *Arch. Toxicol.* **2008**, *82*, 525–530. [CrossRef]
183. Tomasinsig, L.; Zanetti, M. The cathelicidins—Structure, function and evolution. *Curr. Protein Pept. Sci.* **2005**, *6*, 23–34. [CrossRef]
184. Shinnar, A.E.; Butler, K.L.; Park, H.J. Cathelicidin family of antimicrobial peptides: Proteolytic processing and protease resistance. *Bioorg. Chem.* **2003**, *31*, 425–436. [CrossRef]
185. Maier, V.H.; Dorn, K.V.; Gudmundsdottir, B.K.; Gudmundsson, G.H. Characterisation of cathelicidin gene family members in divergent fish species. *Mol. Immunol.* **2008**, *45*, 3723–3730. [CrossRef]
186. Broekman, D.C.; Frei, D.M.; Gylfason, G.A.; Steinarsson, A.; Jornvall, H.; Agerberth, B.; Gudmundsson, G.H.; Maier, V.H. Cod cathelicidin: Isolation of the mature peptide, cleavage site characterisation and developmental expression. *Dev. Comp. Immunol.* **2011**, *35*, 296–303. [CrossRef]
187. Bridle, A.; Nosworthy, E.; Polinski, M.; Nowak, B. Evidence of an antimicrobial-immunomodulatory role of Atlantic salmon cathelicidins during infection with Yersinia ruckeri. *PLoS One* **2011**, *6*, e23417.
188. Maier, V.H.; Schmitt, C.N.; Gudmundsdottir, S.; Gudmundsson, G.H. Bacterial DNA indicated as an important inducer of fish cathelicidins. *Mol. Immunol.* **2008**, *45*, 2352–2358. [CrossRef]
189. Broekman, D.C.; Guethmundsson, G.H.; Maier, V.H. Differential regulation of cathelicidin in salmon and cod. *Fish Shellfish Immunol.* **2013**, *35*, 532–538. [CrossRef]
190. Costa, M.M.; Maehr, T.; Diaz-Rosales, P.; Secombes, C.J.; Wang, T. Bioactivity studies of rainbow trout (*Oncorhynchus mykiss*) interleukin-6: Effects on macrophage growth and antimicrobial peptide gene expression. *Mol. Immunol.* **2011**, *48*, 1903–1916. [CrossRef]
191. Hong, S.; Li, R.; Xu, Q.; Secombes, C.J.; Wang, T. Two types of TNF-alpha exist in teleost fish: Phylogeny, expression, and bioactivity analysis of type-II TNF-alpha3 in rainbow trout oncorhynchus mykiss. *J. Immunol.* **2013**, *191*, 5959–5972. [CrossRef]
192. Shewring, D.M.; Zou, J.; Corripio-Miyar, Y.; Secombes, C.J. Analysis of the cathelicidin 1 gene locus in Atlantic cod (*Gadus morhua*). *Mol. Immunol.* **2011**, *48*, 782–787. [CrossRef]
193. De Bruijn, I.; Belmonte, R.; Anderson, V.L.; Saraiva, M.; Wang, T.; van West, P.; Secombes, C.J. Immune gene expression in trout cell lines infected with the fish pathogenic oomycete *Saprolegnia parasitica*. *Dev. Comp. Immunol.* **2012**, *38*, 44–54. [CrossRef]
194. Chettri, J.K.; Raida, M.K.; Kania, P.W.; Buchmann, K. Differential immune response of rainbow trout (*Oncorhynchus mykiss*) at early developmental stages (larvae and fry) against the bacterial pathogen *Yersinia ruckeri*. *Dev. Comp. Immunol.* **2012**, *36*, 463–474. [CrossRef]
195. Choi, K.Y.; Chow, L.N.; Mookherjee, N. Cationic host defence peptides: Multifaceted role in immune modulation and inflammation. *J. Innate Immun.* **2012**, *4*, 361–370.

196. Park, C.B.; Kim, M.S.; Kim, S.C. A novel antimicrobial peptide from Bufo bufo gargarizans. *Biochem. Biophys. Res. Commun.* **1996**, *218*, 408–413. [CrossRef]
197. Parseghian, M.H.; Luhrs, K.A. Beyond the walls of the nucleus: The role of histones in cellular signaling and innate immunity. *Biochem. Cell Biol.* **2006**, *84*, 589–604. [CrossRef]
198. Noga, E.J.; Ullal, A.J.; Corrales, J.; Fernandes, J.M. Application of antimicrobial polypeptide host defenses to aquaculture: Exploitation of downregulation and upregulation responses. *Comp. Biochem. Physiol. Part D Genomics Proteomics* **2011**, *6*, 44–54. [CrossRef]
199. Robinette, D.; Wada, S.; Arroll, T.; Levy, M.G.; Miller, W.L.; Noga, E.J. Antimicrobial activity in the skin of the channel catfish Ictalurus punctatus: Characterization of broad-spectrum histone-like antimicrobial proteins. *Cell. Mol. Life Sci.* **1998**, *54*, 467–475. [CrossRef]
200. Robinette, D.W.; Noga, E.J. Histone-like protein: A novel method for measuring stress in fish. *Dis. Aquat. Org.* **2001**, *44*, 97–107. [CrossRef]
201. Burrowes, O.J.; Hadjicharalambous, C.; Diamond, G.; Lee, T.C. Evaluation of antimicrobial spectrum and cytotoxic activity of pleurocidin for food applicaitons. *J. Food Sci.* **2004**, *69*, 66–71.
202. Bals, R.; Goldman, M.J.; Wilson, J.M. Mouse b-defensin 1 is a salt-sensitive antimicrobial peptide present in epithelia of the lung and urogenital tract. *Infect. Immun.* **1998**, *66*, 1225–1232.
203. Lee, J.Y.; Yang, S.T.; Lee, S.K.; Jung, H.H.; Shin, S.Y.; Hahm, K.S.; Kim, J.I. Salt-resistant homodimeric bactenecin, a cathelicidin-derived antimicrobial peptide. *FEBS J.* **2008**, *275*, 3911–3920. [CrossRef]
204. Tomita, T.; Hitomi, S.; Nagase, T.; Matsui, H.; Matsuse, T.; Kimura, S.; Ouchi, Y. Effect of ions on antibacterial activity of human beta defensin 2. *Microbiol. Immunol.* **2000**, *44*, 749–754. [CrossRef]
205. Subramanian, S.; Ross, N.W.; MacKinnon, S.L. Myxinidin, a novel antimicrobial peptide from the epidermal mucus of hagfish, *Myxine glutinosa* L. *Mar. Biotechnol. (N. Y.)* **2009**, *11*, 748–757. [CrossRef]
206. Olli, S.; Rangaraj, N.; Nagaraj, R. Effect of selectively introducing arginine and D-amino acids on the antimicrobial activity and salt sensitivity in analogs of human Beta-defensins. *PLoS One* **2013**, *8*, e77031.
207. Mai, J.; Tian, X.L.; Gallant, J.W.; Merkley, N.; Biswas, Z.; Syvitski, R.; Douglas, S.E.; Ling, J.; Li, Y.H. A novel target-specific, salt-resistant antimicrobial peptide against the cariogenic pathogen *Streptococcus mutans*. *Antimicrob. Agents Chemother.* **2011**, *55*, 5205–5213. [CrossRef]
208. Wu, S.P.; Huang, T.C.; Lin, C.C.; Hui, C.F.; Lin, C.H.; Chen, J.Y. Pardaxin, a fish antimicrobial peptide, exhibits antitumor activity toward murine fibrosarcoma *in vitro* and *in vivo*. *Mar. Drugs* **2012**, *10*, 1852–1872. [CrossRef]
209. Wang, W.; Tao, R.; Tong, Z.; Ding, Y.; Kuang, R.; Zhai, S.; Liu, J.; Ni, L. Effect of a novel antimicrobial peptide chrysophsin-1 on oral pathogens and Streptococcus mutans biofilms. *Peptides* **2012**, *33*, 212–219. [CrossRef]
210. Tao, R.; Tong, Z.; Lin, Y.; Xue, Y.; Wang, W.; Kuang, R.; Wang, P.; Tian, Y.; Ni, L. Antimicrobial and antibiofilm activity of pleurocidin against cariogenic microorganisms. *Peptides* **2011**, *32*, 1748–1754. [CrossRef]
211. Pan, C.Y.; Rajanbabu, V.; Chen, J.Y.; Her, G.M.; Nan, F.H. Evaluation of the epinecidin-1 peptide as an active ingredient in cleaning solutions against pathogens. *Peptides* **2010**, *31*, 1449–1458. [CrossRef]
212. Choi, H.; Lee, D.G. The influence of the *N*-terminal region of antimicrobial peptide pleurocidin on fungal apoptosis. *J. Microbiol. Biotechnol.* **2013**, *23*, 1386–1394. [CrossRef]
213. Luders, T.; Birkemo, G.A.; Fimland, G.; Nissen-Meyer, J.; Nes, I.F. Strong synergy between a eukaryotic antimicrobial peptide and bacteriocins from lactic acid bacteria. *Appl. Environ. Microbiol.* **2003**, *69*, 1797–1799. [CrossRef]
214. Patrzykat, A.; Zhang, L.; Mendoza, V.; Iwama, G.K.; Hancock, R.E. Synergy of histone-derived peptides of coho salmon with lysozyme and flounder pleurocidin. *Antimicrob. Agents Chemother.* **2001**, *45*, 1337–1342. [CrossRef]
215. Ivanov, I.E.; Morrison, A.E.; Cobb, J.E.; Fahey, C.A.; Camesano, T.A. Creating antibacterial surfaces with the peptide chrysophsin-1. *ACS Appl. Mater. Interfaces* **2012**, *4*, 5891–5897. [CrossRef]
216. Pan, C.Y.; Lee, S.C.; Rajanbabu, V.; Lin, C.H.; Chen, J.Y. Insights into the antibacterial and immunomodulatory functions of tilapia hepcidin (TH)2–3 against Vibrio vulnificus infection in mice. *Dev. Comp. Immunol.* **2012**, *36*, 166–173. [CrossRef]
217. Souza, A.L.; Diaz-Dellavalle, P.; Cabrera, A.; Larranaga, P., Dalla-Rizza; de-Simone, S.G. Antimicrobial activity of pleurocidin is retained in Plc-2, a C-terminal 12-amino acid fragment. *Peptides* **2013**, *45*, 78–84. [CrossRef]

218. Choi, H.; Lee, D.G. Antimicrobial peptide pleurocidin synergizes with antibiotics through hydroxyl radical formation and membrane damage, and exerts antibiofilm activity. *Biochim. Biophys. Acta* **2012**, *1820*, 1831–1838. [CrossRef]
219. Som, A.; Vemparala, S.; Ivanov, I.; Tew, G.N. Synthetic mimics of antimicrobial peptides. *Biopolymers* **2008**, *90*, 83–93. [CrossRef]
220. Beckloff, N.; Laube, D.; Castro, T.; Furgang, D.; Park, S.; Perlin, D.; Clements, D.; Tang, H.; Scott, R.W.; Tew, G.N.; *et al.* Activity of an antimicrobial peptide mimetic against planktonic and biofilm cultures of oral pathogens. *Antimicrob. Agents Chemother.* **2007**, *51*, 4125–4132. [CrossRef]
221. Hua, J.; Yamarthy, R.; Felsenstein, S.; Scott, R.W.; Markowitz, K.; Diamond, G. Activity of antimicrobial peptide mimetics in the oral cavity: I. Activity against biofilms of Candida albicans. *Mol. Oral Microbiol.* **2010**, *25*, 418–425. [CrossRef]
222. Hua, J.; Scott, R.W.; Diamond, G. Activity of antimicrobial peptide mimetics in the oral cavity: II. Activity against periopathogenic biofilms and anti-inflammatory activity. *Mol. Oral Microbiol.* **2010**, *25*, 426–432. [CrossRef]
223. Hancock, R.E.; Nijnik, A.; Philpott, D.J. Modulating immunity as a therapy for bacterial infections. *Nat. Rev. Microbiol.* **2012**, *10*, 243–254.
224. Terova, G.; Forchino, A.; Rimoldi, S.; Brambilla, F.; Antonini, M.; Saroglia, M. Bio-Mos: An effective inducer of dicentracin gene expression in European sea bass (Dicentrarchus labrax). *Comp. Biochem. Physiol. B Biochem. Mol. Biol.* **2009**, *153*, 372–377. [CrossRef]
225. Chang, C.I.; Pleguezuelos, O.; Zhang, Y.A.; Zou, J.; Secombes, C.J. Identification of a novel cathelicidin gene in the rainbow trout, *Oncorhynchus mykiss*. *Infect. Immun.* **2005**, *73*, 5053–5064. [CrossRef]
226. Sung, W.S.; Lee, J.; Lee, D.G. Fungicidal effect and the mode of action of piscidin 2 derived from hybrid striped bass. *Biochem. Biophys. Res. Commun.* **2008**, *371*, 551–555. [CrossRef]
227. Wang, Y.D.; Kung, C.W.; Chi, S.C.; Chen, J.Y. Inactivation of nervous necrosis virus infecting grouper (*Epinephelus coioides*) by epinecidin-1 and hepcidin 1-5 antimicrobial peptides, and downregulation of Mx2 and Mx3 gene expressions. *Fish Shellfish Immunol.* **2010**, *28*, 113–120. [CrossRef]

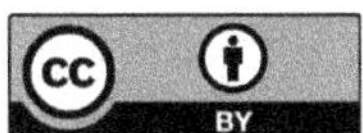

© 2014 by the authors. Licensee MDPI, Basel, Switzerland. This article is an open access article distributed under the terms and conditions of the Creative Commons Attribution (CC BY) license (http://creativecommons.org/licenses/by/4.0/).

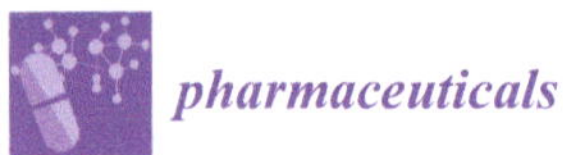

MDPI

Review

Chapter 6:

Host-Defense Peptides with Therapeutic Potential from Skin Secretions of Frogs from the Family Pipidae

J. Michael Conlon * and Milena Mechkarska

Department of Biochemistry, College of Medicine and Health Sciences, United Arab Emirates University, Al Ain 17666, UAE; mpanteva@uaeu.ac.ae

* Author to whom correspondence should be addressed; jmconlon@uaeu.ac.ae; Tel.: +971-3-713-7484; Fax: +971-3-767-2033.

Received: 9 December 2013; in revised form: 7 January 2014; Accepted: 8 January 2014; Published: 15 January 2014

Abstract: Skin secretions from frogs belonging to the genera *Xenopus*, *Silurana*, *Hymenochirus*, and *Pseudhymenochirus* in the family Pipidae are a rich source of host-defense peptides with varying degrees of antimicrobial activities and cytotoxicities to mammalian cells. Magainin, peptide glycine-leucine-amide (PGLa), caerulein-precursor fragment (CPF), and xenopsin-precursor fragment (XPF) peptides have been isolated from norepinephrine-stimulated skin secretions from several species of *Xenopus* and *Silurana*. Hymenochirins and pseudhymenochirins have been isolated from *Hymenochirus boettgeri* and *Pseudhymenochirus merlini*. A major obstacle to the development of these peptides as anti-infective agents is their hemolytic activities against human erythrocytes. Analogs of the magainins, CPF peptides and hymenochirin-1B with increased antimicrobial potencies and low cytotoxicities have been developed that are active (MIC < 5 μM) against multidrug-resistant clinical isolates of *Staphylococcus aureus*, *Escherichia coli*, *Acinetobacter baumannii*, *Stenotrophomonas maltophilia* and *Klebsiella pneumoniae*. Despite this, the therapeutic potential of frog skin peptides as anti-infective agents has not been realized so that alternative clinical applications as anti-cancer, anti-viral, anti-diabetic, or immunomodulatory drugs are being explored.

Keywords: frog skin; magainin; PGLa; caerulein-precursor fragment; xenopsin-precursor-fragment; hymenochirin

---

1. Introduction

The emergence in all regions of the World of strains of pathogenic bacteria and fungi with resistance to commonly used antibiotics constitutes a serious threat to public health and has necessitated a search for novel types of antimicrobial agent to which the microorganisms have not been exposed. Although effective new types of antibiotics against multidrug-resistant Gram-positive bacteria such as methicillin-resistant *Staphylococcus aureus* (MRSA) have been introduced or are in clinical trials, the situation regarding new treatment options for infections produced by multidrug-resistant Gram-negative pathogens such as *Acinetobacter baumannii*, *Pseudomonas aeruginosa*, *Klebsiella pneumoniae*, and *Stenotrophomonas maltophilia* is less encouraging [1]. There is an urgent need for new types of antimicrobial agents with activity against these microorganisms that also possess appropriate pharmacokinetic and toxicological profiles.

Peptides with potent antibacterial and antifungal activity play an important role in the system of innate immunity that predates adaptive immunity and constitutes the first-line defense against invading pathogens for a wide range of vertebrate and invertebrate species. Skin secretions from many species of Anura (frogs and toads) contain cytotoxic peptides, often in very high concentrations, with broad-spectrum antibacterial and antifungal activities and the ability to permeabilize mammalian cells [2,3]. Although usually referred to as antimicrobial peptides, these components are multifunctional, displaying cytokine-mediated immunomodulatory properties as well as anti-cancer, anti-viral, chemoattractive, and insulin-releasing activities. Consequently, it is more informative, therefore, to refer to them as host-defense peptides rather than as exclusively antimicrobial peptides [4]. It is a common fallacy that all anurans produce host-defense peptides in their skin secretions. At the time of writing peptides with antimicrobial activity have been identified in the skins of frogs from species belonging to the Alytidae, Bombinatoridae, Hylidae, Hyperoliidae, Leiopelmatidae, Leptodactylidae, Myobatrachidae, Pipidae, and Ranidae families [2,3]. The sporadic species distribution suggests that production of cytotoxic peptides in the skin may confer some evolutionary advantage to the organism, but is not necessary for survival. It has been suggested that cutaneous symbiotic bacteria may provide the major system of defense against pathogenic microorganisms in the environment with antimicrobial peptides assuming a supplementary role in some species [2]. In the laboratory or in the field, mild electrical stimulation or injections of norepinephrine into the dorsal sac are effective methods of inducing secretion of skin peptides that do not appear to cause harm or undue distress to the animal [5].

Frog skin host-defense peptides vary in size from as small as eight up to 63 amino acid residues. A comparison of their amino acid sequences reveals the lack of any conserved domains that are associated with biological activity. However, with few exceptions, the peptides are cationic, generally with a charge of between +2 and +6 at pH 7 due to the presence of multiple lysine residues, and contain about 50% hydrophobic amino acids. At the time of writing, the Antimicrobial Peptide Database (http://aps.unmc.edu/AP) lists 929 amphibian host-defense peptides, 96% of which have a charge of between +1 and +6 and 90% have between 40% and 70% hydrophobic residues. Circular dichroism and NMR studies have shown that they generally lack stable secondary structure in aqueous solution, but have the propensity to form an amphipathic α-helix in the environment of a phospholipid vesicle or in a membrane-mimetic solvent such as 50% trifluoroethanol-water [2,3]. There is no single mechanism by which peptides produce cell death, but their action does not involve binding to a specific receptor rather a non-specific interaction with the bacterial cell membrane that results in permeabilization and ultimate disintegration [6,7]. Consequently, the frog skin peptides are usually active against microorganisms that are resistant to currently licensed antibiotics due to their markedly different and highly destructive mode of action.

The frog skin host-defense peptides may be grouped together in sets or families on the basis of limited similarities in amino acid sequence. Skin secretions from a single species frequently contain several members of a particular peptide family that are presumed to have arisen from multiple duplications of an ancestral gene. The molecular heterogeneity of the peptides within a particular family is considerable and this variation in primary structure is reflected in a wide variability in antimicrobial potencies and specificities for different microorganisms. It has been suggested that this multiplicity may provide a broader spectrum of defense against the range of pathogenic microorganisms encountered in the environment [8] but conclusive evidence to support this assertion is still required.

A major obstacle to the development of frog skin peptides as therapeutically valuable anti-infective agents, particularly if they are to be administered systemically, is their varying degrees of cytotoxicity to mammalian cells and their short-lives in the circulation. However, effective strategies have been developed to design analogs of the naturally occurring peptides that maintain or increase antimicrobial potency while displaying reduced cytotoxicity to human cells, such as erythrocytes [9–11]. Peptides administered to infected skin or skin lesions can penetrate into the *stratum corneum* to kill microorganisms so that future therapeutic applications are more likely to involve topical rather than systemic administration. This review will examine possible clinical application of well characterized peptides that have been isolated from skin secretions from African clawed frogs belonging to the family Pipidae together with analogs of the naturally occurring peptides that show improved therapeutic potential.

2. The Family Pipidae

The Pipidae are the only principally aquatic group of frogs and, at this time, the taxon comprises 33 well characterized species distributed in five genera: *Hymenochirus, Pipa, Pseudhymenochirus, Silurana,* and *Xenopus* [12]. All are found in Africa south of the Sahara, except for members of the genus *Pipa* which are found in South America. Pipidae is sister-group to Rhinophrynidae (represented by a single species, the Mexican burrowing toad *Rhinophrynus dorsalis*) and the two families are united in the Pipoidea [13]. Phylogenetic relationships within the Pipidae are not entirely clear. Molecular analyses based upon the comparison of the nucleotide sequences of mitochondrial [14–16] and multiple nuclear [17] genes strongly support sister-group relationships between *Silurana* and *Xenopus,* united in the monophyletic clade Xenopodinae. Molecular data also provide support for *Pipa* as sister-group to all other extant pipids [16,18,19]. The origin of the Pipidae is at least Late Jurassic (150 MYA) and it is suggested that the breakup of Gondwanaland led to the establishment of *Pipa* in South America and the remaining genera (*Xenopus* + *Silurana* + *Hymenochirus* + *Pseudhymenochirus*) in Africa [17,20].

The clawed frogs of the genus *Xenopus* currently comprise 19 well characterized species although several unnamed species have been reported [12]. The genus has a complex evolutionary history involving both bifurcating and reticulating modes of speciation [14,15]. Allopolyploidization events, in which two species hybridize and the descendant inherits the complete genome of both ancestors, have given rise to tetraploid, octoploid, and dodecaploid species with no extant *Xenopus* species retaining the diploid status that is thought to be related to the ancestral state existing prior to one or more whole genome duplications. At this time, the ten tetraploid *Xenopus* species have been divided into three species groups on the basis of similarities in morphology, advertisement calls, and/or nucleotide sequences of mitochondrial genes: the *laevis* group includes *X. laevis, X. gilli, X. largeni, X. petersii,* and *X. victorianus;* the *muelleri* group includes *X. muelleri, X. borealis,* and *X. clivii;* and the *fraseri* group includes *X. fraseri* and *X. pygmaeus* [14,21]. It has been proposed that the seven extant octoploid species arose from three distinct allopolyploidization events [22]. Thus, *X. lenduensis* and *X. vestitus* share a common tetraploid ancestor; *X. amieti, X. andrei,* and *X. boumbaensis* form a second group; and *X. itombwensis* and *X. wittei* constitute a third group. Further allopolyploidization events involving a tetraploid species and an octoploid species within the second group have given rise to the dodecaploid species *X. longipes* and *X. ruwenzoriensis.*

The tropical clawed frog *Silurana tropicalis* retains the diploid status (chromosome number 2n = 20) that is thought to be related to the ancestral state but putative allopolyploidization events within the *Silurana* lineage have given rise to the Cameroon clawed frog *S. epitropicalis* with chromosome number 2n = 40 as well as at least two further unnamed tetraploid species [12,23]. The monotypic genus *Pseudhymenochirus* is accepted as sister group to genus *Hymenochirus* (African dwarf frogs) which includes four described species [12]. No allopolyploidization and higher level of ploidy have been reported for species belonging to these two genera [17].

3. Peptides with Antimicrobial Activity

Although peptides with hemolytic activity had been identified in skin secretions of frogs from the genera *Bombina* and *Rana* earlier, *X. laevis* was the first amphibian species in whose skin peptides with antimicrobial activity (magainin-1 and -2) were unambiguously identified [24]. Subsequent analysis of *X. laevis* skin secretions has led to the isolation and characterization of peptide glycine-leucine amide (PGLa) and additional antimicrobial peptides with varying potencies and specificities that are derived from the post-translational processing of the biosynthetic precursors of caerulein and xenopsin [25,26]. These peptides have been termed caerulein precursor fragment (CPF) and xenopsin precursor fragment (XPF). A comparison of the amino acid sequences of procaerulein, promagainin, and proxenopsin, deduced from the nucleotide sequences of cDNAs, reveals significant structural similarity in the N-terminal regions of the precursors suggesting that the peptides may have evolved from a common ancestral gene by a series of duplication events [27]. Orthologs of magainin-1 and -2, PGLa, and CPF, and XPF have been identified in skin secretions of range of frog species belonging to the genus *Xenopus* (*X. amieti* [28], *X. andrei* [29], *X. borealis* [30], *X. clivii* [31], *X. lenduensis* [32], *X. muelleri* and an incompletely characterized species from West Africa referred to as "*Xenopus* new tetraploid 1" and provisionally designated *X. muelleri* West [33], *X. petersii* [32], *X. pygmaeus* [32], and *X. victorianus* [34]). Host-defense peptides have also been isolated from laboratory-generated F1 hybrids of *X. laevis* × *X. muelleri* [35] and *X. laevis* × *X. borealis* [36]. Evolutionary pressure to conserve the primary structures of the antimicrobial peptides from *Xenopus* species has not been strong and the sequences of the procaerulein- and proxenopsin-derived peptides are particularly variable.

Peptides that belong to the PGLa family (PGLa-ST1, originally designated XT-5), the CPF family (CPF-ST1, -ST2, and -ST3, originally designated XT-1, XT-6, and XT-7), and the XPF family (XPF-ST1, -ST2, and -ST3 originally designated XT-2, XT-3, and XT-4) have been isolated from skin secretions of the diploid frog *S. tropicalis* [37]. Although a magainin peptide was not identified in *S. tropicalis* skin secretions, a search of the *S. tropicalis* genome database reveals the presence of a gene encoding a magainin-related peptide (referred to in this article as magainin-ST1) [38]. Peptides belonging to the magainin family (magainin-SE1), the PGLa family (PGLa-SE1 and -SE2), the CPF family (CPF-SE1, -SE2 and -SE3), and the X PF family (XPF-SE1, SE-2, SE-3 and -SE4), have been isolated from skin secretions of the tetraploid from *S. epitropicalis* [39].

More recently, peptidomic analysis of norepinephrine-stimulated skin secretions from the Congo dwarf clawed frog *Hymenochirus boettgeri* [40] and Merlin's clawed frog *Pseudhymenochirus merlini* [41] has led to identification of a family of structurally related host-defense peptides, termed the hymenochirins, with broad-spectrum antimicrobial activity. The hymenochirins show very low structural similarity with the antimicrobial peptides isolated from skin secretions of *Silurana* and *Xenopus* species consistent with the proposed ancient divergence of the Xenopodinae and the sister-group genera *Hymenochirus* and *Pseudhymenochirus* [17,18]. The strongly conserved hymenochirins from *P. merlini* show closest structural similarity to hymenochirin-1 and hymenochirin-5 from *H. boettgeri*. Peptides with novel structural features and broad spectrum antimicrobial activity, termed pseudhymenochirin-1Pa, -1Pb, and -2Pa, were also isolated from *P. merlini* secretions [41]. Unexpectedly, skin secretions from those frogs from the genus *Pipa* examined to date (*Pipa pipa* and *Pipa parva*) do not appear to contain cytotoxic peptides (unpublished data).

3.1. Magainins

The primary structures of the magainin peptides isolated to date from species in the genera *Xenopus* and *Silurana* are shown in Figure 1. Although probably the most intensively studied of all frog skin host-defense peptides, the magainins from the South African clawed frog *X. laevis* have only low or moderate antimicrobial potency against microorganisms. The hemolytic activity against human erythrocytes of magainin-2 in phosphate-buffered saline is low (the concentration producing 50% hemolysis, $LC_{50} > 100$ μM) but the peptide is strongly hemolytic when tested in 1 mM potassium phosphate buffer supplemented with 287 mM glucose ($LC_{50} = 7$ μM) [42]. Several recent studies have investigated in detail the mechanism of action by which magainin-2 produces bacterial cell death [43–45].

Magainin	
X. laevis-1	GIGKFLHSAGKFGKAFVGEIMKS
X. laevis-2	GIGKFLHSAKKFGKAFVGEIMNS
S. tropicalis-ST1	GLKEVAHSAKKFAKGFISGLTGS
S. epitropicalis-SE1	GLKEVLHSTKKFAKGFITGLTGQ
X. petersii-P1	GIGKFLHSAGKFGKAFVGEIMKS
X. petersii-P2	GIGQFLHSAKKFGKAFVGEIMKS
X. borealis-B1	G**KFLHSAGKFGKAFLGEVMIG
X. borealis-B2	GIGKFLHSAGKFGKAFLGEVMKS
X. muelleri-M1	GIGKFLHSAGKFGKAFIGEIMKS
X. muelleri-M2	GFKQFVHSLGKFGKAFVGEMIKPK
X. muelleri West-MW1	GIGKFLHSAGKFGKAFLGEVMKS
X. laevis × *X. muelleri*-LM1	GIGKFLHSAKKFAKAFVGEIMNS
X. clivii-C1	GVGKFLHSAKKFGQALASEIMKS
X. clivii-C2	GVGKFLHSAKKFGQALVSEIMKS
X. pygmaeus-PG1	GVGKFLHAAGKFGKALMGEMMKS
X. pygmaeus-PG2	GVSQFLHSASKFGKALMGEIMKS
X. lenduensis-L1	GIGKFLHSAKKFGKAFVGEVMKS
X. lenduensis-L2	GISQFLHSAKKFGKAFAGEIMKS
X. amieti-AM1	GIKEFAHSLGKFGKAFVGGILNQ
X. amieti-AM2	GVSKILHSAGKFGKAFLGEIMKS
X. andrei-AN1	GIKEFAHSLGKFGKAFVGGILNQ
X. andrei-AN2	GVSKILHSAGKFGKAFLGEIMKS

Figure 1. Primary structures of the magainin peptides isolated from skin secretions of frogs belonging to the genera *Xenopus* and *Silurana*. The amino acid sequence of magainin-ST1 was deduced from the corresponding nucleotide sequence of genomic DNA. In order to maximize structural similarity, gaps denoted by * have been introduced into some sequences. Strongly conserved residues are shaded.

A large number of analogs of magainin-2 have been synthesized with a view to increasing antimicrobial potency while decreasing hemolytic activity [46,47]. These include hybrid peptides comprising fragments of magainin-2 coupled to fragments of other antimicrobial peptides such as cecropin A(1-8)-magainin-2(1-12) which displays strong antimicrobial activity against a range of antibiotic resistant bacterial and fungal strains and low hemolytic activity [48]. Adopting the strategy of increasing cationicity to promote antimicrobial potency has led to the development of the analogue, pexiganan (MSI-78) which represents an analogue of magainin-2 that contains an additional five lysyl residues and an α-amidated C-terminus [49]. It was developed initially as a topical anti-infective agent for the treatment of infected foot ulcers in diabetic patients and as a possible treatment for impetigo. Pexiganan showed broad-spectrum antibacterial activity when tested against 3,109 clinical isolates of Gram-positive and Gram-negative aerobic and anaerobic bacteria [50]. The minimum inhibitory concentration (MIC) at which 90% of isolates were inhibited (MIC_{90}) was less than or equal to 32 μg/mL for several pathogens that are commonly recovered from diabetic foot wounds, including *Staphylococcus* spp., *Streptococcus* spp., *Corynebacterium* spp., *Pseudomonas* spp., *Acinetobacter* spp., *Bacteriodes* spp., *Peptostreptococcus* spp., and *Escherichia coli*. For 92% of the isolates tested, minimum bactericidal concentration (MBC) was the same or within a twofold difference of the MIC, consistent with a bactericidal action. A related study involving 2,515 bacterial isolates from infected foot ulcers from diabetic patients produced similar results with MIC_{90} values for pexiganan of 16 μg/mL or less for a range of Gram-positive aerobes, Gram-negative aerobes and facultative anaerobes [51]. *Proteus* spp. and *Serratia* spp. are also known to colonize foot ulcers but, in common with most frog skin peptides, pexiganan was inactive against strains of *Proteus mirabilis* and *Serratia marcescens*. In phase III multicentre, randomised, double-blind trials in diabetic patients with infected foot ulcers, topical application of pexiganan acetate (1%) achieved clinical cure or improvement in about 90% of patients, a success rate comparable to oral ofloxacin (800 mg/day) used in the control group [52]. The study indicated that the agent was well tolerated. However, the Food and Drug Administration did not approve marketing of this agent on the grounds that efficacy has not been sufficiently demonstrated.

Other examples of activity of magainin-2 and its analogues against important human pathogens include *Helicobacter pylori* [53], *Salmonella typhimurium* [54], the anaerobic periodontal pathogens,

Porphyromonas gingivalis, *Fusobacterium nucleatum*, and *Prevotella loeschei* [55], and *Acanthamoeba polyphagia*, a protozooan responsible for ocular infection in contact lens wearers [56].

3.2. Peptide Glycine-Leucine-Amide (PGLa) Peptides

The primary structures of the PGLa peptides isolated to date from species in the genera *Xenopus* and *Silurana* are shown in Figure 2. Although PGLa from *X. laevis* has often been used as a model peptide to study membrane-peptide interactions, its therapeutic potential as an anti-infective agent has not been extensively investigated. PGLa from *X. laevis* is active against amphotericin B-resistant *Candida albicans*, *Candida krusei*, and *Aspergillus fumigatus* strains and against a fluconazole-resistant *Candida glabrata* isolate [57]. PGLa acts synergistically with magainin-2 both in killing *E. coli* and permeabilizing protein-free liposomes so that the peptides are much more potent when added together than when added alone [58]. The mechanism of action of the peptide alone [59] and in combination with magainin-2 [60] has been studied in detail.

PGLa-AM1 from *X. amieti* shows broad spectrum bactericidal activity with MIC values ≤ 25 μM against reference strains of *E. coli* and *S. aureus* combined with very low toxicity to human red blood cells ($LC_{50} > 500$ μM) [28]. PGLa-AM1 shows potent growth-inhibitory activity against clinical isolates of antibiotic-resistant *A. baumannii*, including strains that are resistant to colistin (MIC in the range 4–32 μM) [61]. The peptide is also active against multiple clinical isolates of antibiotic-resistant *S. maltophilia* (MIC in the range 2–16 μM) (unpublished data).

PGLa-AM1 from *X. amieti* showed potent growth-inhibitory activity against reference stains of both Gram positive (*Streptococcus mutans* MIC = 1.2 μM) and Gram negative (*F. nucleatum* MIC = 1.5 μM) oral bacteria that are associated with tooth decay and periodontal disease. When tested against the opportunistic yeast pathogen *C. albicans*, PGLa-AM1 also proved to be highly effective (MIC = 7.5 μM). PGLa-AM1 showed no cytotoxicity to primary dental pulp fibroblasts at concentrations up to 10 μM and did not stimulate production of the proinflammatory cytokine IL-8 (unpublished data).

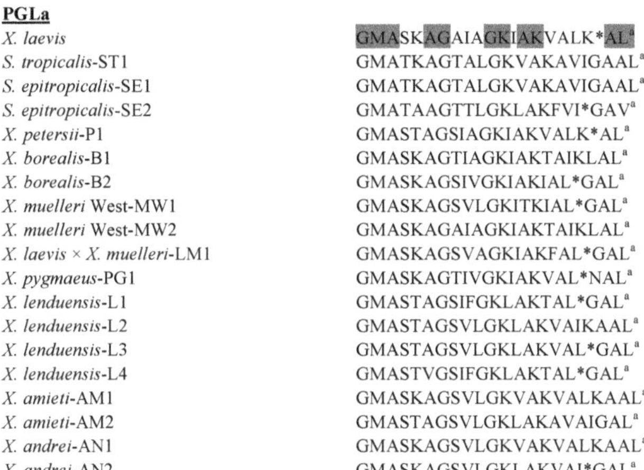

Figure 2. Primary structures of the peptide glycine-leucine-amide (PGLa) peptides isolated from skin secretions of frogs belonging to the genera *Xenopus* and *Silurana*. [a] denotes C-terminal α-amidation. In order to maximize structural similarity, gaps denoted by * have been introduced into some sequences. Strongly conserved residues are shaded.

3.3. Caerulein Precursor Fragment (CPF) Peptides

The primary structures of the CPF peptides and CPF-related peptides isolated to date from species in the genera *Xenopus* and *Silurana* are shown in Figure 3. CPF-C1, the most abundant antimicrobial peptide in skin secretions of *X. clivii*, inhibits the growth of the Gram-negative bacteria *E. coli*, *A. baumannii*, *K. pneumoniae*, and *P. aeruginosa* (MIC in the range 3–25 μM), suggesting potential for development into an anti-infective agent for use against these emerging antibiotic-resistant pathogens [31]. CPF-AM1 from *X. amieti* shows broad spectrum bactericidal activity with MIC values ≤ 25 μM against reference strains of *E. coli* and *S. aureus* combined with moderate toxicity to human red blood cell (LC_{50} = 150 μM) [28]. The peptide shows potent growth-inhibitory activity against clinical isolates of multidrug-resistant *A. baumannii*, including strains that are resistant to colistin (MIC in the range 2–8 μM) [61]. CPF-AM1 is also active against multiple clinical isolates of antibiotic-resistant *S. maltophilia* (MIC in the range 2–8 μM) (unpublished data). Like PGLa-AM1, CPF-AM1 showed potent growth inhibitory activity against reference strains of a range of microorganisms associated with the oral cavity, such as *S. mutans* (MIC = 2.5 μM), *Lactobacillus acidophilus* (MIC = 2.5 μM), *F. nucleatum* (MIC = 2.2 μM), and *C. albicans* (MIC = 9.9 μM) and was not cytotoxic to primary dental pulp fibroblasts at concentrations up to 10 μM (unpublished data).

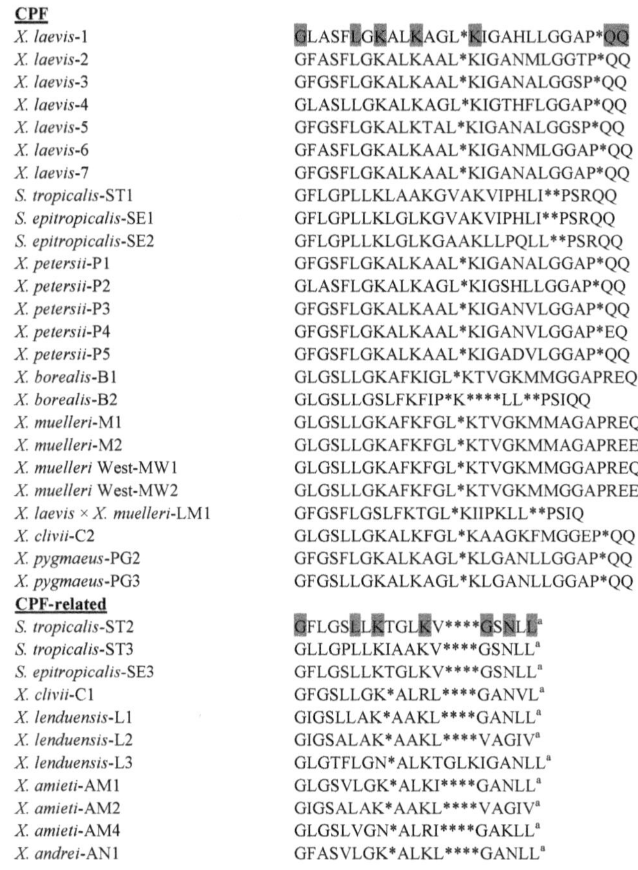

Figure 3. Primary structures of the caerulein precursor fragment (CPF) peptides isolated from skin secretions of frogs belonging to the genera *Xenopus* and *Silurana*. [a] denotes C-terminal α-amidation. In order to maximize structural similarity, gaps denoted by * have been introduced into some sequences. Strongly conserved residues are shaded.

The CPF-related peptide, CPF-ST3 from *S. tropicalis* (formerly described as peptide XT-7 [37]), shows potent broad spectrum antimicrobial activity but is moderately hemolytic against human erythrocytes (LC_{50} = 140 μM) thus limiting its therapeutic applicability. However, the analog [G4K] CPF-ST3 is non-hemolytic (LC_{50} > 500 μM) and retains potent antimicrobial activity [62]. Proton NMR spectroscopy has demonstrated that the reduced toxicity of the analog correlates with a decrease in helicity as well as an increase in cationicity [63]. CPF-SE2 (MIC = 2.5 μM) and CPF-SE3 (MIC = 5 μM) from *S. epitropicalis* show potent growth-inhibitory activity against a range of clinical isolates of MRSA but their utility as systemic anti-infective drugs is again limited by appreciable hemolytic activity against human erythrocytes for CPF-SE2 (LC_{50} = 50 μM) and moderate activity for CPF-SE3 (LC_{50} = 220 μM) [39]. Nevertheless, the peptides may find application as topical agents in treatment of MRSA skin infections and decolonization of MRSA carriers.

3.4. Xenopsin Precursor Fragment (XPF) Peptides

The primary structures of the XPF peptides isolated to date from species in the genera *Xenopus* and *Silurana* are shown in Figure 4. XPF peptides are widely distributed in skin secretions of clawed frogs and have also been identified in the gastrointestinal tract of *X. laevis* [64]. However, the antimicrobial potencies of XPF peptides are generally lower than those of CPF peptides and their potential for development into anti-infective agents has not been well studied. Of those XPF peptides studied to date, XPF-C1 from *X. clivii* shows relatively high growth-inhibitory potency against *E. coli* (MIC = 12.5 μM) but was inactive against *S. aureus* [31].

XPF	
X. laevis-1	GWASKIGQTLGKIAKVGLQGLMQPK
X. laevis-2	GWASKIGQTLGKIAKVGLKELIQPK
S. tropicalis-ST1	GLASTLGSFLGKFAKGGAQAFLQPK
S. tropicalis-ST2	GVWSTVLGGLKKFAKGGLEAIVNPK
S. tropicalis-ST3	GVFLDA***LKKFAKGGMNAVLNPK
S. epitropicalis-SE1	GLFLDT***LKKFAKAGMEAVINPK
S. epitropicalis-SE2	GLASTIGSLLGKFAKGGAQAFLQPK
S. epitropicalis-SE3	GFWTTAAEGLKKFAKAGLASILNPK
S. epitropicalis-SE4	GVWTTILGGLKKFAKGGLEALTNPK
X. borealis-B1	GFKQFVHSM*GKFGKAFVGEIINPK
X. borealis-B2	GWASKIGTQLGKMAKVGLKEFVQS
X. muelleri-M1	GWASKIGQTLGKMAKVGLKDLIQA
X. muelleri West-MW1	GWASKIGQTLGKLAKVGLKEFAQS
X. clivii-C1	GWASKIGQALGKVAKVGLQQFIQPK
X. amieti-AM1	GWASKIAQTLGKMAKVGLQELIQPK
X. andrei-AN1	GWVSKIGQTLGKMAKVGLQELIQPK

Figure 4. Primary structures of the xenopsin precursor fragment (XPF) peptides isolated from skin secretions of frogs belonging to the genera *Xenopus* and *Silurana*. In order to maximize structural similarity, gaps denoted by * have been introduced into some sequences. Strongly conserved residues are shaded.

3.5. Hymenochirins

The primary structures of the hymenochirins isolated to date from *H. boettgeri* and *P. merlini* are shown in Figure 5. Hymenochirin-1B was first isolated from norepinephrine-stimulated skin secretions from the Congo dwarf clawed frog *H. boettgeri* [40]. The peptide is cationic (molecular charge = +6 at pH 7) and has the propensity to adopt an amphipathic α-helical conformation in a membrane-mimetic environment. Hymenochirin-1B displays moderate growth-inhibitory activity against reference strains of Gram-negative (*E. coli* MIC = 25 μM) and Gram-positive bacteria (*S. aureus* MIC = 12.5 μM) and its hemolytic activity against human erythrocytes is relatively low (LC_{50} = 213 μM). Analogs in which the Pro^5, Glu^6 and Asp^9 on the hydrophilic face of the α-helix are substituted by one or more L-lysine residues show increased antimicrobial potency (up to 8-fold) but the peptides are more hemolytic. Increasing the cationicity of hymenochirin-1B while reducing helicity by substitutions with D-lysine generates analogs that are between 2- and 8-fold more potent than the native peptide and are equally or less hemolytic. [E6k,D9k]hymenochirin-1B represents a candidate for drug development as it shows high potency against clinical isolates of MRSA and a range of Gram-negative bacteria, including multidrug-resistant strains of *A. baumannii* and *S. maltophilia* (MIC in the range 0.8–3.1 μM) and New Dehli Metallo-β-Lactamase-1 (NDM-1)-producing clinical isolates of *K. pneumoniae*, *E. coli*, *Enterobacter cloacae* and *Citrobacter freundii* (MIC in the range 3.1–6.25 μM), and low hemolytic activity (LC_{50} = 302 μM) [65].

Hymenochirins	
H. boettgeri-1	IKLSPETKDNLKKVLKGAIKGAIAVAKMV[a]
H. boettgeri-2	LKIPGFVKDTLKKVAKGIFSAVAGAMTPS
H. boettgeri-3	IKIPAVVKDTLKKVAKGVLSAVAGALTQ
H. boettgeri-4	IKIPAFVKDTLKKVAKGVISAVAGALTQ
H. boettgeri-5	IKIPPIVKDTLKKVAKGVLSTIAGALST
P. merlini-1Pa	LKLSPKTKDTLKKVLKGAIKGAIAIASMA[a]
P. merlini-1Pb	LKLSPETKDTLKKVLKGAIKGAIAIASLA[a]
P. merlini-5Pa	ITIPPIVKDTLKKFFKGGIAGVMGKSQ
P. merlini-5Pb	FKIPPIVKDTLKKFFKGGIAGVMGQ
P. merlini-5Pc	ITIPPIIKDTLKKFFKGGIAGVMGKSQ
P. merlini-5Pd	ITIPPIVKDTLKKFFKGGIAGVMGQ
P. merlini-5Pe	ITIPPIVKDTLKKFIKGAISGVM[a]
P. merlini-5Pf	ITIPPIVKDTLKKFFKGGIAGVLGQ
P. merlini-5Pg	ITIPPIVKDTLKKFIKGAISSVM[a]
P. merlini-5Ph	ITIPPIVKNTLKKFIKGAVSALMS
Pseudhymenochirins	
P. merlini-1Pa	IKIPSFFRNILKKVGKEAVSLMAGALKQS
P. merlini-1Pb	IKIPSFFRNILKKVGKEAVSLIAGALKQS
P. merlini-2Pa	GIFPIFAKLLGKVIKVASSLISKGRTE

Figure 5. Primary structures of the hymenochirins isolated from skin secretions of the frogs *Hymenochirus boettgeri* and *Pseudhymenochirus merlini*, and the pseudhymenochirins from *P. merlini*. [a] denotes C-terminal α-amidation. Strongly conserved residues are shaded.

Close upPreliminary data indicate that hymenochirin-1Pa, pseudhymenochirin-1Pb, and pseudhymenochirin-2Pa from *P. merlini* also show potent growth-inhibitory potency against multidrug-resistant clinical isolates of *S. aureus*, *Staphylococcus epidermidis*, *A. baumannii*, and *S. maltophilia* but are more hemolytic than hymenochirin-1B (unpublished data).

4. Peptides with Anti-Cancer Activity

The problems posed by the emergence of multidrug resistance in the treatment of bacterial infections are also encountered in cancer chemotherapy. Because of their non-specific and destructive mechanism of action, cell-penetrating peptides show therapeutic potential for development into anti-cancer agents in cases where the tumor is not responsive to conventional pharmaceutical therapy. In addition, certain cationic antimicrobial peptides can produce tumor cell death by instigating apoptosis via mitochondrial membranes disruption and act as anti-angiogenic factors [66]. Analogs of naturally occurring frog skin host-defense peptides, including those from species within the family Pipidae, have been developed that show selective cytotoxicity against tumor cells and so have potential for development into anti-cancer agents.

Magainin-2 and its C-terminally α-amidated, carboxypeptidase-resistant analog, magainin G show potential as anticancer agents displaying tumoricidal activity against human small cell lung cancer cell lines [67], the RT4, 647V, and 486P bladder cancer cell lines [68], and against suspension cultures of a wide range of hematopoietic cell lines [69]. Out of a range of antimicrobial peptides tested, the magainin-2 analog, pexiganan shows the greatest cytotoxic activity against the U937 human histiocytic lymphoma cell line [70]. The anti-tumor activity of protease-resistant all D-amino acid magainin-2 amide (MSI-238) is markedly superior to the parent compound displaying high potency *in vitro* against non-small cell lung adenocarcinoma A549 cells and *in vivo* against P388 leukemia, S180 ascites, and a spontaneous ovarian tumor [71]. The cytotoxic mechanism of [F5W]magainin-2 against HeLa cells, has been investigated and involves initial interaction of the peptide with cell surface gangliosides [72].

Hymenochirin-1B shows high cytotoxic potency against A549 cells (LC_{50} = 2.5 μM), breast adenocarcinoma MDA-MB-231 cells (LC_{50} = 9.0 μM), colorectal adenocarcinoma HT-29 cells (LC_{50} = 9.7 μM), and hepatocarcinoma HepG2 cells (LC_{50} = 22.5 μM) with appreciably less hemolytic activity against human erythrocytes (LC_{50} = 213 μM) [73]. Structure-activity relationships were investigated by synthesizing analogs of hymenochirin-1B in which Pro^5, Glu^6 and Asp^9 on the hydrophilic face of the peptide helix are replaced by one or more L-lysine or D-lysine residues. The [D9K] analog displays the greatest increase in potency against all four cell lines (up to 6-fold) but hemolytic activity also increases (LC_{50} = 174 μM). The [D9k] and [E6k,D9k] analogs retain relatively high cytotoxic potency against the four tumor cell lines (LC_{50} in the range 2.1–21 μM) but show reduced hemolytic activity (LC_{50} > 300 μM).

CPF-ST3 (peptide XT-7) from *S. tropicalis* shows only moderate cytotoxic potency against HepG2 cells (LC_{50} = 75 μM) but increasing the cationicity of the peptide by appropriate amino acid substitutions by L-lysine that preserve amphipathicity results in a progressive increase in activity ([S15K] CPF-ST3, LC_{50} = 24 μM; ([S15K,N16K]CPF-ST3, LC_{50} = 10 μM; ([P5K,S15K,N16K] CPF-ST3, LC_{50} = 5 μM) [62].

5. Peptides with Anti-Viral Activity

Viruses cannot reproduce independently and instead use host cells for replication. Finding targets for an antiviral drug that would interfere specifically with the virus without harming the host cells poses a challenge for designing of safe and effective antivirals. Viral life cycles vary in their precise details depending on the species of virus but all share a general pattern: binding to a specific receptor on the surface of the host cell, uncoating of the virus inside the cell to release its genome, replication using host-cells machinery, assembly of virus progeny and release of viral particles to infect new host cells. Viruses that have a lipid envelope must also fuse their envelope with the target cell, or with a vesicle that transports them into the cell, before they can uncoat. Certain peptides that are present in frog skin secretions have demonstrated potent antiviral activity, either by directly inactivating the virus particles or by interfering with the initial steps of the viral reproductive cycle such as binding to specific cell surface receptors and subsequent entry into the cytoplasm. These properties, combined the short contact time required to induce killing, have led to their consideration as candidates for development into novel antiviral agents.

Magainin-1 and -2 from *X. laevis* show antiviral properties against herpes simplex virus type 1 (HSV-1) and herpes simplex virus type 2 (HSV-2) but were inactive against the arenavirus, Junin virus The peptides do not appear to inactivate the HSV particles directly but rather target important steps in the viral reproductive cycle [74]. Magainin-2 and PGLa from *X. laevis* markedly reduced the infectivity of channel catfish virus but were less potent against frog virus 3 [75]. Magainin-1 was ineffective against both viruses. Mechanistic studies have shown that an Ala-substituted magainin-2 amide analog directly inactivates vaccinia virus by disrupting and removing the outer membrane envelope [76].

Both CPF-AM1 and PGLa-AM1 from *X. amieti* are capable of destroying more than 90% of extracellular HSV-1 virions within the first 5 min of direct contact (unpublished data). In addition, these two peptides inhibit the viral penetration and replication in Madin-Darby Bovine Kidney (MDBK) cells when applied at non-toxic concentrations (≤200 μM). Similarly, CPF-ST3 (peptide XT-7) can destabilize HSV-1 particles and block virus entry and/or replication with EC_{50} = 87 μM (unpublished data).

For additional amphibian peptides with anti-bacterial, anti-viral and anti-cancer activities, interested readers may refer to the antimicrobial peptide database at http://aps.unmc.edu/AP.

6. Conclusions

The antimicrobial and hemolytic activities of the peptides showing the greatest potential for development into therapeutically valuable anti-infective agents are summarized in Table 1. Over 25 years have passed since the discovery of the magainins in the skin of the African clawed frog, *X. laevis*. Despite displaying potent activity against strains of antibiotic-resistant bacteria and against certain pathogenic fungi and protozoa, the therapeutic potential of frog skin antimicrobial peptides has yet to be realized. Currently, no anti-infective peptide based upon their structures has been adopted in clinical practice. Consequently, interest is moving away from their use as antimicrobials towards other potential clinical applications.

Table 1. Minimum Inhibitory Concentrations (μM) and hemolytic activities against human erythrocytes (μM) of the peptides with greatest therapeutic potential against reference strains and clinical isolates of clinically relevant microorganisms.

Peptide	*E. coli* ATCC 25726	*S. aureus* ATCC 25923	MRSA isolates	*A. baumannii* isolates	*S. maltophilia* isolates	*K. pneumoniae* isolates	LC_{50}
[G4K]CPF-ST3	12.5	6.25	ND	1.6–3.1	ND	ND	>500
PGLa-AM1	12.5	25	ND	4–32	2–16	ND	>500
CPF-AM1	12.5	6.25	ND	2–8	2–8	25	150
CPF-C1	6.25	6.25	ND	3.1	ND	25	140
CPF-SE2	40	2.5	2.5	ND	ND	ND	50
CPF-SE3	40	2.5	5	ND	ND	ND	220
[E6k,D9k] hymenochirin-1B	3.1	1.6	3.1–6.25	1.6	0.8–3.1	3.1–6.25	300

ND: not determined.

Several frog peptides that were first identified on the basis of their abilities to inhibit growth of bacteria have been shown to stimulate release of insulin from BRIN-BD11clonal β-cells and improve glucose tolerance in mice and so show potential for treatment of patients with Type 2 diabetes (reviewed in [77]). For example, CPF-1, CPF-3, CPF-5 and CPF-6 from *X. laevis* and CPF-SE1 from *S. epitropicalis* produced a significant increase in the rate of insulin release from BRIN-BD11 cells at concentrations as low as 0.03 nM. Similarly, magainin-AM1, magainin-AM2, CPF-AM1, and PGLa-AM1 stimulated release of the incretin peptide, GLP-1 from GLUTag cells with magainin-AM2 exhibiting the greatest potency (minimum concentration producing a significant stimulation = 1 nM) and CPF-AM1 producing the maximum stimulatory response (3.2-fold of basal rate at a concentration of 3 μM) [78].

Several frog skin peptides with cytotoxic properties have subsequently been shown to possess complex cytokine-mediated immunomodulatory activities. Effects on the production of both pro-inflammatory and anti-inflammatory cytokines have been observed (reviewed in [79]). Endotoxemic complications, such as severe sepsis and septic shock, following infection by Gram-negative bacteria are caused by release of lipopolysaccharide from bacterial membrane into the bloodstream and result in high levels of mortality. The importance of agents that modulate the immune function of the host in the treatment of sepsis is recognized [80]. The [E6k,D9k] analog of hymenochirin-1B increases the production of anti-inflammatory cytokine IL-10 from both unstimulated and concanavalin A-stimulated human peripheral blood mononuclear cells without increasing the rate of production of the pro-inflammatory cytokines TNF-α and IL-17 suggesting a possible therapeutic role in attenuating the inflammatory response triggered by bacteria [65].

Acknowledgments: The work carried out in the authors' laboratory was supported by grants from U.A.E. University and the Terry Fox Fund for Cancer Research.

Conflicts of Interest: The authors declare no conflict of interest.

References

1. Savard, P.; Perl, T.M. A call for action: Managing the emergence of multidrug-resistant *Enterobacteriaceae* in the acute care settings. *Curr. Opin. Infect. Dis.* **2012**, *25*, 371–377. [CrossRef]
2. Conlon, J.M. The contribution of skin antimicrobial peptides to the system of innate immunity in anurans. *Cell Tissue Res.* **2011**, *343*, 201–212. [CrossRef]
3. Conlon, J.M. Structural diversity and species distribution of host-defense peptides in frog skin secretions. *Cell. Mol. Life Sci.* **2011**, *68*, 2303–2315. [CrossRef]
4. Yeung, A.T.Y.; Gellatly, S.L.; Hancock, R.E. Multifunctional cationic host defence peptides and their clinical applications. *Cell. Mol. Life Sci.* **2011**, *68*, 2161–2176. [CrossRef]
5. Gammill, W.M.; Fites, J.S.; Rollins-Smith, L.A. Norepinephrine depletion of antimicrobial peptides from the skin glands of *Xenopus laevis*. *Dev. Comp. Immunol.* **2012**, *37*, 19–27. [CrossRef]
6. Almeida, P.F.; Pokorny, A. Mechanisms of antimicrobial, cytolytic, and cell-penetrating peptides: From kinetics to thermodynamics. *Biochemistry* **2009**, *48*, 8083–8093. [CrossRef]
7. Huang, Y.; Huang, J.; Chen, Y. Alpha-helical cationic antimicrobial peptides: Relationships of structure and function. *Protein Cell* **2010**, *1*, 143–152. [CrossRef]
8. Tennessen, J.A.; Woodhams, D.C.; Chaurand, P.; Reinert, L.K.; Billheimer, D.; Shyr, Y.; Caprioli, R.M.; Blouin, M.S.; Rollins-Smith, L.A. Variations in the expressed antimicrobial peptide repertoire of northern leopard frog (*Rana pipiens*) populations suggest intraspecies differences in resistance to pathogens. *Dev. Comp. Immunol.* **2009**, *33*, 1247–1257. [CrossRef]
9. Conlon, J.M.; Al-Ghaferi, N.; Abraham, B.; Leprince, J. Strategies for transformation of naturally-occurring amphibian antimicrobial peptides into therapeutically valuable anti-infective agents. *Methods* **2007**, *42*, 349–357. [CrossRef]
10. Jiang, Z.; Vasil, A.I.; Hale, J.D.; Hancock, R.E.; Vasil, M.L.; Hodges, R.S. Effects of net charge and the number of positively charged residues on the biological activity of amphipathic alpha-helical cationic antimicrobial peptides. *Biopolymers* **2008**, *90*, 369–383. [CrossRef]
11. Matsuzaki, K. Control of cell selectivity of antimicrobial peptides. *Biochim. Biophys. Acta* **2009**, *1788*, 1687–1692. [CrossRef]
12. Frost, D.R. Amphibian Species of the World: An Online Reference, Version 5.6. 2013, Electronic Database. American Museum of Natural History: New York, USA. Available online: http://research.amnh.org/herpetology/amphibia/index.php (accessed on 13 January 2014).
13. Frost, D.R.; Grant, T.; Faivovich, J.; Bain, R.H.; Haas, A.; Haddad, C.F.B.; de Sá, R.O.; Channing, A.; Wilkinson, M.; Donnellan, S.C.; *et al.* The amphibian tree of life. *Bull. Am. Mus. Nat. Hist.* **2006**, *297*, 1–370.
14. Evans, B.J.; Kelley, D.B.; Tinsley, R.C.; Melnick, D.J.; Cannatella, D.C. A mitochondrial DNA phylogeny of African clawed frogs: Phylogeography and implications for polyploid evolution. *Mol. Phylogenet. Evol.* **2004**, *33*, 197–213. [CrossRef]
15. Evans, B.J. Genome evolution and speciation genetics of clawed frogs (*Xenopus* and *Silurana*). *Front. Biosci.* **2008**, *13*, 4687–4706. [CrossRef]
16. Irisarri, I.; Vences, M.; San Mauro, D.; Glaw, F.; Zardoya, R. Reversal to air-driven sound production revealed by a molecular phylogeny of tongueless frogs, family Pipidae. *BMC Evol. Biol.* **2011**, *11*. [CrossRef]
17. Bewick, A.J.; Chain, F.J.; Heled, J.; Evans, B.J. The pipid root. *Syst. Biol.* **2012**, *61*, 913–926. [CrossRef]
18. Roelants, K.; Bossuyt, F. Archaeobatrachian paraphyly and pangaean diversification of crown- group frogs. *Syst. Biol.* **2005**, *54*, 111–126. [CrossRef]
19. Roelants, K.; Gower, D.J.; Wilkinson, M.; Loader, S.P.; Biju, S.D.; Guillaume, K.; Moriau, L.; Bossuyt, F. Global patterns of diversification in the history of modern amphibians. *Proc. Natl. Acad. Sci. USA* **2007**, *104*, 887–892.
20. Báez, A.M. The Fossil Record of the Pipidae. In *The Biology of Xenopus*; Tinsley, R.C., Kobel, H.R., Eds.; Clarendon Press: Oxford, UK, 1996; pp. 329–347.
21. Kobel, H.R.; Loumont, C.; Tinsley, R.C. The Extant Species. In *The Biology of Xenopus*; Tinsley, R.C., Kobel, H.R., Eds.; Clarendon Press: Oxford, UK, 1996; pp. 9–33.

22. Evans, B.J.; Greenbaum, E.; Kusamba, C.; Carter, T.F.; Tobias, M.L.; Mendel, S.A.; Kelley, D.B. Description of a new octoploid frog species (Anura: Pipidae: *Xenopus*) from the Democratic Republic of the Congo, with a discussion of the biogeography of African clawed frogs in the Albertine Rift. *J. Zool.* **2011**, *283*, 276–290.
23. Tymowska, J.; Fischberg, M. A comparison of the karyotype, constitutive heterochromatin, and nucleolar organizer regions of the new tetraploid species *Xenopus epitropicalis* Fischberg and Picard with those of *Xenopus tropicalis* Gray (Anura, Pipidae). *Cytogenet. Cell Genet.* **1982**, *34*, 49–157.
24. Zasloff, M. Magainins, a class of antimicrobial peptides from *Xenopus* skin: Isolation, characterization of two active forms and partial cDNA sequence of a precursor. *Proc. Natl. Acad. Sci. USA* **1987**, *84*, 5449–5453.
25. Gibson, B.W.; Poulter, L.; Williams, D.H.; Maggio, J.E. Novel peptide fragments originating from PGLa and the caerulein and xenopsin precursors from *Xenopus laevis*. *J. Biol. Chem.* **1986**, *261*, 5341–5349.
26. Soravia, E.; Martini, G.; Zasloff, M. Antimicrobial properties of peptides from Xenopus granular gland secretions. *FEBS Lett.* **1988**, *228*, 337–340. [CrossRef]
27. Hunt, L.T.; Barker, W.C. Relationship of promagainin to three other prohormones from the skin of *Xenopus laevis*: A different perspective. *FEBS Lett.* **1988**, *233*, 282–288. [CrossRef]
28. Conlon, J.M.; Al-Ghaferi, N.; Ahmed, E.; Meetani, M.A.; Leprince, J.; Nielsen, P.F. Orthologs of magainin, PGLa, procaerulein-derived, and proxenopsin-derived peptides from skin secretions of the octoploid frog *Xenopus amieti* (Pipidae). *Peptides* **2010**, *31*, 989–994. [CrossRef]
29. Mechkarska, M.; Ahmed, E.; Coquet, L.; Leprince, J.; Jouenne, T.; Vaudry, H.; King, J.D.; Takada, K.; Conlon, J.M. Genome duplications within the Xenopodinae do not increase the multiplicity of antimicrobial peptides in *Silurana paratropicalis* and *Xenopus andrei* skin secretions. *Comp. Biochem. Physiol. D Genomics Proteomics* **2011**, *6*, 206–212. [CrossRef]
30. Mechkarska, M.; Ahmed, E.; Coquet, L.; Leprince, J.; Jouenne, T.; Vaudry, H.; King, J.D.; Conlon, J.M. Antimicrobial peptides with therapeutic potential from skin secretions of the Marsabit clawed frog *Xenopus borealis* (Pipidae). *Comp. Biochem. Physiol. C Toxicol. Pharmacol.* **2010**, *152*, 467–472. [CrossRef]
31. Conlon, J.M.; Mechkarska, M.; Ahmed, E.; Leprince, J.; Vaudry, H.; King, J.D.; Takada, K. Purification and properties of antimicrobial peptides from skin secretions of the Eritrea clawed frog *Xenopus clivii* (Pipidae). *Comp. Biochem. Physiol. C Toxicol. Pharmacol.* **2011**, *153*, 350–354. [CrossRef]
32. King, J.D.; Mechkarska, M.; Coquet, L.; Leprince, J.; Jouenne, T.; Vaudry, H.; Takada, K.; Conlon, J.M. Host-defense peptides from skin secretions of the tetraploid frogs *Xenopus petersii* and *Xenopus pygmaeus*, and the octoploid frog *Xenopus lenduensis* (Pipidae). *Peptides* **2012**, *33*, 35–43. [CrossRef]
33. Mechkarska, M.; Ahmed, E.; Coquet, L.; Leprince, J.; Jouenne, T.; Vaudry, H.; King, J.D.; Conlon, J.M. Peptidomic analysis of skin secretions demonstrates that the allopatric populations of *Xenopus muelleri* (Pipidae) are not conspecific. *Peptides* **2011**, *32*, 1502–1508. [CrossRef]
34. King, J.D.; Mechkarska, M.; Meetani, M.A.; Conlon, J.M. Peptidomic analysis of skin secretions provides insight into the taxonomic status of the African clawed frogs *Xenopus victorianus* and *Xenopus laevis sudanensis* (Pipidae). *Comp. Biochem. Physiol. D Genomics Proteomics* **2013**, *8*, 250–254. [CrossRef]
35. Mechkarska, M.; Meetani, M.; Michalak, P.; Vaksman, Z.; Takada, K.; Conlon, J.M. Hybridization between the tetraploid African clawed frogs *Xenopus laevis* and *Xenopus muelleri* (Pipidae) increases the multiplicity of antimicrobial peptides in the skin secretions of female offspring. *Comp. Biochem. Physiol. D Genomics Proteomics* **2012**, *7*, 285–291. [CrossRef]
36. Mechkarska, M.; Prajeep, M.; Leprince, J.; Vaudry, H.; Meetani, M.A.; Evans, B.J.; Conlon, J.M. A comparison of host-defense peptides in skin secretions of female *Xenopus laevis* × *Xenopus borealis* and *X. borealis* × *X. laevis* F1 hybrids. *Peptides* **2013**, *45*, 1–8. [CrossRef]
37. Ali, M.F.; Soto, A.; Knoop, F.C.; Conlon, J.M. Antimicrobial peptides isolated from skin secretions of the diploid frog, *Xenopus tropicalis* (Pipidae). *Biochim. Biophys. Acta* **2001**, *1550*, 81–89.
38. Roelants, K.; Fry, B.G.; Ye, L.; Stijlemans, B.; Brys, L.; Kok, P.; Clynen, E.; Schoofs, L.; Cornelis, P.; Bossuyt, F. Origin and functional diversification of an amphibian defense peptide arsenal. *PLoS Genet.* **2013**, *9*, e1003662.
39. Conlon, J.M.; Mechkarska, M.; Prajeep, M.; Sonnevend, A.; Coquet, L.; Leprince, J.; Jouenne, T.; Vaudry, H.; King, J.D. Host-defense peptides in skin secretions of the tetraploid frog *Silurana epitropicalis* with potent activity against methicillin-resistant *Staphylococcus aureus* (MRSA). *Peptides* **2012**, *37*, 113–119. [CrossRef]
40. Mechkarska, M.; Prajeep, M.; Coquet, L.; Leprince, J.; Jouenne, T.; Vaudry, H.; King, J.D.; Conlon, J.M. The hymenochirins: A family of antimicrobial peptides from the Congo dwarf clawed frog *Hymenochirus boettgeri* (Pipidae). *Peptides* **2012**, *35*, 269–275. [CrossRef]

41. Conlon, J.M.; Prajeep, M.; Mechkarska, M.; Coquet, L.; Leprince, J.; Jouenne, T.; Vaudry, H.; King, J.D. Characterization of the host-defense peptides from skin secretions of Merlin's clawed frog *Pseudhymenochirus merlini*: Insights into phylogenetic relationships among the Pipidae. *Comp. Biochem. Physiol. D Genomics Proteomics* **2013**, *8*, 352–357. [CrossRef]
42. Helmerhorst, E.J.; Reijnders, M.; van't Hof, W.; Veerman, C.; Nieuw-Amerongen, A.V. A critical comparison of the hemolytic and fungicidal activities of cationic antimicrobial peptides. *FEBS Lett.* **1999**, *449*, 105–110.
43. Imura, Y.; Choda, N.; Matsuzaki, K. Dagainin 2 in action: Distinct modes of membrane permeabilization in living bacterial and mammalian cells. *Biophys. J.* **2008**, *95*, 5757–5765. [CrossRef]
44. Tamba, Y.; Ariyama, H.; Levadny, V.; Yamazaki, M. Kinetic pathway of antimicrobial peptide magainin 2-induced pore formation in lipid membranes. *J. Phys. Chem. B* **2010**, *114*, 12018–12026. [CrossRef]
45. Epand, R.F.; Maloy, W.L.; Ramamoorthy, A.; Epand, R.M. Probing the "charge cluster mechanism" in amphipathic helical cationic antimicrobial peptides. *Biochemistry* **2010**, *49*, 4076–4084. [CrossRef]
46. Zasloff, M.; Martin, B.; Chen, H.C. Antimicrobial activity of synthetic magainin peptides and several analogues. *Proc. Natl. Acad. Sci. USA* **1988**, *85*, 910–913. [CrossRef]
47. Cuervo, J.H.; Rodriguez, B.; Houghten, R.A. The magainins: Sequence factors relevant to increased antimicrobial activity and decreased hemolytic activity. *Pept. Res.* **1988**, *1*, 81–86.
48. Shin, S.Y.; Kang, J.H.; Lee, M.K.; Kim, S.Y.; Kim, Y.; Hahm, K.S. Cecropin A—Magainin 2 hybrid peptides having potent antimicrobial activity with low hemolytic effect. *Biochem. Mol. Biol. Int.* **1998**, *44*, 1119–1126.
49. Fuchs, P.C.; Barry, A.L.; Brown, S.D. *In vitro* antimicrobial activity of MSI-78, a magainin analog. *Antimicrob. Agents Chemother.* **1998**, *42*, 1213–1216.
50. Ge, Y.; MacDonald, D.L.; Holroyd, K.J.; Thornsberry, C.; Wexler, H.; Zasloff, M. *In vitro* antibacterial properties of pexiganan, an analog of magainin. *Antimicrob. Agents Chemother.* **1999**, *43*, 782–788.
51. Ge, Y.; MacDonald, D.; Henry, M.M.; Hait, H.I.; Nelson, K.A.; Lipsky, B.A.; Zasloff, M.A.; Holroyd, K.J. *In vitro* susceptibility to pexiganan of bacteria isolated from infected diabetic foot ulcers. *Diagn. Microbiol. Infect. Dis.* **1999**, *35*, 45–53. [CrossRef]
52. Lipsky, B.A.; Holroyd, K.J.; Zasloff, M. Topical *versus* systemic antimicrobial therapy for treating mildly infected diabetic foot ulcers: A randomized, controlled, double-blinded, multicenter trial of pexiganan cream. *Clin. Infect. Dis.* **2008**, *47*, 1537–1545. [CrossRef]
53. Iwahori, A.; Hirota, Y.; Sampe, R.; Miyano, S.; Takahashi, N.; Sasatsu, M.; Kondo, I.; Numao, N. On the antibacterial activity of normal and reversed magainin 2 analogs against *Helicobacter pylori*. *Biol. Pharm. Bull.* **1997**, *20*, 805–808. [CrossRef]
54. Macias, E.A.; Rana, F.; Blazyk, J.; Modrzakowski, M.C. Bactericidal activity of magainin 2: Use of lipopolysaccharide mutants. *Can. J. Microbiol.* **1990**, *36*, 582–584. [CrossRef]
55. Genco, C.A.; Maloy, W.L.; Kari, U.P.; Motley, M. Antimicrobial activity of magainin analogues against anaerobic oral pathogens. *Int. J. Antimicrob. Agents* **2003**, *21*, 75–78. [CrossRef]
56. Schuster, F.L.; Jacob, L.S. Effects of magainins on ameba and cyst stages of *Acanthamoeba polyphaga*. *Antimicrob. Agents Chemother.* **1992**, *36*, 1263–1271. [CrossRef]
57. Helmerhorst, E.J.; Reijnders, I.M.; van't Hof, W.; Simoons-Smit, I.; Veerman, E.C.; Amerongen, A.V. Amphotericin B- and fluconazole-resistant *Candida* spp., *Aspergillus fumigatus*, and other newly emerging pathogenic fungi are susceptible to basic antifungal peptides. *Antimicrob. Agents Chemother.* **1999**, *43*, 702–704.
58. Westerhoff, H.V.; Zasloff, M.; Rosner, J.L.; Hendler, R.W.; de Waal, A.; Vaz Gomes, A.; Jongsma, P.M.; Riethorst, A.; Juretić, D. Functional synergism of the magainins PGLa and magainin-2 in *Escherichia coli*, tumor cells and liposomes. *Eur. J. Biochem.* **1995**, *228*, 257–264. [CrossRef]
59. Lohner, K.; Prossnigg, F. Biological activity and structural aspects of PGLa interaction with membrane mimetic systems. *Biochim. Biophys. Acta* **2009**, *1788*, 1656–1666. [CrossRef]
60. Strandberg, E.; Zerweck, J.; Wadhwani, P.; Ulrich, A.S. Synergistic insertion of antimicrobial magainin-family peptides in membranes depends on the lipid spontaneous curvature. *Biophys. J.* **2013**, *104*, L9–L11. [CrossRef]
61. Conlon, J.M.; Sonnevend, A.; Pál, T.; Vila-Farrés, X. Efficacy of six frog skin-derived antimicrobial peptides against colistin-resistant strains of the *Acinetobacter baumannii* group. *Int. J. Antimicrob. Agents* **2012**, *39*, 317–320. [CrossRef]
62. Conlon, J.M.; Galadari, S.; Raza, H.; Condamine, E. Design of potent, non-toxic antimicrobial agents based upon the naturally occurring frog skin peptides, ascaphin-8 and peptide XT-7. *Chem. Biol. Drug Des.* **2008**, *72*, 58–64. [CrossRef]

63. Subasinghage, A.P.; Conlon, J.M.; Hewage, C.M. Development of potent anti-infective agents from *Silurana tropicalis*: Conformational analysis of the amphipathic, alpha-helical antimicrobial peptide XT-7 and its non-haemolytic analogue [G4K]XT-7. *Biochim. Biophys. Acta* **2010**, *1804*, 1020–1028. [CrossRef]
64. Moore, K.S.; Bevins, C.L.; Brasseur, M.M.; Tomassini, N.; Turner, K.; Eck, H.; Zasloff, M. Antimicrobial peptides in the stomach of *Xenopus laevis*. *J. Biol. Chem.* **1991**, *266*, 19851–19857.
65. Mechkarska, M.; Prajeep, M.; Radosavljevic, G.D.; Jovanovic, I.P.; Al Baloushi, A.; Sonnevend, A.; Lukic, M.L.; Conlon, J.M. An analog of the host-defense peptide hymenochirin-1B with potent broad-spectrum activity against multidrug-resistant bacteria and immunomodulatory properties. *Peptides* **2013**, *50*, 153–159. [CrossRef]
66. Mader, J.S.; Hoskin, D.W. Cationic antimicrobial peptides as novel cytotoxic agents for cancer treatment. *Expert Opin. Investig. Drugs* **2006**, *15*, 933–946. [CrossRef]
67. Ohsaki, Y.; Gazdar, A.F.; Chen, H.C.; Johnson, B.E. Antitumor activity of magainin analogues against human lung cancer cell lines. *Cancer Res.* **1992**, *52*, 3534–3538.
68. Lehmann, J.; Retz, M.; Sidhu, S.S.; Suttmann, H.; Sell, M.; Paulsen, F.; Harder, J; Unteregger, G.; Stöckle, M. Antitumor activity of the antimicrobial peptide magainin II against bladder cancer cell lines. *Eur. Urol.* **2006**, *50*, 141–147. [CrossRef]
69. Cruciani, R.A.; Barker, J.L.; Zasloff, M.; Chen, H.C.; Colamonici, O. Antibiotic magainins exert cytolytic activity against transformed cell lines through channel formation. *Proc. Natl. Acad. Sci. USA* **1991**, *88*, 3792–3796.
70. Koszałka, P.; Kamysz, E.; Wejda, M.; Kamysz, W.; Bigda, J. Antitumor activity of antimicrobial peptides against U937 histiocytic cell line. *Acta. Biochim. Pol.* **2011**, *58*, 111–117.
71. Baker, M.A.; Maloy, W.L.; Zasloff, M.; Jacob, L.S. Anticancer efficacy of magainin 2 and analogue peptides. Anticancer efficacy of magainin 2 and analogue peptides. *Cancer Res.* **1993**, *53*, 3052–3057.
72. Miyazaki, Y.; Aoki, M.; Yano, Y.; Matsuzaki, K. Interaction of antimicrobial peptide magainin 2 with gangliosides as a target for human cell binding. *Biochemistry* **2012**, *51*, 10229–10235. [CrossRef]
73. Attoub, S.; Arafat, H.; Mechkarska, M.; Conlon, J.M. Anti-tumor activities of the host-defense peptide hymenochirin-1B. *Regul. Pept.* **2013**, *115*, 141–149.
74. Albiol Matanic, V.C.; Castilla, V. Antiviral activity of antimicrobial cationic peptides against Junin virus and herpes simplex virus. *Int. J. Antimicrob. Agents* **2004**, *23*, 382–389. [CrossRef]
75. Chinchar, V.G.; Bryan, L.; Silphadaung, U.; Noga, E.; Wade, D.; Rollins-Smith, L. Inactivation of viruses infecting ectothermic animals by amphibian and piscine antimicrobial peptides. *Virology* **2004**, *323*, 268–275. [CrossRef]
76. Dean, R.E.; O'Brien, L.M.; Thwaite, J.E.; Fox, M.A.; Atkins, H.; Ulaeto, D.O. A carpet-based mechanism for direct antimicrobial peptide activity against vaccinia virus membranes. *Peptides* **2010**, *31*, 1966–1972. [CrossRef]
77. Srinivasan, D.; Mechkarska, M.; Abdel-Wahab, Y.H.; Flatt, P.R.; Conlon, J.M. Caerulein precursor fragment (CPF) peptides from the skin secretions of *Xenopus laevis* and *Silurana epitropicalis* are potent insulin-releasing agents. *Biochimie* **2013**, *95*, 429–435. [CrossRef]
78. Ojo, O.O.; Conlon, J.M.; Flatt, P.R.; Abdel-Wahab, Y.H. Frog skin peptides (tigerinin-1R, magainin-AM1, -AM2, CPF-AM1, and PGla-AM1) stimulate secretion of glucagon-like peptide 1 (GLP-1) by GLUTag cells. *Biochem. Biophys. Res. Commun.* **2013**, *431*, 14–18. [CrossRef]
79. Pantic, J.M.; Mechkarska, M.; Lukic, M.L.; Conlon, J.M. Effects of tigerinin peptides on cytokine production by mouse peritoneal macrophages and spleen cells and by human peripheral blood mononuclear cells. *Biochimie* **2014**, in press.
80. Kotsaki, A.; Giamarellos-Bourboulis, E.J. Emerging drugs for the treatment of sepsis. *Expert Opin. Emerg. Drugs* **2012**, *17*, 379–391. [CrossRef]

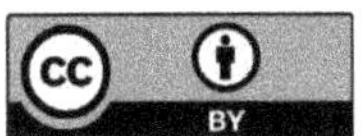

© 2014 by the authors. Licensee MDPI, Basel, Switzerland. This article is an open access article distributed under the terms and conditions of the Creative Commons Attribution (CC BY) license (http://creativecommons.org/licenses/by/4.0/).

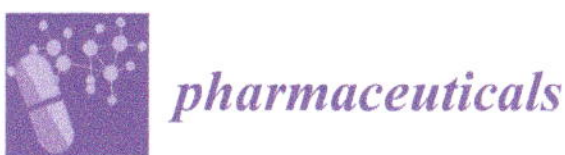

pharmaceuticals

MDPI

Review

Chapter 7: Antimicrobial Peptides in Reptiles

Monique L. van Hoek

National Center for Biodefense and Infectious Diseases, and School of Systems Biology, George Mason University, MS1H8, 10910 University Blvd, Manassas, VA 20110, USA; mvanhoek@gmu.edu; Tel.: +1-703-993-4273; Fax: +1-703-993-7019

Received: 6 March 2014; in revised form: 9 May 2014; Accepted: 12 May 2014; Published: 10 June 2014

Abstract: Reptiles are among the oldest known amniotes and are highly diverse in their morphology and ecological niches. These animals have an evolutionarily ancient innate-immune system that is of great interest to scientists trying to identify new and useful antimicrobial peptides. Significant work in the last decade in the fields of biochemistry, proteomics and genomics has begun to reveal the complexity of reptilian antimicrobial peptides. Here, the current knowledge about antimicrobial peptides in reptiles is reviewed, with specific examples in each of the four orders: Testudines (turtles and tortosises), Sphenodontia (tuataras), Squamata (snakes and lizards), and Crocodilia (crocodilans). Examples are presented of the major classes of antimicrobial peptides expressed by reptiles including defensins, cathelicidins, liver-expressed peptides (hepcidin and LEAP-2), lysozyme, crotamine, and others. Some of these peptides have been identified and tested for their antibacterial or antiviral activity; others are only predicted as possible genes from genomic sequencing. Bioinformatic analysis of the reptile genomes is presented, revealing many predicted candidate antimicrobial peptides genes across this diverse class. The study of how these ancient creatures use antimicrobial peptides within their innate immune systems may reveal new understandings of our mammalian innate immune system and may also provide new and powerful antimicrobial peptides as scaffolds for potential therapeutic development.

Keywords: antimicrobial peptides; antibacterial; reptile; biofilm; broad-spectrum; Gram-positive; Gram-negative

---

1. Introduction

Reptiles are among the oldest amniotes. They are cold-blooded (ectothermic) vertebrates with dry and scaly skin that usually lay soft-shelled eggs with amniotic membranes. They thrive in diverse environments, ranging as far north as Hudson's Bay in Canada, and as far south as Cape Horn, Chile. They range from very small geckos to enormous crocodiles and have survived millennia of evolution. They are highly adapted to their environment, including their innate immune systems, allowing them to be such successful animals. Antimicrobial peptides are part of the innate immune system, and may contribute to the survival of these animals in microbe-filled, challenging environment. This paper will review the known and predicted antimicrobial peptides of reptiles. A set of known host defense antimicrobial peptides is collected in the Antimicrobial Peptide Database [1,2] and the examples from reptiles have been annotated (Table 1). Recently, many reptilian genomes have been sequenced. From these genomes, potential antimicrobial peptide genes have been predicted here by bioinformatics analysis (Tables 2–8), which should be synthesized and tested for activity in future work. Overall, the Reptile class thrives in diverse and challenging environments, partly due to their robust innate immune system, and our hypothesis is that antimicrobial peptides contribute to the evolutionary success of reptiles as they do in mammals and other species.

Table 1. Known reptile antimicrobial peptides identified in the Antimicrobial Peptide Database (APD2) [2].

Peptide name	Sequence	APD Identified	Source Organism	Comment Reference	Activity (*)
		Cathelicidin			
OH-CATH	KRFKKFFKKLKNSVKK RAKKFFKKPRVIGVSIPF	AP00895	*O. Hannah* (Snake)	Derivatives: OH-CATH30; OH-CM6 [3,4]	G+, G−
Derivative OH-CATH30	KFFKKLKNSVKKRA KKFFKKPRVIGVSIPF			[5,6]	G+, G−
Derivative OH-CM6	KFFKKLKKAVKKGFKKFAKV			[3,4]	G+, G−
BF-CATH	KRFKKFFKKLKKSVKK RAKKFFKKPRVIGVSIPF	AP00896	*Bungarus fasciatus* (Snake)	[7]	G+, G−, F, Cancer cells
Derivative BF-30	KFFRKLKKSVKKRAK EFFKKPRVIGVSIPF	AP01239	*B. fasciatus*	[8–10]	G+, G−
Derivative BF-15	KFFRKLKKSVVKRFK		*B. fasciatus*	[8]	G+, G−
NA-CATH	KRFKKFFKKLKNSVKKRA KKFFKKPKVIGVTFPF	AP00897	*N. atra* (Snake)	[3]	G+, G−
		Waprin			
Omwaprin	KDRPKKPGLCPPRPQKPCVK ECKNDDSCPGQQKCCN YGCKDECRDPIFVG	AP01589	*Oxyuranus microlepidotus* (Snake)	4S = S [11,12]	G+
		Proline Rich			
Lethal peptide I/Waglerin	GGKPDLRPCHPP CHYIPRPKPR	AP00238	*Trimeresurus wagleri*, Wagler's pit viper (Snake)	P24335, [13]	Tx
		β-Defensin or defensin-like			
TBD-1 (Turtle β-defensin 1)	YDLSKNCRLRGGICYIGK CPRRFFRSGSCSRGNVCCLRFG	AP01380	Turtle	3S = S [14]	G+, G−, F
Pelovaterin	DDTPSSRCGSGGWGPCLPI VDLLCIVHVTVGCSGGFGCCRIG	AP01381	Turtle	2JR3 BBBh2o [15,16]	G−
TEWP (turtle egg-white protein)	EKKCPGRCTLKCGKHER PTLPYNCGKYICCVPVKVK	AP01382	Turtle	2B5B XXQ [17–19]	G-, V
		Crotamine defensin-like toxin			
Crotamine	YKQCHKKGGHCFPKEKICLPP SSDFGKMDCRWRWKCCKKGSG	AP01650	Snake Venom	1Z99, 3S = S ZZP [20,21]	G+, G−, F, P, Mammalian and Cancer cells

(*) Activity abbreviations: G+, G−, inhibiting both G+ and G− bacteria; G+, Gram-positive bacteria only, G−, Gram-negative bacteria only; V, antiviral; F, antifungal; P: antiparasitic, Tx: Toxin activity to mammals.

2. Four Orders of Reptiles

The structural and sequence diversity of antimicrobial peptides is impressive (see below), but it is useful to first review the phylogenetic and physiological diversity of the Reptilia class in order to appreciate all the ecosystems and environments that they live in and the prey that they eat.

All living reptiles fall within the kingdom Animalia, the phylum Chordata, the class Reptilia, and the clade Sauropsida [22]. There are four orders within the class Reptilia: turtles and tortoises (Testudines), tuataras (Sphenodontia), snakes and lizards (Squamata), and crocodilans (Crocodilia). Each order will be briefly introduced below. Many reptile species are endangered, including the painted turtle, and the Siamese crocodile. Although considered by phylogenetic analysis to be "monophyletic" with avians (Sauropsida; See Cladogram, Figure 1), reptiles are still generally considered to be separate from birds. Some researchers use the term avian reptile and non-avian reptile to distinguish the two groups [23]. Within the non-avian reptilians, the crocodilians are considered to be the most closely related to the avian branch. Interestingly, this evolutionary connection is reflected in the antimicrobial profile in that neither avians nor reptilians encode α-defensin antimicrobial peptides, for example, which are a critical part of mammalian innate immunity. In contrast, avians do not appear to express hepcidin peptides, while reptiles do, highlighting a potential difference.

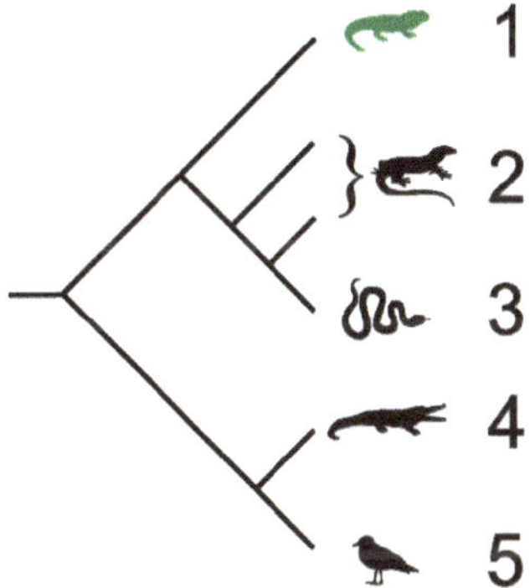

Figure 1. Cladogram showing the relationships of extant members of the Sauria (Sauropsida) which includes birds and reptiles. Branch lengths are not representative of divergence time. 1. Tuataras; 2. Lizards; 3. Snakes; 4. Crocodiles; 5. Birds. Cladogram by Benchill, licensed under the Creative Commons Attribution 3.0 Unported license [24].

2.1. Testudines (Turtles and Tortises)

The testudine order includes the turtles and tortosises. The western painted turtle (*Chrysemys picta bellii*) is a small turtle of North America, commonly found in ponds and other slow-moving fresh water [25].

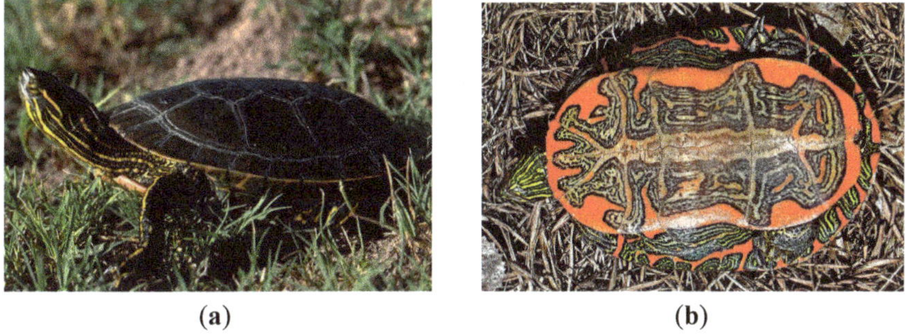

(a) **(b)**

Figure 2. Western Painted Turtle *Chrysemys picta bellii*. (**a**) Western painted turtle. Photo by Gary M. Stolz, U.S. Fish and Wildlife Service in the Public domain [26]. (**b**) Underside of a Western Painted Turtle. Photo by Matt Young [27].

This intensely colorful turtle (Figure 2) has existed for approximately 15 million years, according to the fossil record [25]. The genomes of three turtles have recently been sequenced, including the green sea turtle (*Chelonia mydas*) and the Chinese softshell turtle *Pelodiscus sinensis* [28], as well as the western painted turtle, *Chrysemys picta bellii* [29,30]. Interestingly, these papers place the turtles as a sister group to crocodiles and birds, which is different than their prior morphological classification [31]. The precise evolutionary relationship of the testudine class with other reptiles is a matter of current debate [32–36]. Their genomes appear to encode cathelicidin antimicrobial peptides that are "snake-like" but encode defensin type peptides (gallinacin-like) that may be more similar to "avian" antimicrobial peptides.

2.2. *Sphenodontia (Tuataras)*

The family Sphenodontidae (within Lepidosauromorpha) contains the genus of Sphenodon, which has one species, *S. puctatus* (previously thought to have three species including *S. guntheri*, and *S. diversum*, now considered sub-species) all commonly referred to as tuatara lizards [37,38], although they are not classified as lizards. The tuatara (Figure 3) is the farthest removed from the avian lineage in terms of evolution and is considered to be the most "ancient" extant reptile, in existence in its current form for 100 million years.

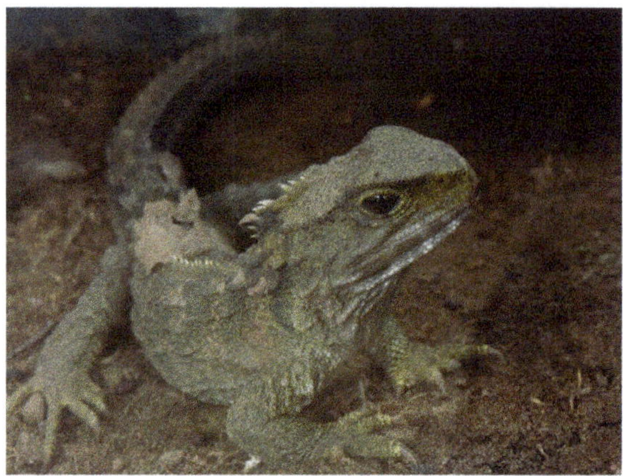

Figure 3. *Sphenodon punctatus*, Tuatara, Nga Manu, Waikanae, New Zealand. Photo by PhillipC [39].

The tuatara lives only on the costal islands of New Zealand [40]. There are currently significant efforts underway to sequence the tuatara genome [41]. However, until the genomes and transcriptomes can be analyzed for antimicrobial peptides and verified from tuatara samples, there are no known antimicrobial peptides from the tuatara.

2.3. *Squamata (Snakes and Lizards)*

The Squamata order of Lepidosauromorpha includes lizards and snakes. In the group of snakes which although limbless are considered tetrapod vertebrates and are descended from four legged ancestors, we will consider elapid snakes and pythons. Elapid snakes are venomous, fanged snakes commonly found in warm climates. Pythons are nonvenomous snakes that are found in Africa, Asia and Australia. The King cobra (*Ophiophagus (O.) hannah*) is one of the longest venomous snakes [42], with lengths up to 18 ft (Figure 4a). The genus *Naja* is a group of venomous elapid snakes in southern Africa and South Asia, including the species *Naja (N.) atra*, the Chinese King cobra (Figure 4b). The Banded Krait (*Bungarus (B.) fasciatus*) is commonly found in Southeast Asia and India and has distinctive banding markings (Figure 4c). The Burmese python (*Python bivittatus*) is typically found in tropical areas including Southeast Asia and is one of the largest snakes, typically reaching 12 ft long. This snake is also found as an invasive species in the Florida Everglades in the Southeast United States [43]. Snakes encode well-studied cathelicidin peptides that appear to be generally similar throughout the reptiles, despite the well-known sequence diversity of cathelicidin antimicrobial peptides in general.

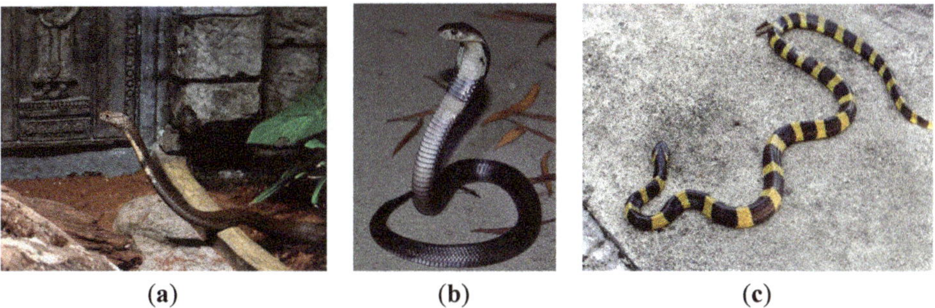

Figure 4. Elapid snakes (**a**) The King cobra (*O. hannah*) [44] (**b**) A juvenile Chinese cobra *(N. atra)* [45] (**c**) Banded Krait *(B. fasciatus)* [46].

The Squamata order also includes the lizards. Unlike snakes, lizards have four legs and external ears. There are more than 6,000 species of lizards, making it the largest group of reptiles. Lizards inhabit a wide range of ecological niches, from hot, dry desserts to cool, moist forests. The main groups of lizards include Gekkota, Iguania, Scincomorpha and Platynota (Varanoidea). Although the tuatara looks much like a lizard, it is excluded from the lizard group. The Gekkota suborder includes geckos, while skinks fall into the suborder Scincomorpha. Monitor lizards, Komodo dragons and Gila monsters are classified as Platynota (Varanoidea). The suborder Iguania includes chameleons, anoles and iguanas. The Carolina green anole lizard (*Anolis carolinensis)* is a small tree-living lizard, often green or brown, commonly found in the southeastern United States. It has intense green, blue and white coloring, especially evident on the male, and has a pink dewlap on its throat (Figure 5). The Anole lizard genome encodes for many β-defensin antimicrobial peptide genes and lysozyme genes.

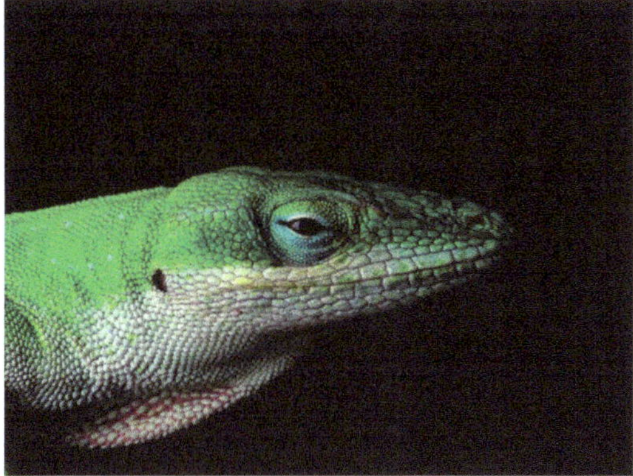

Figure 5. Male Carolina Anole with partially expanded dewlap [47].

The genomes of several members of the Squamata have recently been sequenced including the anole lizard [23], the elapid snakes *O. hannah* [15], *B. fasciatus*, and *N. atra* [30]. High-throughput sequencing and mass-spectrometry proteomics has been recently performed on snake venom, which should provide a deep view of proteins and peptides produced in the venom [48]. Antimicrobial peptides have been identified in the anole (defensins) [49], as well as cathelicidins in all three species of elapid snakes (see below) [3]. Very recently, the python genome has been sequenced [30]. Genome projects are also underway for other reptiles, such as the common garter snake (*Thamnophis sirtalis*) [23].

2.4. Crocodilia (Crocodilians)

The order of crocodilians (Crocodilia) within the group Archosauromorpha includes alligators and caimans (family Alligatoridae), crocodiles (family Crocodylidae), and gharials (gavials, family Gavialidae) (Figure 6). Most species live in fresh-water, but a few have also adapted to salt-water conditions. These animals are evolutionarily ancient, and along with birds, are considered the only surviving relatives of dinosaurs (Archosauria). Within their semi-aquatic ecosystems, these large animals are the apex predators, using their powerful jaws to capture large and small prey [50]. They are cold-blooded and egg-laying. They can be found around the world, in the Americas, in Asia, South America, and Africa [51]. The ancestors of alligators and crocodiles first emerged in the Late Cretaceous era, and the modern alligators and crocodiles are estimated to be as much as 83 million years old.

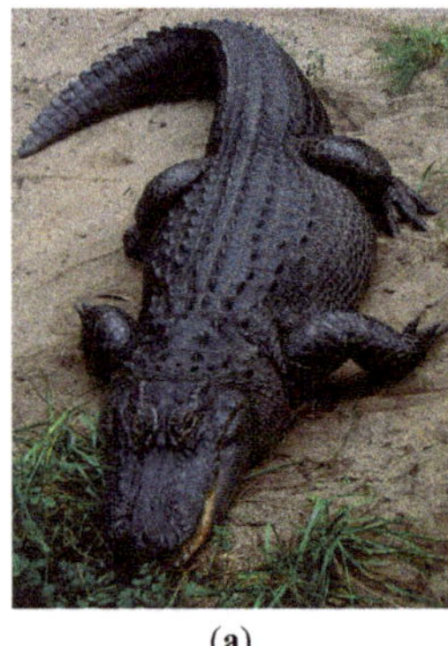

(a)

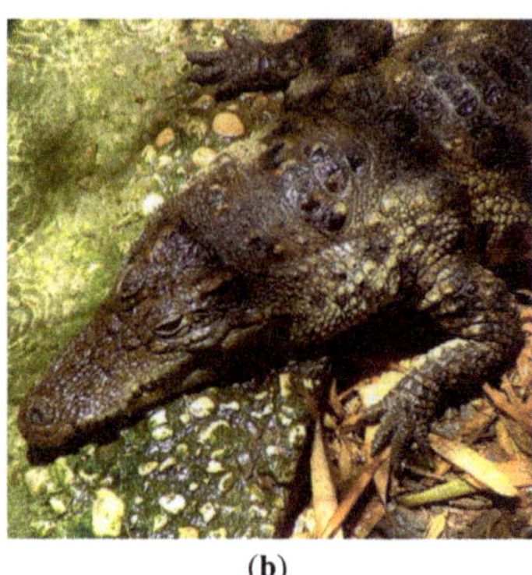

(b)

Figure 6. Crocodilians. (**a**) The American alligator, *Alligator mississippiensis* [52]. (**b**) The Siamese crocodile, *Crocodylus siamesnsis* [53].

Today, the American alligator is commonly found all around the Gulf of Mexico and Southeastern United States, having made a comeback from near extinction due to overhunting. The meat and skins of farmed alligators are now harvested for consumption and use. This large animal is typically 8–11 ft long and 200–500 lbs depending on gender and age [54]. The alligator has a broad snout and the top teeth come down over the bottom lips, unlike the crocodile. Alligators inhabit swamps such as the Great Dismal Swamp, rivers and streams, ponds and lakes, with a preference for fresh water over brackish water, and intolerance for salt water. Alligators can be infected by *Mycoplasma alligatoris* [55] as well as other bacterial pathogens. In terms of temperature preference, alligators are more cold tolerant than most other crocodilian species, accounting for their location as far north as South Carolina in the United States [54].

The Siamese crocodile (*Crocodylus siamensis*) [56,57] is a critically endangered freshwater crocodilian found in Southeast Asia (Cambodia, Vietnam, Thailand, Indonesia and Burma for example). Like most crocodiles, it is a tropical animal with low tolerance for the cold [3]. This animal is smaller than the alligator, typically about 7 ft long and 80–150 lbs when fully grown, although larger specimens have been recorded [4]. These animals are being intensively studied as part of their conservation, and are bred in captivity, and thus are accessible to researchers for DNA or blood samples [58–60].

Crocodilians such as alligators can carry a high burden of fecal coliforms from their aquatic environment [61], yet despite their potentially near-constant exposure to potential pathogens, alligators and other crocodilians do not seem to be susceptible to infection by these organisms, either systemically or on their skin, via wounds or lesions. This has led to the idea that these animals may have highly potent antimicrobial components to their immune systems [57,62–67]. Several crocodilian genomes have been published [68] or are underway [69]. The peptides that have been discovered in crocodilians are outlined in the sections below and include lysozyme, defensin, hepcidin, hemocidin and other antimicrobial peptides. Several important crocodilian genomes have been sequenced, including the Chinese alligator (*Alligator sinensis*), the American alligator (*Alligator mississippiensis*), the saltwater crocodile (*Crocodylus porosus*) and the Indian gharial (*Gavialis gangeticus*) [69,70]. It will be very interesting to compare freshwater species to saltwater species in terms of their innate immune response profiles, as the environmental organisms will be significantly different between the two types of water.

3. Antimicrobial Peptides of Reptiles

Reptiles are highly adapted to their environments, which often include many bacteria, allowing them to be such successful animals. Antimicrobial peptides are part of the innate immune system, and may contribute to the survival of reptiles. However, to date there has been no direct data in reptiles such as gene knock-out experiments to demonstrate their importance to overall survival, development and resistance to infection, as has been done in mice [71]. There has been some suggestion that β-defensin peptides are associated with fur color in dogs [72,73], but again no studies of this kind have yet been done on reptiles. This area of research presents many opportunities for scientists to explore the role of antimicrobial peptides in these animals. This paper will review the known (Table 1) and predicted antimicrobial peptides of reptiles. Recently, new reptilian genomes have been sequenced. From these genomes, additional antimicrobial peptide genes have been predicted here by bioinformatics analysis (Tables 2–8), which should be synthesized and tested for activity.

Antimicrobial peptides are well-characterized peptides, and exhibit significant structure-function specificity. Following the identification of magainin peptides in amphibians in 1987 [74], scientists have been exploring the diversity of peptides expressed in different animals, looking for new structures and new functions of antimicrobial peptides. The structure and function of each of the major classes of antimicrobial peptides is described below, in addition to the data pertaining to its known or predicted expression in reptiles.

3.1. *Defensin Peptides in Reptiles*

Defensins are one of the major classes of antimicrobial peptides in higher vertebrates. These 3–4 kDa cationic peptides are characterized by having six cysteines arranged in three disulfide bonds, with the characteristic pairing of the bonds highly characteristic for each type of defensin. Defensins have predominantly β-sheet characteristic with some α-helices. Defensins are encoded in the genome and are processed from a pro-defensin molecule by proteases [75].

3.1.1. Three Sub-Classes of Defensins

Defensins are known to be critical components of innate immunity in many animals [76]. The three main sub-classes of defensins are α, β- and θ-defensins. In humans, α-defensins are commonly found in neutrophils and other leukocytes (for example, Human Neutrophil peptide HNP-1 = α-defensin 1), and are important in the ability of white blood cells to deal with pathogens [77]. The β-defensins are defined as having a Cys1-Cys5, Cys2-Cys4, and Cys3-Cys6 bonding pattern of cysteines. In humans, β-defensins are commonly expressed in epithelial cells, and are widely expressed in the body [78]. The expression of these cationic antimicrobial peptides are often induced following bacterial or viral infection as part of the innate immune response, except for hBD1 which appears to be constitutively expressed in humans. The third class of defensins is the θ-defensins. θ-Defensins are not known outside of primates, and are not expressed in humans [21] but are very active antiviral peptides [76].

Within the reptiles, there are no known genes for α-defensins, and only the β-defensins appear to be expressed, similar to what is found in avians. Within some species of reptiles, β-defensin genes and peptides have been identified, for example in the red-eared slider turtle [79]. Lizards are known to be highly resistant to infection, and recently genes encoding up to 32 different β-defensin-like peptides were identified in the *Anole carolinensis* genome [49]. Indeed, using an antibody that reacts to AcBD15 (one of those β-defensin-like peptides in anole), staining was observed in some (but not all) of the granules of heterophilic and basophilic granulocytes in lizards, a snake, a turtle and the tuatara, but not alligator nor chicken granulocytes. Cells from other tissues such as epidermis were negative for staining. Alibardi *et al.* describe that not all the granules within a granulocyte stained with the antibody, suggesting that there may be different types of granules as is seen in mammalian neutrophils [22].

Similarly, turtle leukocytes were found to contain TBD-1, the first β-defensin identified in reptile leukocytes [14]. In the turtle system, TBD-1 was also identified in other tissues, such as the skin [18,80, 81]. These fascinating and unique results suggest that further study of the antimicrobial peptidome of reptilian granulocytes should be performed.

3.1.2. Inducible Expression of β-Defensins in Wounded Lizards

The first extensive report of an *in vivo* role for β-defensin peptide expression was in the anole lizard (Table 2). It has long been known that lizards can lose their tails as a method of predator escape, and that these tail then regenerate from the wound site. In this process, a wound is formed, which does not typically get infected. β-Defensin peptides are found to be expressed both within the azurophilic granulocytes in the wound-bed as well as in the associated epithelium [82,83], and are observed in phagosomes containing degraded bacteria. While there is a distinct lack of inflammation in the wound, which is associated with regeneration, there is a high level of expression of AcBD15 and AcBD27 (two of the most highly expressed β-defensins in that tissue) [84,85]. Overall, there appears to be a fascinating role of AcBD15 and AcBD27 in the wound healing and regeneration in the anole lizard.

Table 2. Predicted defensin-like protein genes in multiple reptilian species.

Organism	Peptide annotation	aa	Locus- Accession #
Alligator mississippiensis	Gallinacin-14-like	58	XP_006270781.1
Alligator sinensis	Gallinacin-14-like	58	XP_006033878.1
Anolis carolinensis	β-Defensin-like protein 5	62	CBY85058.1
Anolis carolinensis	β-Defensin-like protein 8	65	CBY85059.1
Anolis carolinensis	β-Defensin-like protein 9	66	CBY85060.1
Anolis carolinensis	β-Defensin-like protein 10	67	CBY85061.1
Anolis carolinensis	β-Defensin-like protein 15	63	CCA62931.1
Anolis carolinensis	β-Defensin-like protein 21	89	CBY85062.1
Anolis carolinensis	β-Defensin-like protein 22	95	CBY85063.1
Anolis carolinensis	β-Defensin-like protein 27	81	CBY85064.1
Anolis carolinensis	Gallinacin-10-like	68	XP_003225602.1
Anolis carolinensis	Gallinacin-13-like	60	XP_003225598.1
Anolis carolinensis	Hypothetical protein LOC100555370		XP_003227809.1
Anolis carolinensis	Hypothetical protein LOC100555565		XP_003227810.1
Anolis carolinensis	Hypothetical protein LOC100555756		XP_003227811.1
Anolis carolinensis	Hypothetical protein LOC100562305		XP_003225604.1
Anolis carolinensis	Hypothetical protein LOC100562502	65	XP_003225605.1
Anolis carolinensis	Hypothetical protein LOC100562898		XP_003225607.1
Anolis carolinensis	Hypothetical protein LOC100563098		XP_003225608.1
Chrysemys picta bellii	β-Defensin 1-like	80	XP_005308390.1
Chrysemys picta bellii	Gallinacin-5-like		XP_005290738.1
Chrysemys picta bellii	Gallinacin-5-like, partial		XP_005314963.1
Chrysemys picta bellii	Gallinacin-14-like	58	XP_005308403.1
Pelodiscus sinensis	Gallinacin-1 α-like		XP_006137072.1
Pelodiscus sinensis	Lingual antimicrobial peptide-like isoform X2		XP_006127561.1
Bothrops neuwiedi	β-Defensin-like protein		AGF25392.1
Bothrops jararacussu	β-Defensin-like protein		AGF25388.1
Bothrops leucurus	β-Defensin-like protein		AGF25389.1
Bothrops matogrossensis	β-Defensin-like protein		AGF25391.1, AGF25390.1
Bothrops diporus	β-Defensin-like protein		AGF25384.1
Bothrops pauloensis	β-Defensin-like protein		AGF25393.1
Bothrops jararaca	β-Defensin-like protein		AGF25386.1, AGF25387.1
Bothrops atrox	β-Defensin-like protein		AGF25383.1
Bothrops erythromelas	β-defensin-like protein		AGF25385.1

3.1.3. Expression of β-Defensins in Reptile Eggs

Reptile eggs are a good biological sample for the purification of peptides and proteins, since there is so much material within each egg. Recently, it was found that while the β-defensin-like peptide pelovaterin (Table 1) identified in the eggshell of the Chinese soft-shelled turtle does indeed have antimicrobial activity, these peptides may also play an additional role in the formation of the eggshell, through aggregation [15]. This is similar to the role of the gallin defensin-like peptide in avian eggs [86–90].

3.2. Cathelicidin Peptides in Reptiles

Cathelicidins are a second major class of antimicrobial peptides in higher eukaryotes. They are characterized as being antimicrobial peptides derived by proteolytic cleavage from a pre-propeptide that includes the cathelin domain in mammals and less-well conserved cathelin domain in other eukaryotes [91,92]. In humans, cathelicidins are stored in the azurophilic granules of neutrophils as the inactive prepropeptide, and are processed by enzymes (neutrophil elastase [93] or a serine protease [19]) to the mature active peptide [94]. In humans and higher vertebrates, the active cathelicidin peptide is always encoded on Exon 4 of the cathelicidin encoding gene [91,95,96]. Four cathelicidin-like peptides have been identified in the chicken (*Gallus gallus domesticus*) [97], including fowlicidin-1, -2 and -3 (also known as chCATH-1, chCATH-2/CMAP27, chCATH-3) [98], and chCATH-B1/chCATH-4 [99]. In humans, the hCAP18 cathelicidin is processed by proteinase 3 inside the granule [19] or neutrophil elastase in the extracellular space [4] to its active form. In the case of chicken cathelicidin, the pre-pro-cathelin domain peptide is cleaved by a serine protease to release the mature peptide following stimulation of heterophils with LPS [100].

3.3. Cathelicidin Peptides in Snakes

Cathelicidin peptides have been identified and characterized in the snake family (Table 1) [1,2], although there may be similar genes in other reptiles by genomic analysis (see below). Highly related cathelicidins were identified in *B. fasciatus*, *O. hannah* and *N. atra* [3] (Table 3). We identified additional genes for antimicrobial peptides by BLAST searching the genomes of the pit vipers (*Bothrops atrox*, *Trimeresurus wagler* and *Crotalus durissus*) [13] and the Eastern brown snake (*Pseudonaja textilis*) (Table 3). The genes of these cathelicidins have the general structure of the cathelicidin genes, including a poorly conserved cathelin domain and the c-terminal active peptide. The snake cathelicidins have been well studied. The functional cathelicidin peptide of the snake family is highly divergent from the functional cathelicidin peptide of humans, for example, confirming the "general rule" of cathelicidins, which is that the active peptides are highly divergent, but the pre-pro-regions in the gene and the peptide are more highly conserved [101].

3.3.1. King Cobra (*Ophiophagus (O.) Hannah*)

Zhao *et al.* determined the hemolytic and antimicrobial activity of the predicted *O. hannah* cathelicidin, OH-CATH [3] (Table 1). The OH-CATH peptide proved to be an excellent inhibitor of bacterial growth and demonstrated broad-spectrum activity against bacterial isolates including multi-drug resistant strains. The OH-CATH peptide displayed greater potency than the human cathelicidin LL-37 against a variety of known human bacterial pathogens and the antimicrobial potency of OH-CATH was not significantly impacted by the concentration of salt in the media. They demonstrated that OH-CATH showed no hemolytic activity against erythrocytes, even at a concentration of 200 μg/mL, suggesting low cytotoxicity of the peptide to eukaryotic cells [3]. Additional studies with smaller fragments of OH-CATH (Table 1) have also been tested and found to be active both *in vitro* and *in vivo*, even against antibiotic resistant bacteria [4,6]. Their strong antimicrobial activity and lack of hemolytic activity make the reptile cathelicidins strong candidates for development into new therapeutics.

Table 3. Known and predicted cathelicidin open reading frames in multiple snake species. The active antimicrobial peptides NA-CATH, BF-CATH and OH-CATH are highlighted.

Protein name [Organism]	Accession		Sequence
Cathelicidin-NA antimicrobial peptide [Naja atra]	B6S2X0.1	1 81 157	MEGFFWKTLLVVGALTISGTSSFPHKPLTYEEAVDLAVSVYN SKSGEDSLYRLLEAVPALKWDALSESNQELNFSVKETV 80 CQMAEERSLEECDFQEAGAVMGCTGYYFFGESPPVLVLTCK SVGNE-EEQKQEEGNEEEKEVEKEEKEEDQKDQPKR 156 VKRFKKFFKKLKNSVKKRAKKFFKKPKVIGVTFPF191
Cathelicidin-BF antimicrobial peptide [Bungarus fasciatus]	B6D434.1	1 81 157	MEGFFWKTLLVVGALAIAGTSSLPHKPLIYEEAVDLAVSIYN SKSGEDSLYRLLEAVSPPKWDPLSESNQELNFTMKETV 80 CLVAEERSLEECDFQEDGAIMGCTGYYFFGESPPVLVLTCK PVGEE-EEQKQEEGNEEEKEVEKEEKEEDEKDQPRR 156 VKRFKKFFRKLKKSVKKRAKEFFKKPRVIGVSIPF 191
Cathelicidin-OH antimicrobial peptide [Ophiophagus hannah]	B6S2X2.1	1 81 157	MEGFFWKTLLVVGALAIGGTSSLPHKPLTYEEAVDLAVSIYNS KSGEDSLYRLLEAVPPPEWDPLSESNQELNFTIKETV 80 CLVAEERSLEECDFQEDGVVMGCTGYYFFGESPPVVVLTCKP VGEE-GEQKQEEGNEEEKEVEEEEQEEDEKDQPRR 156 VKRFKKFFKKLKNSVKKRAKKFFKKPRVIGVSIPF 191
cathelicidin-like peptide precursor [Bothrops atrox]	AGS36140.1	1 79 155	MQGFFWKTWLVVALC–GTSSSLAHRPLSYGEALELALSIYNSK AGEESLFRLLEAVPQPEWDPLSEGSQQLNFTIKETV 78 CQVEEERPLEECGFQEDGVVLECTGYYFFGETPPVVVLTCVPV GGV-EEEEEDE-EEQKAEVEKDEKEDEEKDRPKR 154 VKRFKKFFKKLKNSVKKRVKKFFRKPRVIGVTFPF 189
cathelicidin-related antimicrobial peptide isoform precursor [Pseudonaja textilis]	AGS36144.1	1 81 150	MEGFFWKTWLVVAAFAIGGTSSLPHKPLTYEEAVDLAVSTYN GKSGEESLYRLLEAVPPPKWDPLSESNQELNLTIKETV 80 CLVAEERSLEECDFQDDGAVMGCTGYFFFGESPPVLVLTCEPL GED-EEQNQEEE——EEEEKEEDEKDQPRR 149 VKRFKKFFMKLKKSVKKRVMKFFKKPMVIGVTFPF 184
cathelicidin-related antimicrobial peptide precursor [Pseudonaja textilis]	AGS36143.1	1 81 150	MDGFFWKTWLVVAALAIGGTSSLPHKPLTYEEAVDLAVSTYN GKSGEESLYRLLEAVPPPKWDPLSESNQELNLTIKETV 80 CLVAEERSLEECDFQDDGAVMGCTGYFFFGESPPVLVLTCEP LGED-EEQNQEEE——-EEEEKEEDEKDQPRR 149 VKRFKKFFRKLKKSVKKRVKKFFKKPRVIGVTIPF 184
cathelicidin-like peptide precursor [Bothrops lutzi]	AGS36141.1	1 79 155	MQGFFWKTLLVVALC—GTSSSLAHRPLSYGEALELALSVYNS KAGEESLFRLLEAVPQPEWDPLSEGSQQLNFTIKETV 78 CQVEEERPLEECGFQEDGVVLECTGYYFFGETPPVVVLTCVP VGGV-EEEEEDE-EEQKAEVEKDEKEDEEKDRPKR 154 VKRFKKFFKKLKNNVKKRVKKFFRKPRVIGVTIPF 189
cathelicidin-like peptide precursor [Lachesis muta rhombeata]	AGS36142.1	1 79 160	MQGFFWKTWLVLAVC–GTPASLAHRPLSYGEALELAVSVYN GKAGEASLYRLLEAVPQPEWDPSSEGSQQLNFTLKETA 78 CQVEEERSLEECGFQEDGVVLECTGYYFFGETPPVVVLSCVP VGGVeEEEEEEE-EEQKAEAENDEKEDEEKDQPKR 159 160 VKRFKKFFKKVKKSVKKRLKKIFKKPMVIGVTFPF 194
cathelicidin-like peptide precursor [Crotalus durissus terrificus]	AGS36138.1	1 79 160	MQGFFWKTWLVLAVC—GTPASLAHRPLSYGEALELAVSVYN GKAGEASLYRLLEAVPQPEWDPSSEGSQQLNFTLKETA 78 CQVEEERSLEECGFQEDGVVLECTGYYFFGETPPVVVLSCVP VGGVeEEEEEEE-EEQKAEAENDEKGDEEKDQPKR 159 VKRFKKFFKKVKKSVKKRLKKIFKKPMVIGVTIPF 194

3.3.2. Chinese King Cobra *(Naja (N.) Atra)*

The genus *Naja* is a group of venomous elapid snakes in the southern Africa and South Asia, including the species *N. atra*, the Chinese King cobra. The cathelicidin peptide from the Chinese King cobra, *N. atra* (NA-CATH) (Table 1), has been well studied. The full-length NA-CATH peptide was synthesized and was found to be antimicrobial against a wide variety of bacteria [102–105]. Smaller fragments of this peptide have been identified and found to be effective [102–105].

Interestingly, while the human cathelicidin peptide (LL-37) was found to exert antibiofilm activity against bacterial pathogens such as *Pseudomonas* [103] and *Staphylococcus* [105], NA-CATH did not exhibit antibiofilm effect against *Pseudomonas*, despite similar overall biophysical properties (length, size, charge) to LL-37.

The smallest identified fragment of NA-CATH is an 11-amino acid peptide, called ATRA, which imperfectly repeats in the NA-CATH sequence (Figure 7a) [102]. Variants of the ATRA peptide have been found to be very informative regarding the role of charged residues and proline residues in the activity of small antimicrobial peptides [102]. The peptide ATRA-1 is almost identical to the ATRA-2 peptide, with the exception of the 3d (A/F) and 10th (L/P) residues. Variants of these peptides were made to switch out the 3rd and 10th position amino acids, such that ATRA-1A contains alanine at position 3 rather than phenylalanine (F). Another variant was ATRA-1P, which contains proline at position 10 rather than leucine (L). All the peptides were the same length, similar molecular weight, and the same net charge. It was found for multiple gram-negative bacteria that ATRA-1P was almost as ineffective as ATRA-2, while ATRA-1A was as effective as ATRA-1 [102]. These results suggested that the introduction of a proline in ATRA-1P may have affected the charge distribution on that peptide, which then may disrupt the antibacterial activity of the peptide (Figure 7b,c).

Further studies have examined the D-amino acid enantiomer of the ATRA peptides [106], and found that D-ATRA-1A is as effective as ATRA-1A, and as it is protease resistant, potentially has a longer half-life. The ATRA peptides have also been demonstrated to be highly antimicrobial both *in vitro* and *in vivo* against both gram-negative bacteria such as *Escherichia coli* K12 strain and *Aggregatibacter actinomycetemcomitans*-Y4 [102], *Pseudomonas aeruginosa* [103] and *Francisella novicida* [104]. ATRA peptides are also antimicrobial against the gram-positive bacteria *Staphylococcus aureus* [105].

3.3.3. Banded Krait *(B. fasciatus)*

The cathelicidin peptide from *B. fasciatus* (BF-CATH, Table 1, Table 3) is also very well studied. The full-length BF-CATH peptide has been shown to have antimicrobial activity against a variety of bacteria including antibiotic resistant bacteria [7,107]. Smaller fragments of BF-CATH have also been expressed and studied [10,108] (Table 1). For example, BF-30 showed significant activity against drug-resistant *E. coli* and *S. aureus* both *in vitro* and *in vivo* [109]. BF-15 is a shorter version of BF-CATH with lower hemolytic activity, and broad-spectrum antimicrobial activity even against antibiotic-resistant bacteria [8].

Peptide Description	Peptide Sequence
NA-CATH Active Peptide	**KRFKKFFKKLK**NSVK**KRAKKFFKKPK**VIGVTFPF
ATRA-1	**KRFKKFFKKLK**
ATRA-2	------------------------------ **KRAKKFFKKPK**
ATRA-1A	**KAFKKFFKKLK**
ATRA-1P	**KRFKKFFKKPK**

(a) Sequence of the Chinese King Cobra *Naja atra* cathelicidin and ATRA derivatives.

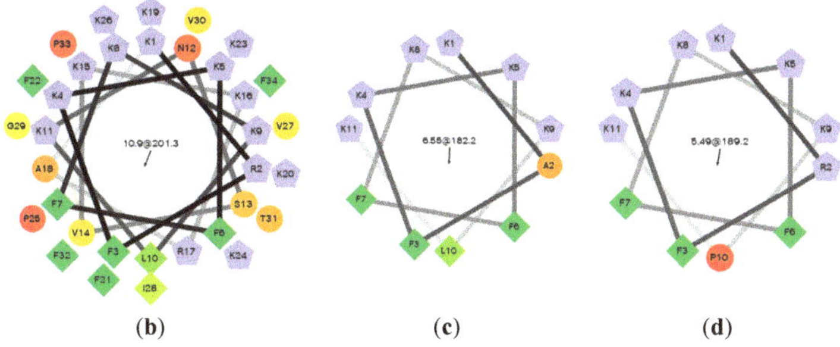

(b) **(c)** **(d)**

Figure 7. *Naja atra* cathelicidin peptide analysis. (**a**) Sequences of the NA-CATH active peptide and derivatives [102–105]. (**b**) Helical wheel projection of NA-CATH. (**c**) Analysis of the active ATRA-1A peptide (**d**) Analysis of the inactive ATRA-1P peptide. From Rzlab.ucr.edu/scripts/wheel/wheel.cgi: "The hydrophilic residues are presented as circles, hydrophobic residues as diamonds, potentially negatively charged as triangles, and potentially positively charged as pentagons. Hydrophobicity is color coded as well: the most hydrophobic residue is green, and the amount of green is decreasing proportionally to the hydrophobicity, with zero hydrophobicitycoded as yellow. Hydrophilic residues are coded red with pure red being the most hydrophilic (uncharged) residue, and the amount of red decreasing proportionally to the hydrophilicity. The potentially charged residues are light blue."

3.3.4. Predicted Cathelicidins in Other Snake Species

By performing BLAST analysis with the elapid snake cathelicidins against other snake sequences in the database, we identified cathelicidin-like gene sequences in the venomous pit viper, *Bothrops atrox*, and the Eastern brown snake, *Pseudonaja textilis* (Table 3). These genes should be further studied to verify that cathelicidin-like peptides are produced and to determine the activity of these peptides.

3.4. Cathelicidin Peptides in Lizards

Cathelicidin-like peptides Ac-CATH-1, Ac-CATH-2a, Ac-CATH -2b, and Ac-CATH -3 have been reported in the genome of the Carolina anole lizard (*Anolis carolinensis*) [110] (Table 4). In addition, cathelicidin 1 and 2 antibody reactive peptides have been identified by immunocytochemistry staining within granules of heterophilic and basophilic granulocytes [111]. This study also identified cathelicidin-antibody staining material in wound epidermis and associated with bacteria within wounds [111].

Table 4. Predicted active cathelicidin peptides in the anole lizard [91,92].

Organism	Peptide annotation
Anolis carolinensis	Ac-CATH-1 MGRITRSRWGRFWRGAKRFVKKHGVSIALAGLRFG (+10)
Anolis carolinensis	Ac-CATH-2a/b DPQMTRFRGLGHFFKGFGRGFIWGLNH (+3)
Anolis carolinensis	Ac-CATH-3—no active peptide encoded.

3.5. Cathelicidin Peptides in Turtles

Analysis of the recently published genomes revealed that there are many cathelicin-like genes in turtles. While no active cathelicidin peptides have been demonstrated yet in the turtle (Table 1), there are at many predicted cathelicidin-like peptide genes (Table 5). Many of these are annotated as being similar to the snake cathelicidins (eg OH-CATH).

Table 5. Predicted cathelicidin pre-pro-protein genes in multiple turtle species.

Organism	Peptide annotation	Locus- Accession #
Chrysemys picta bellii	Cathelicidin-OH antimicrobial peptide-like	XM_005295113.1
Chrysemys picta bellii	Cathelicidin-OH antimicrobial peptide-like	XP_005295170.1
Chrysemys picta bellii	Cathelicidin-2-like	XP_005295171.1
Chrysemys picta bellii	Uncharacterized LOC101951069	XR_255838.1
Chrysemys picta bellii	Uncharacterized LOC101951243	XR_255839.1
Pelodiscus sinensis	Cathelicidin-2-like	XM_006114422.1
Pelodiscus sinensis	Cathelicidin-2-like	XM_006114419.1
Pelodiscus sinensis	Cathelicidin-OH antimicrobial peptide-like transcript variant X1	XM_006129620.1
Pelodiscus sinensis	Cathelicidin-OH antimicrobial peptide-like transcript variant X2	XM_006129621.1
Pelodiscus sinensis	Cathelicidin-OH antimicrobial peptide-like	XM_006129625.1
Pelodiscus sinensis	Cathelicidin-BF antimicrobial peptide-like	XP_006114480.1
Pelodiscus sinensis	Cathelicidin-BF antimicrobial peptide-like	XM_006114418.1
Pelodiscus sinensi	Cathelicidin-2-like	XP_006114484.
Pelodiscus sinensis	Cathelicidin-2-like	XP_006114481.1
Pelodiscus sinensis	Cathelicidin-OH antimicrobial peptide-like isoform X1	XP_006129682.1
Pelodiscus sinensis	Cathelicidin-OH antimicrobial peptide-like isoform X2	XP_006129683.1
Pelodiscus sinensis	Cathelicidin-OH antimicrobial peptide-like	XP_006129687.1
Chelonia mydas	Hypothetical protein UY3_13361	EMP29519.1
Chelonia mydas	Hypothetical protein UY3_13360	EMP29518.1

3.6. Cathelicidin Peptides in Crocodilians

Analysis of the databases revealed that there are many cathelicidin-like genes in alligators. While no active cathelicidin peptides have been demonstrated yet in the alligator (Table 1), there are at many predicted cathelicidin-like peptide genes (Table 6). Many of these genes are annotated as being similar to the snake cathelicidins (e.g., OH-CATH).

Table 6. Predicted cathelicidin pre-pro-protein genes in Alligator species.

Organism	Peptide annotation	Locus- Accession #
Alligator mississippiensis	Cathelicidin-2-like	XM_006262429.1
Alligator mississippiensis	Cathelicidin-2-like	XP_006262491.1
Alligator mississippiensis	Cathelicidin-OH antimicrobial peptide-like	XM_006262431.1
Alligator mississippiensis	Cathelicidin-OH antimicrobial peptide-like	XM_006262430.1
Alligator mississippiensis	Cathelicidin-OH antimicrobial peptide-like	XP_006262492.1
Alligator mississippiensis	Cathelicidin-OH antimicrobial peptide-like	XP_006262493.1
Alligator sinensis	Cathelicidin-2-like	XM_006026412.1
Alligator sinensis	Cathelicidin-2-like	XP_006026474.1
Alligator sinensis	Cathelicidin-2-like	XP_006026475.1
Alligator sinensis	Cathelicidin-3-like	XM_006026409.1
Alligator sinensis	Cathelicidin-3-like	XP_006026471.1
Alligator sinensis	Cathelicidin-OH antimicrobial peptide-like	XM_006037224.1
Alligator sinensis	Cathelicidin-OH antimicrobial peptide-like	XM_006026410.1
Alligator sinensis	Cathelicidin-OH antimicrobial peptide-like	XM_006026411.1
Alligator sinensis	Cathelicidin-OH antimicrobial peptide-like	XM_006037211.1
Alligator sinensis	Cathelicidin-OH antimicrobial peptide-like	XP_006037286.1
Alligator sinensis	Cathelicidin-OH antimicrobial peptide-like	XP_006026472.1
Alligator sinensis	Cathelicidin-OH antimicrobial peptide-like	XP_006037273.1
Alligator sinensis	Cathelicidin-OH antimicrobial peptide-like	XP_006026487.1

3.7. *Liver-Derived Peptides in Reptiles*

3.7.1. Hepcidin (HAMP1)

Hepcidin antimicrobial peptides are liver-expressed peptides containing eight cysteines (four disulfide bonds) that are broadly antimicrobial, binds iron and is involved in ferroportin binding [112, 113]. A gene encoding a hepcidin-like peptide (E8ZAD0_CROSI) was recently proposed to be encoded by the Siamese crocodile (*Crocodylus siamensis*). A 26 aa peptide (Cshepc), representing the predicted active peptide (FNSHFPICSYCCNCCRNKGCGLCCRT), was expressed in yeast, and the unpurified product was found to have antimicrobial activity against both Gram-positive bacteria such as *S. aureus* and *Bacillus subtilis*, as well as Gram-negative bacteria *Escherichia coli* and *Aeromonas sobria* [114]. Hepcidin-like sequences were also identified in the anole lizard, although interestingly hepcidins appear to be missing in most avians [115].

3.7.2. LEAP-2, Liver Expressed Antimicrobial Peptide-2

Another liver-expressed peptide, LEAP-2, is expressed in many different organisms, has broad-spectrum antibacterial and antifungal activity, and can be induced following bacterial challenge [116–118]. This 40 aa, 4-cysteine, cationic peptide differs significantly from hepcidin in sequence and predicted structure [119], but is also predominantly expressed in the liver.

The Leap-2 gene is annotated in many of the sequenced reptiles (Table 7), including *Pelodiscus sinensis, Chrysemys picta bellii, Alligator sinensis, Alligator mississippiensis*, as identified by a BLAST analysis we performed with the LEAP-2 from *Anolis carolinensis*. The antimicrobial activity or biological role of this peptide in reptiles has not been studied.

Table 7. Predicted LEAP-2 pre-propeptide amino-acid sequences identified in reptiles.

Species	Predicted LEAP-2 full sequence	Accession Number
Anolis carolinensis	MTPLKITAVILICSALLFQTQGASLYPPNSQLVRQR RMTPFWRGISRPIGASCRDNSECSTRLCRSKHCSLRTSQE	XP_003217432.1
Alligator sinensis	MHWLKVIAVMLLFALHLFQIHCASLHQPNSQPKRQRRM TPFWRGVSSLRPIGASCRDDIECVTMLCRKSHCSLRTSRE	XP_006023615.1
Alligator mississippiensis	MHWLKVIAVMLLFALHLFQIHCASLHQPNSQPKRQRRM TPFWRGVSSLRPIGASCKDDGECITMRCRKSHCSLRTSRE	XP_006263463.1
Pelodiscus sinensis	MQCLKVIALLLFCAALLTQTHCASLHHSSSQLTRQRRMTP FWRGISLRPIGALCRHDNECISMLCRKNRCSLRISCE	XP_006128591.1
Chrysemys picta belli	MQYLKVIAVLLLCAALLSQIHSASLHRPSSHLTRQRRMTPF WRGISLRPIGAICRDDSECVSRLCRKNHCSIRISRA	XP_005302895.1

3.8. Lysozyme in Reptiles

Lysozyme is a very important part of innate immunity in most animals. In humans, it is packaged into neutrophil granules, released in tears and other secretions, and is very effective against a broad spectrum of bacteria. Not surprisingly, reptiles have also been found to use lysozyme as part of their innate immune response. In the crocodilians, a lysozyme-like enzyme was identified with broad-spectrum antibacterial activity [67]. Lysozyme proteins very similar to chicken lysozymes (~130 aa) have been identified from some species of turtles, including the soft shelled turtle (*Trionyx sinensis*), the Asiatic soft shelled turtle (*Amyda cartilagenea*) and the green sea turtle (*Chelonia mydas*) [17,19,120–122], although the antimicrobial activity of these molecules has not yet been proven. Lysozyme peptide has also been identified from *Crocodylus siamensis* [67]. Lysozyme-like genes were identified by analysis of reptile genomes (Table 8).

3.9. Crotamine Peptides in Reptiles

Defensins are one example of cysteine-stabilized polypeptides with antimicrobial function. A similar family of peptides is the crotamine toxin family isolated from rattlesnakes with a similar gamma-core motif to defensins [123,124], which is considered a cell-penetrating peptide The sequence of crotamine is YKQ**C**HKKGGH**C**FPKEKI**C**LPPSSDFGKMD**C**RWRWK**CC**KKGSG (+8) [2]. This cationic peptide contains nine lysines (underlined), three disulfide bonds (6 cysteines, shown in bold) and has a defensin-like fold (Figure 8).

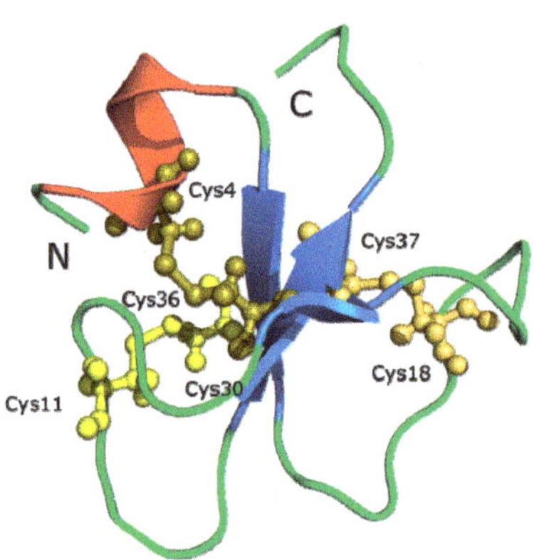

Figure 8. The crotamine chemical structure. Crotamine, a Na+ channel-affecting toxin from *Crotalus durissus terrificus* venom (PDB 1H5O) [125].

Table 8. Selected predicted lysozyme genes identified in reptiles.

Reptile name	Enzyme Name	Accession Number
Softshell turtle lysozyme C(SSTL)	Lysozyme C (1,4-β-N-acetylmuramidase C)	Q7LZQ1.3
Asiatic softshell turtle lysozyme C (ASTL)	Lysozyme C	P85345.1
Pelodiscus sinensis	Lysozyme	ADR51676.1
Pelodiscus sinensis	PREDICTED: lysozyme g-like isoform X2	XP_006113603.1
Pelodiscus sinensis	PREDICTED: lysozyme g-like isoform X1	XP_006113602.1
Pelodiscus sinensis	PREDICTED: lysozyme g-like	XP_006113601.1
Chelonia mydas	Lysozyme C	EMP38935.1
Chelonia mydas	Lysozyme G	EMP27176.1
Chrysemys picta bellii	PREDICTED: lysozyme C-like	XP_005314893.1
Chrysemys picta bellii	PREDICTED: lysozyme C-like	XP_005312037.1
Chrysemys picta bellii	PREDICTED: lysozyme g-like protein 2	XP_005283410.1
Chrysemys picta bellii	PREDICTED: lysozyme G-like	XP_005283294.1
Ophiophagus hannah	Lysozyme C, partial	ETE58503.1
Anolis carolinensis	Lysozyme C, milk isozyme-like	XP_003225844.1, XP_003216710.1, XP_003216704.1
Anolis carolinensis	Lysozyme C II-like	XP_003224512.1
Anolis carolinensis	Lysozyme g-like	XP_003227178.1
Alligator sinensis	Lysozyme C-like	XP_006027022.1, XP_006027021.1
Alligator sinensis	Lysozyme G-like	XP_006026406.1, XP_006026397.1, XP_006026395.1, XP_006026396.1

Some reptiles are known to express crotamine-like peptides, and The X-ray structure of crotamine, from the Brazilian snake *Crotalus durissus terrificus*, was recently solved (PDB 4GV5_A) [126]. We found that some species of reptiles have genes that are annotated as crotamine-like (Table 9).

Table 9. Crotamine-like peptide genes in reptiles.

Reptile	AA	Name	Accession numbers
Uromastyx aegyptia	67	crotamine-Uro-1	AGI97143.1
Crotalus durissus terrificus	65	crotamine	AAF34911.1, AAF34910.1, AAC02995.1, AAC06241.1
Crotalus durissus	34	crotamine	ACA63453.1, ACA63452.1, ACA63451.1, ACA63450.1, ACA63449.1, ACA63448.1, ACA63447.1, ACA63446.1
Crotalus oreganus helleri	65	crotamine 7	AEU60015.1
Crotalus oreganus helleri	65	crotamine 6	AEU60014.1
Crotalus oreganus helleri	65	crotamine 5	AEU60013.1
Crotalus oreganus helleri	70	crotamine 4	AEU60012.1
Crotalus oreganus helleri	70	crotamine 3	AEU60011.1
Crotalus oreganus helleri	83	crotamine 2	AEU60010.1
Crotalus oreganus helleri	70	crotamine 1	AEU60009.1
Pogona barbata	102	CLP-POGL1	AAZ75614.1
Pogona barbata	67	CLP-POGL2	AAZ75615.1
Pogona barbata	61	CLP-POGU3	AAZ75613.1
Pogona barbata	98	CLP-POGU2	AAZ75612.1
Pogona barbata	76	CLP-POGU1	AAZ75611.1
Varanus tristis	83	crotamine-Var-5	AGI97148.1
Varanus glauerti	83	crotamine-Var-4	AGI97147.1
Varanus glauerti	83	crotamine-Var-3	AGI97146.1
Varanus glauerti	83	crotamine-Var-2	AGI97145.1
Varanus glauerti	83	crotamine-Var-1	AGI97144.1

It has been a matter of some debate whether crotamine peptides are antimicrobial or if they just contain a similar cysteine-stabilized core structure. Recently, it was demonstrated that crotamine toxin is expressed similarly on epithelial or mucosal surfaces, and displays some antimicrobial activity against *Bacillus subtilis*, and was able to permeabilize *Staphylococcus aureus* cells, for example [20]. In addition, crotamine has been shown to be antifungal [127]. Thus, it seems that crotamine should be considered as an antimicrobial peptide of reptiles.

3.10. Other Peptides in Reptiles

3.10.1. Leucrocin

There are a handful of peptides identified in reptiles that were not easily classified in the categories above. One interesting example is the peptide leucrocin, an antibacterial compound from white blood cells of the Siamese crocodile (*Crocodylus siamensis*). Unlike Crocosin [65], which does not appear to be peptide based, leucrocins are very small peptides with antibacterial activity. The amino acid sequence of Leucrocin I is NGVQPKY, and of Leucrocin II is NAGSLLSGWG [66]. No known genes encode for these peptides, so their source is unclear. Recently, a synthetic peptide based on the Leucrocin sequence was found to have broad-spectrum antibacterial activity [128].

3.10.2. Omwaprin

Another example of an unusual antimicrobial peptide in reptiles is omwaprin, which is a member of the waprin family of venom proteins (Sequence shown in Table 1) [11,12], and was isolated from the Australian inland taipan (*Oxyuranus microlepidotus*), considered the most venomous snake (a member of the Elapid family of snakes). This 50 aa peptide has relatively salt-tolerant antibacterial activity against gram-positive bacteria and was found to be non-toxic to mice upon injection. Its activity was found to be highly dependent upon the four disulfide-bonds, similar to the hepcidins and defensins [11]. Thus, except for its large size, this peptide appears to have many favorable properties as a potential therapeutic candidate.

3.10.3. Hemocidin

Fragments of hemoglobin have been found to have some antimicrobial activity, and have been referred to as hemocidins [129–131]. In the study of the Siamese crocodile, 13 fragments of crocodile hemoglobin were found to have antimicrobial activity, including peptides similar to hemoglobin β subunit [59,60]. Recently, the hemoglobin α- and β-chains of crocodilian species (*Crocodylus siamensis, Alligator mississippiensis, Crocodylus niloticus* and *Caiman crocodilus*) have been reported [132]. The *in vivo* relevance of these peptides in the crocodile remains to be determined, but it represents a potential other class of antimicrobial peptides from reptiles that should be investigated.

3.10.4. Other Peptides

Other peptides have been identified in reptiles that do not fall into the various classes of antimicrobial peptides described above. These include a short, synthetic tryptophan-rich cationic antimicrobial peptide, pEM-2 (KKWRWWLKALAKK) that was shown to have broad-spectrum bactericidal activities, and was identified as a fragment of myotoxin II, a snake venom Lys49 phospholipase A2 [133,134]. Synthetic variants of this peptide were shown to have improved antimicrobial activity, salt resistance and reduced hemolytic activity [135,136]. These peptides have led to other advances in rational design of synthetic peptides, including peptides with exclusively arginine and tryptophan residues [137].

Gomes et al isolated, but did not sequence, a small 1370 Da peptide from the venom of a pit viper (*Borthrops jaracaca*), which showed very good activity against different fungi and yeast [138].

Another group identified an antimicrobial peptide derived from *N. atra* venom, the vgf-1 peptide, and found that this peptide had significant antimicrobial activity against drug-resistant clinical strains of *Mycobacterium tuberculosis* [139].

4. Conclusions

Reptiles are evolutionarily ancient, found in diverse and microbially challenging environments and appear to have robust immune systems. Some reptiles, especially lizards, have unique properties such as tail regeneration. All of these features suggest that reptiles may express many interesting antimicrobial peptides. A few reptilian antimicrobial peptides have been isolated and studied which demonstrate broad-spectrum antimicrobial and antifungal activity. These include members of the cathelicidin and defensin and lysozyme class.

Antimicrobial peptides are known in three of the four orders of reptiles: the testudines, crocodilians, and the squamata. No peptides are known from the sphenodontia (tuataras), as this organism has just been sequenced [41]. Reptile neutrophils appear to have granules that contain both cathelicidin-like peptides as well as β-defensin peptides, although unlike mammals, there are no genes encoding α-defensins. β-defensin-like peptides and lysozyme are also found in reptile eggs. These peptides are expressed in wounds, such as when lizards lose their tails. Detailed study of the Chinese cobra Naja atra cathelicidin peptides has revealed smaller peptides that could be useful for therapeutic applications.

Overall, reptiles reflect the diversity of antimicrobial peptides within higher organisms. They appear to express cathelicidins and β-defensins, and express hepcidins unlike avians. Additional classes of antimicrobial peptides such as lysozyme, LEAP-2 and crotamine also appear to be highly expressed in reptiles. With the advent of high-throughput genomics, new reptilian genomes have been sequenced and their transcriptomes determined. Analysis of these sequences has revealed that there are additional genes that may encode AMPs in reptiles. Future studies may reveal the in vivo role of antimicrobial peptides in reptiles. In the face of the emerging challenges due to antibiotic resistant bacteria, new and useful molecules that could be developed into future antibiotics may potentially be found in the reptilian AMPs.

Acknowledgments: MVH was partially supported by HDTRA1-12-C-0039, Translational Peptides for Personnel Protection.

Conflicts of Interest: The author declares no conflict of interest.

References

1. Wang, G. Antimicrobial Peptide Database. Available online: http://aps.unmc.edu/AP (accessed on 9 May 2014).
2. Wang, G.; Li, X.; Wang, Z. APD2: The updated antimicrobial peptide database and its application in peptide design. *Nucleic Acids Res.* **2009**, *37*, D933–D937. [CrossRef]
3. Zhao, H.; Gan, T.X.; Liu, X.D.; Jin, Y.; Lee, W.H.; Shen, J.H.; Zhang, Y. Identification and characterization of novel reptile cathelicidins from elapid snakes. *Peptides* **2008**, *29*, 1685–1691. [CrossRef]
4. Li, S.A.; Lee, W.H.; Zhang, Y. Efficacy of OH-CATH30 and its analogs against drug-resistant bacteria *in vitro* and in mouse models. *Antimicrob. Agents Chemother.* **2012**, *56*, 3309–3317. [CrossRef]
5. Zhang, B.Y.; Li, S.M.; Gao, Z.H.; Shen, J.H. Protective effects of snake venom antimicrobial peptide OH-CATH on *E. coli* induced rabbit urinary tract infection models. *Dong Wu Xue Yan Jiu* **2013**, *34*, 27–32.
6. Zhang, Y.; Zhao, H.; Yu, G.Y.; Liu, X.D.; Shen, J.H.; Lee, W.H.; Zhang, Y. Structure-function relationship of king cobra cathelicidin. *Peptides* **2010**, *31*, 1488–1493. [CrossRef]
7. Wang, Y.; Hong, J.; Liu, X.; Yang, H.; Liu, R.; Wu, J.; Wang, A.; Lin, D.; Lai, R. Snake cathelicidin from Bungarus fasciatus is a potent peptide antibiotics. *PloS One* **2008**, *3*, e3217.
8. Chen, W.; Yang, B.; Zhou, H.; Sun, L.; Dou, J.; Qian, H.; Huang, W.; Mei, Y.; Han, J. Structure-activity relationships of a snake cathelicidin-related peptide, BF-15. *Peptides* **2011**, *32*, 2497–2503. [CrossRef]

9. Wang, H.; Ke, M.; Tian, Y.; Wang, J.; Li, B.; Wang, Y.; Dou, J.; Zhou, C. BF-30 selectively inhibits melanoma cell proliferation via cytoplasmic membrane permeabilization and DNA-binding *in vitro* and in B16F10-bearing mice. *Eur. J. Pharmacol.* **2013**, *707*, 1–10.
10. Zhou, H.; Dou, J.; Wang, J.; Chen, L.; Wang, H.; Zhou, W.; Li, Y.; Zhou, C. The antibacterial activity of BF-30 *in vitro* and in infected burned rats is through interference with cytoplasmic membrane integrity. *Peptides* **2011**, *32*, 1131–1138. [CrossRef]
11. Nair, D.G.; Fry, B.G.; Alewood, P.; Kumar, P.P.; Kini, R.M. Antimicrobial activity of omwaprin, a new member of the waprin family of snake venom proteins. *Biochem. J.* **2007**, *402*, 93–104. [CrossRef]
12. Banigan, J.R.; Mandal, K.; Sawaya, M.R.; Thammavongsa, V.; Hendrickx, A.P.; Schneewind, O.; Yeates, T.O.; Kent, S.B. Determination of the X-ray structure of the snake venom protein omwaprin by total chemical synthesis and racemic protein crystallography. *Protein Sci.* **2010**, *19*, 1840–1849. [CrossRef]
13. Schmidt, J.J.; Weinstein, S.A.; Smith, L.A. Molecular properties and structure-function relationships of lethal peptides from venom of Wagler's pit viper, *Trimeresurus wagleri*. *Toxicon* **1992**, *30*, 1027–1036. [CrossRef]
14. Stegemann, C.; Kolobov, A., Jr.; Leonova, Y.F.; Knappe, D.; Shamova, O.; Ovchinnikova, T.V.; Kokryakov, V.N.; Hoffmann, R. Isolation, purification and de novo sequencing of TBD-1, the first beta-defensin from leukocytes of reptiles. *Proteomics* **2009**, *9*, 1364–1373. [CrossRef]
15. Lakshminarayanan, R.; Vivekanandan, S.; Samy, R.P.; Banerjee, Y.; Chi-Jin, E.O.; Teo, K.W.; Jois, S.D.; Kini, R.M.; Valiyaveettil, S. Structure, self-assembly, and dual role of a beta-defensin-like peptide from the Chinese soft-shelled turtle eggshell matrix. *J. Am. Chem. Soc.* **2008**, *130*, 4660–4668. [CrossRef]
16. Lakshminarayanan, R.; Chi-Jin, E.O.; Loh, X.J.; Kini, R.M.; Valiyaveettil, S. Purification and characterization of a vaterite-inducing peptide, pelovaterin, from the eggshells of Pelodiscus sinensis (Chinese soft-shelled turtle). *Biomacromolecules* **2005**, *6*, 1429–1437. [CrossRef]
17. Thammasirirak, S.; Ponkham, P.; Preecharram, S.; Khanchanuan, R.; Phonyothee, P.; Daduang, S.; Srisomsap, C.; Araki, T.; Svasti, J. Purification, characterization and comparison of reptile lysozymes. *Comp. biochem. Phys. Toxicol. Pharmacol.* **2006**, *143*, 209–217.
18. Chattopadhyay, S.; Sinha, N.K.; Banerjee, S.; Roy, D.; Chattopadhyay, D.; Roy, S. Small cationic protein from a marine turtle has beta-defensin-like fold and antibacterial and antiviral activity. *Proteins* **2006**, *64*, 524–531. [CrossRef]
19. Ponkham, P.; Daduang, S.; Kitimasak, W.; Krittanai, C.; Chokchaichamnankit, D.; Srisomsap, C.; Svasti, J.; Kawamura, S.; Araki, T.; Thammasirirak, S. Complete amino acid sequence of three reptile lysozymes. *Comp. Biochem. Phys. Toxicol. Pharmacol.* **2010**, *151*, 75–83. [CrossRef]
20. Yount, N.Y.; Kupferwasser, D.; Spisni, A.; Dutz, S.M.; Ramjan, Z.H.; Sharma, S.; Waring, A.J.; Yeaman, M.R. Selective reciprocity in antimicrobial activity *versus* cytotoxicity of hBD-2 and crotamine. *Proc. Natl. Acad. Sci. USA* **2009**, *106*, 14972–14977. [CrossRef]
21. Coronado, M.A.; Georgieva, D.; Buck, F.; Gabdoulkhakov, A.H.; Ullah, A.; Spencer, P.J.; Arni, R.K.; Betzel, C. Purification, crystallization and preliminary X-ray diffraction analysis of crotamine, a myotoxic polypeptide from the Brazilian snake Crotalus durissus terrificus. *Acta Crystallogr. F* **2012**, *68*, 1052–1054. [CrossRef]
22. Modesto, S.P.; Anderson, J.S. The phylogenetic definition of reptilia. *Syst. Biol.* **2004**, *53*, 815–821. [CrossRef]
23. Alfoldi, J.; Di Palma, F.; Grabherr, M.; Williams, C.; Kong, L.; Mauceli, E.; Russell, P.; Lowe, C.B.; Glor, R.E.; Jaffe, J.D.; *et al.* The genome of the green anole lizard and a comparative analysis with birds and mammals. *Nature* **2011**, *477*, 587–591. [CrossRef]
24. Cladogram by Benchill, licensed under the Creative Commons Attribution 3.0 Unported license. Available online: http://en.wikipedia.org/wiki/File:Tuatara_cladogram.svg (accessed on 9 May 2014).
25. Ernst, C.H.; Lovich, J.E. *Turtles of the United States and Canada*, 2nd ed.; Johns Hopkins University Press: Baltimore, MD, USA, 2009; pp. 185–259.
26. Photo from Oregon Department of Fish & Wildlife, licensed under the Creative Commons Attribution-Share Alike 2.0 Generic license. Photo by Gary M. Stolz/U. S. Fish and Wildlife Service in the Public domain. Available online: http://en.wikipedia.org/wiki/FileA4_Western_painted_turtle.jpg (accessed on 9 May 2014).
27. Underside of a Western Painted Turtle. Photo by Matt Young, l.u.t.C.C.A.-S.A.G.l. Available online: http://en.wikipedia.org/wiki/File:B4_Western_painted_turtle_underside.jpg (accessed on 9 May 2014).
28. Wang, Z.; Pascual-Anaya, J.; Zadissa, A.; Li, W.; Niimura, Y.; Huang, Z.; Li, C.; White, S.; Xiong, Z.; Fang, D.; *et al.* The draft genomes of soft-shell turtle and green sea turtle yield insights into the development and evolution of the turtle-specific body plan. *Nat. Genet.* **2013**, *45*, 701–706. [CrossRef]

29. Jiang, J.J.; Xia, E.H.; Gao, C.W.; Gao, L.Z. The complete mitochondrial genome of western painted turtle, *Chrysemys picta bellii* (Chrysemys, Emydidae). *Mitochondrial DNA* **2014**. [CrossRef]
30. Shaffer, H.B.; Minx, P.; Warren, D.E.; Shedlock, A.M.; Thomson, R.C.; Valenzuela, N.; Abramyan, J.; Amemiya, C.T.; Badenhorst, D.; Biggar, K.K.; *et al.* The western painted turtle genome, a model for the evolution of extreme physiological adaptations in a slowly evolving lineage. *Genome Biol.* **2013**, *14*, R28. [CrossRef]
31. Gilbert, S.F.; Corfe, I. Turtle origins: Picking up speed. *Dev. Cell* **2013**, *25*, 326–328. [CrossRef]
32. Zardoya, R.; Meyer, A. Complete mitochondrial genome suggests diapsid affinities of turtles. *Proc. Natl. Acad. Sci. USA* **1998**, *95*, 14226–14231. [CrossRef]
33. Iwabe, N.; Hara, Y.; Kumazawa, Y.; Shibamoto, K.; Saito, Y.; Miyata, T.; Katoh, K. Sister group relationship of turtles to the bird-crocodilian clade revealed by nuclear DNA-coded proteins. *Mol. Biol. Evol.* **2005**, *22*, 810–813. [CrossRef]
34. Roos, J.; Aggarwal, R.K.; Janke, A. Extended mitogenomic phylogenetic analyses yield new insight into crocodylian evolution and their survival of the Cretaceous-Tertiary boundary. *Mol. Phylogenet. Evol.* **2007**, *45*, 663–673. [CrossRef]
35. Katsu, Y.; Matsubara, K.; Kohno, S.; Matsuda, Y.; Toriba, M.; Oka, K.; Guillette, L.J., Jr.; Ohta, Y.; Iguchi, T. Molecular cloning, characterization, and chromosome mapping of reptilian estrogen receptors. *Endocrinology* **2010**, *151*, 5710–5720.
36. Lyson, T.R.; Sperling, E.A.; Heimberg, A.M.; Gauthier, J.A.; King, B.L.; Peterson, K.J. MicroRNAs support a turtle + lizard clade. *Biol. Lett.* **2012**, *8*, 104–107. [CrossRef]
37. Jones, M.E.; Cree, A. Tuatara. *Curr. Biol.* **2012**, *22*, R986–R987. [CrossRef]
38. Hay, J.M.; Sarre, S.D.; Lambert, D.M.; Allendorf, F.W.; Daugherty, C.H. Genetic diversity and taxonomy: A reassessment of species designation in tuatara (Sphenodon: Reptilia). *Conserv. Genet.* **2010**, *11*, 1063–1081.
39. Photo by PhillipC, licensed under the Creative Commons Attribution 2.0 Generic license. Available online: http://en.wikipedia.org/wiki/File:Sphenodon_punctatus_in_Waikanae,_New_Zealand.jpg (accessed on 9 May 2014).
40. Ramstad, K.M.; Nelson, N.J.; Paine, G.; Beech, D.; Paul, A.; Paul, P.; Allendorf, F.W.; Daugherty, C.H. Species and cultural conservation in New Zealand: maori traditional ecological knowledge of tuatara. *Conserv. Biol.* **2007**, *21*, 455–464. [CrossRef]
41. Miller, H.C.; Biggs, P.J.; Voelckel, C.; Nelson, N.J. De novo sequence assembly and characterisation of a partial transcriptome for an evolutionarily distinct reptile, the tuatara (*Sphenodon punctatus*). *BMC Genomics* **2012**, *13*, 439. [CrossRef]
42. Vonk, F.J.; Casewell, N.R.; Henkel, C.V.; Heimberg, A.M.; Jansen, H.J.; McCleary, R.J.; Kerkkamp, H.M.; Vos, R.A.; Guerreiro, I.; Calvete, J.J.; *et al.* The king cobra genome reveals dynamic gene evolution and adaptation in the snake venom system. *Proc. Natl. Acad. Sci. US A* **2013**, *110*, 20651–20656. [CrossRef]
43. Pyron, R.A.; Burbrink, F.T.; Guiher, T.J. Claims of potential expansion throughout the U.S. by invasive python species are contradicted by ecological niche models. *PloS One* **2008**, *3*, e2931. [CrossRef]
44. Photo by Greg Hume, licensed under the Creative Commons Attribution 2.0 Generic license. Available online: http://en.wikipedia.org/wiki/File:King_Cobra_25.jpg (accessed on 9 May 2014).
45. Found inside a water catchment on Lantau. 2011, Photo by: Thomas Brown. This file is licensed under the Creative Commons Attribution 2.0 Generic license. Available online: http://en.wikipedia.org/wiki/File: Naja_atra_juvenile.jpg (accessed on 9 May 2014).
46. Photo by AshLin. Photo of Banded Krait captured in Binnaguri, N.B., India on 19 Sep 2006. This file is licensed under the Creative Commons Attribution-Share Alike 2.5 Generic license. Available online: http://en.wikipedia.org/wiki/File:AB_054_Banded_Krait.JPG (accessed on 9 May 2014).
47. Photo by PiccoloNamek at en.wikipedia, licensed under the Creative Commons Attribution-Share Alike 3.0 Unported license. Available online: http://en.wikipedia.org/wiki/File:Anolis_carolinensis.jpg (accessed on 9 May 2014).
48. Aird, S.D.; Watanabe, Y.; Villar-Briones, A.; Roy, M.C.; Terada, K.; Mikheyev, A.S. Quantitative high-throughput profiling of snake venom gland transcriptomes and proteomes (*Ovophis okinavensis* and *Protobothrops flavoviridis*). *BMC Genomics* **2013**, *14*, 790. [CrossRef]

49. Dalla Valle, L.; Benato, F.; Maistro, S.; Quinzani, S.; Alibardi, L. Bioinformatic and molecular characterization of beta-defensins-like peptides isolated from the green lizard Anolis carolinensis. *Dev. Comp. Immunol.* **2012**, *36*, 222–229. [CrossRef]
50. Erickson, G.M.; Gignac, P.M.; Steppan, S.J.; Lappin, A.K.; Vliet, K.A.; Brueggen, J.D.; Inouye, B.D.; Kledzik, D.; Webb, G.J. Insights into the ecology and evolutionary success of crocodilians revealed through bite-force and tooth-pressure experimentation. *PloS One* **2012**, *7*, e31781. [CrossRef]
51. Shirley, M.H.; Vliet, K.A.; Carr, A.N.; Austin, J.D. Rigorous approaches to species delimitation have significant implications for African crocodilian systematics and conservation. *Proc. Biol. Sci.* **2014**, *281*, 20132483.
52. An American Alligator (One of two) in captivity at the Columbus Zoo, Powell, Ohio. This file is licensed under the Creative Commons Attribution-Share Alike 3.0 Unported license. Available online: http://en.wikipedia.org/wiki/File:American_Alligator.jpg (accessed on 9 May 2014).
53. A Siamese Crocodile (Crocodylus siamensis) at the Jerusalem Biblical Zoo. This file is licensed under the Creative Commons Attribution-Share Alike 3.0 Unported license. Available online: http://commons.wikimedia.org/wiki/File:Siamese_Crocodile-Biblical_Zoo.JPG (accessed on 9 May 2014).
54. Lance, V.A. Alligator physiology and life history: The importance of temperature. *Exp. Gerontol.* **2003**, *38*, 801–805. [CrossRef]
55. Brown, D.R.; Schumacher, I.M.; Nogueira, M.F.; Richey, L.J.; Zacher, L.A.; Schoeb, T.R.; Vliet, K.A.; Bennett, R.A.; Jacobson, E.R.; Brown, M.B. Detection of antibodies to a pathogenic mycoplasma in American alligators (*Alligator mississippiensis*), broad-nosed Caimans (*Caiman latirostris*), and Siamese crocodiles (*Crocodylus siamensis*). *J. Clin. Microbiol.* **2001**, *39*, 285–292. [CrossRef]
56. Meganathan, P.R.; Dubey, B.; Batzer, M.A.; Ray, D.A.; Haque, I. Molecular phylogenetic analyses of genus Crocodylus (Eusuchia, Crocodylia, Crocodylidae) and the taxonomic position of *Crocodylus porosus*. *Mol. Phylogenet. Evol.* **2010**, *57*, 393–402. [CrossRef]
57. Kommanee, J.; Preecharram, S.; Daduang, S.; Temsiripong, Y.; Dhiravisit, A.; Yamada, Y.; Thammasirirak, S. Antibacterial activity of plasma from crocodile (*Crocodylus siamensis*) against pathogenic bacteria. *Ann. Clin. Microbiol. Antimicrob.* **2012**, *11*, 22. [CrossRef]
58. Theansungnoen, T.; Yaraksa, N.; Daduang, S.; Dhiravisit, A.; Thammasirirak, S. Purification and Characterization of Antioxidant Peptides from Leukocyte Extract of *Crocodylus siamensis*. *Protein J.* **2014**, *33*, 24–31.
59. Srihongthong, S.; Pakdeesuwan, A.; Daduang, S.; Araki, T.; Dhiravisit, A.; Thammasirirak, S. Complete amino acid sequence of globin chains and biological activity of fragmented crocodile hemoglobin (*Crocodylus siamensis*). *Protein J.* **2012**, *31*, 466–476.
60. Jandaruang, J.; Siritapetawee, J.; Thumanu, K.; Songsiriritthigul, C.; Krittanai, C.; Daduang, S.; Dhiravisit, A.; Thammasirirak, S. The effects of temperature and pH on secondary structure and antioxidant activity of *Crocodylus siamensis* hemoglobin. *Protein J.* **2012**, *31*, 43–50.
61. Johnston, M.A.; Porter, D.E.; Scott, G.I.; Rhodes, W.E.; Webster, L.F. Isolation of faecal coliform bacteria from the American alligator (*Alligator mississippiensis*). *J. Appl. Microbiol.* **2010**, *108*, 965–973. [CrossRef]
62. Merchant, M.E.; Mills, K.; Leger, N.; Jerkins, E.; Vliet, K.A.; McDaniel, N. Comparisons of innate immune activity of all known living crocodylian species. *Com. Biochem. Physiol. Part B* **2006**, *143*, 133–137.
63. Merchant, M.E.; Leger, N.; Jerkins, E.; Mills, K.; Pallansch, M.B.; Paulman, R.L.; Ptak, R.G. Broad spectrum antimicrobial activity of leukocyte extracts from the American alligator (*Alligator mississippiensis*). *Vet. Immunol. Immunopathol.* **2006**, *110*, 221–228. [CrossRef]
64. Merchant, M.E.; Roche, C.; Elsey, R.M.; Prudhomme, J. Antibacterial properties of serum from the American alligator (*Alligator mississippiensis*). *Comp. biochem. Physiol. Part B* **2003**, *136*, 505–513. [CrossRef]
65. Preecharram, S.; Jearranaiprepame, P.; Daduang, S.; Temsiripong, Y.; Somdee, T.; Fukamizo, T.; Svasti, J.; Araki, T.; Thammasirirak, S. Isolation and characterisation of crocosin, an antibacterial compound from crocodile (*Crocodylus siamensis*) plasma. *Nihon chikusan Gakkaiho* **2010**, *81*, 393–401.
66. Pata, S.; Yaraksa, N.; Daduang, S.; Temsiripong, Y.; Svasti, J.; Araki, T.; Thammasirirak, S. Characterization of the novel antibacterial peptide Leucrocin from crocodile (*Crocodylus siamensis*) white blood cell extracts. *Dev. Comp. Immunol.* **2011**, *35*, 545–553.
67. Pata, S.; Daduang, S.; Svasti, J.; Thammasirirak, S. Isolation of Lysozyme like protein from crocodile leukocyte extract (*Crocodylus siamensis*). *KMITL Sci. Technol. J.* **2007**, *7*, 70–85.
68. Castoe, T.A.; Pollock, D.D. Chinese alligator genome illustrates molecular adaptations. *Cell res.* **2013**, *23*, 1254–1255. [CrossRef]

69. St John, J.A.; Braun, E.L.; Isberg, S.R.; Miles, L.G.; Chong, A.Y.; Gongora, J.; Dalzell, P.; Moran, C.; Bed'hom, B.; Abzhanov, A.; *et al.* Sequencing three crocodilian genomes to illuminate the evolution of archosaurs and amniotes. *Genome Biol.* **2012**, *13*, 415. [CrossRef]
70. Wan, Q.H.; Pan, S.K.; Hu, L.; Zhu, Y.; Xu, P.W.; Xia, J.Q.; Chen, H.; He, G.Y.; He, J.; Ni, X.W.; *et al.* Genome analysis and signature discovery for diving and sensory properties of the endangered Chinese alligator. *Cell Res.* **2013**, *23*, 1091–1105. [CrossRef]
71. Chromek, M.; Arvidsson, I.; Karpman, D. The antimicrobial peptide cathelicidin protects mice from Escherichia coli O157:H7-mediated disease. *PloS One* **2012**, *7*, e46476. [CrossRef]
72. Oguro-Okano, M.; Honda, M.; Yamazaki, K.; Okano, K. Mutations in the melanocortin 1 receptor, beta-defensin103 and agouti signaling protein genes, and their association with coat color phenotypes in Akita-inu dogs. *J. Vet. Med. Sci.* **2011**, *73*, 853–858. [CrossRef]
73. Schmutz, S.M.; Berryere, T.G. Genes affecting coat colour and pattern in domestic dogs: A review. *Anim. Genet.* **2007**, *38*, 539–549. [CrossRef]
74. Zasloff, M. Magainins, a class of antimicrobial peptides from Xenopus skin: isolation, characterization of two active forms, and partial cDNA sequence of a precursor. *Proc. Natl. Acad. Sci. USA* **1987**, *84*, 5449–5453. [CrossRef]
75. Wilson, C.L.; Schmidt, A.P.; Pirila, E.; Valore, E.V.; Ferri, N.; Sorsa, T.; Ganz, T.; Parks, W.C. Differential Processing of {alpha}- and {beta}-Defensin Precursors by Matrix Metalloproteinase-7 (MMP-7). *J. Biol. Chem.* **2009**, *284*, 8301–8311.
76. Zhao, L.; Lu, W. Defensins in innate immunity. *Curr. Opin. Hematol.* **2014**, *21*, 37–42. [CrossRef]
77. Lehrer, R.I.; Lu, W. alpha-Defensins in human innate immunity. *Immunol. Rev.* **2012**, *245*, 84–112. [CrossRef]
78. Garcia, J.R.; Jaumann, F.; Schulz, S.; Krause, A.; Rodriguez-Jimenez, J.; Forssmann, U.; Adermann, K.; Kluver, E.; Vogelmeier, C.; Becker, D.; *et al.* Identification of a novel, multifunctional beta-defensin (human beta-defensin 3) with specific antimicrobial activity. Its interaction with plasma membranes of Xenopus oocytes and the induction of macrophage chemoattraction. *Cell Tissue Res.* **2001**, *306*, 257–264. [CrossRef]
79. Kaplinsky, N.J.; Gilbert, S.F.; Cebra-Thomas, J.; Lillevali, K.; Saare, M.; Chang, E.Y.; Edelman, H.E.; Frick, M.A.; Guan, Y.; Hammond, R.M.; *et al.* The Embryonic Transcriptome of the Red-Eared Slider Turtle. *PloS one* **2013**, *8*, e66357.
80. Lorenzo, A. Immunolocalization of a beta-defensin (Tu-BD-1) in the skin and subdermal granulocytes of turtles indicate the presence of an antimicrobial skin barrier. *Ann. Anat.* **2013**, *195*, 554–561. [CrossRef]
81. Benato, F.; Dalla Valle, L.; Skobo, T.; Alibardi, L. Biomolecular identification of beta-defensin-like peptides from the skin of the soft-shelled turtle Apalone spinifera. *J. Exp. Zool. Part B* **2013**, *320*, 210–217. [CrossRef]
82. Alibardi, L. Ultrastructural immunolocalization of beta-defensin-27 in granulocytes of the dermis and wound epidermis of lizard suggests they contribute to the anti-microbial skin barrier. *Anat. Cell Biol.* **2013**, *46*, 246–253. [CrossRef]
83. Alibardi, L. Histochemical, Biochemical and Cell Biological aspects of tail regeneration in lizard, an amniote model for studies on tissue regeneration. *Prog. Histochem. Cytochem.* **2014**, *48*, 143–244. [CrossRef]
84. Alibardi, L. Granulocytes of reptilian sauropsids contain beta-defensin-like peptides: a comparative ultrastructural survey. *J. Morphol.* **2013**, *274*, 877–886. [CrossRef]
85. Alibardi, L.; Celeghin, A.; Dalla Valle, L. Wounding in lizards results in the release of beta-defensins at the wound site and formation of an antimicrobial barrier. *Dev. Comp. Immunol.* **2012**, *36*, 557–565. [CrossRef]
86. Abdel Mageed, A.M.; Isobe, N.; Yoshimura, Y. Immunolocalization of avian beta-defensins in the hen oviduct and their changes in the uterus during eggshell formation. *Reproduction* **2009**, *138*, 971–978. [CrossRef]
87. Gong, D.; Wilson, P.W.; Bain, M.M.; McDade, K.; Kalina, J.; Herve-Grepinet, V.; Nys, Y.; Dunn, I.C. Gallin; an antimicrobial peptide member of a new avian defensin family, the ovodefensins, has been subject to recent gene duplication. *BMC Immunol.* **2010**, *11*, 12.
88. Herve, V.; Meudal, H.; Labas, V.; Rehault Godbert, S.; Gautron, J.; Berges, M.; Guyot, N.; Delmas, A.F.; Nys, Y.; Landon, C. 3D NMR structure of hen egg gallin (chicken ovo-defensin) reveals a new variation of the beta-defensin fold. *J. Biol. Chem.* 2014.
89. Herve-Grepinet, V.; Rehault-Godbert, S.; Labas, V.; Magallon, T.; Derache, C.; Lavergne, M.; Gautron, J.; Lalmanach, A.C.; Nys, Y. Purification and characterization of avian beta-defensin 11, an antimicrobial peptide of the hen egg. *Antimicrob. Agents Chemother.* **2010**, *54*, 4401–4409. [CrossRef]

90. Mine, Y.; Oberle, C.; Kassaify, Z. Eggshell matrix proteins as defense mechanism of avian eggs. *J. Agric. Food Chem.* **2003**, *51*, 249–253. [CrossRef]
91. Kosciuczuk, E.M.; Lisowski, P.; Jarczak, J.; Strzalkowska, N.; Jozwik, A.; Horbanczuk, J.; Krzyzewski, J.; Zwierzchowski, L.; Bagnicka, E. Cathelicidins: family of antimicrobial peptides. A review. *Mol. Biol. Reports* **2012**, *39*, 10957–10970. [CrossRef]
92. Lehrer, R.I.; Ganz, T. Cathelicidins: A family of endogenous antimicrobial peptides. *Curr. Opin. Hematol.* **2002**, *9*, 18–22. [CrossRef]
93. Cole, A.M.; Shi, J.; Ceccarelli, A.; Kim, Y.H.; Park, A.; Ganz, T. Inhibition of neutrophil elastase prevents cathelicidin activation and impairs clearance of bacteria from wounds. *Blood* **2001**, *97*, 297–304. [CrossRef]
94. Tongaonkar, P.; Golji, A.E.; Tran, P.; Ouellette, A.J.; Selsted, M.E. High fidelity processing and activation of the human alpha-defensin HNP1 precursor by neutrophil elastase and proteinase 3. *PloS One* **2012**, *7*, e32469.
95. Nizet, V.; Gallo, R.L. Cathelicidins and innate defense against invasive bacterial infection. *Scand. J. Infect. Dis.* **2003**, *35*, 670–676. [CrossRef]
96. Zanetti, M.; Gennaro, R.; Scocchi, M.; Skerlavaj, B. Structure and biology of cathelicidins. *Adv. Exp. Med. Biol.* **2000**, *479*, 203–218.
97. van Dijk, A.; Molhoek, E.M.; Bikker, F.J.; Yu, P.L.; Veldhuizen, E.J.; Haagsman, H.P. Avian cathelicidins: Paradigms for the development of anti-infectives. *Vet. Microbiol.* **2011**, *153*, 27–36. [CrossRef]
98. Van Dijk, A.; Veldhuizen, E.J.; van Asten, A.J.; Haagsman, H.P. CMAP27, a novel chicken cathelicidin-like antimicrobial protein. *Vet. Immunol. Immunopathol.* **2005**, *106*, 321–327. [CrossRef]
99. Xiao, Y.; Cai, Y.; Bommineni, Y.R.; Fernando, S.C.; Prakash, O.; Gilliland, S.E.; Zhang, G. Identification and functional characterization of three chicken cathelicidins with potent antimicrobial activity. *J. Biol. Chem.* **2006**, *281*, 2858–2867.
100. Van Dijk, A.; Tersteeg-Zijderveld, M.H.; Tjeerdsma-van Bokhoven, J.L.; Jansman, A.J.; Veldhuizen, E.J.; Haagsman, H.P. Chicken heterophils are recruited to the site of Salmonella infection and release antibacterial mature Cathelicidin-2 upon stimulation with LPS. *Mol. Immunol.* **2009**, *46*, 1517–1526. [CrossRef]
101. Sorensen, O.E.; Borregaard, N. Cathelicidins–nature's attempt at combinatorial chemistry. *Comb. Chem. High Throughput Screen.* **2005**, *8*, 273–280. [CrossRef]
102. De Latour, F.A.; Amer, L.S.; Papanstasiou, E.A.; Bishop, B.M.; van Hoek, M.L. Antimicrobial activity of the Naja atra cathelicidin and related small peptides. *Biochem. Biophys. Res. Commun.* **2010**, *396*, 825–830. [CrossRef]
103. Dean, S.N.; Bishop, B.M.; van Hoek, M.L. Susceptibility of Pseudomonas aeruginosa Biofilm to Alpha-Helical Peptides: D-enantiomer of LL-37. *Front. Microbiol.* **2011**, *2*, 128.
104. Amer, L.S.; Bishop, B.M.; van Hoek, M.L. Antimicrobial and antibiofilm activity of cathelicidins and short, synthetic peptides against Francisella. *Biochem. Biophys. Res. Commun.* **2010**, *396*, 246–251. [CrossRef]
105. Dean, S.N.; Bishop, B.M.; van Hoek, M.L. Natural and synthetic cathelicidin peptides with anti-microbial and anti-biofilm activity against *Staphylococcus aureus*. *BMC Microbiol.* **2011**, *11*, 114. [CrossRef]
106. Juba, M.; Porter, D.; Dean, S.; Gillmor, S.; Bishop, B. Characterization and performance of short cationic antimicrobial peptide isomers. *Biopolymers* **2013**, *100*, 387–401. [CrossRef]
107. Wang, Y.; Zhang, Z.; Chen, L.; Guang, H.; Li, Z.; Yang, H.; Li, J.; You, D.; Yu, H.; Lai, R. Cathelicidin-BF, a snake cathelicidin-derived antimicrobial peptide, could be an excellent therapeutic agent for acne vulgaris. *PloS One* **2011**, *6*, e22120.
108. Hao, Q.; Wang, H.; Wang, J.; Dou, J.; Zhang, M.; Zhou, W.; Zhou, C. Effective antimicrobial activity of Cbf-K16 and Cbf-A7 A13 against NDM-1-carrying Escherichia coli by DNA binding after penetrating the cytoplasmic membrane *in vitro*. *J. Pept. Sci.* **2013**, *19*, 173–180. [CrossRef]
109. Wang, J.; Li, B.; Li, Y.; Dou, J.; Hao, Q.; Tian, Y.; Wang, H.; Zhou, C. BF-30 effectively inhibits ciprofloxacin-resistant bacteria *in vitro* and in a rat model of vaginosis. *Arch. Pharm. Res.* **2013**. [CrossRef]
110. Dalla Valle, L.; Benato, F.; Paccanaro, M.C.; Alibardi, L. Bioinformatic and molecular characterization of cathelicidin-like peptides isolated from the green lizard Anolis carolinensis (Reptilia: Lepidosauria: Iguanidae). *Ital. J. Zool.* **2013**, *80*, 177–186. [CrossRef]
111. Alibardi, L. Ultrastructural immunolocalization of chatelicidin-like peptides in granulocytes of normal and regenerating lizard tissues. *Acta Histochem.* 2013.
112. Park, C.H.; Valore, E.V.; Waring, A.J.; Ganz, T. Hepcidin, a urinary antimicrobial peptide synthesized in the liver. *J. Biol. Chem.* **2001**, *276*, 7806–7810.

113. Rodriguez, R.; Jung, C.L.; Gabayan, V.; Deng, J.C.; Ganz, T.; Nemeth, E.; Bulut, Y. Hepcidin induction by pathogens and pathogen-derived molecules is strongly dependent on interleukin-6. *Infect. Immun.* **2014**, *82*, 745–752. [CrossRef]
114. Hao, J.; Li, Y.W.; Xie, M.Q.; Li, A.X. Molecular cloning, recombinant expression and antibacterial activity analysis of hepcidin from Simensis crocodile (*Crocodylus siamensis*). *Comp. Biochem. Phys. Part B* **2012**, *163*, 309–315. [CrossRef]
115. Hilton, K.B.; Lambert, L.A. Molecular evolution and characterization of hepcidin gene products in vertebrates. *Gene* **2008**, *415*, 40–48.
116. Sang, Y.; Ramanathan, B.; Minton, J.E.; Ross, C.R.; Blecha, F. Porcine liver-expressed antimicrobial peptides, hepcidin and LEAP-2: cloning and induction by bacterial infection. *Dev. Comp. Immunol.* **2006**, *30*, 357–366. [CrossRef]
117. Hocquellet, A.; Odaert, B.; Cabanne, C.; Noubhani, A.; Dieryck, W.; Joucla, G.; le Senechal, C.; Milenkov, M.; Chaignepain, S.; Schmitter, J.M.; *et al.* Structure-activity relationship of human liver-expressed antimicrobial peptide 2. *Peptides* **2010**, *31*, 58–66. [CrossRef]
118. Henriques, S.T.; Tan, C.C.; Craik, D.J.; Clark, R.J. Structural and functional analysis of human liver-expressed antimicrobial peptide 2. *Chembiochem* **2010**, *11*, 2148–2157. [CrossRef]
119. Krause, A.; Sillard, R.; Kleemeier, B.; Kluver, E.; Maronde, E.; Conejo-Garcia, J.R.; Forssmann, W.G.; Schulz-Knappe, P.; Nehls, M.C.; Wattler, F.; *et al.* Isolation and biochemical characterization of LEAP-2, a novel blood peptide expressed in the liver. *Protein Sci.* **2003**, *12*, 143–152. [CrossRef]
120. Araki, T.; Yamamoto, T.; Torikata, T. Reptile lysozyme: the complete amino acid sequence of soft-shelled turtle lysozyme and its activity. *Biosci. Biotechnol. Biochem.* **1998**, *62*, 316–324. [CrossRef]
121. Chijiiwa, Y.; Kawamura, S.; Torikata, T.; Araki, T. Amino acid sequence and activity of green turtle (*Chelonia mydas*) lysozyme. *Protein J.* **2006**, *25*, 336–344. [CrossRef]
122. Prajanban, B.O.; Shawsuan, L.; Daduang, S.; Kommanee, J.; Roytrakul, S.; Dhiravisit, A.; Thammasirirak, S. Identification of five reptile egg whites protein using MALDI-TOF mass spectrometry and LC/MS-MS analysis. *J. Proteomics* **2012**, *75*, 1940–1959. [CrossRef]
123. Radis-Baptista, G.; Kerkis, I. Crotamine, a small basic polypeptide myotoxin from rattlesnake venom with cell-penetrating properties. *Curr. Pharm. Design* **2011**, *17*, 4351–4361. [CrossRef]
124. Kerkis, I.; Silva Fde, S.; Pereira, A.; Kerkis, A.; Radis-Baptista, G. Biological versatility of crotamine—A cationic peptide from the venom of a South American rattlesnake. *Expert Opin. Investig. Drugs* **2010**, *19*, 1515–1525. [CrossRef]
125. Structure of crotamine, a Na+ channel affecting toxin from Crotalus durissus terrificus venom (PDB 1H5O). This image is licensed under the Creative Commons Attribution-Share Alike 3.0 Unported license. Available online: http://en.wikipedia.org/wiki/File:Crotamin_1H5O.png (accessed on 9 May 2014).
126. Radis-Baptista, G.; Kubo, T.; Oguiura, N.; Prieto da Silva, A.R.; Hayashi, M.A.; Oliveira, E.B.; Yamane, T. Identification of crotasin, a crotamine-related gene of Crotalus durissus terrificus. *Toxicon* **2004**, *43*, 751–759. [CrossRef]
127. Yamane, E.S.; Bizerra, F.C.; Oliveira, E.B.; Moreira, J.T.; Rajabi, M.; Nunes, G.L.; de Souza, A.O.; da Silva, I.D.; Yamane, T.; Karpel, R.L.; *et al.* Unraveling the antifungal activity of a South American rattlesnake toxin crotamine. *Biochimie* **2013**, *95*, 231–240.
128. Yaraksa, N.; Anunthawan, T.; Theansungnoen, T.; Daduang, S.; Araki, T.; Dhiravisit, A.; Thammasirirak, S. Design and synthesis of cationic antibacterial peptide based on Leucrocin I sequence, antibacterial peptide from crocodile (*Crocodylus siamensis*) white blood cell extracts. *J. Antibiot.* **2013**, *67*, 205–212.
129. Mak, P. Hemocidins in a functional and structural context of human antimicrobial peptides. *Front. Biosci.* **2008**, *13*, 6859–6871.
130. Sheshadri, P.; Abraham, J. Antimicrobial properties of hemoglobin. *Immunopharm. Immunotoxicol.* **2012**, *34*, 896–900. [CrossRef]
131. Parish, C.A.; Jiang, H.; Tokiwa, Y.; Berova, N.; Nakanishi, K.; McCabe, D.; Zuckerman, W.; Xia, M.M.; Gabay, J.E. Broad-spectrum antimicrobial activity of hemoglobin. *Bioorg. Med. Chem.* **2001**, *9*, 377–382.
132. Anwised, P.; Kabbua, T.; Temsiripong, T.; Dhiravisit, A.; Jitrapakdee, S.; Araki, T.; Yoneda, K.; Thammasirirak, S. Molecular cloning and expression of alpha-globin and beta-globin genes from crocodile (*Crocodylus siamensis*). *Protein J.* **2013**, *32*, 172–182.

133. Santamaria, C.; Larios, S.; Quiros, S.; Pizarro-Cerda, J.; Gorvel, J.P.; Lomonte, B.; Moreno, E. Bactericidal and antiendotoxic properties of short cationic peptides derived from a snake venom Lys49 phospholipase A2. *Antimicrob. Agents Chemother.* **2005**, *49*, 1340–1345. [CrossRef]
134. Santamaria, C.; Larios, S.; Angulo, Y.; Pizarro-Cerda, J.; Gorvel, J.P.; Moreno, E.; Lomonte, B. Antimicrobial activity of myotoxic phospholipases A2 from crotalid snake venoms and synthetic peptide variants derived from their C-terminal region. *Toxicon* **2005**, *45*, 807–815. [CrossRef]
135. Yu, H.Y.; Huang, K.C.; Yip, B.S.; Tu, C.H.; Chen, H.L.; Cheng, H.T.; Cheng, J.W. Rational design of tryptophan-rich antimicrobial peptides with enhanced antimicrobial activities and specificities. *Chembiochem* **2010**, *11*, 2273–2282. [CrossRef]
136. Chu, H.L.; Yu, H.Y.; Yip, B.S.; Chih, Y.H.; Liang, C.W.; Cheng, H.T.; Cheng, J.W. Boosting salt resistance of short antimicrobial peptides. *Antimicrob. Agents Chemother.* **2013**, *57*, 4050–4052. [CrossRef]
137. Deslouches, B.; Steckbeck, J.D.; Craigo, J.K.; Doi, Y.; Mietzner, T.A.; Montelaro, R.C. Rational design of engineered cationic antimicrobial peptides consisting exclusively of arginine and tryptophan, and their activity against multidrug-resistant pathogens. *Antimicrob. Agents Chemother.* **2013**, *57*, 2511–2521. [CrossRef]
138. Gomes, V.M.; Carvalho, A.O.; Da Cunha, M.; Keller, M.N.; Bloch, C., Jr.; Deolindo, P.; Alves, E.W. Purification and characterization of a novel peptide with antifungal activity from Bothrops jararaca venom. *Toxicon* **2005**, *45*, 817–827. [CrossRef]
139. Xie, J.P.; Yue, J.; Xiong, Y.L.; Wang, W.Y.; Yu, S.Q.; Wang, H.H. In vitro activities of small peptides from snake venom against clinical isolates of drug-resistant Mycobacterium tuberculosis. *Int. J. Antimicrob. Agents* **2003**, *22*, 172–174. [CrossRef]

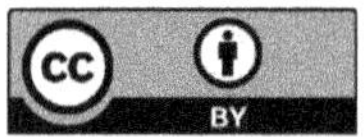

© 2014 by the author. Licensee MDPI, Basel, Switzerland. This article is an open access article distributed under the terms and conditions of the Creative Commons Attribution (CC BY) license (http://creativecommons.org/licenses/by/4.0/).

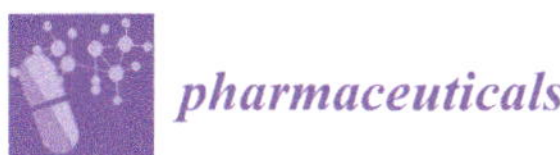

MDPI

Review

Chapter 8:

Avian Antimicrobial Host Defense Peptides: From Biology to Therapeutic Applications

Guolong Zhang [1,2,3,*] and Lakshmi T. Sunkara [1]

1 Department of Animal Science, Oklahoma State University, Stillwater, OK 74078, USA
2 Department of Biochemistry and Molecular Biology, Oklahoma State University, Stillwater, OK 74078, USA
3 Department of Physiological Sciences, Oklahoma State University, Stillwater, OK 74078, USA
* Author to whom correspondence should be addressed; glenn.zhang@okstate.edu; Tel.: +1-405-744-6619; Fax: +1-405-744-7390.

Received: 6 February 2014; in revised form: 18 February 2014; Accepted: 19 February 2014; Published: 27 February 2014

Abstract: Host defense peptides (HDPs) are an important first line of defense with antimicrobial and immunomoduatory properties. Because they act on the microbial membranes or host immune cells, HDPs pose a low risk of triggering microbial resistance and therefore, are being actively investigated as a novel class of antimicrobials and vaccine adjuvants. Cathelicidins and β-defensins are two major families of HDPs in avian species. More than a dozen HDPs exist in birds, with the genes in each HDP family clustered in a single chromosomal segment, apparently as a result of gene duplication and diversification. In contrast to their mammalian counterparts that adopt various spatial conformations, mature avian cathelicidins are mostly α-helical. Avian β-defensins, on the other hand, adopt triple-stranded β-sheet structures similar to their mammalian relatives. Besides classical β-defensins, a group of avian-specific β-defensin-related peptides, namely ovodefensins, exist with a different six-cysteine motif. Like their mammalian counterparts, avian cathelicidins and defensins are derived from either myeloid or epithelial origin expressed in a majority of tissues with broad-spectrum antibacterial and immune regulatory activities. Structure-function relationship studies with several avian HDPs have led to identification of the peptide analogs with potential for use as antimicrobials and vaccine adjuvants. Dietary modulation of endogenous HDP synthesis has also emerged as a promising alternative approach to disease control and prevention in chickens.

Keywords: host defense peptides; antimicrobial resistance; antibiotic alternatives; chicken

---

1. Introduction

Host defense peptides (HDPs), also known as antimicrobial peptides, constitute a large group of small peptides that have been discovered in virtually all forms of life [1–3]. Natural HDPs are generally positively charged and comprised of less than 100 amino acid residues with amphipathic properties. HDPs represent an important first-line of defense particularly in those species whose adaptive immune system is lacking or primitive. Most HDPs are encoded by distinct genes, and a large number of structurally different HDPs normally exist in a single species. A majority of HDPs are strategically synthesized in the host phagocytic and mucosal epithelial cells that regularly encounter the microorganisms from the environment. Synthesized initially as precursors, HDPs are generally processed by host proteases to release mature peptides upon infection and inflammation [1,2].

Mature HDPs are broadly active against Gram-negative and Gram-positive bacteria, mycobacteria, fungi, viruses, and even cancerous cells [1,2]. Relying primarily on the physical membrane-lytic mechanisms, HDPs kill bacteria with a low risk of triggering resistance [4]. Additionally, HDPs were recently found to interact specifically with several membrane-bound or intracellular receptors with a profound ability to modulate the host response to inflammation and infection [5–7]. Because of antimicrobial and immunomodulatory activities, HDPs are being actively explored for antimicrobial therapy particularly against drug-resistant microbes [8]. A number of HDPs have been found with preferential expression in the male reproductive tract and several are linked to sperm maturation and might have potential for infertility treatment [9,10].

2. Classification of HDPs

HDPs are structurally diversified. Based on the secondary structure, HDPs are classified into α-helical, β-sheet, αβ, and non-αβ families [1–3,11]. In general, α-helical peptides are amphipathic, often with a bend around the central region disrupting an otherwise fairly perfect cylindrical structure. The β-sheet HDPs are usually formed by the presence of disulfide bonds with amphipathic patches scattered on the surface. The αβ-peptides consist of both α-helical and β-sheet structures, whereas non-αβ HDPs are free of α-helical and β-sheet structures, often unstructured, and rich in proline, arginine or histidine residues.

2.1. Cathelicidins

Among an ever increasing number of HDPs that have been reported, two major families, namely cathelicidins and defensins, exist in vertebrate animals [12–14] (Figure 1). Cathelicidins have been reported in a variety of vertebrate species including fish, amphibians, reptiles, birds, and mammals [12,15]. Multiple cathelicidins normally exist in each species, except for euarchontogliers (e.g., primates, rabbits, and rodents) and carnivorans (e.g., cats and dogs). Cathelicidins are named for the presence of a cathelin-like domain in the N-terminal region of the peptide precursor (Figure 1). Although the signal peptide and cathelin-like domain of cathelicidins are extremely conserved across species, mature peptide sequences at the C-terminal region are highly diversified even within a species. Neutrophilic granule proteins (NGPs) are a group of cathelicidin-related HDPs that have been reported in rabbits, rodents, and many other mammalian species [16–18]. Although they apparently have evolved from cathelicidins, NGPs are conserved throughout the entire sequence, including the C-terminal region. Given rabbit NGP, also known as p15, is biologically active without proteolytic cleavage [19], it is possible that other NGPs may not be processed to become biologically active.

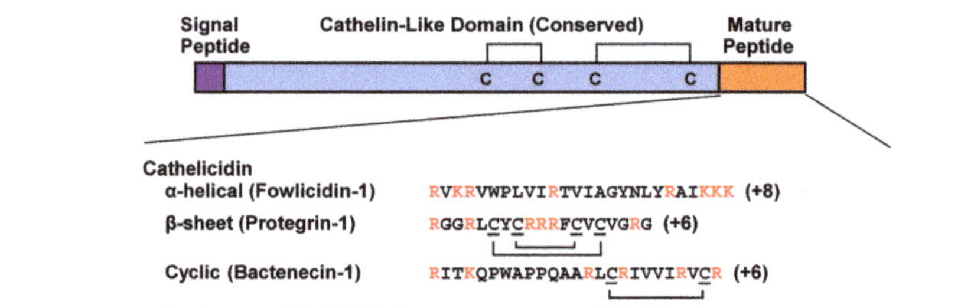

Figure 1. *Cont.*

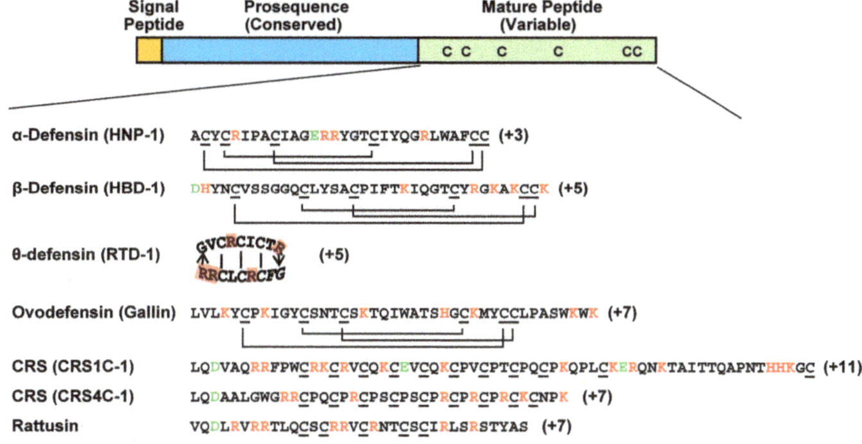

Figure 1. Schematic drawing of vertebrate cathelicidin and defensin precursor peptides. (**A**) Cathelicidins and cathelicidin-related peptides known as NGPs are highly conserved in the cathelin-like domain that contains two disulfide bridges. Unlike cathelicidins whose C-terminal segments are highly variable across species and proteolytically cleaved from the cathelicidin-like domain to become biologically active, NGPs are conserved throughout the entire sequence and functionally active without being processed. (**B**) The defensin family includes classical α-, β-, and θ-defensins with indicated disulfide bonds as well as four subfamilies of defensin-related peptides with unknown disulfide bonding patterns. Avian-specific ovodefensins contain six cysteines but with a different spacing pattern from that of classical defensins. Rodent-specific CRS1C, CRS4C, and rattusin also exist with 11, 9, and 5 cysteine residues, respectively, that presumably form intermolecular disulfide bonds. Positively and negatively charged amino acids are indicated in red and green, respectively.

2.2. *Defensins*

Vertebrate defensins are further classified into three subfamilies including α-, β-, and θ-defensins that are characterized by the presence of six cysteines with different spacing and bonding patterns (Figure 1) [9,13,14]. The α-defensins are mammalian-specific with a C1-C6, C2-C4, and C3-C5 cysteine-bridging pattern, whereas β-defensins are universal in vertebrates with a C1-C5, C2-C4, and C3-C6 bridging pattern. The θ-defensins, on the other hand, have only been discovered in primates, with a pseudogene present in the human genome [20]. The six cysteines of θ-defensins form a cyclic structure by a head-to-tail ligation of two truncated α-defensins [20]. Three additional subfamilies of α-defensin-related peptides have also been found in rodents [21,22]. Two groups of cryptdin-related sequence (CRS) peptides, namely CRS1C and CRS4C, appear to exist only in mice with 11 and nine cysteines, respectively [21]. A unique rat-specific rattusin was recently reported to consist of five cysteines [22]. Although rodent defensin-related sequences are located within the α-defensin gene cluster and highly similar to α-defensins in the signal and pro-sequences, the disulfide bridging patterns of the C-terminal mature peptides are totally different among them (Figure 1). Albeit with no reported tertiary structures, these defensin-related peptides are likely to form homo- or hetero-dimers or oligomers because of the presence of an odd number of cysteines. Another group of β-defensin-related molecules, recently classified as ovodefensins, appear to be specific in birds [23]. Albeit with six cysteines in the C-terminal mature region forming a disulfide bonding pattern identical to β-defensins [24], avian ovodefensins consist of a different cysteine spacing pattern (Figure 1).

3. Discovery of Avian HDPs

Both the cathelicidin and defensin families of HDPs exist in birds [25,26]. However, NGPs appear to be specific to mammals and no NGP-like cathelicidins have been reported in any avian species. Only β-defensins have been discovered in birds, and no α- or θ-defensins exist. Rodent-specific rattusin or CRS peptides are also absent in birds. However, ovodefensins are uniquely present in several avian species [23]. Excellent reviews are available on the general knowledge of avian HDPs [27,28], and this review will focus on their biology and therapeutic applications, with more emphasis on the similarities and differences between avian and mammalian HDPs.

3.1. Avian Cathelicidins

Four distinct cathelicidin genes have been reported in birds. The first two avian cathelicidins (CATH1 and CATH2) were reported in chickens in 2004 and 2005, respectively [29,30]. The same two peptides, together with a third chicken cathelicidin (CATH3), were also independently reported as fowlicidin 1–3 [18]. The fourth chicken cathelicidin, known as CATH-B1, was discovered to be preferentially expressed in the bursa of Fabricius [31], a specialized organ for hematopoiesis and B cell development in birds. All four chicken cathelicidins were found to cluster densely together within a 7.5-kb distance toward one end of chromosome 2 [18,31]. All four chicken cathelicidin genes adopt a 4-exon, 3-intron structure, typical for a mammalian cathelicidin. The first three exons encode the 5′-untranslated region, signal peptide, and a majority of the cathelin-like domain, while the last exon encodes primarily the mature peptides, in addition to the 3′-untranslated region [18,31]. Chicken CATH1–3 share similar exon sizes and a typical cathelin-like domain with mammalian cathelicidins, whereas CATH-B1 consists of an alternatively spliced and unusually large first exon and an uncharacteristic cathelin-like domain [31].

Alignment of four chicken cathelicidin peptide sequences revealed that they are similar to each other and also homologous to mammalian cathelicidins in the signal peptide and cathelin-like domain (Figure 2). Among them, CATH1 and CATH3 are most closely related with >90% identity throughout the entire sequence, while CATH-B1 is a distant member, sharing only 40% with CATH1 (Figure 2). The orthologs of chicken CATH1–3 were also recently reported in several other avian species such as the common quail and common pheasant [32,33]. With recent completion of genome sequencing for the turkey, mallard duck, rock dove (*Columba livia*), ground tit (*Pseudopodoces humilis*), saker falcon (*Falco cherrug*), Peregrine Falcon (*Falco peregrinus*), and budgerigar (*Melopsittacus undulatus*), a number of avian cathelicidin sequences have been predicted and become available in GenBank.

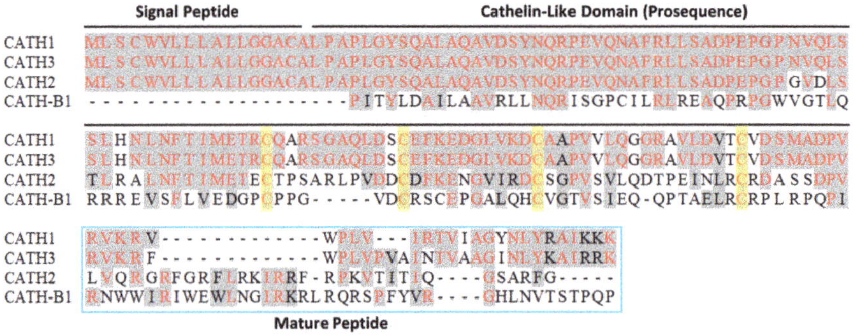

Signal Peptide — **Cathelin-Like Domain (Prosequence)**

```
CATH1    MLSCWVLLLALLGGACALPAPLGYSQALAQAVDSYNQRPEVQNAFRLLSADPEPGPNVQLS
CATH3    MLSCWVLLLALLGGACALPAPLGYSQALAQAVDSYNQRPEVQNAFRLLSADPEPGPNVQLS
CATH2    MLSCWVLLLALLGGACALPAPLGYSQALAQAVDSYNQRPEVQNAFRLLSADPEPGPGVDLS
CATH-B1  -------------------PITYLDAILAAVRLLNQRISGPCILRLREAQPRPGWVGTLQ

CATH1    SLHNLNFTIMETRCQARSGAQLDSCEFKEDGLVKDCAAPVVLQGGRAVLDVTCVDSMADPV
CATH3    SLHNLNFTIMETRCQARSGAQLDSCEFKEDGLVKDCAAPVVLQGGRAVLDVTCVDSMADPV
CATH2    TLRALNFTIMETECTPSARLPVDDCDFKENGVIRDCSGPVSVLQDTPEINLRCRDASSDPV
CATH-B1  RRREVSFLVEDGPCPPG-----VDCRSCEPGALQHCVGTVSIEQ-QPTAELRCRPLRPQPI

CATH1    RVKRV-------------WPLV---IRTVIAGYNLYRAIKKK
CATH3    RVKRF-------------WPLVPVAINTVAAGINLYKAIRRK
CATH2    LVQRGRFGRFLRKIRRF-RPKVTITIQ----GSARFG-----
CATH-B1  RNWWIRIWEWLNGIRKRLRQRSPFYVR----GHLNVTSTPQP
```

Mature Peptide

Figure 2. Amino acid sequence alignment of four chicken cathelicidins. Conserved sequences are shaded and identical residues are in red. Dashes are created to maximize the alignment. Each cathelicidin precursor consists of a conserved signal peptide sequence, a cathelin-like domain, and a variable C-terminal mature peptide sequence. Four cysteines in the cathelin-like domain are highlighted in yellow. Note that an N-terminal, 117-amino acid segment of CATH-B1 was omitted for clarity.

3.2. Avian β-Defensins

More than a dozen unique β-defensin genes are present, and no α- or θ-defensins exist in birds. The first two avian β-defensins, known as gallinacins 1–2, were isolated in 1994 from chicken heterophils [34], an equivalent of mammalian neutrophils. The turkey orthologs of gallinacins 1–2 were also independently purified from heterophil granules later in the same year [34]. With the completion of the chicken genome sequencing, a large number of additional chicken β-defensin genes were independently reported by Lynn, *et al.* [29] and Xiao, *et al.* [35], respectively. Because of different numbering systems used by the two groups, a new standard nomenclature for chicken β-defensins was proposed [36]. To be consistent with the mammalian defensin nomenclature, the term "gallinacin" was suggested to be dropped and a new term "avian β-defensin (AvBD)" be adopted [36]. The AvBD numbering system was proposed to follow Xiao's [35]. With deposition of a new chicken β-defensin, *i.e.*, AvBD14 (under the GenBank accession no. AM402954), after initial two publications, the chicken genome now appears to encode a total of 14 distinct β-defensin genes (AvBD1–14) packed within a 85-kb distance toward one end of chromosome 3 [36]. In contrast with most mammalian β-defensin genes, which primarily consist of two exons, at least five AvBDs (AvBD1, 2, 6, 7, and 8) are comprised of a minimum of four exons [35]. The remaining AvBD genes contain three exons, while AvBD12 and -14 appear to have only two exons.

Sequencing alignment of all 14 chicken β-defensins revealed that they are highly conserved at the N-terminal signal peptide region (Figure 3). The spacing pattern of six cysteines are also conserved at the C-terminal segment. Additionally, two glycines, with one preceding the second cysteine and the other preceding the fourth cysteine, are also largely conserved (Figure 3). Most other residues are quite diverse among AvBDs. In contrast to mammalian α-defensins with a long, often negatively charged prosequence, β-defensins including AvBDs consist of a short prosequence, which is even absent in a few cases. The C-terminal tails of AvBDs after the last cysteine are generally short, consisting mostly of 3-6 amino acids. AvBD3, 11 and 13 are exceptions. AvBD3 and AvBD13 have up to 30 residues after the last cysteine [35], while AvBD11 contains two tandem, but different six-cysteine motifs at the C-terminus [35]. As a result, mature AvBD11 may form six, instead of three, intramolecular disulfide bonds. AvBD11 is the only known β-defensin with such a sequence, and functional significance for the existence of such two defensin motifs remain to be studied. A number of AvBDs have also been found in several other species of birds including the turkey, ostrich, king penguin, zebra finch, duck, and goose [37–43]. Many additional AvBD sequences have also been predicted and deposited in GenBank.

```
         Signal Peptide   Prosequence          Mature Peptide
AvBD1    MRIVYLLLPFILL-LAQGAAGSSQA-LGRKSDCFRKSGFCAFL-KCPSL-TLIS--GKCSRF-YLCCKRIWG-----
AvBD3    MRIVYLLIPFFLL-FLQGAAGTA-------TQCRIRGGFCRVG-SCRFP-HIAI--GKCATF-ISCCGRAYEVDALN
AvBD2    MRILYLLFSLLFL-ALQVSPGLSSP-RRDMLFC--KGGSCHFG-GCPSH-LIKV--GSCFGF-RSCCKWPWNA----
AvBD6    MRILYLLLSVLFV-VLQGVAGQPYF-SSPIHACRYQRGVCIPG-PCRWP-YYRV--GSCGSGLKSCCVRNRWA----
AvBD7    MRILYLLLSVLFV-VLQGVAGQPFI-PRPIDTCRLRNGICFPG-ICRRP-YYWI--GTCNNGIGSCCARGWRS----
AvBD14   MG-IFLLFLVLLA-VPQAAP------ESDTVTCRKMKGKCSFL-LCPFF-KRSS--GTCYNGLAKCCRPFW------
AvBD9    MRILFFLVAVLFF-LFQAAPAYSQE-DADTLACRQSHGSCSFV-ACRAP-SVDI--GTCRGGKLKCCKWAPSS----
AvBD10   MKILCLLFAVLLF-LFQAAPGSADPLFPDTVACRTQGNFCRAG-ACPPT-FTIS--GQCHGGLLNCCAKIPAQ----
AvBD4    MKILCFFIVLLFV-AVHGAVGFSRS-PRYHMQCGYRGTFCTPG-KCPYG-NAYL--GLCRPK-YSCCRWL-------
AvBD11   MKLFSCLMALLLF-LLQAVPGLGLP-RDT-SRCVGYHGYCIRSKVCPKP-FAAF--GTCSWRQKTCCVDTTSD-FHT
AvBD8    MKILYLLLAVLLT-VLQSSLGFMRV-PNNEAQCEQAGGICSKD-HCFHLHTRAF--GHCQRG-VPCCRTVYD-----
AvBD5    MQILPLLFAVLLL-MLRAEPGLSLA-RGLPQDCERRGGFCSHK-SCPPG-IGRI--GLCSKE-DFCCRSRWYS----
AvBD13   MRILQLLFAIVVILLLQDAPARGFS---DSQLCRNNHGHCRRL--CFHM-ESWA--GSCMNGRLRCCRFSTKQPFSN
AvBD12   MRNLCFVFIFISL-LAHGSTH-------GPDSCNHDRGLCRVG-NCNPG-EYLA--KYCFEPVILCCKPLSPTPTKT
Gallin1  MRFLYLIFSVFLL-VSLATPGYGLV----LKYC-PKIGYCSNT--CSKT-QIWATSHGC---KMYCCLPASWKWK--
Gallin2  MRFLCLVFAVLLL-VSLAAPGYGLV----LKYC-PKIGYCSNT--CSKT-QIWATSHGC---KMYCCLPASWKWK--
Gallin3  MRFLCLVFAVLLL-VSLAAPGYGLV----LKYC-PKIGYCSNT--CSKT-QIWATSHGC---KMYCCLPANWKWK--
```

Figure 3. Amino acid sequence alignment of chicken β-defensins and ovodefensins. Conserved sequences are shaded and identical residues are in red. Dashes are created to maximize the alignment. Each β-defensin precursor is comprised of a conserved signal peptide, an optional short prosequence, and a C-terminal mature sequence consisting of six cysteines. Note that the cysteine spacing patterns are different between chicken ovodefensins (known as gallin 1–3) and classical β-defensins. Additional C-terminal tail sequences of AvBD3, 11, and 13 were omitted for simplicity.

Besides classical β-defensins, chickens have also been found to express three closely related β-defensin-related peptides, namely gallin 1–3 [23,44,45]. In fact, multiple peptides with a similar cysteine-spacing pattern have been reported earlier in the mallard duck, turkey, and black swan [46–48]. This group of peptides were in turn classified as ovodefensins because of their preferential expression in the oviduct with abundant presence in egg white [23]. Ovodefensins appear to be avian-specific, containing a six-cysteine motif of C-$X_{3\text{-}5}$-C-X_3-C-X_{11}-C-$X_{3\text{-}4}$-CC, as opposed to that of C-$X_{4\text{-}8}$-C-$X_{3\text{-}5}$-C-$X_{9\text{-}13}$-C-$X_{4\text{-}7}$-CC in classical avian β-defensins (Figure 3).

4. Evolution of Avian HDPs

4.1. *Avian Cathelicidins*

Phylogenetic analysis of all publically available avian cathelicidins revealed that they are clustered into three distinct clades, namely CATH1/3, CATH2, and CATH-B1 (Figure 4), suggesting that these three clades of cathelicidin genes have evolved before divergence of these bird species from each other, unlike mammalian cathelicidin genes, a majority of which were duplicated after species separation [18]. Surprisingly, an initial analysis of the zebra finch (*Taeniopygia guttata*) genome failed to identify any cathelicidin sequences [39]. If that is the case, it will be interesting to know why the cathelicidin genes were lost in zebra finch, although it is likely that the genome segments containing the cathelicidin genes failed to be sequenced, because the entire genome were only sequenced to 5.5 × coverage to encompass 94% of the genome [49]. Consistent with our assumption, scores of gaps are present in the syntenic cathelicidin region in the current zebra finch genome assembly (WUGSC 3.2.4/taeGut1) released in July 2008.

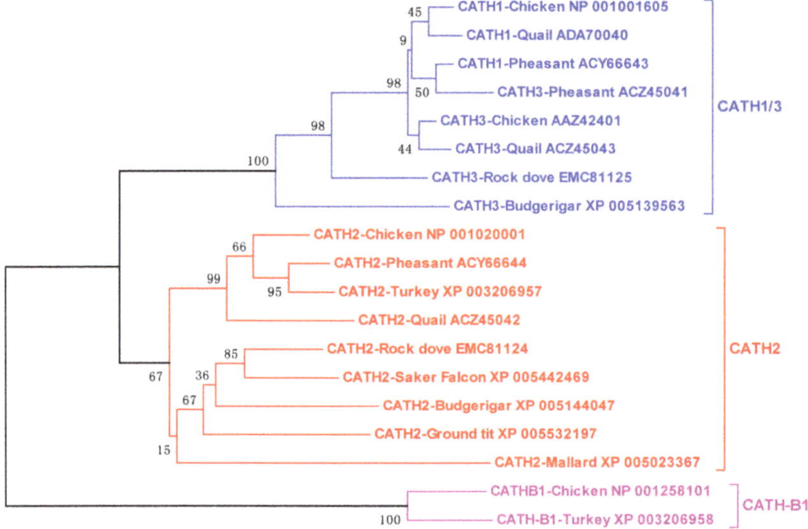

Figure 4. Phylogenetic analysis of avian cathelicidins. The phylogenetic tree was constructed with the full-length amino acid sequences using the neighbor-joining method, and the reliability of each branch was assessed by using 1,000 bootstrap replications. Numbers on the branches indicate the percentage of 1,000 bootstrap samples supporting the branch. The species and GenBank accession number of each sequence are indicated.

4.2. *Avian β-Defensins*

Phylogenetic analysis of all available avian β-defensins and related peptide sequences revealed the presence of cross-species, gene-specific clusters for most genes, implying that a majority have evolved before the split of the bird species from each other (Figure 5), reminiscent of avian cathelicidin genes. However, species-specific AvBD genes do exist. For example, AvBD14 appears specific to chickens, because no orthologs have been found in any other avian species, despite the availability of several avian genome sequences. Supported by a bootstrap value of 52 (Figure 5), it is likely that AvBD14 duplicated from AvBD13 after the separation of chickens from other birds. Zebra finch lacks the AvBD6 gene [39,40], although it is present in the chicken, turkey, goose, and mallard duck genomes. The AvBD1 gene is conserved in the chicken, turkey, goose, quail, and ostrich, but has apparently duplicated and diversified into three paralogous genes (AvBD123, 124, and 125) in the zebra finch [39,40] (Figure 5). Likewise, the AvBD3 gene has also expanded to a total of eight paralogous genes in the zebra finch genome [39,40] (Figure 5).

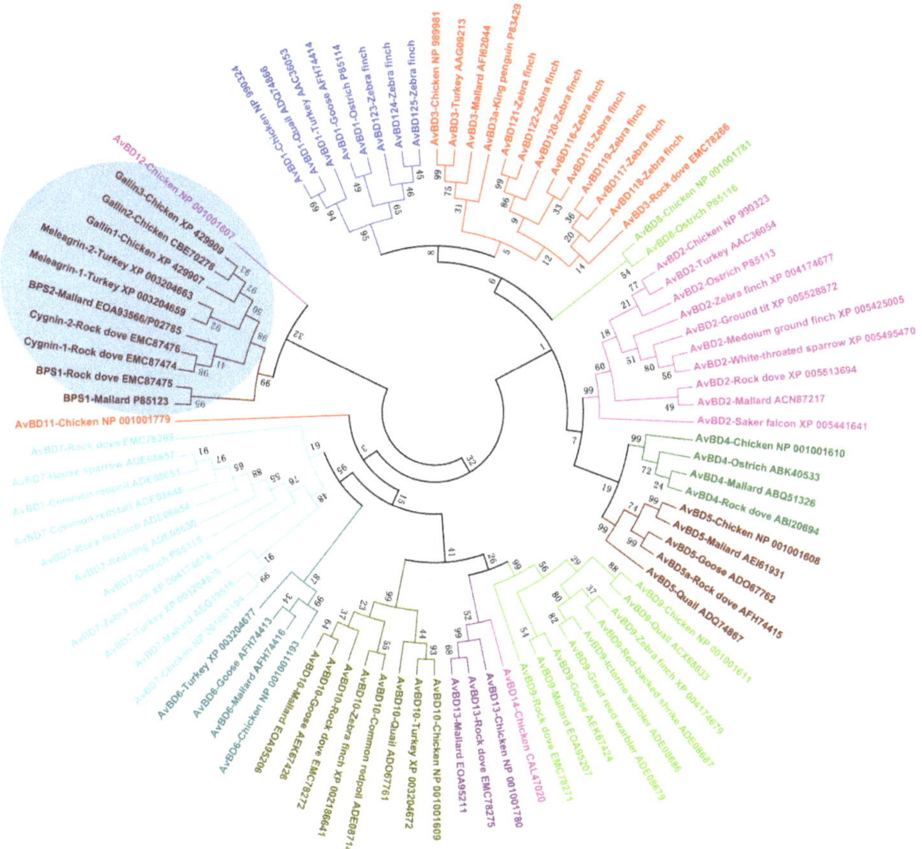

Figure 5. Phylogenetic analysis of avian defensins (see Figure 4 legend for details).

Ovodefensins clearly form a distinct clade, which is further divided into two subgroups (Figure 5). Small basic protein 1 (BPS1) in the mallard duck or rock dove is separated from the remaining ovodefensins. A closer examination of their amino acid sequences indicated that BPS1 consists of a cysteine-spacing pattern of C-X_3-C-X_3-C-X_{11}-C-X_4-CC, as opposed to C-X_5-C-X_3-C-X_{11}-C-X_3-CC in other ovodefensins. It remains to see whether these two subgroups of ovodefensins are present only in certain species of birds. It is also important to know how they are functionally different from each other and from classical defensins.

Importantly, ovodefensins are clustered with AvBD12 as supported by a bootstrap value of 32 (Figure 5), suggesting that ovodefensins might have duplicated and diversified from AvBD12 as a result of gene duplication after separations of birds from other animal species. Consistent with the notion that ovodefensins are derived from classical AvBDs, three chicken ovodefensin/gallin genes are located in tandem on chromosome 3, approximately 260 kb centromeric to the AvBD gene cluster on the current chicken genome assembly. To further support a possible origination of gallins from AvBD12, the gallin genes consist of two exons separated by an intron, which is identical to the genomic structure of the AvBD12 and AvBD14 genes, whereas all other AvBD genes are comprised of at least three exons [35].

5. Expression and Regulation of Avian HDPs

5.1. Tissue Expression Pattern

Like mammalian counterparts, avian cathelicidins and β-defensins are derived from the bone marrow and/or epithelial cells, with the majority expressing in a wide variety of tissues. CATH1–3 are primarily of myeloid origin, while CATH-B1, a distant member of avian cathelicidins, is derived from epithelial cells. Chicken CATH1–3 mRNAs are predominantly expressed in the bone marrow, but also throughout the mucosal tissues of the digestive, respiratory, and urogenital tracts [29,30,50]. On the other hand, chicken CATH-B1 mRNA shows a more restricted expression pattern, with preferential expression in the secretory epithelial cells of the bursa of Fabricius [31,50]. Consist with the role of cathelicidins in the first line of host defense, abundant CATH1–3 proteins can be detected in the granules of heterophils, as in the case of chicken CATH2 [51], whereas mature CATH-B1 protein is secreted from the epithelial cells and concentrated on the basolateral surfaces of the M cells in the bursal lymphoid follicles [31].

Myeloid avian β-defensins include AvBD1, 2, and 4–7, whereas the remaining AvBD8–14 are mainly of epithelial origin, although both myeloid and epithelial AvBDs are also expressed in a majority of other tissues [29,35,52]. In agreement with their myeloid origin, AvBD1 and AvBD2 mRNAs have been found abundantly in the bone marrow and their proteins in heterophil granules in the chickens, turkey, and ostrich [34,42,53]. It will be interesting to know the tissue expression pattern of those species-specific AvBDs such as AvBD115–125 in the zebra finch [40]. However, because they are orthologous to AvBD1 and AvBD3 (Figure 5), they are expected to share a similar expression pattern to AvBD1 and AvBD3.

Human cathelicidin LL-37 has been found in seminal plasma associated with sperm and prostasomes [54]. A majority of β-defensins in rats (and likely in other mammalian species as well) are expressed preferentially in the male reproductive system and the epididymis and testis in particular [55]. Like their mammalian counterparts, many avian cathelicidins and β-defensins are expressed adequately in the male and female reproductive organs, particularly in the testis, epididymis, ovary, and oviduct [29,35,50,56], suggesting a possible role in reproduction. Ovodefensins have been found to be among the major components of egg white in the chicken, turkey, and duck [44–48]. Consistently, chicken ovodefensin gallin 1–3 mRNA and proteins are the most abundantly expressed in tubular gland cells in the magnum of the chicken oviduct [23], a segment that secretes egg white.

5.2. Developmental Regulation

The expression of chicken cathelicidins and β-defensins has been studied during the pre- and post-hatch periods and found to be developmentally regulated. At the embryonic stage, most chicken cathelicidin and AvBD mRNAs were detected as early as embryonic day 3 (E3), except for CATH-B1 and AvBD11, which did not appear until day E9 [57]. All four cathelicidin mRNA expression was generally increased as embryos develops, whereas the 14 β-defensins were differentially expressed [57]. AvBD3, 4, 5, 10, 11, 12, and 14 were largely enhanced during the embryonic development, whereas the remaining chicken β-defensins showed a biphasic expression pattern. In the case of AvBD2, 6, and 7, their expression was increased on day E6 relative to that in day E3, decreased on day E9, and then increased gradually with the age of embryos [57].

After hatch, chicken cathelicidins and β-defensins are also developmentally regulated in both gene- and tissue-specific patterns. During the first 28 days, CATH1–3 showed an age-dependent increase both in the cecal tonsil and lung, whereas all four cathelicidins were peaked in the bursa on day 4 after hatching, with a gradual decline by day 28 [50]. On the other hand, CATH1–3 showed a peak expression in the cecum on day 28, while the highest expression of CATH-B1 was seen in both the lung and cecal tonsil on day 14 [50]. AvBD1 and AvBD2 mRNA gradually reduced in different segments of the intestinal tract in the first week post-hatch, but restored and increased gradually in the following week [58]. In the reproductive tract, more than a half of AvBDs increased during the sexual maturation in the vagina, ovary, and epididymis of chickens, whereas others showed little no expression [56,59,60].

5.3. Regulation by Infection and Inflammation

HDPs are critically involved in the first line of host defense. Dysregulation of the HDP synthesis often leads to immune deficiency or autoimmunity such as Crohn's disease and psoriasis in humans [61, 62]. Many, but not all, HDPs are induced upon infection and inflammation in humans and mice. On the other hand, certain pathogens suppress HDP synthesis as a strategy to evade the immune system [63–65]. A number of studies have been conducted on the transcriptional response of cathelicidins and β-defensins in chickens and several other avian species. Like their mammalian relatives, multiple AvBDs are inducible in response to microbial products (e.g., lipopolysaccharides and CpG DNA), live bacteria, viruses or parasites in the intestinal, reproductive, and respiratory tracts [38,56,59,60,66,67]. However, it appears that many avian HDP genes are regulated differently in different tissues in response to different stimuli. For example, chicken CATH1 was induced in the cecal tonsil [66], but not the jejunum of chickens in response to *Salmonella* infections [51]. On the other hand, chicken CATH1 was down-regulated by *Campylobacter jejuni* or *Eimeria praecox* [68–70], perhaps as a mechanism of immune evasion.

5.4. Regulation by Dietary Compounds

Because suppressing HDP expression is a microbial strategy for immune subversion, inducing the synthesis of endogenous HDPs will conversely augment the host capacity to fight off infections [71–73]. Unlike infection or injury that triggers HDP expression with an unwanted and often exaggerated inflammatory response, butyrate and vitamin D3 have been found to be highly potent in augmenting HDP synthesis without provoking inflammation in humans [74–78]. Several other compounds like dietary histone deacetylase inhibitors, retinoic acid, forskolin, and sugars are also capable of inducing HDP expression in humans [79–83].

In chickens, butyrate has been revealed as a strong inducer of HDP expression *in vitro* and *in vivo*. Among all 14 AvBDs and 4 cathelicidins, half of them were induced with others largely unchanged in chicken cells in response to butyrate [84]. Butyrate was further shown to enhance the antibacterial activity of chicken monocytes, and supplementation of butyrate in the feed enhanced clearance of *Salmonella enteritidis* in the cecum of chickens following an experimental infection [84]. Among all saturated free fatty acids with 1–18 carbons, butyrate was the most potent in stimulating HDP expression in chicken cells [85]. Furthermore, butyrate synergizes with the agonists of the cyclic adenosine monophosphate (cAMP) signaling pathway in inducing HDP expression [86]. Feeding with butyrate and a plant extract containing forskolin, which is an adenylyl cyclase agonist, showed a strong synergy in augmenting HDP expression in the crop and jejunum of chickens [86]. Mitogen-activated protein kinase signaling pathways were revealed to be critically involved in the HDP-inducing synergy between butyrate and forskolin [86]. The results indicated the potential for use of these dietary compounds in promoting HDP synthesis, host immunity, and disease resistance.

6. Biological Activities of Avian HDPs

6.1. Antimicrobial Activities

The antibacterial efficacy of all four chicken cathelicidins and many defensins have been evaluated. Like their mammalian counterparts, most chicken HDPs are capable of killing a broad spectrum of Gram-positive and Gram-negative bacteria, and fungi including antibiotic-resistant strains generally in the low micromolar range. For example, chicken CATH1–3 are broadly active with the minimum inhibitory concentration (MIC) values mostly between 0.5 and 2 μM against a range of bacteria [18, 87], and CATH-B1 also has the MIC values between 0.5 and 2.5 μM against *E. coli, S. aureus*, and *P. aeruginosa* [31]. However, many HDPs showed varying efficiencies against different pathogens. Chicken AvBD1 and AvBD2 kill 90% *S. enteriditis, C. jejuni*, and *Candida albicans* at <4 μM, but showed a much reduced efficiency against *Pasteurella multocida* [41]. Similarly, AvBD9 is active against most Gram-positive and Gram-negative bacteria tested with the MIC values in the range of 2–4 μM, but with a minimum activity against *S. typhimurium* (>30 μM) [88]. On the other hand, AvBD13 was found to be minimally active against a range of bacteria examined, with the MIC values in the range of 50–100 μM [89]. The antibacterial activity of chicken CATH1–3 is not affected by the presence of physiological concentrations of salt [18]; however, that of chicken defensins is greatly reduced by salt [26], reminiscent of mammalian defensins [13]. In the case of CATH1–3, AvBD2, and presumably most other avian HDPs, non-specific membrane disruption and lysis is a major bactericidal mechanism [87,90,91].

Ovodefensins are unique in that they generally lack an obvious antibacterial activity as seen with turkey meleagrin as well as duck BPS1 and BPS2 [46,48]. Chicken gallin is the only ovodefensin with known antibacterial activities, but appears to have a narrow range. Among several common Gram-negative and Gram-positive bacteria tested, chicken gallin1/2 showed an activity only against *E. coli*, but not *Salmonella, S. aureus* or *Listeria monocytogenes* [24]. It is hence very unlikely that the major biological function of ovodefensins is antibacterial.

6.2. Immunomodulatory Activities

Besides having direct microbicidal activities, HDPs have increasingly been appreciated to play a profound role in regulating host immune responses to infections. Many peptides are shown to be actively involved in chemotaxis and activation of immune cells, regulation of dendritic cell differentiation, induction of angiogenesis and re-epithelialization, modulation of cytokine and chemokine gene expression, and potentiation of antigen-specific adaptive immune response [5,92,93]. Importantly, many HDPs directly bind to and neutralize bacterial membrane components such as lipopolysaccharides (LPS), lipotechoic acid, and peptidoglycan and suppress the production of proinflammatory cytokines induced by bacteria and membrane components [94,95].

In chickens, CATH1 was shown to possess excellent immunomodulatory properties with a strong capacity to specifically chemoattract neutrophils without affecting the migration of monocytes or lymphocytes [96]. Furthermore, CATH1 and CATH2 activates macrophages or peripheral blood mononuclear cells by inducing synthesis of an array of cytokines and chemokines at moderate levels, which is distinct from that induced by LPS [96,97], CATH1–3 were shown to bind to LPS directly, with 50% binding occurring at approximately 10 μM [18,87]. Moreover, three peptides at 10–20 μM substantially abrogated LPS-induced production of proinflammatory cytokines in macrophages and peripheral blood mononuclear cells [18,87,97]. CATH1 was further found to augment adaptive immune response when administered into mice together with chicken ovalbumin, a model antigen [96]. In the case of human cathelicidin LL-37, glyceraldehyde 3-phosphate dehydrogenase (GAPDH) and sequestosome-1/p62 were recently identified as intracellular receptors to mediate cytokine/chemokine production in monocytes [98,99]. It will be interesting to examine whether chicken cathelicidins also utilize the same receptors to modulate the macrophage response.

7. Structures-Activity Relationships of Avian HDPs

7.1. Structural Features

To date, the tertiary structures of three chicken cathelicidins (CATH1–3), two β-defensins (chicken AvBD2 and penguin AvBD103a/spheniscin-2), and a chicken ovodefensin (gallin1/2) have been determined by nuclear magnetic resonance (NMR) in solutions. Unlike mammalian cathelicidins that adopt various conformations, all three chicken cathelicidins are largely α-helical with a mild kink or rather extensive bend around the center in aqueous solutions [87,90,100] (Figure 6). A mild kink in CATH1 and CATH3 is induced by the presence of a glycine residue, whereas an extensive bend in CATH2 is caused by proline (Figure 6A). Additionally, all three chicken cathelicidins consist of a flexible unstructured segment at the N-terminal region [87,90,100]. Unlike typical amphipathic α-helical HDPs, no obvious segregation of hydrophobic residues from hydrophilic residues is seen with either CATH1 or CATH2; instead, the positively charged residues are mostly concentrated at both ends (Figure 6B). On the other hand, CATH2 are rather amphipathic throughout the entire α-helix. Three truncated analogs of chicken CATH1 consisting of amino acid residues 1–16, 8–26, and 5–26 were also revealed to adopt similar confirmations to the full-length peptide in the presence of LPS or zwitterionic dodecylphosphocholine micelles [101,102].

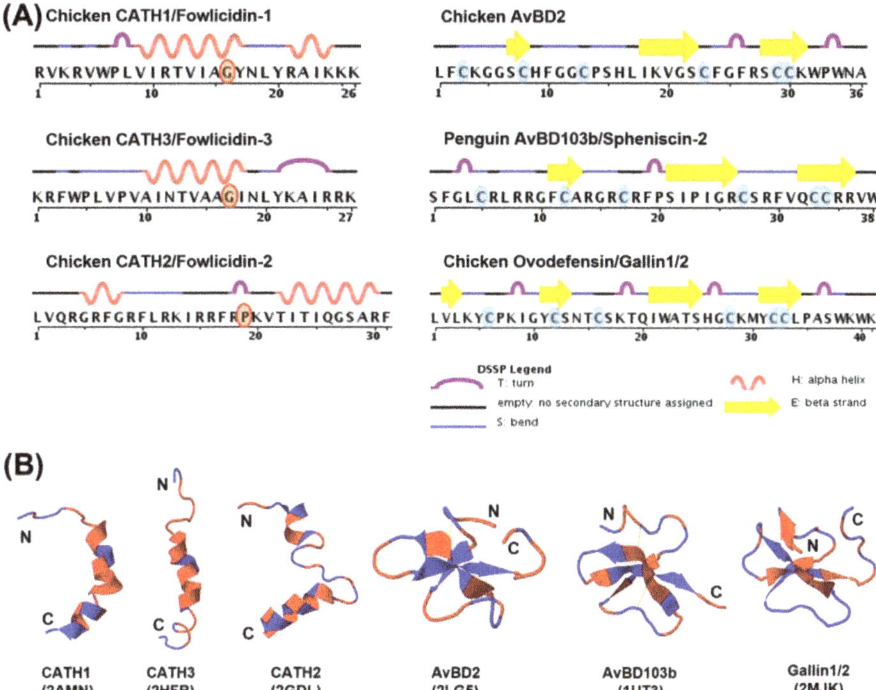

Figure 6. Structures of avian cathelicidins and β-defensins. (**A**) Secondary structural features of cathelicidins and β-defensins. (**B**) Tertiary ribbon structures of cathelicidins and β-defensins. Polar residues are indicated in blue and nonpolar residues in red. Disulfide bonds of β-defensins are shown in yellow. Protein Data Bank identification number for each molecule is indicated in parenthesis.

Both penguin AvBD103a and chicken AvBD2 adopt a triple-stranded, antiparallel β-sheet structure stabilized by three pairs of intramolecular disulfide bonds [91,103] (Figure 6B), typical of mammalian β-defensins. Penguin AvBD103a also consists of an α-helical segment at the N-terminal region with a hydrophobic patch on the surface [103]. However, AvBD2 lacks either the α-helical or an obvious amphipathic feature [91]. A β-bulge that is formed by the G-X-C motif around the fourth cysteine and highly conserved in both mammalian α- and β-defensins is also present in both AvBD2 and AvBD103a (Figure 6B). Albeit with a different cysteine-spacing pattern, chicken gallin1/2 also consists of a characteristic β-defensin fold with three antiparallel β-sheets [24]. However, unlike classical β-defensins, gallin1/2 is comprised of two additional β-sheets formed separately by Val^{2}-Leu^{3} at the N-terminal end and Thr^{24}-Ser^{25} preceding the fourth cysteine [24] (Figure 6).

7.2. Structure-Activity Relationships

Structure-activity relationship (SAR) studies with α-helical HDPs indicated that the antimicrobial potency and target specificity are strongly influenced by structural and physicochemical parameters, such as cationicity (net charge), helicity, amphipathicity, and hydrophobicity [11,104,105]. However, in general there is no simple correlation between any of these physicochemical properties and peptide functions. A delicate balance of these parameters often dictates the antimicrobial potency and target selectivity [11,104,105]. Within a certain range, an improvement in these parameters is often positively correlated with the antimicrobial activity of peptides, but sometimes is accompanied by unwanted enhancement in cytotoxicity as well [104–107]. In several cases, the antimicrobial domain of the peptides is located separately from the domain responsible for cytotoxicity [108,109], meaning that the peptide derivatives devoid of the lytic domain could be identified with improved therapeutic potential.

In the case of β-sheet HDPs and defensins in particular, antimicrobial and immunomodulatory activities are strongly influenced by structural integrity, cationicity, and hydrophobicity [11,110,111]. The presence of three intramolecular disulfide bonds in many cases is dispensable for the antibacterial activity, but essential for other activities such as chemotactic activity [112] and the ability to resist proteolysis [113]. On the contrary, the antibacterial activity of human β-defensin-1 drastically increases when the peptide is reduced [114]. In fact, some defensins may be naturally reduced in the intestinal tract by thioredoxin, a redox enzyme [114]. Cationicity of defensins is believed to dictate the killing of Gram-negative bacteria, whereas hydrophobicity appears to confer the activity against Gram-positive bacteria [111].

In avian species, a series of SAR studies with chicken CATH1, CATH2, and AvBD2 have yielded some very interesting observations. Investigations of chicken CATH1 analogs with either N- or C-terminal deletions revealed that the cationic residues at both N- and C-terminal regions are dispensable for the antibacterial, LPS-binding, and cytotoxic activities, whereas the C-terminal helix (Arg^{21}-Lys^{25}) is essential for all three activities [100]. Tryptophan at position 6 (Trp^{6}) is critical in both LPS binding and cytotoxicity [100,115], but is dispensable for neutrophil chemotaxis [96]. Furthermore, an omission of Trp^{6} in CATH1 also resulted in an obvious reduction in its ability to kill bacteria [115] and induce chemokine synthesis in macrophages [96]. Replacing the kink-causing glycine (Gly^{16}) with a helix-stabilizing residue, leucine, resulted in no obvious difference in either antibacterial, LPS-binding or cytotoxic activity [100], indicating that enhancing the helicity of α-helical HDPs may not necessarily result in an improvement in the antibacterial potency. Simultaneous substitutions of multiple amino acid residues to make CATH1 nearly perfectly amphipathic surprisingly caused a loss of the antibacterial potency against certain bacteria and undesirably, an increase in hemolytic activities [100]. Collectively, these findings suggested that a fine tuning of various structural and physicochemical parameters including cationicity, helicity, hydrophobicity, and amphipathicity, rather than a simple alteration of one, will result in an enhancement in the therapeutic potential of α-helical HDPs, which is in agreement with earlier findings [11,104,105].

Studies with a series of CATH2 analogs with deletions of either N- or C-terminal residues showed that neither α-helical segment *per se* is sufficient to bind LPS, kill bacteria or lyse mammalian cells [90].

Inclusion of four additional amino acids in the central bending region (Arg^{15}-Arg^{18}) beyond either N- or C-terminal α-helical segment to the α-helical segment was associated with a significant enhancement in both antibacterial and LPS-neutralizing activities [90]. To directly evaluate the functional significance of the central bending segment, a substitution of leucine for proline greatly reduced the antibacterial and hemolytic activities. The abilities to neutralize LPS-induced cytokine production and to stimulate chemokine synthesis in peripheral blood mononuclear cells were also significantly impaired by such a proline-to-leucine substitution [97], implying that the bending is critically important in the peptide interactions with membranes as well as the cell activation receptors. Interestingly, a gradual increase in cationicity, helicity and amphipathicity among all peptide analogs led to a gradual enhancement in antibacterial potency and LPS neutralization [90]. Furthermore, substitution of multiple tryptophans for phenylalanines in an N-terminal, 15-amino acid fragment of CATH2 led to an improvement in antibacterial and LPS-neutralizing activities [116]. Head-to-tail cyclization of this CATH2 variant further increased its serum stability with a reduced cytotoxicity [117]. The same study also revealed that D-amino acid substitutions rendered the peptide completely resistant to trypsin proteolysis [117].

In the case of chicken AvBD2, D-enantiomerization resulted in little difference in the activity against both Gram-positive and Gram-negative bacteria, suggesting that membrane is the primary target [91]. However, unlike many mammalian defensins whose structural integrity has a minimum impact on the antibacterial activity, reducing AvBD2 led to a drastic loss in the activity against Gram-positive bacteria, but was less prominent against Gram-negative bacteria [91]. Substitution of alanine for a conserved lysine following the sixth cysteine resulted in an obvious N-terminal structural modification and a marked decrease in the antibacterial activity against both Gram-positive and Gram-negative bacteria [91]. Surprisingly, a reduction of disulfide bonds rendered the lysine-alanine substituted AvBD2 nearly completely inactive in killing bacteria [91]. Therefore, conformational changes (and subsequent changes in hydrophobicity and/or amphipathicity) are likely the underlying mechanism behind many of the alterations in the antibacterial activity of AvBD2.

8. Potential Therapeutic Applications

HDPs including avian HDPs can be potentially used in a variety of applications such as antimicrobial therapy (Figure 7). Additionally, HDPs hold promise in augmenting the efficacy of vaccines as adjuvants. Although a number of avian HDPs are expressed in both male and female reproductive tracts and believed to promote sperm maturation and fertility like their mammalian counterparts [10,118], experimental evidence is yet to prove the link. Therefore, the potential role and application of avian HDPs in infertility treatment will not be discussed here. To reduce the cost of delivering synthetic peptides and minimize peptide degradation, endogenous HDPs can also be induced by certain cost-effective dietary compounds to help the host better fight off infections (Figure 7).

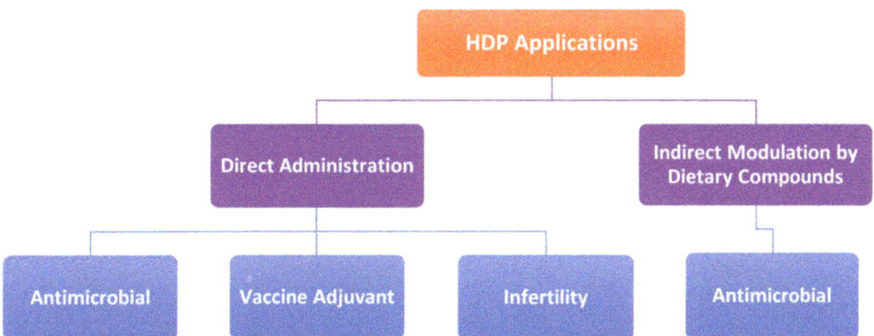

Figure 7. Potential therapeutic applications of host defense peptides (HDPs). Synthetic HDPs can be directly administered exogenously as antimicrobials, vaccine adjuvants or infertility drugs. Alternatively, endogenous HDPs can modulated by dietary compounds for antimicrobial therapies.

8.1. Antimicrobial Therapies

HDPs are active against a broad range of bacteria, mycobacteria, fungi, and parasites [1,8]. Rather than relying on a single or a limited number of intracellular targets like most currently available antibiotics, HDPs kills microbes primarily through physical electrostatic interactions and membrane disruption. Therefore, it is difficult for microbes to gain resistance to HDPs [1,8]. At the same time, most HDPs have the capacity to recruit and activate immune cells and facilitate the resolution of inflammation [6,8]. In fact, the antibacterial and immunomodulatory properties of HDPs can be harnessed separately for antimicrobial therapy, particularly against antibiotic-resistant strains [6,8]. A few HDPs have been evaluated clinically for their antibacterial efficacy, and several more are currently at different stages of human trials. Because of a relatively low efficacy as compared with many of the conventional antibiotics, all clinical trials with HDPs have met a limited success [119]. As a result, no HDPs have been approved by the FDA to date. More efforts are being shifted toward exploring the immune regulatory activities of HDPs. Excitedly, several small HDPs with no or weak antibacterial activities have been proved to be highly efficient in protecting animals from infections by recruiting and activating neutrophils and/or monocytes [95,120]. Because they act on the host but not on the pathogens, these immunomodulatory peptides have the potential to control a broad spectrum of pathogens without triggering resistance.

In avian species, only chicken CATH1 has been evaluated for its *in vivo* antibacterial efficacy. A single intraperitoneal administration of a C-terminal, 21-amino acid CATH1 peptide analog, known as fowlicidin-1 (6–26), led to a 50% increase in the survival of mice from a lethal dose of methicillin-resistant *S. aureus* (MRSA), concomitant with a reduction in the bacterial titer in both peritoneal fluids and spleens of mice [115]. Additionally, fowlicidin-1(6–26) is more potent in inducing neutrophil chemotaxis and macrophage activation than human cathelicidin LL-37 and a *de novo* synthesized peptide, IDR-1 [96]. Because of its ability to induce neutrophil chemotaxis and macrophage activation, fowlicidin-1(6–26) protected 50% mice if given 4 days prior to an otherwise lethal MRSA infection, and 100% mice survived if the peptide was received 1 or 2 days before infection [96]. This is the first HDP that has been shown to protect animals from bacterial infections beyond a 48-h window. Therefore, fowlicidin-1(6–26) represents an attractive candidate for further exploration as a novel antimicrobial for both therapeutic and prophylactic applications. Rational design and functional screening of additional CATH1-related peptides may lead to identification of new peptide analogs with improved safety and therapeutic potential, particularly against antibiotic-resistant pathogens.

It is worth noting that many HDPs and defensins in particular have obvious antiviral effects by acting as lectins or by modulating host cell responses. Enveloped and non-enveloped viruses such as human immunodeficiency virus (HIV-1), influenza A virus (IAV), cytomegalovirus (CMV), herpes simplex virus (HSV-1 and HSV-2), vesicular stomatitis virus (VSV) , adenovirus, and papillomavirus (HPV) have been shown to be sensitive to human α-, β- and/or θ-defensins [121,122]. In some cases, defensins can directly inactivate viruses by disrupting envelop lipid bilayers, aggregating viral glycoproteins or blocking the binding of viruses to host cell receptors [122]. In other cases, the antiviral effects of defensins are indirectly mediated by modifying host cell responses such as inhibition of protein kinase C (PKC) activation or down-regulation of host cell receptor expression [122]. Limited work exists on the antiviral activities of avian HDPs. Only a few duck β-defensins were recently shown to inhibit the replication of duck hepatitis virus (DHV) [37,67]. However, the antiviral mechanisms or the susceptibility of other viruses to avian HDPs remains unknown, but warrant further investigations.

8.2. Vaccine Adjuvants

HDPs have been shown to profoundly impact the development of adaptive immune response by regulating the migration, maturation, and activation of different immune cell types including dendritic cells and T and B lymphocytes [5,8,123]. Several HDPs are capable of enhancing antigen-specific adaptive immune response when co-administered with vaccines [123]. HDPs have been found to synergize with other adjuvants like CpG DNA and polyphosphazene in potentiating adaptive immune response [124–126]. The adjunvanticity of chicken AvBD1, duck AvBD2, and chicken CATH1 have been experimentally verified. When fused with the infectious bursal disease virus (IBDV) VP2 gene in a DNA vaccine, chicken AvBD1 increased the VP2-specific antibody titers, $CD4^+$ and $CD8^+$ T cell populations, and conferred better protection against an infectious bursal disease virus (IBDV) challenge in chickens [127]. Duck AvBD2 was shown to be chemotactic to T- and B-lymphocytes *in vitro*, with the ability to suppress the mRNA expression of an inhibitory receptor, namely dendritic cell immunoreceptor (DCIR), in duck splenocytes [128]. Chicken CATH1, when co-administered with chicken ovalbumin (OVA), was found to enhance both IgG_1 and IgG_{2a} titers to OVA in mice [96]. Because CATH 1 was more potent than LL-37 or IDR-1 in inducing surface expression of CD86, a co-stimulatory molecule, on macrophages [96], CATH1 may be more efficient in promoting antigen presentation and adaptive immunity and therefore, represent an excellent candidate as an adjuvant or a component of an adjuvant complex.

8.3. *Direct Administration* vs. *Indirect Modulation*

The production cost and stability are two major obstacles for *in vivo* applications of many peptide-based drugs. Purification from natural sources or chemical synthesis are inefficient and cost-prohibitive for large-scale production of HDPs. Although recombinant expression of HDPs has been achieved in bacteria and yeasts, an inclusion of a fusion protein is often needed to reduce the peptide toxicity to the host and aid in the peptide solubility [129]. In order to achieve the maximum activity, an extra proteolytic cleavage step and additional production costs are often unavoidable. Given a short half-life of most natural peptides *in vivo*, it is desirable to retard the peptide degradation by chemical modifications that often involves the use of D-amino acids, cyclization or peptidomimetics [130]. However, it remains unknown how those modifications would impact the immunomodulatory functions of HDPs, which appear to be receptor-dependent.

To overcome the high manufacturing cost and minimize degradation of HDPs for *in vivo* applications, it is advantageous to develop convenient and cost-effective strategies to specifically induce the synthesis of endogenous HDPs. Several dietary compounds including short-chain fatty acids and vitamin D_3 have shown promise in stimulating HDP synthesis in humans without triggering inflammatory response [131,132]. Dietary supplementation of HDP-inducing compounds has emerged as a novel antibiotic-alternative approach to antimicrobial therapy [131,132]. In chickens, butyrate, structural analogs of butyrate, and cAMP signaling agonists have been shown to be potent inducers of HDPs [84–86]. Desirably, butyrate and cAMP agonists are synergistic in augmenting HDP gene expression and bacterial clearance in chickens [86], suggesting their potential as alternatives to antibiotics for disease control and prevention. However, dietary regulation of HDPs often exhibit gene-, cell-, and species-specific patterns. HDP genes are differentially regulated in response to a dietary compound, with some being induced and others unaltered. In chickens, approximately a half number of chicken HDPs are induced by butyrate [84]. Some HDPs are regulated in a cell-specific pattern. For example, chicken AvBD9 gene increased by more than 5000-fold in HD11 macrophages, but with only a less than 10-fold induction in cecal intestinal cells after a 24-h exposure to 4 mM butyrate [84]. The same compound that show a strong HDP-inducing activity in one animal species, may completely lose its ability to induce HDPs in another species. A case in point is vitamin D3, which strongly augments cathelicidin gene expression in human but not mouse cells [75,76]. Therefore, it is important to evaluate the HDP-inducing efficacy of individual compounds in different species.

9. Conclusions

Birds harbor approximately 20 unique cathelicidins and β-defensin genes in each species. It appears that most have evolved before divergence of birds from each other. Unlike mammalian cathelicidins that adopt different tertiary structures, avian cathelicidins are mostly α-helical, with a hinge around the central region and a flexible N-terminal segment. Besides classical β-defensins, a group of avian-specific, β-defensin-related peptides, namely ovodefensins, exist with a different cysteine-spacing pattern. However, the overall three-dimensional structure of ovodenfensins resemble that of β-defensins. Coupled with their close chromosomal proximity with the β-defensin gene cluster, ovodefensins were clearly diversified from a β-defensin ancestral gene, possibly AvBD12, after separation of the birds from other vertebrate species. Several avian HDPs have been shown to possess potent, broad-spectrum antibacterial activities with a strong ability to modulate the host response to infection and inflammation. Structure-activity relationship studies have led to the identification of a few avian HDPs and their analogs as promising candidates as antimicrobials or vaccine adjuvants. Because avian HDPs can be induced by dietary compounds such as short-chain fatty acids and cAMP signaling agonists, dietary modulation of endogenous HDP synthesis may have potential to be further explored as a novel, cost-effective antimicrobial strategy.

Acknowledgments: Invaluable contributions from the past and current members of the Zhang Laboratory are greatly appreciated. The research on host defense peptides in the Zhang Laboratory is supported by the U.S. Department of Agriculture grant (2008-35204-04544), Oklahoma Center for the Advancement of Science and Technology grants (AR12.2-077 and HR12-051), and Oklahoma Agricultural Experiment Station project (H-2811).

Conflicts of Interest: The authors declare no conflict of interest.

References

1. Zasloff, M. Antimicrobial peptides of multicellular organisms. *Nature* **2002**, *415*, 389–395. [CrossRef]
2. Pasupuleti, M.; Schmidtchen, A.; Malmsten, M. Antimicrobial peptides: Key components of the innate immune system. *Crit. Rev. Biotechnol.* **2012**, *32*, 143–171. [CrossRef]
3. Wang, G. Database-Guided Discovery of Potent Peptides to Combat HIV-1 or Superbugs. *Pharmaceuticals (Basel)* **2013**, *6*, 728–758. [CrossRef]
4. Brogden, K.A. Antimicrobial peptides: Pore formers or metabolic inhibitors in bacteria? *Nat. Rev. Microbiol.* **2005**, *3*, 238–250. [CrossRef]
5. Yang, D.; Biragyn, A.; Hoover, D.M.; Lubkowski, J.; Oppenheim, J.J. Multiple roles of antimicrobial defensins, cathelicidins, and eosinophil-derived neurotoxin in host defense. *Annu. Rev. Immunol.* **2004**, *22*, 181–215. [CrossRef]
6. Choi, K.Y.; Chow, L.N.; Mookherjee, N. Cationic host defence peptides: Multifaceted role in immune modulation and inflammation. *J. Innate Immun.* **2012**, *4*, 361–370.
7. Hilchie, A.L.; Wuerth, K.; Hancock, R.E. Immune modulation by multifaceted cationic host defense (antimicrobial) peptides. *Nat. Chem. Biol.* **2013**, *9*, 761–768. [CrossRef]
8. Hancock, R.E.; Nijnik, A.; Philpott, D.J. Modulating immunity as a therapy for bacterial infections. *Nat. Rev. Microbiol.* **2012**, *10*, 243–254. [CrossRef]
9. Semple, F.; Dorin, J.R. β-Defensins: Multifunctional modulators of infection, inflammation and more? *J. Innate Immun.* **2012**, *4*, 337–348. [CrossRef]
10. Tollner, T.L.; Bevins, C.L.; Cherr, G.N. Multifunctional glycoprotein DEFB126—A curious story of defensin-clad spermatozoa. *Nat. Rev. Urol.* **2012**, *9*, 365–375. [CrossRef]
11. Takahashi, D.; Shukla, S.K.; Prakash, O.; Zhang, G. Structural determinants of host defense peptides for antimicrobial activity and target cell selectivity. *Biochimie* **2010**, *92*, 1236–1241. [CrossRef]
12. Zanetti, M. Cathelicidins, multifunctional peptides of the innate immunity. *J. Leukoc. Biol.* **2004**, *75*, 39–48. [CrossRef]
13. Selsted, M.E.; Ouellette, A.J. Mammalian defensins in the antimicrobial immune response. *Nat. Immunol.* **2005**, *6*, 551–557. [CrossRef]
14. Ganz, T. Defensins: Antimicrobial peptides of innate immunity. *Nat. Rev. Immunol.* **2003**, *3*, 710–720. [CrossRef]
15. Kosciuczuk, E.M.; Lisowski, P.; Jarczak, J.; Strzalkowska, N.; Jozwik, A.; Horbanczuk, J.; Krzyzewski, J.; Zwierzchowski, L.; Bagnicka, E. Cathelicidins: Family of antimicrobial peptides. *A review. Mol. Biol Rep.* **2012**, *39*, 10957–10970. [CrossRef]
16. Levy, O.; Ooi, C.E.; Elsbach, P.; Doerfler, M.E.; Lehrer, R.I.; Weiss, J. Antibacterial proteins of granulocytes differ in interaction with endotoxin. Comparison of bactericidal/permeability-increasing protein, p15s, and defensins. *J. Immunol.* **1995**, *1995*, 5403–5410.

17. Moscinski, L.C.; Hill, B. Molecular cloning of a novel myeloid granule protein. *J. Cell. Biochem.* **1995**, *59*, 431–442. [CrossRef]
18. Xiao, Y.; Cai, Y.; Bommineni, Y.R.; Fernando, S.C.; Prakash, O.; Gilliland, S.E.; Zhang, G. Identification and functional characterization of three chicken cathelicidins with potent antimicrobial activity. *J. Biol Chem.* **2006**, *281*, 2858–2867.
19. Zarember, K.A.; Katz, S.S.; Tack, B.F.; Doukhan, L.; Weiss, J.; Elsbach, P. Host defense functions of proteolytically processed and parent (unprocessed) cathelicidins of rabbit granulocytes. *Infect. Immun.* **2002**, *70*, 569–576. [CrossRef]
20. Lehrer, R.I. Primate defensins. *Nat. Rev. Microbiol.* **2004**, *2*, 727–738. [CrossRef]
21. Andersson, M.L.; Karlsson-Sjoberg, J.M.; Putsep, K.L. CRS-peptides: Unique defense peptides of mouse Paneth cells. *Mucosal Immunol.* **2012**, *5*, 367–376. [CrossRef]
22. Patil, A.A.; Ouellette, A.J.; Lu, W.; Zhang, G. Rattusin, an intestinal alpha-defensin-related peptide in rats with a unique cysteine spacing pattern and salt-insensitive antibacterial activities. *Antimicrob. Agents Chemother.* **2013**, *57*, 1823–1831. [CrossRef]
23. Gong, D.; Wilson, P.W.; Bain, M.M.; McDade, K.; Kalina, J.; Herve-Grepinet, V.; Nys, Y.; Dunn, I.C. Gallin; an antimicrobial peptide member of a new avian defensin family, the ovodefensins, has been subject to recent gene duplication. *BMC Immunol.* **2010**, *11*, 12. [CrossRef]
24. Herve, V.; Meudal, H.; Labas, V.; Rehault Godbert, S.; Gautron, J.; Berges, M.; Guyot, N.; Delmas, A.F.; Nys, Y.; Landon, C. 3D NMR structure of hen egg gallin (chicken ovo-defensin) reveals a new variation of the beta-defensin fold. *J. Biol. Chem.* **2014**, in press.
25. Van Dijk, A.; Molhoek, E.M.; Bikker, F.J.; Yu, P.L.; Veldhuizen, E.J.; Haagsman, H.P. Avian cathelicidins: Paradigms for the development of anti-infectives. *Vet. Microbiol.* **2011**, *153*, 27–36. [CrossRef]
26. Van Dijk, A.; Veldhuizen, E.J.; Haagsman, H.P. Avian defensins. *Vet. Immunol Immunopathol.* **2008**, *124*, 1–18. [CrossRef]
27. Sugiarto, H.; Yu, P.L. Avian antimicrobial peptides: The defense role of beta-defensins. *Biochem. Biophys. Res. Commun.* **2004**, *323*, 721–727. [CrossRef]
28. Cuperus, T.; Coorens, M.; van Dijk, A.; Haagsman, H.P. Avian host defense peptides. *Dev. Comp. Immunol.* **2013**, *41*, 352–369. [CrossRef]
29. Lynn, D.J.; Higgs, R.; Gaines, S.; Tierney, J.; James, T.; Lloyd, A.T.; Fares, M.A.; Mulcahy, G.; O'Farrelly, C. Bioinformatic discovery and initial characterisation of nine novel antimicrobial peptide genes in the chicken. *Immunogenetics* **2004**, *56*, 170–177. [CrossRef]
30. Van Dijk, A.; Veldhuizen, E.J.; van Asten, A.J.; Haagsman, H.P. CMAP27, a novel chicken cathelicidin-like antimicrobial protein. *Vet. Immunol. Immunopathol.* **2005**, *106*, 321–327. [CrossRef]
31. Goitsuka, R.; Chen, C.L.; Benyon, L.; Asano, Y.; Kitamura, D.; Cooper, M.D. Chicken cathelicidin-B1, an antimicrobial guardian at the mucosal M cell gateway. *Proc. Natl. Acad. Sci. USA* **2007**, *104*, 15063–15068. [CrossRef]
32. Feng, F.; Chen, C.; Zhu, W.; He, W.; Guang, H.; Li, Z.; Wang, D.; Liu, J.; Chen, M.; Wang, Y.; Yu, H. Gene cloning, expression and characterization of avian cathelicidin orthologs, Cc-CATHs, from Coturnix coturnix. *FEBS J.* **2011**, *278*, 1573–1584.
33. Wang, Y.; Lu, Z.; Feng, F.; Zhu, W.; Guang, H.; Liu, J.; He, W.; Chi, L.; Li, Z.; Yu, H. Molecular cloning and characterization of novel cathelicidin-derived myeloid antimicrobial peptide from Phasianus colchicus. *Dev. Comp. Immunol.* **2011**, *35*, 314–322. [CrossRef]
34. Evans, E.W.; Beach, G.G.; Wunderlich, J.; Harmon, B.G. Isolation of antimicrobial peptides from avian heterophils. *J. Leukoc. Biol.* **1994**, *56*, 661–665.
35. Xiao, Y.; Hughes, A.L.; Ando, J.; Matsuda, Y.; Cheng, J.F.; Skinner-Noble, D.; Zhang, G. A genome-wide screen identifies a single beta-defensin gene cluster in the chicken: Implications for the origin and evolution of mammalian defensins. *BMC Genomics* **2004**, *5*, 56. [CrossRef]
36. Lynn, D.J.; Higgs, R.; Lloyd, A.T.; O'Farrelly, C.; Herve-Grepinet, V.; Nys, Y.; Brinkman, F.S.; Yu, P.L.; Soulier, A.; Kaiser, P.; *et al.* Avian beta-defensin nomenclature: A community proposed update. *Immunol. Lett.* **2007**, *110*, 86–89. [CrossRef]
37. Ma, D.; Zhang, K.; Zhang, M.; Xin, S.; Liu, X.; Han, Z.; Shao, Y.; Liu, S. Identification, expression and activity analyses of five novel duck beta-defensins. *PLoS One* **2012**, *7*, e47743.

38. Ma, D.; Zhang, M.; Zhang, K.; Liu, X.; Han, Z.; Shao, Y.; Liu, S. Identification of three novel avian beta-defensins from goose and their significance in the pathogenesis of Salmonella. *Mol. Immunol.* **2013**, *56*, 521–529. [CrossRef]
39. Cormican, P.; Lloyd, A.T.; Downing, T.; Connell, S.J.; Bradley, D.; O'Farrelly, C. The avian Toll-Like receptor pathway—Subtle differences amidst general conformity. *Dev. Comp. Immunol.* **2009**, *33*, 967–973. [CrossRef]
40. Hellgren, O.; Ekblom, R. Evolution of a cluster of innate immune genes (beta-defensins) along the ancestral lines of chicken and zebra finch. *Immunome Res.* **2010**, *6*, 3. [CrossRef]
41. Evans, E.W.; Beach, F.G.; Moore, K.M.; Jackwood, M.W.; Glisson, J.R.; Harmon, B.G. Antimicrobial activity of chicken and turkey heterophil peptides CHP1, CHP2, THP1, and THP3. *Vet. Microbiol.* **1995**, *47*, 295–303. [CrossRef]
42. Sugiarto, H.; Yu, P.L. Identification of three novel ostricacins: An update on the phylogenetic perspective of beta-defensins. *Int. J. Antimicrob. Agents* **2006**, *27*, 229–235. [CrossRef]
43. Thouzeau, C.; Le Maho, Y.; Froget, G.; Sabatier, L.; Le Bohec, C.; Hoffmann, J.A.; Bulet, P. Spheniscins, avian beta-defensins in preserved stomach contents of the king penguin, Aptenodytes patagonicus. *J. Biol Chem.* **2003**, *278*, 51053–51058.
44. Mann, K. The chicken egg white proteome. *Proteomics* **2007**, *7*, 3558–3568. [CrossRef]
45. Mann, K.; Mann, M. In-depth analysis of the chicken egg white proteome using an LTQ Orbitrap Velos. *Proteome Sci* **2011**, *9*, 7. [CrossRef]
46. Odani, S.; Koide, T.; Ono, T.; Takahashi, Y.; Suzuki, J. Covalent structure of a low-molecular-mass protein, meleagrin, present in a turkey (Meleagris gallopavo) ovomucoid preparation. *J. Biochem.* **1989**, *105*, 660–663.
47. Simpson, R.J.; Morgan, F.J. Isolation and complete amino acid sequence of a basic low molecular weight protein from black swan egg white. *Int. J. Pept. Protein Res.* **1983**, *22*, 476–481.
48. Naknukool, S.; Hayakawa, S.; Ogawa, M. Multiple biological functions of novel basic proteins isolated from duck egg white: Duck basic protein small 1 (dBPS1) and 2 (dBPS2). *J. Agric. Food Chem.* **2011**, *59*, 5081–5086. [CrossRef]
49. Warren, W.C.; Clayton, D.F.; Ellegren, H.; Arnold, A.P.; Hillier, L.W.; Kunstner, A.; Searle, S.; White, S.; Vilella, A.J.; Fairley, S.; *et al.* The genome of a songbird. *Nature* **2010**, *464*, 757–762. [CrossRef]
50. Achanta, M.; Sunkara, L.T.; Dai, G.; Bommineni, Y.R.; Jiang, W.; Zhang, G. Tissue expression and developmental regulation of chicken cathelicidin antimicrobial peptides. *J. Anim. Sci. Biotechnol.* **2012**, *3*, 15. [CrossRef]
51. Van Dijk, A.; Tersteeg-Zijderveld, M.H.; Tjeerdsma-van Bokhoven, J.L.; Jansman, A.J.; Veldhuizen, E.J.; Haagsman, H.P. Chicken heterophils are recruited to the site of Salmonella infection and release antibacterial mature Cathelicidin-2 upon stimulation with LPS. *Mol. Immunol.* **2009**, *46*, 1517–1526. [CrossRef]
52. Zhao, C.; Nguyen, T.; Liu, L.; Sacco, R.E.; Brogden, K.A.; Lehrer, R.I. Gallinacin-3, an inducible epithelial beta-defensin in the chicken. *Infect. Immun.* **2001**, *69*, 2684–2691. [CrossRef]
53. Harwig, S.S.; Swiderek, K.M.; Kokryakov, V.N.; Tan, L.; Lee, T.D.; Panyutich, E.A.; Aleshina, G.M.; Shamova, O.V.; Lehrer, R.I. Gallinacins: Cysteine-rich antimicrobial peptides of chicken leukocytes. *FEBS Lett.* **1994**, *342*, 281–285. [CrossRef]
54. Andersson, E.; Sorensen, O.E.; Frohm, B.; Borregaard, N.; Egesten, A.; Malm, J. Isolation of human cationic antimicrobial protein-18 from seminal plasma and its association with prostasomes. *Hum. Reprod.* **2002**, *17*, 2529–2534. [CrossRef]
55. Patil, A.A.; Cai, Y.; Sang, Y.; Blecha, F.; Zhang, G. Cross-species analysis of the mammalian beta-defensin gene family: Presence of syntenic gene clusters and preferential expression in the male reproductive tract. *Physiol. Genomics* **2005**, *23*, 5–17. [CrossRef]
56. Anastasiadou, M.; Avdi, M.; Michailidis, G. Expression of avian beta-defensins and Toll-like receptor genes in the rooster epididymis during growth and Salmonella infection. *Anim. Reprod. Sci.* **2013**, *140*, 224–231. [CrossRef]
57. Meade, K.G.; Higgs, R.; Lloyd, A.T.; Giles, S.; O'Farrelly, C. Differential antimicrobial peptide gene expression patterns during early chicken embryological development. *Dev. Comp. Immunol.* **2009**, *33*, 516–524. [CrossRef]
58. Bar-Shira, E.; Friedman, A. Development and adaptations of innate immunity in the gastrointestinal tract of the newly hatched chick. *Dev. Comp. Immunol.* **2006**, *30*, 930–941. [CrossRef]

59. Anastasiadou, M.; Avdi, M.; Theodoridis, A.; Michailidis, G. Temporal changes in the expression of avian beta-defensins in the chicken vagina during sexual maturation and Salmonella infection. *Vet. Res. Commun.* **2013**, *37*, 115–122. [CrossRef]
60. Michailidis, G.; Avdi, M.; Argiriou, A. Transcriptional profiling of antimicrobial peptides avian beta-defensins in the chicken ovary during sexual maturation and in response to Salmonella enteritidis infection. *Res. Vet. Sci.* **2012**, *92*, 60–65. [CrossRef]
61. Gersemann, M.; Wehkamp, J.; Stange, E.F. Innate immune dysfunction in inflammatory bowel disease. *J. Intern. Med.* **2012**, *271*, 421–428. [CrossRef]
62. Gilliet, M.; Lande, R. Antimicrobial peptides and self-DNA in autoimmune skin inflammation. *Curr. Opin. Immunol.* **2008**, *20*, 401–407. [CrossRef]
63. Islam, D.; Bandholtz, L.; Nilsson, J.; Wigzell, H.; Christensson, B.; Agerberth, B.; Gudmundsson, G. Downregulation of bactericidal peptides in enteric infections: A novel immune escape mechanism with bacterial DNA as a potential regulator. *Nat. Med.* **2001**, *7*, 180–185. [CrossRef]
64. Bergman, P.; Johansson, L.; Asp, V.; Plant, L.; Gudmundsson, G.H.; Jonsson, A.B.; Agerberth, B. Neisseria gonorrhoeae downregulates expression of the human antimicrobial peptide LL-37. *Cell. Microbiol.* **2005**, *7*, 1009–1017. [CrossRef]
65. Chakraborty, K.; Ghosh, S.; Koley, H.; Mukhopadhyay, A.K.; Ramamurthy, T.; Saha, D.R.; Mukhopadhyay, D.; Roychowdhury, S.; Hamabata, T.; Takeda, Y.; *et al.* Bacterial exotoxins downregulate cathelicidin (hCAP-18/ LL-37) and human beta-defensin 1 (HBD-1) expression in the intestinal epithelial cells. *Cell. Microbiol.* **2008**, *10*, 2520–2537. [CrossRef]
66. Akbari, M.R.; Haghighi, H.R.; Chambers, J.R.; Brisbin, J.; Read, L.R.; Sharif, S. Expression of antimicrobial peptides in cecal tonsils of chickens treated with probiotics and infected with Salmonella enterica serovar typhimurium. *Clin. Vaccine Immunol.* **2008**, *15*, 1689–1693. [CrossRef]
67. Ma, D.; Lin, L.; Zhang, K.; Han, Z.; Shao, Y.; Liu, X.; Liu, S. Three novel Anas platyrhynchos avian beta-defensins, upregulated by duck hepatitis virus, with antibacterial and antiviral activities. *Mol. Immunol.* **2011**, *49*, 84–96. [CrossRef]
68. Meade, K.G.; Narciandi, F.; Cahalane, S.; Reiman, C.; Allan, B.; O'Farrelly, C. Comparative *in vivo* infection models yield insights on early host immune response to Campylobacter in chickens. *Immunogenetics* **2009**, *61*, 101–110. [CrossRef]
69. Van Dijk, A.; Herrebout, M.; Tersteeg-Zijderveld, M.H.; Tjeerdsma-van Bokhoven, J.L.; Bleumink-Pluym, N.; Jansman, A.J.; Veldhuizen, E.J.; Haagsman, H.P. Campylobacter jejuni is highly susceptible to killing by chicken host defense peptide cathelicidin-2 and suppresses intestinal cathelicidin-2 expression in young broilers. *Vet. Microbiol.* **2012**, *160*, 347–354. [CrossRef]
70. Sumners, L.H.; Miska, K.B.; Jenkins, M.C.; Fetterer, R.H.; Cox, C.M.; Kim, S.; Dalloul, R.A. Expression of Toll-like receptors and antimicrobial peptides during Eimeria praecox infection in chickens. *Exp. Parasitol.* **2011**, *127*, 714–718. [CrossRef]
71. Raqib, R.; Sarker, P.; Bergman, P.; Ara, G.; Lindh, M.; Sack, D.A.; Nasirul Islam, K.M.; Gudmundsson, G.H.; Andersson, J.; Agerberth, B. Improved outcome in shigellosis associated with butyrate induction of an endogenous peptide antibiotic. *Proc. Natl. Acad. Sci. USA* **2006**, *103*, 9178–9183. [CrossRef]
72. Liu, P.T.; Stenger, S.; Tang, D.H.; Modlin, R.L. Cutting edge: Vitamin D-mediated human antimicrobial activity against Mycobacterium tuberculosis is dependent on the induction of cathelicidin. *J. Immunol.* **2007**, *179*, 2060–2063.
73. Sarker, P.; Ahmed, S.; Tiash, S.; Rekha, R.S.; Stromberg, R.; Andersson, J.; Bergman, P.; Gudmundsson, G.H.; Agerberth, B.; Raqib, R. Phenylbutyrate counteracts Shigella mediated downregulation of cathelicidin in rabbit lung and intestinal epithelia: A potential therapeutic strategy. *PLoS One* **2011**, *6*, e20637.
74. Schauber, J.; Svanholm, C.; Termen, S.; Iffland, K.; Menzel, T.; Scheppach, W.; Melcher, R.; Agerberth, B.; Luhrs, H.; Gudmundsson, G.H. Expression of the cathelicidin LL-37 is modulated by short chain fatty acids in colonocytes: Relevance of signalling pathways. *Gut* **2003**, *52*, 735–741. [CrossRef]
75. Wang, T.T.; Nestel, F.P.; Bourdeau, V.; Nagai, Y.; Wang, Q.; Liao, J.; Tavera-Mendoza, L.; Lin, R.; Hanrahan, J.W.; Mader, S.; *et al.* Cutting edge: 1,25-dihydroxyvitamin D3 is a direct inducer of antimicrobial peptide gene expression. *J. Immunol.* **2004**, *173*, 2909–2912.

76. Gombart, A.F.; Borregaard, N.; Koeffler, H.P. Human cathelicidin antimicrobial peptide (CAMP) gene is a direct target of the vitamin D receptor and is strongly up-regulated in myeloid cells by 1,25-dihydroxyvitamin D3. *FASEB J.* **2005**, *19*, 1067–1077. [CrossRef]
77. Schauber, J.; Dorschner, R.A.; Yamasaki, K.; Brouha, B.; Gallo, R.L. Control of the innate epithelial antimicrobial response is cell-type specific and dependent on relevant microenvironmental stimuli. *Immunology* **2006**, *118*, 509–519.
78. Steinmann, J.; Halldorsson, S.; Agerberth, B.; Gudmundsson, G.H. Phenylbutyrate induces antimicrobial peptide expression. *Antimicrob. Agents Chemother.* **2009**, *53*, 5127–5133. [CrossRef]
79. Schauber, J.; Iffland, K.; Frisch, S.; Kudlich, T.; Schmausser, B.; Eck, M.; Menzel, T.; Gostner, A.; Luhrs, H.; Scheppach, W. Histone-deacetylase inhibitors induce the cathelicidin LL-37 in gastrointestinal cells. *Mol. Immunol.* **2004**, *41*, 847–854.
80. Elloumi, H.Z.; Holland, S.M. Complex regulation of human cathelicidin gene expression: Novel splice variants and 5'UTR negative regulatory element. *Mol. Immunol.* **2008**, *45*, 204–217. [CrossRef]
81. Schwab, M.; Reynders, V.; Loitsch, S.; Steinhilber, D.; Schroder, O.; Stein, J. The dietary histone deacetylase inhibitor sulforaphane induces human beta-defensin-2 in intestinal epithelial cells. *Immunology* **2008**, *125*, 241–251.
82. Chakraborty, K.; Maity, P.C.; Sil, A.K.; Takeda, Y.; Das, S. cAMP stringently regulates human cathelicidin antimicrobial peptide expression in the mucosal epithelial cells by activating cAMP-response element-binding protein, AP-1, and inducible cAMP early repressor. *J. Biol. Chem.* **2009**, *284*, 21810–21827. [CrossRef]
83. Cederlund, A.; Kai-Larsen, Y.; Printz, G.; Yoshio, H.; Alvelius, G.; Lagercrantz, H.; Stromberg, R.; Jornvall, H.; Gudmundsson, G.H.; Agerberth, B. Lactose in human breast milk an inducer of innate immunity with implications for a role in intestinal homeostasis. *PLoS One* **2013**, *8*, e53876.
84. Sunkara, L.T.; Achanta, M.; Schreiber, N.B.; Bommineni, Y.R.; Dai, G.; Jiang, W.; Lamont, S.; Lillehoj, H.S.; Beker, A.; Teeter, R.G.; *et al.* Butyrate enhances disease resistance of chickens by inducing antimicrobial host defense peptide gene expression. *PLoS One* **2011**, *6*, e27225.
85. Sunkara, L.T.; Jiang, W.; Zhang, G. Modulation of antimicrobial host defense peptide gene expression by free fatty acids. *PLoS One* **2012**, *7*, e49558.
86. Sunkara, L.T.; Zeng, X.; Curtis, A.R.; Zhang, G. Cyclic AMP synergizes with butyrate in promoting beta-defensin 9 expression in chickens. *Mol. Immunol.* **2014**, *57*, 171–180.
87. Bommineni, Y.R.; Dai, H.; Gong, Y.X.; Soulages, J.L.; Fernando, S.C.; Desilva, U.; Prakash, O.; Zhang, G. Fowlicidin-3 is an alpha-helical cationic host defense peptide with potent antibacterial and lipopolysaccharide-neutralizing activities. *FEBS J.* **2007**, *274*, 418–428. [CrossRef]
88. Van Dijk, A.; Veldhuizen, E.J.; Kalkhove, S.I.; Tjeerdsma-van Bokhoven, J.L.; Romijn, R.A.; Haagsman, H.P. The beta-defensin gallinacin-6 is expressed in the chicken digestive tract and has antimicrobial activity against food-borne pathogens. *Antimicrob. Agents Chemother.* **2007**, *51*, 912–922. [CrossRef]
89. Higgs, R.; Lynn, D.J.; Gaines, S.; McMahon, J.; Tierney, J.; James, T.; Lloyd, A.T.; Mulcahy, G.; O'Farrelly, C. The synthetic form of a novel chicken beta-defensin identified in silico is predominantly active against intestinal pathogens. *Immunogenetics* **2005**, *57*, 90–98.
90. Xiao, Y.; Herrera, A.I.; Bommineni, Y.R.; Soulages, J.L.; Prakash, O.; Zhang, G. The central kink region of fowlicidin-2, an alpha-helical host defense peptide, is critically involved in bacterial killing and endotoxin neutralization. *J. Innate Immun.* **2009**, *1*, 268–280.
91. Derache, C.; Meudal, H.; Aucagne, V.; Mark, K.J.; Cadene, M.; Delmas, A.F.; Lalmanach, A.C.; Landon, C. Initial insights into structure-activity relationships of avian defensins. *J. Biol. Chem.* **2012**, *287*, 7746–7755. [CrossRef]
92. McPhee, J.B.; Hancock, R.E. Function and therapeutic potential of host defence peptides. *J. Pept. Sci.* **2005**, *11*, 677–687. [CrossRef]
93. Bowdish, D.M.; Davidson, D.J.; Hancock, R.E. A re-evaluation of the role of host defence peptides in mammalian immunity. *Curr. Protein Pept. Sci.* **2005**, *6*, 35–51.
94. Bowdish, D.M.; Hancock, R.E. Anti-endotoxin properties of cationic host defence peptides and proteins. *J. Endotoxin Res.* **2005**, *11*, 230–236. [CrossRef]

95. Scott, M.G.; Dullaghan, E.; Mookherjee, N.; Glavas, N.; Waldbrook, M.; Thompson, A.; Wang, A.; Lee, K.; Doria, S.; Hamill, P.; *et al.* An anti-infective peptide that selectively modulates the innate immune response. *Nat. Biotechnol.* **2007**, *25*, 465–472.
96. Bommineni, Y.R.; Pham, G.H.; Sunkara, L.T.; Achanta, M.; Zhang, G. Immune regulatory activities of fowlicidin-1, a cathelicidin host defense peptide. *Mol. Immunol.* **2014**, *59*, 55–63.
97. Van Dijk, A.; Molhoek, E.M.; Veldhuizen, E.J.; Bokhoven, J.L.; Wagendorp, E.; Bikker, F.; Haagsman, H.P. Identification of chicken cathelicidin-2 core elements involved in antibacterial and immunomodulatory activities. *Mol. Immunol.* **2009**, *46*, 2465–2473.
98. Yu, H.B.; Kielczewska, A.; Rozek, A.; Takenaka, S.; Li, Y.; Thorson, L.; Hancock, R.E.; Guarna, M.M.; North, J.R.; Foster, L.J.; *et al.* Sequestosome-1/p62 is the key intracellular target of innate defense regulator peptide. *J. Biol. Chem.* **2009**, *284*, 36007–36011. [CrossRef]
99. Mookherjee, N.; Lippert, D.N.; Hamill, P.; Falsafi, R.; Nijnik, A.; Kindrachuk, J.; Pistolic, J.; Gardy, J.; Miri, P.; Naseer, M.; *et al.* Intracellular receptor for human host defense peptide LL-37 in monocytes. *J. Immunol.* **2009**, *183*, 2688–2696.
100. Xiao, Y.; Dai, H.; Bommineni, Y.R.; Soulages, J.L.; Gong, Y.X.; Prakash, O.; Zhang, G. Structure-activity relationships of fowlicidin-1, a cathelicidin antimicrobial peptide in chicken. *FEBS J.* **2006**, *273*, 2581–2593.
101. Bhunia, A.; Mohanram, H.; Bhattacharjya, S. Lipopolysaccharide bound structures of the active fragments of fowlicidin-1, a cathelicidin family of antimicrobial and antiendotoxic peptide from chicken, determined by transferred nuclear Overhauser effect spectroscopy. *Biopolymers* **2009**, *92*, 9–22. [CrossRef]
102. Saravanan, R.; Bhattacharjya, S. Oligomeric structure of a cathelicidin antimicrobial peptide in dodecylphosphocholine micelle determined by NMR spectroscopy. *Biochim. Biophys. Acta* **2011**, *1808*, 369–381.
103. Landon, C.; Thouzeau, C.; Labbe, H.; Bulet, P.; Vovelle, F. Solution structure of spheniscin, a beta-defensin from the penguin stomach. *J. Biol. Chem.* **2004**, *279*, 30433–30439.
104. Tossi, A.; Sandri, L.; Giangaspero, A. Amphipathic, alpha-helical antimicrobial peptides. *Biopolymers* **2000**, *55*, 4–30. [CrossRef]
105. Dathe, M.; Wieprecht, T. Structural features of helical antimicrobial peptides: Their potential to modulate activity on model membranes and biological cells. *Biochim. Biophys. Acta* **1999**, *1462*, 71–87.
106. Nagaoka, I.; Kuwahara-Arai, K.; Tamura, H.; Hiramatsu, K.; Hirata, M. Augmentation of the bactericidal activities of human cathelicidin CAP18/LL-37-derived antimicrobial peptides by amino acid substitutions. *Inflamm. Res.* **2005**, *54*, 66–73. [CrossRef]
107. Chen, Y.; Mant, C.T.; Farmer, S.W.; Hancock, R.E.; Vasil, M.L.; Hodges, R.S. Rational design of alpha-helical antimicrobial peptides with enhanced activities and specificity/therapeutic index. *J. Biol. Chem.* **2005**, *280*, 12316–12329. [CrossRef]
108. Skerlavaj, B.; Gennaro, R.; Bagella, L.; Merluzzi, L.; Risso, A.; Zanetti, M. Biological characterization of two novel cathelicidin-derived peptides and identification of structural requirements for their antimicrobial and cell lytic activities. *J. Biol. Chem.* **1996**, *271*, 28375–28381.
109. Shin, S.Y.; Park, E.J.; Yang, S.T.; Jung, H.J.; Eom, S.H.; Song, W.K.; Kim, Y.; Hahm, K.S.; Kim, J.I. Structure-activity analysis of SMAP-29, a sheep leukocytes-derived antimicrobial peptide. *Biochem. Biophys. Res. Commun.* **2001**, *285*, 1046–1051. [CrossRef]
110. Taylor, K.; Barran, P.E.; Dorin, J.R. Structure-activity relationships in beta-defensin peptides. *Biopolymers* **2008**, *90*, 1–7. [CrossRef]
111. Lehrer, R.I.; Lu, W. alpha-Defensins in human innate immunity. *Immunol. Rev.* **2012**, *245*, 84–112.
112. Wu, Z.; Hoover, D.M.; Yang, D.; Boulegue, C.; Santamaria, F.; Oppenheim, J.J.; Lubkowski, J.; Lu, W. Engineering disulfide bridges to dissect antimicrobial and chemotactic activities of human beta-defensin 3. *Proc. Natl. Acad. Sci. USA* **2003**, *100*, 8880–8885.
113. Maemoto, A.; Qu, X.; Rosengren, K.J.; Tanabe, H.; Henschen-Edman, A.; Craik, D.J.; Ouellette, A.J. Functional analysis of the alpha-defensin disulfide array in mouse cryptdin-4. *J. Biol. Chem.* **2004**, *279*, 44188–44196.
114. Schroeder, B.O.; Wu, Z.; Nuding, S.; Groscurth, S.; Marcinowski, M.; Beisner, J.; Buchner, J.; Schaller, M.; Stange, E.F.; Wehkamp, J. Reduction of disulphide bonds unmasks potent antimicrobial activity of human beta-defensin 1. *Nature* **2011**, *469*, 419–423. [CrossRef]
115. Bommineni, Y.R.; Achanta, M.; Alexander, J.; Sunkara, L.T.; Ritchey, J.W.; Zhang, G. A fowlicidin-1 analog protects mice from lethal infections induced by methicillin-resistant Staphylococcus aureus. *Peptides* **2010**, *31*, 1225–1230.

116. Molhoek, E.M.; van Dijk, A.; Veldhuizen, E.J.; Dijk-Knijnenburg, H.; Mars-Groenendijk, R.H.; Boele, L.C.; Kaman-van Zanten, W.E.; Haagsman, H.P.; Bikker, F.J. Chicken cathelicidin-2-derived peptides with enhanced immunomodulatory and antibacterial activities against biological warfare agents. *Int. J. Antimicrob. Agents* **2010**, *36*, 271–274. [CrossRef]
117. Molhoek, E.M.; van Dijk, A.; Veldhuizen, E.J.; Haagsman, H.P.; Bikker, F.J. Improved proteolytic stability of chicken cathelicidin-2 derived peptides by D-amino acid substitutions and cyclization. *Peptides* **2011**, *32*, 875–880.
118. Zhou, Y.S.; Webb, S.; Lettice, L.; Tardif, S.; Kilanowski, F.; Tyrrell, C.; Macpherson, H.; Semple, F.; Tennant, P.; Baker, T.; *et al.* Partial deletion of chromosome 8 beta-defensin cluster confers sperm dysfunction and infertility in male mice. *PLoS Genet.* **2013**, *9*, e1003826. [CrossRef]
119. Hancock, R.E.; Sahl, H.G. Antimicrobial and host-defense peptides as new anti-infective therapeutic strategies. *Nat. Biotechnol.* **2006**, *24*, 1551–1557. [CrossRef]
120. Nijnik, A.; Madera, L.; Ma, S.; Waldbrook, M.; Elliott, M.R.; Easton, D.M.; Mayer, M.L.; Mullaly, S.C.; Kindrachuk, J.; Jenssen, H.; *et al.* Synthetic cationic peptide IDR-1002 provides protection against bacterial infections through chemokine induction and enhanced leukocyte recruitment. *J. Immunol.* **2010**, *184*, 2539–2550. [CrossRef]
121. Klotman, M.E.; Chang, T.L. Defensins in innate antiviral immunity. *Nat. Rev. Immunol.* **2006**, *6*, 447–456.
122. Wilson, S.S.; Wiens, M.E.; Smith, J.G. Antiviral mechanisms of human defensins. *J. Mol. Biol.* **2013**, *425*, 4965–4980. [CrossRef]
123. Nicholls, E.F.; Madera, L.; Hancock, R.E. Immunomodulators as adjuvants for vaccines and antimicrobial therapy. *Ann. N. Y. Acad. Sci.* **2010**, *1213*, 46–61.
124. Yang, J.; Mao, M.; Zhang, S.; Li, H.; Jiang, Z.; Cao, G.; Cao, D.; Wang, X.; Zhang, L. Innate defense regulator peptide synergizes with CpG ODN for enhanced innate intestinal immune responses in neonate piglets. *Int. Immunopharmacol.* **2012**, *12*, 415–424. [CrossRef]
125. Kovacs-Nolan, J.; Mapletoft, J.W.; Latimer, L.; Babiuk, L.A.; Hurk, S. CpG oligonucleotide, host defense peptide and polyphosphazene act synergistically, inducing long-lasting, balanced immune responses in cattle. *Vaccine* **2009**, *27*, 2048–2054. [CrossRef]
126. Kindrachuk, J.; Jenssen, H.; Elliott, M.; Townsend, R.; Nijnik, A.; Lee, S.F.; Gerdts, V.; Babiuk, L.A.; Halperin, S.A.; Hancock, R.E. A novel vaccine adjuvant comprised of a synthetic innate defence regulator peptide and CpG oligonucleotide links innate and adaptive immunity. *Vaccine* **2009**, *27*, 4662–4671.
127. Zhang, H.H.; Yang, X.M.; Xie, Q.M.; Ma, J.Y.; Luo, Y.N.; Cao, Y.C.; Chen, F.; Bi, Y.Z. The potent adjuvant effects of chicken beta-defensin-1 when genetically fused with infectious bursal disease virus VP2 gene. *Vet. Immunol. Immunopathol.* **2010**, *136*, 92–97. [CrossRef]
128. Soman, S.S.; Nair, S.; Issac, A.; Arathy, D.S.; Niyas, K.P.; Anoop, M.; Sreekumar, E. Immunomodulation by duck defensin, Apl_AvBD2: *In vitro* dendritic cell immunoreceptor (DCIR) mRNA suppression, and B- and T-lymphocyte chemotaxis. *Mol. Immunol.* **2009**, *46*, 3070–3075. [CrossRef]
129. Li, Y. Recombinant production of antimicrobial peptides in Escherichia coli: A review. *Protein Expr Purif.* **2011**, *80*, 260–267. [CrossRef]
130. Rotem, S.; Mor, A. Antimicrobial peptide mimics for improved therapeutic properties. *Biochim. Biophys. Acta* **2009**, *1788*, 1582–1592.
131. Campbell, Y.; Fantacone, M.L.; Gombart, A.F. Regulation of antimicrobial peptide gene expression by nutrients and by-products of microbial metabolism. *Eur. J. Nutr.* **2012**, *51*, 899–907. [CrossRef]
132. Van der Does, A.M.; Bergman, P.; Agerberth, B.; Lindbom, L. Induction of the human cathelicidin LL-37 as a novel treatment against bacterial infections. *J. Leukoc. Biol.* **2012**, *92*, 735–742. [CrossRef]

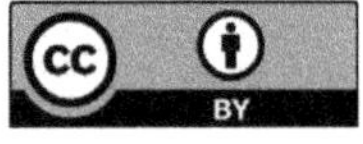

© 2014 by the authors. Licensee MDPI, Basel, Switzerland. This article is an open access article distributed under the terms and conditions of the Creative Commons Attribution (CC BY) license (http://creativecommons.org/licenses/by/4.0/).

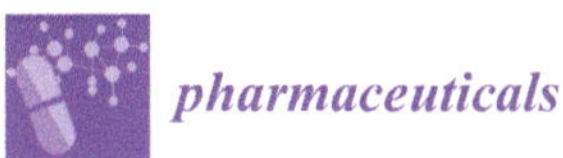

MDPI

Review

Chapter 9:

Human Antimicrobial Peptides and Proteins

Guangshun Wang

Department of Pathology and Microbiology, College of Medicine, University of Nebraska Medical Center, 986495 Nebraska Medical Center, Omaha, NE 68198-6495, USA; gwang@unmc.edu; Tel.: +1-402-559-4176; Fax: +1-402-559-4077

Received: 17 January 2014; in revised form: 15 April 2014; Accepted: 29 April 2014; Published: 13 May 2014

Abstract: As the key components of innate immunity, human host defense antimicrobial peptides and proteins (AMPs) play a critical role in warding off invading microbial pathogens. In addition, AMPs can possess other biological functions such as apoptosis, wound healing, and immune modulation. This article provides an overview on the identification, activity, 3D structure, and mechanism of action of human AMPs selected from the antimicrobial peptide database. Over 100 such peptides have been identified from a variety of tissues and epithelial surfaces, including skin, eyes, ears, mouths, gut, immune, nervous and urinary systems. These peptides vary from 10 to 150 amino acids with a net charge between −3 and +20 and a hydrophobic content below 60%. The sequence diversity enables human AMPs to adopt various 3D structures and to attack pathogens by different mechanisms. While α-defensin HD-6 can self-assemble on the bacterial surface into nanonets to entangle bacteria, both HNP-1 and β-defensin hBD-3 are able to block cell wall biosynthesis by binding to lipid II. Lysozyme is well-characterized to cleave bacterial cell wall polysaccharides but can also kill bacteria by a non-catalytic mechanism. The two hydrophobic domains in the long amphipathic α-helix of human cathelicidin LL-37 lays the basis for binding and disrupting the curved anionic bacterial membrane surfaces by forming pores or via the carpet model. Furthermore, dermcidin may serve as ion channel by forming a long helix-bundle structure. In addition, the C-type lectin RegIIIα can initially recognize bacterial peptidoglycans followed by pore formation in the membrane. Finally, histatin 5 and GAPDH(2-32) can enter microbial cells to exert their effects. It appears that granulysin enters cells and kills intracellular pathogens with the aid of pore-forming perforin. This arsenal of human defense proteins not only keeps us healthy but also inspires the development of a new generation of personalized medicine to combat drug-resistant superbugs, fungi, viruses, parasites, or cancer. Alternatively, multiple factors (e.g., albumin, arginine, butyrate, calcium, cyclic AMP, isoleucine, short-chain fatty acids, UV B light, vitamin D, and zinc) are able to induce the expression of antimicrobial peptides, opening new avenues to the development of anti-infectious drugs.

Keywords: antimicrobial chemokines; antimicrobial neuropeptides; antimicrobial proteins; cathelicidin LL-37; defensins; dermcidin; hepcidins; histatins; RNases

---

1. Introduction

Host defense antimicrobial peptides (AMPs) are key components of the innate immune system shared by both invertebrates and vertebrates. Invertebrates such as insects and crustaceans do not have adaptive immune systems and innate defense systems serve as the only protective mechanism. It is now appreciated that innate immune systems also play an indispensable role in vertebrates by directly killing invading microbes in the early stage. Later, vertebrate AMPs can also help augment the adaptive immune system to further handle infections. Thus, host defense peptides may have dual role: rapid microbial killing and subsequent immune modulation [1–6].

The universality of AMPs is evidenced by the identification of these molecules in a variety of organisms. Over 2,300 such peptides have been isolated and characterized according to the online updated Antimicrobial Peptide Database (APD) [7,8]. As of April 2014, there are 233 AMPs from bacteria (*i.e.*, bacteriocins), six from protozoa, 12 from fungi, 306 from plants, and 1,801 host defense peptides from animals. AMPs are usually gene-coded and can be constitutively expressed or induced to fend off invading pathogens. In addition, some bacteria use a second mechanism to assemble peptide antibiotics by using a multiple-enzyme system, leading to distinct chemical modifications not observed in gene-coded cases. Most of the AMPs are cationic and short with less than 50 amino acids. Such features are ideal to target the negatively charged surface of bacteria [1–6].

AMPs also protect humans from microbial infection. They have been identified in a variety of exposed tissues or surfaces such as skin, eyes, ears, mouth, airways, lung, intestines, and the urinary tract. While human cathelicidin LL-37 is detected in the skin of new born infants [9], human beta-defensin 2 (hBD-2) is frequently expressed in older individuals. Human S100 proteins, hBD-2, human beta-defensin 3 (hBD-3), and cathelicidin are significantly higher in fetal keratinocytes than in postnatal skin cells [10]. In addition, psoriasin (S100A7), RNase 7, and hBD-3 are differentially expressed in healthy human skin [11]. When the skin barrier is broken, psoriasin is up-regulated [12]. Lysozyme and lactoferrin have been found in human tears [13]. In addition, β-defensins are expressed in human middle ear epithelial cells [14]. Drosomycin-like defensin (DLD) [15] is produced in human oral epithelial cells as part of host defense against fungal infection. Defensins, cathelicidins, and histatins are important in preventing oral cavity [16]. Apart from antimicrobial activity, human AMPs such as cathelicidins and defensins possess other functions such as immune modulation, apoptosis, and wound healing [1–6]. It is now recognized that certain defensins also play a critical role in sperm fertilization [17–19]. By the time this manuscript was completed, 103 human AMPs were found in the APD [7,8]. A selected set of these peptides is provided in Table 1. The lengths of these human peptides range from 10 (neurokinin A) to 149 amino acids (RegIIIα). Their net charges vary from −3 (β-amyloid peptide) to +20 (antimicrobial chemokine CXCL9). On average, human AMPs have 55 amino acids with a net charge of +5.6. Thus, both the average length and net charge for the current list of human AMPs are higher than those averages from all the AMPs (32.4 residues and net charge +3.2). An important reason for this is the inclusion of human antimicrobial proteins (> 100 amino acids) with high net charges (on average +10). The sequence diversity of human AMPs directly determines their structural and functional diversity. This review article highlights the discovery, activity, structure, mechanism of action, and therapeutic strategies of human host defense peptides selected from the APD.

Table 1. Discovery timeline of select human antimicrobial peptides and proteins [1].

Year	Name	Sequence	Source	Activity [2]	Ref.
1922	Lysozyme	KVFERCELARTLKRLGMDGYRGISL ANWMCLAKWESGYNTRATNYNAG DRSTDYGIFQINSRYWCNDGKTPGA VNACHLSCSALLQDNIADAVACAKR VVRDPQGIRAWVAWRNRCQNRDV RQYVQGCGV	saliva, tears, intestine	G, F	[20]
1985	α-Defensin HNP-1	ACYCRIPACIAGERRYGTCIYQGRL WAFCC	Neutrophils, bone marrow	G, V, F, P, C	[21]
1985	α-Defensin HNP-2	CYCRIPACIAGERRYGTCIYQGRL WAFCC	Neutrophils, bone marrow	G, V, F, C	[21]
1985	α-Defensin HNP-3	DCYCRIPACIAGERRYGTCIYQGRLW AFCC	Neutrophils, bone marrow	G, V, F, C	[21]
1988	Histatin 1	DSHEKRHHGYRRKFHEKHHSH REFPFYGDYGSNYLYDN	saliva	F	[22]

Table 1. *Cont.*

Year	Name	Sequence	Source	Activity [2]	Ref.
1988	Histatin 3	DSHAKRHHGYKRKFHEKHHSHR GYRSNYLYDN	saliva	G, F	[22]
1989	α-Defensin HNP-4	VCSCRLVFCRRTELRVGNCLIGGVSFT YCCTRV	neutrophils	G, V, F	[23]
1990	RNase 2	KPPQFTWAQWFETQHINMTSQQCTNA MQVINNYQRRCKNQNTFLLTTFANVVN VCGNPNMTCPSNKTRKNCHHSGSQVP LIHCNLTTPSPQNISNCRYAQTPANMFY IVACDNRDQRRDPPQYPVVPVHLDRII	eosinophils	V, P	[24]
1990	RNase 3 (Eosinophil cationic protein, ECP)	RPPQFTRAQWFAIQHISLNPPRCTIAM RAINNYRWRCKNQNTFLRTTFANVVN VCGNQSIRCPHNRTLNNCHRSRFRVPL LHCDLINPGAQNISNCTYADRPGRRFY VVACDNRDPRDSPRY PVVPVHLDTTI	neutrophils	G, V, P	[24]
1992	α-Defensin HD-5	ATCYCRTGRCATRESLSGVCEISGRL YRLCCR	Paneth cells/intestine, female reproductive system	G, V, F	[25]
1993	α-Defensin HD-6	AFTCHCRRSCYSTEYSYGTCTVM GINHRFCCL	Paneth cells/intestine	V, F	[26]
1995	β-Defensin hBD-1	DHYNCVSSGGQCLYSACPIFTKIQ GTCYRGKAKCCK	Kidney, Skin, salivary glands	G, F, C	[27]
1995	Cathelicidin LL-37	LLGDFFRKSKEKIGKEFKRIVQRIK DFLRNLVPRTES	neutrophils; skin	G, V, F, P, C	[28–30]
1997	β-Defensin hBD-2	GIGDPVTCLKSGAICHPVFCPRRY KQIGTCGLPGTKCCKKP	skin, lung, epithelia, uterus, salivary glands	G, V, F	[31]
1998	Granulysin	GRDYRTCLTIVQKLKKMVDKPTQRS VSNAATRVCRTGRSRWRDVCRNFM RRYQSRVTQGLVAGETA QQICEDLR	cytolytic T and NK cells	G, F, P, C	[32]
1999	Ubiquicidin	KVHGSLARAGKVRGQTPKVAKQEK KKKKTGRAKRRMQYNRRFVNVVPT FGKKKGPNANS	macrophages	G	[33]
2000	Thrombocidin-1 (TC-1)	AELRCMCIKTTSGIHPKNIQSLEVIG KGTHCNQVEVIATLKDGRKICLDPD APRIKKIVQKKLAGDES	human blood platelets	G, F	[34]
2000	Hepcidin 25 (LEAP-1)	DTHFPICIFCCGCCHRSKCGMCCKT	plasma, Urine/Liver	G, F	[35]
2000	Neuropeptide α-MSH	SYSMEHFRWGKPV	brain	G+, V, F	[36]
2001	β-Defensin hBD-3	GIINTLQKYYCRVRGGRCAVLSCL PKEEQIGKCSTRGRKCCRRKK	Skin, salivary glands	G, V, F	[37]
2001	β-Defensin hBD-4	FELDRICGYGTARCRKKCRSQEYRI GRCPNTYACCLRKWDESLLNRTKP	testis, lung, kidney, neutrophils	G	[38]
2001	Dermcidin	SSLLEKGLDGAKKAVGGLGKLGK DAVEDLESVGKGAVHDVKDVLDSV	eccrine sweat/skin	G, F	[39]
2002	RNase 7	KPKGMTSSQWFKIQHMQPSPQACN SAMKNINKHTKRCKDLNTFLHEPFSS VAATCQTPKIACKNGDKNCHQSHGA VSLTMCKLTSGKYPNCRYKEKRQNK SYVVACKPPQKKDSQQFHLVPVHLDRVL	urinary tract; respiratory tract; skin	G, F	[40]
2003	RNase 5 (angiogenin)	QDNSRYTHFLTQHYDAKPQGRDDR YCESIMRRRGPTSPCKDINTFIHGNK RSIKAICENKNGNPHRENLRISKSSFQ VTTCKLHGGSPWPPCQYRATAGFRN VVVACENGLPVHLDQSIFRRPRP	Liver, skin, intestine	G+, F	[41]

Table 1. *Cont.*

Year	Name	Sequence	Source	Activity [2]	Ref.
2003	Chemokine CCL20	SNFDCCLGYTDRILHPKFIVGFTRQL ANEGCDINAIIFHTKKKLSVCANPK QTWVKYIVRLLSKKVKNM	skin	G, F, P	[42]
2003	Chemokine CXCL9	TPVVRKGRCSCISTNQGTIHLQSLK DLKQFAPSPSCEKIEIIATLKNGVQT CLNPDSADVKELIKKWEKQVSQKK KQKNGKKHQKKKVLKVRKSQRSR QKKTT	blood	G, P	[42]
2005	Psoriasin (S100A7)	MSNTQAERSIIGMIDMFHKYTRRD DKIDKPSLLTMMKENFPNFLSACD KKGTNYLADVFEKKDKNEDKKID FSEFLSLLGDIATDYHKQSHGAA PCSGGSQ	Skin, salivary glands, breast	G-	[43]
2006	RegIIIα	EEPQRELPSARIRCPKGSKAYG SHCYALFLSPKSWTDADLACQ KRPSGNLVSVLSGAEGSFVSSL VKSIGNSYSYVWIGLHDPTQG TEPNGEGWEWSSSDVMNYFA WERNPSTISSPGHCASLSRSTAF LRWKDYNCNVRLPYVCKFTD	intestine	G+	[44]
2008	Substance P	RPKPQQFFGLM	the nervous system	G, F	[45]
2008	Drosomycin-like defensin (DLD)	CLAGRLDKQCTCRRSQPSRRS GHEVGRPSPHCGPSRQCGCHMD	oral epithelial cells, skin	F	[46]
2009	Elafin	AQEPVKGPVSTKPGSCPIILIRCA MLNPPNRCLKDTDCPGIKKCCE GSCGMACFVPQ	γδ T cells	G, F, V	[47]
2010	β-amyloid peptide 1-42	DAEFRHDSGYEVHHQKLVFFAE DVGSNKGAIIGLMVGGVVI	brain	G, F	[48]
2011	Chemerin	ELTEAQRRGLQVALEEFHKHPP VQWAFQETSVESAVDTPFPAGI FVRLEFKLQQTSCRKRDWKKP ECKVRPNGRKRKCLACIKLGS EDKVLGRLVHCPIETQVLREAE EHQETQCLRVQRAGEDPHSFY FPGQFAFS	skin	G, F	[49]
2012	Amylin	KCNTATCATQRLANFLVHSS NNFGAILSSTNVGSNTY	pancreatic β-cells	G	[50]
2012	KDAMP	RAIGGGLSSVGGGSSTIKY	eyes	G-	[51]
2013	DEFB114	DRCTKRYGRCKRDCLESEKQ IDICSLPRKICCTEKLYEEDDMF	epididymis	G, F	[19]

[1] Data from the APD [7,8]. For a complete list of human AMPs, please visit the APD website (*http://aps.unmc.edu/AP*) and search in the name field using "human". [2] In the APD, antimicrobial activities against different types of microbes are annotated as below: G, bacteria; G+, Gram-positive bacteria only; G-, Gram-negative bacteria only; F, fungi; V, viruses; P, parasites; C, cancer cells.

2. Identification of Human Antimicrobial Peptides

Antimicrobial substances might have been noticed long time ago [1–6]. Human lysozyme (130 amino acids), discovered in saliva by Alexander Fleming in 1922 [20], is recognized as the first antimicrobial protein [6]. However, the isolation and characterization of many more AMPs with defined amino acid sequences did not start until the 1980s (please refer to the annual AMP discovery plot in ref. [52]). Two major methods were utilized for AMP identification. Initially, chromatographic approaches were used to isolate and characterize new peptides. With the recognition of peptide sequence motifs, bioinformatic approaches were later developed to identify AMPs at the genomic level. In the following, we describe the discovery of the major families of human antibacterial peptides identified during 1985 and 2013.

2.1. Human Defensins

Host defense peptides are usually expressed as precursor proteins and the mature form is released by protease processing. In 1985, the Lehrer group isolated a family of the mature form of α-defensins from human blood [21]. Based on the source, property and size, these peptides were named as human neutrophil peptides (HNP-1, HNP-2, and HNP-3). The three defensins have nearly identical amino acid sequences (Table 1). Compared to HNP-2, both HNP-1 and HNP-3 contain only one additional amino acid residue at the N-terminus: alanine for HNP-1 and aspartate for HNP-3. This additional acidic residue in HNP-3 may make HNP-3 less active than HNP-1 or HNP-2 in killing *Staphylococcus aureus*, *Pseudomonas aeruginosa*, and *Escherichia coli*. A fourth human neutrophil defensin, HNP-4, was reported in 1989 [23]. It was also purified to homogeneity by chromatographic methods. HNP-4 has a distinct peptide sequence with 33 amino acids. *In vitro*, purified HNP-4 was shown to kill *E. coli*, *Streptococcus faecalis*, and *Candida albicans*. Lehrer and colleagues found that HNP-1, HNP-2, and HNP-3 are abundant in bone marrow, and can be detected in peripheral blood leukocytes, spleen and thymus by RT-PCR [53].

In 1989, Ouellette and colleagues identified α-defensin genes from mouse Paneth cells [54]. Bevins hypothsized that such orthologs also exist in human epithelial cells as part of the host defense mechanism. A genetic approach was developed to map additional defensin genes based on the high conservation of the nucleotide sequences in the signal coding region as well as the untranslated 5′ region. Using the probes from the conserved regions, they cloned the gene of HD-5 from human Paneth cells [25]. Likewise, HD-6 was identified [26]. These peptides are tissue-specific as they are only expressed in the Paneth cells of human intestines. The six human α-defensins (Table 1) share the same disulfide bond pattern. If we number the six cysteines in Roman numbers: I, II, III, to VI, the three disulfide bonds in α-defensins are C^{I}–C^{VI}, C^{II}–C^{IV}, and C^{III}–C^{V}. Interestingly, alpha defensins have been found in the neutrophils of rabbits, rats, hamsters, and guinea pigs, but not in mice or pigs [55].

Members from the human β-defensin family were discovered in the 1990s. Different from α-defensins, the three disulfide bonds in β-defensins are C^{I}–C^{V}, C^{II}–C^{IV}, and C^{III}–C^{VI}. Also, β-defensins have a slightly longer sequence to allow for an additional helical region. The first human β defensin (hBD-1) was reported by Bensch *et al.* from human plasma in 1995 [27]. Quantitative mRNA analysis revealed kidney as the major source for hBD-1 [56]. In addition, different truncated forms of hBD-1 were also isolated and found to be active against *E. coli*. The activity of hBD-1 might have been compromised in cystic fibrosis (CF) lung due to its salt-sensitive activity against *P. aeruginosa* [57]. Subsequently, hBD-2 was identified from lesional psoriatic skin using the whole *E. coli* affinity column [32]. This material was selected for AMP isolation based on the fact that patients with lesional psoriatic skin have fewer skin infections than expected. This peptide is effective in killing Gram-negative bacteria *E. coli*, *P. aeruginosa*, and yeast *C. albicans*, but is only bacteriostatic against Gram-positive *S. aureus*. Like hBD-1, the activity of HBD-2 is also salt-sensitive [58]. In 2001, both hBD-3 and hBD-4 were documented [37,38]. Based on this disulfide bond linkage pattern, hBD-3 was also identified by using a bioinformatic approach [59,60]. In contrast to hBD-1 and hBD-2, hBD-3 remained active against *S. aureus* and vancomycin-resistant *Enterococcus faecium* at physiological salt concentrations [37]. Bioinformatic studies led to the identification of 28 additional human and 43 mouse β-defensin genes in the respective genome [61]. Several of these β-defensins (hBD-6, hBD-26, hBD-27, hBD-28, and DEFB114) are indeed antimicrobial *in vitro* [62–64]. This sequence motif-based peptide prediction may be applied to any other species with a completed genome.

In insects, the activation of TOLL directly leads to the expression of drosomycin against fungal infection [65]. In 2008, human drosomycin-like defensin was detected in oral mucosa [46,66], indicating that this ancient innate defense mechanism is conserved. Sequence alignment in the APD revealed 40% similarity to insect drosomycin, which comprises one α-helical and three β-strands. Therefore, such a combined structure resembles human β-defensins to some extent. This peptide appears to be specifically effective against filamentous fungi (e.g., *Aspergillus* spp) as it did not kill tested yeast, Gram-positive or Gram-negative bacteria. Although the connection pattern of the six cysteines has not yet elucidated, the resulting three disulfide bonds are critical for the antifungal activity of human drosomycin-like defensing [46].

It is interesting to mention that a different type of defensins (called θ-defensins) has been identified from non-human primates [66,67]. These 18-residue defensins are circular due to the formation of a peptide bond between the N- and C-terminal ends. Like α- and β-defensins, they are also stabilized by three sets of disulfide bonds (C^{I}–C^{VI}, C^{II}–C^{V}, and C^{III}–C^{IV}). These defensins are generated by liganding two truncated α-defensins. These genes are not expressed in humans due to the existence of a premature stop codon. Like monkey θ-defensins, synthetic peptides corresponding to these human counterpart pseudogenes are HIV-1 inhibitory [68–70]. It is uncertain whether the loss of θ-defensins made humans generally more susceptible to HIV-1 infection.

2.2. *Human Histatins: Two Genes Multiple Peptides*

Histatins are a family of AMPs rich in histidines. In 1988, histatins 1, 3, and 5 were isolated from human saliva by size-exclusion chromatography followed by HPLC separation [22]. All three histatins exhibit the ability to kill the pathogenic yeast, *C. albicans*. Subsequently, other histatins were also isolated [71]. However, only histatins 1 and 3 are gene encoded [22,72], since others are the cleaved products of these two peptides. The histatin genes are located on chromosome 4, band q13 and exclusively expressed in human salivary secretions [73].

2.3. *Human Cathelicidins: One Gene Multiple Peptides*

The significance of cathelicidins in protecting humans from infection is established by data from animal models [74–76]. Cathelicidin peptides were first isolated in 1989 [77]. The precursor proteins of cathelicidins share a highly conserved N-terminal "cathelin" domain, but have drastically different antimicrobial sequences, ranging from Pro- and Arg-rich peptides, helical peptides, to disulfide-linked sequences [78]. The word "cathelicidin" was originally used to refer to the entire precursor protein. However, it is now accepted as the family name for mature AMPs from the C-terminal region. Another term hCAP-18 is abbreviated from human cationic protein of 18 kDa, representing the precursors prior to the release of cathelicidin peptides. However, these terms are interchangeably used in the literature.

Based on the conserved sequences in the cathelicidin precursors, Agerberth and colleagues cloned the only human cathelicidin gene and predicted the antimicrobial peptide as FALL-39 in analogy to PR-39 discovered in cattle [28]. Using the probes designed based on rabbit CAP-18, Larrick *et al.* also cloned the C-terminal antimicrobial peptide [29]. In the same year, Cowland *et al.* isolated a 19 kDa precursor protein hCAP-18 from human neutrophils [30]. Subsequently, the European group isolated the natural form of the mature human cathelicidin peptide from neutrophils [79]. Since the isolated peptide contains 37 amino acids and starts with a pair of leucines, it was named LL-37, which is two residues shorter than the initially predicted peptide FALL-39 [28]. Interestingly, ALL-38, another form of human cathelicidin peptides, was also characterized in 2003 [80]. This alterative form contains one more alanine at the N-terminus than LL-37. ALL-38 was generated in female vagina due to the action of gastricsin on sperm hCAP-18. Antimicrobial assays revealed a similar activity spectrum for LL-37 and ALL-38 against a panel of bacteria, including *E. coli*, *S. aureus*, *P. aeruginosa*, and *Bacillus megaterium*. Thus, ALL-38, as well as other active peptides such as SgI-29 [81], plays a defense role in the human reproductive system. In addition, LL-37 fragments were isolated from human skin by chromatographic approaches [82]. These fragments have varying activities compared to intact LL-37. Hence, a single human cathelicidin gene has been processed into different forms of active peptides [83]. This phenomenon, however, is not unique to humans. There is precedence that multiple AMPs are programmed in a single plant gene [84]. One possibility for this is that different cathelicidin fragments provide a means to expanding the functional space of the single human cathelicidin gene. A different model is utilized by sheep, horses, and cattle, which produce multiple cathelicidins with varying functions [85–88].

2.4. Human Dermcidin

Besides human cathelicidin LL-37 [89], dermcidin, an anionic defense peptide, was found in human sweat [39]. Unlike human defensins and cathelicidins that are induced under inflammatory and injured conditions, dermcidin is constitutively expressed in human sweat [90]. Furthermore, dermcidin variants as well as fragments were also detected. It appears that the level of dermcidin did not vary between healthy people and infected patients [91]. In addition, dermcidin may be related to other human diseases such as cancer and atherosclerosis [92,93].

2.5. Human Hepcidins

Human liver expressed antimicrobial peptide-1 (LEAP-1) was discovered from human blood ultrafiltrate in 2000 [35]. The same peptide was also found by Ganz *et al.* from human urine and named as hepcidin 25 [94]. This liver-synthesized peptide is especially rich in cysteines (32%), leading to four disulfide bonds in a 25-residue peptide. In 2009, the connection pattern of the four disulfide bonds was revised to C7–C22, C10–C13, C11–C19, and C14–C22 [95]. This antimicrobial peptide also plays an important role in ferrous use [96] and single-residue mutations in this molecule are associated with severe juvenile hemochromatosis, a genetic disease of severe iron overload [97]. Unlike LEAP-1, antimicrobial peptide LEAP-2, however, is not involved in the regulation of iron use [98].

2.6. Human AMPs Derived from Known Proteins

Some AMPs are derived from known proteins. Park *et al.* isolated buforin I from amphibians in 1996 [99]. Sequence comparison revealed that buforin I is a cleaved fragment of histone H2A. Of interest, this mRNA was also detected in humans, suggesting a possible role of this peptide in antimicrobial defense [100].

The human airways are essential for the exchange of molecules with the environment. It is necessary to guard this channel to prevent the infection of microbes in the air. In 2001, Ganz and colleagues isolated calcitermin primarily targeting Gram-negative bacteria. This 15-residue peptide is derived from the C-terminus of calgranulin C (a S100 protein). It contains three histidines (His9, His11, and His13) at the N-terminus and has the potential to adopt a helical conformation in membranes. These histidines may explain its enhanced activity in acidic buffers (pH 5.4) and in the presence of micromolar concentrations of $ZnCl_2$ [101].

Another example for protein-derived AMPs is KDAMP, keratin-derived AMPs, which were identified from bactericidal lysate fractions of human corneal epithelial cells. These molecules are rich in glycines [51]. The glycines appear to be important for killing *P. aeruginosa* as substitution of a string of glycines with alanines reduced peptide potency. A search of the APD reveals that glycine-rich (>25%) AMPs have also been identified in bacteria, plants, insects, spiders, nematodes, crustaceans, fish, and amphibians. Thus, glycine-rich peptides constitute a common molecular design for host defense [102–110].

2.7. Antimicrobial Chemokines and AMPs from Human Immune Cells

The fact that some AMPs possess chemotactic effects inspired the evaluation of antimicrobial activity of chemokines, which are known for chemotaxis. In 2000, Krijgsveld *et al.* found antimicrobial thrombocidins, peptides derived from CXC chemokines in human blood platelets [34]. In 2003, Oppenheim and colleagues identified 20 antimicrobial chemokines [42] and additional two members (CCL27 and CCL28) were also reported by Hieshima and colleagues [111]. In 2011, antimicrobial activity of chemotactic chemerin was also reported [49]. Further studies are required to establish the *in vivo* relevance of the *in vitro* activity of these chemokines. The common nature of chemokines and AMPs, however, bridges the innate and adaptive immune systems.

Antimicrobial peptides have also been found in other immune cells. In 1999, Hiemstra *et al.* identified ubiquicidin from ribosomal protein S30 in various tissues. This peptide is active against *Listeria monocytogenes, S. aureus, Salmonella typhimurium, and E. coli.* Considering the fact that *L. monocytogenes* can live within cells, the expression of ubiquicidin in macrophages would limit the replication of this bacterium. Interestingly, ribosomal protein S30 is identical in rats, mice and humans [33]. In 1998, granulysin (74 amino acids) was detected in human cytotoxic T cells and natural killer (NK) cells [32]. Similar proteins called NK-lysins are found in other animals [112]. Granulysin is active against Gram-positive and Gram-negative bacteria, and fungi, including mycobacteria. Thus, the human adaptive immune system has incorporated an innate defense molecule for direct disruption of tumor cells or invading microbes. In addition, human $\gamma\delta$ T cells produce antimicrobial peptide elafin [47]. Like human secretory leucoprotease inhibitor (SLPI), elafin was initially identified as a protease inhibitor. Elafin shows an inhibitory effect on bacteria, fungi, and viruses [113].

2.8. Antimicrobial Neuropeptides

Antibacterial peptides were also isolated from the neuroendocrine system from cattle. Secretolytin corresponds to the C-terminal fragment (residues 614–626) of bovine chromogranin B [114]. This peptide displayed activity against *M. luteus* and reduced the growth of *B. megaterium*. Vasostatin-1 is a 76-residue N-terminal fragment of bovine chromogranin A. This peptide is active against both Gram-positive bacteria and fungi [115]. It is conserved in humans, pigs, horses, mice, rats, and frogs. Catestatin is a 21-residue AMP derived from human chromogranin A [116]. Subsequently, cattle enkelytin, the C-terminal fragment corresponding to residues 209–237 of proenkephalin-A was also found to be antibacterial [117]. A similar proenkephalin system exists in humans although the processing machinery can differ [118]. Thus, these neuropeptides also play a communication role between neuroendocrine and the immune system [119].

In 1998, human neuropeptide Y (36 residues) was demonstrated to have antimicrobial activity [120]. Interestingly, the antifungal activity of this peptide against *C. albicans* increased several folds by truncating N-terminal 12 residues, implying the importance of the helical region 14–32. A more recent study, however, only observed activity against *E. coli,* but not *C. albicans* [121]. Future studies will clarify whether the peptide has direct antimicrobial effects. In 1999, adrenomedullin, usually expressed on surface epithelial cells, was reported to have antibacterial activity against all the tested bacteria, but not *C. albicans* [122]. Alpha-MSH was added to the human AMP list in 2000 as well [36]. These findings extended host defense peptides to the nervous system [123]. Since then, more antimicrobial neuropeptides have been documented [45,124]. Some of these neuropeptides may become leads for developing new antibiotics. For example, alarin is a human brain neuropeptide with activity against only Gram-negative bacteria such as *E. coli,* but not Gram-positive bacteria such as *S. aureus* [124]. In particular, α-MSH showed *in vitro* antifungal activity against *C. albicans* at fM to pM [125], much lower than nM for some bacterial lantibiotics and μM for many cationic peptides.

2.9. Beta-Amyloid Peptides

Beta-amyloid peptides have long been thought to be the culprit of Alzheimer's disease. It is believed that the β-sheet form, not the helical form of the peptide, is toxic. A recent demonstration of antimicrobial activity for β-amyloid peptides adds a new research dimension to this worrisome disease [48]. Further studies along this line could be useful to provide novel insight into the mechanism of this human disease. In 2012, amylin (human islet amyloid polypeptide, hIAPP) was found bactericidal, too [50]. Transformation of amylin into toxic fibrils can disrupt cell membranes and lead to β-cell death, perhaps one of the causative factors of type 2 diabetes mellitus. The aggregated form of amylin is likely to exert its cytotoxicity by damaging cell membranes [126]. It is noticeable that, when in excess, bacteria microcin E492 can form fibrils as a storage form and lose antimicrobial activity [127]. Is there anything in common here from bacteria to humans? Perhaps, this is one mechanism that nature attempts to remove the toxic effects of an over expressed protein, including antimicrobial peptide.

2.10. Human Antimicrobial Proteins

There are 14 antimicrobial proteins (>100 amino acids) in the APD database as of March 2014 [8]. This includes the first antimicrobial protein lysozyme [20]. Several eosinophil proteins were purified in 1990. Both eosinophil-derived neurotoxin (EDN, or RNase 2) and eosinophil cationic protein (ECP, or RNase 3) possess anti-parasitic activity against *Brugia pahangi* and *Brugia malayi* [24]. These two ribonucleases are also active against respiratory syncytial virus (RSV) with a single-stranded RNA [128]. In addition, RNase 3 has a unique bacterial agglutinating activity [129]. In 2002, RNase 7 was identified from human skin [40]. Remarkably, it is active against bacteria such as *Mycobacterium vaccae* and yeast, even at 4 °C [130]. Recombinant RNase 7 exhibited antimicrobial activity against uropathogens (*E. coli, P. aeruginosa, Klebsiella pneumonia, Proteus mirabilis, E. faecalis*, and *Staphylococcus saprophyticus*) [131,132]. In fact, RNase 7 is the most abundant innate defense peptide in the human urinary tract [132], although the contributions of other human AMPs cannot be ignored [56,133–135]. Human RNase 5, (also known as angiogenin or ANG) with weak RNase activity, is initially implicated in angiogenesis. It appears that the nucleus location is necessary for angiogenesis [136]. In 2003, RNase 5 was found to have a toxic effect on Gram-positive bacteria and fungi [41]. However, another study found little activity using a commercial material [137]. In 2006, RNase 8 was found to inhibit *M. vaccae* [138,139]. Therefore, of the eight human ribonucleases, RNases 2, 3, 5, 7, and 8 appear to play a role in host defense.

Psoriasin is another human protein with multiple functions. It is identical to S100A7, a protein member of the S100 family. Psoriasin was initially characterized as a Ca^{2+} binding protein with chemotactic property from human skin psoriatic lesions [140,141]. Subsequently, psoriasin was found in cancer lesions, making it a potential cancer biomarker [142]. However, the antimicrobial activity of psoriasin against *E. coli* was not demonstrated until 2005 [43].

Three RegIII (regenerating gene family protein III) proteins were initially identified in mice [143]. RegIIIα, a RegIIIγ homolog protein, was found in humans. Different from RegIIIβ from mice, human RegIIIα only inhibited the growth of Gram-positive bacteria such as *L. monocytogenes, Listeria innocua*, and *E faecalis* [44].

3. Antimicrobial and Anticancer Activities of Human Antimicrobial Peptides

3.1. Antibacterial Activities

Antibacterial activities of human AMPs have been mentioned in the preceding section. This section provides an overview of the activity spectrum of these peptides. Based on the APD [8], the majority of human AMPs (90 out of 103) can inhibit the growth of bacteria. They display a broad-spectrum activity against a variety of Gram-positive and Gram-negative bacteria. However, three human AMPs kill primarily Gram-positive bacteria. RNase 5 has an effect on *S. pneumonia* [41], while α-MSH is inhibitory to *S. aureus* [36]. A third AMP, RegIIIα, is active against *L. monocytogenes, L. innocua*, and *E. faecalis* [44]. In addition, ten human AMPs are inhibitory mainly to Gram-negative bacteria. These include hBD-26, hBD-27, human calcitermin, psoriasin/S100A7, CCL8, CCL13, CCL19, alarin, HMGN2, and KDAMP peptides [42,43,51,63,101]. They may control different Gram-negative pathogens. For example, both calcitermin and HMGN2 were active against *E. coli* and *P. aeruginosa* [101,144]. Alarin is active against *E. coli*, while the KDAMP peptides are primarily active against *P. aeruginosa*. Thus, these peptides may form the basis for developing new antimicrobials with a desired antibacterial activity spectrum.

3.2. Antiviral Activity

Of the 103 human AMPs, 16 are virucidal. They include the six well-characterized human α-defensins (HNP-1, HNP-2, HMP-3, HNP-4, HD-5, and HD-6), three β-defensins (hBD-1, hBD-2, and hBD-3), cathelicidin LL-37, histatin 5, α-MSH, elafin, SLPI, CXCL12, RNase 2, and RNase 3. Elafin is the major antiviral protein in cervicovaginal lavage fluid [113]. Both RNase 2 and RNase 3 inhibit respiratory syncytial viruses (RSV) [145,146]. SLPI levels in saliva and semen, but not breast milk, approximate the level required for HIV-1 inhibition *in vitro* [147]. Although HNP-1 is a lectin that binds to gp120 and CD4, it shows an inhibitory effect after HIV-1 entry [148]. It also inhibits non-enveloped BK virus infection by aggregating virions and blocks binding to host cells [149]. Of the four human β-defensins, hBD-2 and hBD-3 can be induced by viral infection and block HIV replication by directly neutralizing the virions and through modulation of the CXCR4 coreceptor [150]. Human cathelicidin LL-37 is also inhibitory to HIV-1 [151,152]. Wang *et al.* further dissected the active region of LL-37. While the central fragment GI-20 showed an optimal therapeutic index, the LL-37 core peptide FK-13 contains the minimal anti-HIV sequence [152]. In the histatin family, only a histatin-5-derived peptide has an effect on HIV-1 [153]. For a systematic review of AMPs with known anti-HIV activity, interested readers may refer to a recent review article [154].

3.3. *Antifungal Activity*

In the APD, 58 human AMPs are fungicidal [8]. Typical examples are human α-defensins, cathelicidin LL-37, hepcidins, and histatins. In the case of LL-37, protease processing into fragments such as KS-30 and RK-31 is essential in inhibiting *C. albicans* [155]. In addition, the antifungal activity of LL-37 depends on both media and pH. Both LL-25 and RK-31 can rapidily enter the cell cytoplasm [156]. It is likely that these LL-37 fragments target intracellular molecules. It appears that such cathelicidin fragments in human sweat play a role in human skin innate defense against fungal infection [155].

3.4. *Antiparasitic Activity*

Some human AMPs also have antiparasitic properties. These include HNP-1, LL-37, granulysin, CCL2, CCl20, CCL28, CXCL4 (hPF4), CXCL6, CXCL9, CXCL10, RNase 2, and RNase 3. RNases 2 and 3 might be the earliest AMP examples from humans that were demonstrated to have antiparasitic activity [24]. Other more recent examples are HNP-1 against the promastigotes and amastigotes forms of *Leishmania major* [157], chemokine CCL28 against *Leishmania mexicana* [158], LL-37 against *Entamoeba histol* ytica [159], and Platelet factor 4 (hPF4) against malarial parasite *Plasmodium falciparum* [160]. These examples verify that human defense peptides also play a role in controlling parasite infections.

3.5. *Anticancer Activity*

There is a growing interest in developing AMPs into anticancer peptides. Magainins, cecropins, and defensins were all shown to have anticancer effects [161–163]. Many other AMPs possess this activity as well and some were discussed in previous review articles [164–166]. A more complete and updated list of anticancer AMPs can be searched in the APD database [8]. The 166 anticancer peptides cover multiple sources, including animals (105 peptides), plants (48 AMPs), bacteria (seven bacteriocins), fungi (one peptide), and laboratory synthesis (five peptides).

The anticancer activities of human AMPs have not been widely evaluated since only six members are annotated as anticancer in the APD [8]. They are HNP-1, HNP-2, HNP-3, hBD-1, LL-37, and granulysin. Indeed, reduced expression of granulysin in patients is correlated with the progression of cancer [167]. However, the level of granulysin increased substantially in cancer cells [168]. Similar observations have been made with human defensins and LL-37. While HNP-1 inhibits the growth of human lung adenocarcinoma xenograft in nude mice [169], the same molecule can be overexpressed in tumors [170,171]. HBD-1 can suppress urological and prostate cancers [172,173]. In oral squamous cell carcinoma, hBD-1 also suppressed tumor proliferation, whereas hBD-2 and hBD-3 showed an opposite effect [174]. Likewise, human cathelicidin LL-37 is overexpressed in breast, ovarian, and lung cancers, but it suppresses tumorigenesis in gastric cancer [175]. Such a complex involvement of AMPs in various cancers deserves additional studies. In particular, it is important to elucidate the factors that trigger the overexpression of AMPs in certain cancer cells.

Our current knowledge, however, may be utilized to our advantage. For instance, the over-expression of human cathelicidin LL-37 or defensins may serve as useful biomarkers for cancer diagnosis [176–178]. In addition, the fragments of LL-37 with demonstrated anticancer effects *in vitro* [179] and *in vivo* [180] might constitute useful templates for designing new anti-tumor drugs, especially those resistant to existing therapeutics. Anticancer AMPs can work by different mechanisms. The effects may result from a direct bacterial killing when bacteria could be the culprit of cancer (e.g., gastric cancer) [175]. AMPs may selectively kill cancer cells in part due to exposed anionic phosphatidylserines (PS) [181]. It is also possible that some AMPs kill cancer cells indirectly by inducing apoptosis (see below).

3.6. Cytotoxic Effects of Human AMPs

It is accepted that many AMPs target bacterial membranes. While bacteria are abundant in anionic lipids such as phosphatidylglycerols (PG) and cardiolipin (CL) [83], human cells comprise zwitterionic phosphocholines (PC) and cholesterol. The differences in membranes of bacterial and human cells to a large extent determine cell selectivity of cationic AMPs. Indeed, among the 103 human AMPs, only three peptides are annotated to have cytotoxic effects on mammalian cells. In the case of LL-37, we found it possible to reduce the peptide cytotoxicity by decreasing peptide hydrophobicity [179,182]. The relatively low cytotoxicity of human AMPs makes them attractive templates for engineering new antimicrobials.

In addition to membrane differences, human cells could use other mechanisms to reduce or remove the potential toxic effect of AMPs on themselves. By expressing a peptide called p33 on the cell surface, the toxic effects of human LL-37 is masked [183]. Instread of directly secreting AMPs, humans also release exosomes (nanovesicles enriched in host defense peptides) into the urinary tract to keep it sterile [184]. It may be speculated that such exosomes, similar to artificial AMP-containing liposomes, could be an effective way to reduce cytotoxicity to human cells.

3.7. Other Biological Functions of Human AMPs

In addition to antimicrobial and anticancer activities, many human AMPs possess other functions such as chemotaxis, apoptosis, and wound healing:

Chemotactic activity. Currently, 35 human AMPs have chemotactic properties. Examples are defensins and cathelicidin LL-37. Antimicrobial chemokines were originally identified for chemotactic activity. A clear difference between chemokines and AMPs is the concentration needed for action. While the chemotactic effect needs peptides in the nM-pM range, antimicrobial action usually requires μM peptides [185]. Another difference between chemotactic and antimicrobial activities lies in the molecular target. While AMPs usually target membranes of invading bacteria, the chemotactic effects require the association of peptides to host cell receptors. As one example, human LL-37 achieves its chemotactic ability to monocytes, macrophages, neutrophils, and T cells by binding formyl peptide receptor-like 1 (FPRL-1) [186].

Apoptosis. Apoptosis is the process of programmed cell death. Different factors can trigger cell apoptosis. AMPs are one of these factors. Interestingly, apoptosis may be induced or suppressed by the same peptide depending on the biological context. Human LL-37 induces apoptosis in vascular smooth muscle cells, primary airway epithelial cells, oral squamous cell carcinoma SAS-H1 cells, intact rat aorta rings and cultured rat aorta smooth muscle cells, Jurkat T-cells and A549 cells [187–191], while it suppresses this process in keratinocytes and neutrophils [192,193]. As a consequence, elucidation of the mechanism to control apoptosis may offer new therapeutic strategies. A recent interesting finding is that inhibition of human LL-37-induced apoptosis by administrating urothelial glycosaminoglycan (GAG) analogs can prevent the development of interstitial cystitis (IC) in a mouse model [194]. LL-37 could suppress the lipopolysaccharides (LPS)-induced apoptosis of endothelial cells, thereby attenuating lethal sepsis/endotoxin shock [195]. In the case of colon cancer, however, activation of apoptosis suppresses tumorigenesis [196]. It seems that apoptosis requires the major antimicrobial region FK-16 (*i.e.*, corresponding to residues 17-32) of human cathelicidin LL-37 [179,180].

Wound healing. Human host defense peptides can also promote wound healing, a process of injury repairs. Salivary histatin 2 can enhance fibroblast cell migration, whereas human LL-37 at 1 μM can induce cell migration and promote proliferation [197]. It is proposed that these peptides play a role in fast wound coverage.

In summary, antimicrobial activity is a common property of human AMPs, although the *in vivo* relevance has not firmly established for each polypeptide. Furthermore, human AMPs can perform other functions depending on the biological context, peptide concentration, proteases, and the metabolic state. Under diseased conditions, AMPs may have an opposite effect (e.g., cancer suppression *vs.* progression). Understanding the elegant balance of AMPs in these processes in the healthy state as well as the factors that could tilt the balance to a diseased state may yield useful means for cancer treatment.

4. Three-Dimensional Structures of Human Antimicrobial Peptides

Three-dimensional structure of human host defense AMPs are helpful to understand the function of AMPs described above. Many short and linear antimicrobial peptides do not have a folded structure free in solution. However, they may become structured upon interactions with host cells by binding to a specific receptor to trigger the biological responses to microbial invasion. In addition, such AMPs may also adopt a defined structure upon association with bacterial targets such as membranes. The bound structure in either category is not trivial to determine. Membrane-mimetic models are normally utilized to determine the membrane-bound structures of receptors or AMPs. These models include organic solvents, detergent/lipid micelles, lipid bicelles, nanodiscs, and lipid bilayers [198,199]. The known 3D structures of these short peptides are primarily determined by multi-dimensional solution nuclear magnetic resonance (NMR) spectroscopy [199]. Some AMPs possess a folded structure in aqueous solutions primarily due to the structural stabilization of disulfide bonds. The structures of these small proteins can be determined by NMR or X-ray crystallographic methods. When both methods are applied, similar structures are usually found. In addition, NMR measurements can gain insight into protein dynamics (*i.e.*, motions). Among the 103 human AMPs annotated in the APD database, 42 have a known 3D structure (27 determined by NMR and 15 by X-ray) [8].

Although there are different classification schemes [1–6,200], the structures of natural AMPs fall into four large families (α, β, αβ, and non-αβ) [201]. Peptides in the α family contain α-helical structure as the major secondary structure. Typical examples are human cathelicidin LL-37, histatins, dermcidin, and granulysin. The β family is characterized by at least a pair of two β-strands in the structure. Human α-defensins, hepcidins, and SLPI use this type of structure. The αβ family contains both α and β secondary structures, whereas the non-αβ family has neither α nor β structure (also called extended structures). While there are multiple structural examples for the αβ family (Table 2), no structural example has been found for the non-αβ family of human AMPs. In the following, we highlight atomic structures of human AMPs from the α, β, and αβ families. These structures are annotated in the APD database [8] and structural coordinates can be obtained from the Protein Data Bank (PDB) [202] via the APD links.

Table 2. Properties of selected human antimicrobial peptides with known 3D structure [1].

APD ID	Peptide name	Length	Net charge	Pho%	Boman index	Structure class
2257	Lysozyme	130	+8	40	2.28	α
505	Histatin 5	24	+5	8	4.81	α
780	Lactoferricin	49	+10	36	3.14	α
310	LL-37	37	+6	35	2.99	α
433	Dermcidin	47	−2	38	1.11	α
1161	Granulysin	74	+11	33	3.5	α
2072	Psoriasin/S100A7	101	−1	32	2.3	α
1676	β-Amyloid peptide 1-42	42	−3	45	0.77	α
176	HNP-1	30	+3	53	1.07	β
177	HNP-2	29	+3	51	1.17	β
178	HNP-3	30	+2	50	1.42	β
179	HNP-4	33	+4	51	1.4	β

Table 2. *Cont.*

APD ID	Peptide name	Length	Net charge	Pho%	Boman index	Structure class
180	HD-5	32	+4	40	2.6	β
181	HD-6	32	+2	40	1.71	β
192	Hepcidin 20	20	+3	60	0.46	β
193	Hepcidin 25 (LEAP-1)	25	+2	52	0.89	β
2095	SLPI	107	+12	34	1.87	β
451	hBD-1	36	+4	36	1.3	αβ
524	hBD-2	41	+7	36	0.9	αβ
283	hBD-3	45	+11	33	2.87	αβ
811	LEAP-2	40	+4	40	2.94	αβ
2067	RNase 5	125	+11	28	2.99	αβ
2073	RNase 7	128	+16	32	2.16	αβ
2071	RegIIIα	149	+1	33	1.77	αβ
2085	CCL1	73	+10	41	2.25	αβ
2086	CCL8	75	+6	37	2.27	αβ
2088	CCL13	75	+11	36	1.89	αβ
2075	CCL20	69	+8	43	1.34	αβ
2187	CCL27	56	+1	41	1.57	αβ
2076	CXCL1	73	+6	38	1.51	αβ
2080	CXCL10	77	+11	36	2.25	αβ

[1] Obtained from the Antimicrobial Peptide Database (*http://aps.unmc.edu/AP*) [8]. Peptide hydrophobic amino acid content (percent) is represented by pho% in the table. Protein-binding potential [1] was re-named as Boman index in the APD database in 2003.

4.1. The α-Helical Family: Histatins, Cathelicidins, Dermcidin, and Granulysin

Histatins. Histatins 1, 3, and 5 are active against *C. albicans* and their candidacidal activities are in the following order: histatin 5 > histatin 3 > histatin 1 [203]. Rai *et al.* investigated the relationship between sequence length and activity using histatin 5 as the template. They found that the C-terminal sequence is important [204]. P-113 with 12 residues corresponding to residues 4–15 of histatin 5 retained anti-candida activity [205]. Using histatin 3 as a model, Zuo *et al.* found increased activity when the active sequence was expressed in tandem (repeated once) [206]. However, duplication of the functional domain of histatin 5 did not enhance candidacidal activity [207]. These results suggest that active domain duplication is not necessary a universal strategy for activity enhancement. Histatin 5 can adopt a helical conformation in the presence of membrane-mimetic agents [204]. However, this helical structure did not appear to be essential for candidacidal activity as peptides with a less helical structure (achieved by proline insertion) can be equally active [208]. Histatin 5 contains a consensus sequence, HEXXH, which is known to bind Zinc. Zinc binding can lead to vesicle fusion and helical conformation as well [209]. Zinc binding actually potentiates peptide activity against gram-positive bacteria *E. faecalis* [210]. An analog of histatin 5 was found to bind DNA and have nuclease activity due to the synergistic oxidative and hydrolytic activities of the metal-peptide complex [211].

Human cathelicidin LL-37. To understand the structural basis of antimicrobial activity, 3D triple-resonance NMR spectroscopy was used to solve a high-quality structure for human LL-37 in the presence of sodium dodecyl sulfate (SDS) micelles [182]. LL-37 has a long helix covering residues 2–31, whereas the C-terminal tail is disordered and does not superimpose well to each other (Figure 1A). This structure is fully consistent with the backbone dynamics measured by an independent NMR experiment. This amphipathic helical region determined in SDS micelles is responsible for binding to bacterial outer and inner membranes. Interestingly, the LL-37 tail appeared to be involved in peptide aggregation [212], which influences LL-37 activity [213]. The N-terminal region of LL-37 is less important for antibacterial activity since LL-23, a natural fragment of LL-37, is only active against susceptible *E. coli* or *S. aureus* strains. The weak activity of LL-23 is attributed to a hydrophilic residue Ser9 that splits the hydrophobic face into two clusters [214]. This Ser9 residue also segregates the hydrophobic surface of LL-37 into two hydrophobic domains. It is established that the central helix

(Figure 1B) of human LL-37 is critical for antibacterial, anti-biofilm, and antiviral activity (reviewed in ref [83]).

Dermcidin. Unlike cationic cathelicidin LL-37 (net charge +6), dermcidin (DCD-1) has a net charge of −2. This peptide also prefers anionic membranes, however. DCD-1L, a variant with one additional leucine at the C-terminus, showed an enhanced affinity for membranes than DCD-1. In the membrane bound state, DCD-1L has a helical conformation. It is located on the membrane surface and can aggregate in the presence of zinc [215]. This oligomeric structure of dermcidin has recently been determined by X-ray crystallography [216]. A hexameric helix-bundle structure (Figure 1C) is proposed to insert into bacterial membrane as an ion channel. In the crystal, the Zn^{2+} coordinates with a group of acidic amino acids. It should be pointed out that the 3D structure of DCD-1L was also determined previously by 3D NMR spectroscopy using a ^{15}N-labeled peptide in a 50% trifluoenthanol (TFE) solution. Four helical regions were identified (α1: 5–7; α2: 10–12; α3: 26–33; and α4: 36–45) [217]. In this case, TFE might have disrupted the oligomeric structure of dermcidin. There are precedents for such an effect of TFE. For example, the oligomeric structure of a K^+ channel did not survive in TFE but retained in membrane-mimetic micelles such as SDS (reviewed in ref. [198]). These examples emphasize the importance of determining the 3D structure of AMPs in a proper environment.

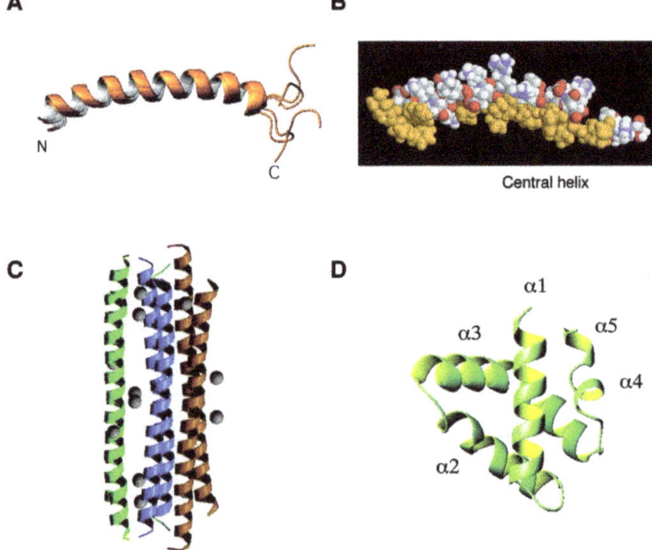

Figure 1. Three-dimensional structures of human antimicrobial peptides from the α-helical family: (**A**) and (**B**) human cathelicidin LL-37 determined by NMR spectroscopy (PDB ID: 2K6O); (**C**) dermcidin determined by X-ray crystallography (PDB ID, 2YMK); and (**D**) granulysin determined by X-ray diffraction (PDB ID: 1L9L). In the case of LL-37, an ensemble of five structures is shown to better view the disordered C-terminal tail (A), whereas a space-filling model is given to show the segregation of the hydrophobic surface (gold) into two domains (B) [182]. The longer one corresponds to the central helix which is important for antimicrobial, anti-biofilm and antiviral activities [83]. Images were generated by using the software MOLMOL [218]. Further details can be found in the text.

Granulysin. Incorporation of AMPs into cytotoxic T cells might have conferred the ability to lyse cells. The crystal structure of granulysin is shown in Figure 1D. There are five helical regions (α1: 2–17; α2: 23–35); α3: 39–61; α4: 66–69; α5: 71–73) [219]. The sequences of human granulysin (74 amino acids) and other NK-lysins share a low degree of similarity (~35%), but homologous modeling reveals antimicrobial features (active helices and basic residue positions) are conserved [112]. Although granulysin only contains two disulfide bonds, it belongs to the saposin-like protein family [220]. Saposin-like proteins comprise several helices usually stabilized by three disulfide bonds [221]. Twelve AMPs in the APD [8] from amoebozoa, nematodes, and large animals such as pigs are annotated to share the saposin-like protein fold [112]. To be antimicrobial, however, neither the entire sequence nor the protein fold is needed. For example, synthetic peptides and analogs derived from helices 3 and 4 are active against *Vibrio cholera* [222]. In addition, the peptide based on the helix-bend-helix motif (residues 31–50) displayed similar antimicrobial activity against Propionibacterium acnes (a key therapeutic target in acne) when synthesized entirely using D-amino acids [223]. Because short peptides can be readily synthesized, they provide useful alternatives for topical treatment of such bacterial infections.

4.2. The β Family: α-Defensins

Alpha-defensins. Structurally, α-defensins consist of three β-strands that form a β-sheet. In the crystal, a dimeric structure is found for human HNP-1, where two copies of the molecule pack together. HNP-2 and HNP-3 have a similar structure. Thus, it is primarily due to the single amino acid difference in these defensins (Table 1) that influences peptide activity. With a more hydrophobic sequence, HNP-4 is more potent against *E. coli* and *C. albicans* than other human α-defensins [23]. Using a kinetic 96-well turbidimetric procedure, the relative potencies of six human α-defensins were compared. In the case of Gram-positive *S. aureus*, the activity is in the following order: HNP-2 > HNP-1 > HNP-3 > HNP-4. In contrast, their relative potencies against Gram-negative *E. coli* is HNP-4 > HNP-2 > HNP-1 = HNP-3 [224]. Thus, the antibacterial activities of these defensins are also bacteria dependent. This likely reflects the distinct differences in membranes of these organisms. The poor antibacterial activity of HNP-3 is not surprising considering the presence of an acidic aspartate at the N-terminus of the peptide, making it unfavorable to target the negatively charged surface of bacteria. HD-5 displayed a rather potent activity, which is comparable to HNP-2 against *S. aureus* and HNP-4 against *E. coli*. The higher activities of HNP-4 and HD-5 against *E. coli* are correlated with their higher net charge of +4 (Table 2). HD-6 has a poor antibacterial activity. In the crystal, it forms a tetrameic structure (Figure 2B) [123].

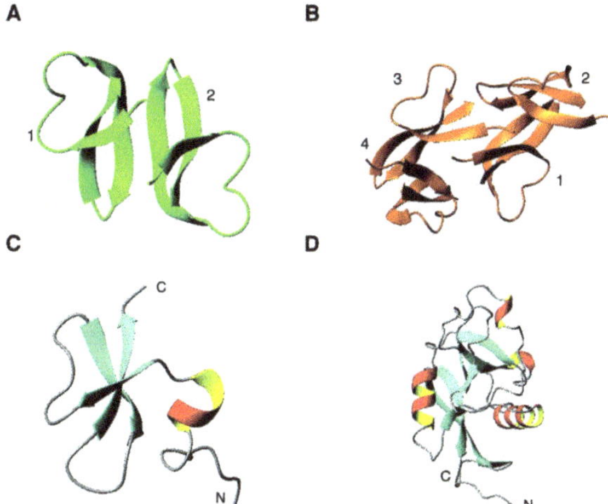

Figure 2. Select 3D structures of human antimicrobial peptides from the β and αβ families: (**A**) HNP-1 (dimeric crystal structure, PDB ID: 3GNY); (**B**) HD-6 (tetrameric crystal structure, PDB ID: 1ZMQ); (**C**) hBD-3 (NMR structure, PDB ID: 1KJ6) and RegIIIα (crystal structure, PDB ID: 4MTH). See the text for further details.

4.3. *The αβ Family: β-Defensins, Antimicrobial Chemokines, RNases, and RegIIIα*

Beta-defensins. Human β-defensins comprise both α and β structures in the same 3D fold. Figure 2C shows the NMR structure of human β-defensin 3 (hBD-3), which starts with a helical structure followed by three beta strands [225]. NMR translational diffusion studies revealed a dimer for hBD-3, but a monomer for both hBD-1 and hBD-2 in solution. The stronger antibacterial activity of hBD-3 than either hBD-1 or hBD-2 was attributed to the dimeric structure as well as higher charge density on the protein surface [225]. Interestingly, the disulfide-linked form of hBD-1 is poorly active and became highly potent against bacteria and fungus *C. albicans* under reduced conditions where the disulfide-linked structure was disrupted [226]. It seems that the folded hBD-1 is the stored form, which can be transformed into an active form when needed.

Antimicrobial chemokines. Chemokines interact with receptors to realize chemotactic functions. They share a similar fold consisting of a three-stranded sheet followed by one α-helix at the C-terminus [227–229]. The N-terminal region is frequently disordered (Figure 3A–C).

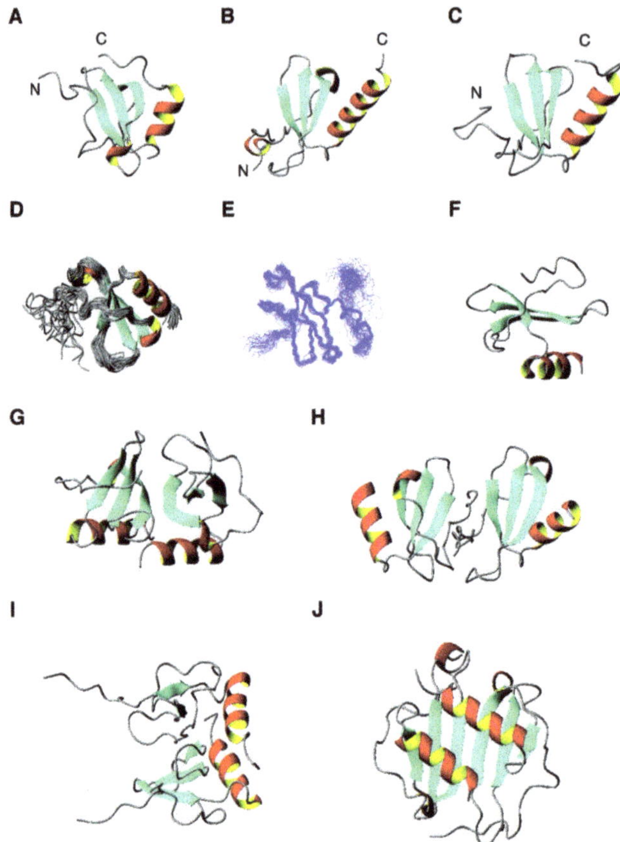

Figure 3. 3D structures of human chemokines with antimicrobial activity. Shown are (**A**) CCL1 (NMR structure, PDB ID: 1EL0); (**B**) CCL8 (crystal structure, PDB ID: 1ESR); (**C**) CCL11 (NMR structure, PDB ID: 2EOT); (**D**) CCL21 (NMR structure, PDB ID: 2L4N); (**E**) CCL27 (NMR structure, PDB ID: 2KUM); (**F**) CXCL12 (NMR structure, PDB ID: 2KOL); (G) CCL20 (crystal structure, PDB ID: 1M8A); (**H**) CCL13 (crystal structure, PDB ID: 2RA4); (**I**) CXCL1 (NMR structure, PDB ID: 1MSH); (**J**) CXCL10 (crystal structure, PDB ID: 1O80).

This can be best seen using a superimposed structural ensemble for CCL20 or CCL27 [230,231] determined by NMR (Figure 3D,E). The β-sheet appears to separate the N-terminal domain that interacts with cell receptors and the C-terminal domain that contains the antimicrobial helix for targeting bacterial membranes (Figure 3F) [232]. Some chemokines can also form oligomers. The dimeric forms of CCL20, CCL13, CXCL1, and CXCL10 [233–236] are shown in panels G to J of Figure 3. The dimer interface is normally composed of the C-terminal helix and strand 3. In the case of CCL13, however, it is the N-terminal region that occupies the interface (Figure 3H). Yung *et al.* found a direct binding of antimicrobial chemokines CXCL9 (net charge of +20) and CXCL10 (net charge +11) to the cell wall of *S. aureus* likely via the positively charged patches on these protein surfaces [237].

Under certain situations, the antimicrobial peptide is generated by further processing of a precursor protein. For example, antimicrobial thrombocidin-1 (TC-1) is produced by truncating two residues from the C-terminus of the parent protein NAP-2 (*i.e.*, neutrophil-activating peptide-2), which is poorly active. NMR analysis revealed that the C-terminus of TC-1 is mobile. In contrast, the C-terminus of NAP-2 is less mobile. It was proposed that the additional two residues locked the C-terminus via electrostatic interactions [238]. The additional Asp residue could have masked the positively-charged surface of the C-terminal helix that targets bacterial membranes. Likewise, insertion of an acidic Glu to the N-terminal region of GF-17, a peptide corresponding to the major antimicrobial region of human cathelicidin LL-37 [179], substantially reduced the peptide activity [239].

RNases. The structures of RNase 3 (Figure 4, panels A and B) and RNase 5 (panels C and D) were solved by both X-ray diffraction and multi-dimensional NMR spectroscopy. Although RNase 3 is dimeric in the crystal, the protein fold determined by the two techniques is similar. In addition, NMR studies revealed two conformations for His114 of RNase 5 in solution [240]. The structures of RNase 2 and RNase 7 are given in Figure 4 (panels E and F). Unlike chemokines discussed above, the antimicrobial region has been mapped to the N-terminus of RNase 7 [130,241]. In particular, a cluster of lysines were identified as key elements for antibacterial activity (bold in Table 1). It is proposed recently that the N-terminal antimicrobial function is conserved in the ribonuclease family [242]. One may wonder why a protein is created for bacterial defense if only part of the chain is required to kill pathogens. One possibility is the stability gain as part of the protein. Another possibility is that a folded protein structure allows for the incorporation of a variety of active sites on the protein surface. In certain cases, such functional sites may be overlapping [243]. In the case of RNase 7, the adjacent active site and antimicrobial residues allows us to propose a yet-to-be-proved "peel-and-kill" model. In other words, binding to bacteria by the cationic amino acids is followed by digestion of pathogenic nucleic acids. The multiple active sites also enable functional regulation. For example, an endogenous molecule can bind to RNase 7 and regulates its antimicrobial activity [244]. This could be one of the unique features of antimicrobial proteins distinct from small antimicrobial peptides.

Antimicrobial lectin RegIIIα. RegIIIα (or HIP/PAP) is a C-type lectin that binds peptidoglycan carbohydrates of Gram-positive bacterial cell walls. The structural basis of this binding has been elucidated (Figure 2D) [245]. Different from other C-type calcium-dependent lectins, the binding of RegIIIα to peptidoglycans is calcium independent (*i.e.*, lacking calcium-binding motif). The binding, however, requires the "EPN" motif and depends on sugar chain length. However, it seems that this peptidoglycan binding serves as an early recognition step for the peptide action as it can create a pore on bacterial membranes. The structure of the oligomeric form of the protein has recently been determined by combining X-ray structure and electron microscopy data, providing insight into the lethal step of bacterial killing by this intestine lectin [246].

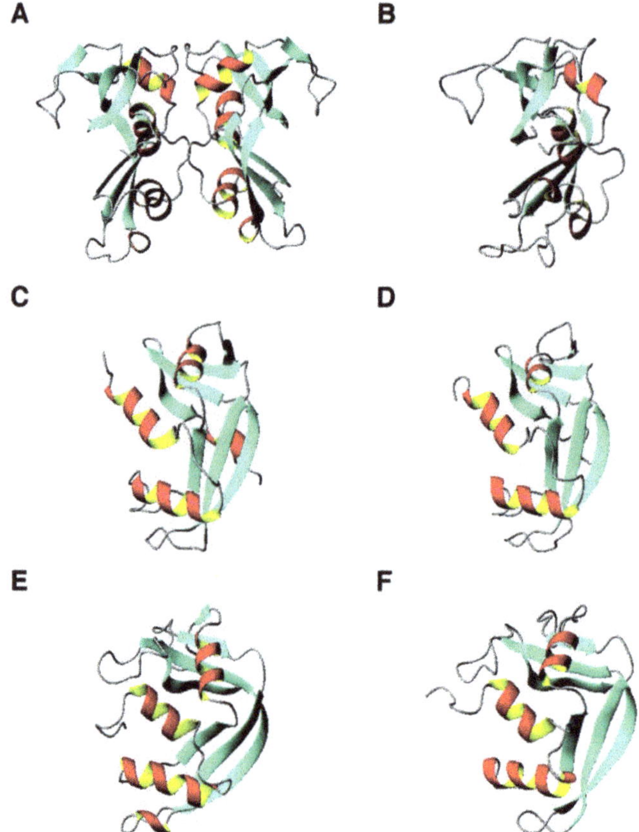

Figure 4. 3D structures of human ribonucleases with antimicrobial activity. Shown are (**A**) RNase 3 (dimeric crystal structure, PDB ID: 4A2O); (**B**) RNase 3 (NMR structure, PDB ID: 2KB5); (**C**) RNase 5 (crystal structure, PDB ID: 1B1I); (**D**) RNase 5 (NMR structure, PDB ID: 1AWZ); (**E**) RNase 2 (crystal structure, PDB ID: 2BZZ); and (**F**) RNase 7 (NMR structure, PDB ID: 2HKY).

5. Mechanism of Action of Human Antimicrobial Peptides

It is generally believed that cationic AMPs target anionic bacterial membranes. In the past years, significant advances have been made in elucidating the molecular targets of human AMPs. As described below, human AMPs can interact with a variety of molecular targets either on the cell surface (including membranes) or within the cells.

5.1. Targeting Bacterial Cell Wall

The molecular targets of AMPs are not limited to bacterial membranes. The assembly of HD-6 on bacterial surface entangles bacteria, providing a new defense mechanism for human innate immunity [123]. HNP-1 targets lipid II to block the biosynthesis of bacterial cell walls [247]. Böhling *et al.* found a close correlation of the hBD-3 activity with cell wall components [248]. A subsequent study corroborated the binding of hBD-3 to lipid II as well [249]. In the APD [7,8], there are 18 AMPs that use this mechanism to combat bacteria. Examples are nisins, mersacidin from bacteria, plectasin from fungi, Cg-Def, an oyster defensin [250–252]. Hence, blocking bacterial cell wall synthesis is a widely deployed innate defense mechanism. It is possible to identify small molecule mimetics that bind bacterial cell walls [253,254]. Although not discussed here, other defensins can directly recognize specific lipids in fungal membranes [255–257].

RegIII proteins are a family of lectins that can specifically recognize the carbohydrate portion of bacteria. While RegIIIα targets the peptidoglycan carbohydrate backbone for Gram-positive bacterial killing [245], mouse RegIIIβ associates with the lipid A portion of Gram-negative bacterial LPS [258]. In the case of murine RegIIIβ, amino acid residues in two structural motifs termed "loop 1" and "loop 2" are important for peptidoglycan and lipid A binding (Arg-135, Asp-142) and for the bactericidal activity (Glu-134, Asn-136, and Asp-142).

It is well known that human lysozyme not only binds a single peptidoglycan chain but also cuts the sugar repeats, thereby inhibiting bacterial cell wall synthesis [259]. In addition, some AMPs can associate with cell surface proteins to interfere with the docking and entry of viruses such as human immunodeficiency virus type 1 (HIV-1). For example, the association of SLPI with human annexin II can avoid the attachment of viral lipid phosphatidylserine (PS) to the same protein in human macrophages [260].

5.2. *Targeting Bacterial Inner Membranes*

Human cathelicidin LL-37 is a representative member in the helical family. It is proposed that LL-37 disrupts bacterial membranes. The membrane disruption of LL-37 involves at least three steps. First, the cationic peptide can recognize and coat the anionic surface of bacteria. With a classic amphipathic helical structure, this cationic peptide prefers to target anionic bacterial membranes. Second, LL-37 binds to the outer membranes and cross the outer membrane. Third, the peptide reaches the inner membrane. It initially binds to the inner membrane parallel to the surface, which is the basis for the carpet model [261]. At elevated concentrations, the peptide may disrupt the membranes by micellization. Alternatively, the peptide might take a vertical position to form a pore [262].

The ability of hepcidin 25 (hep-25) and its isoform hepcidin 20 (hep-20) to perturb bacterial membranes is markedly pH-dependent. The membrane disruption is more evident at acidic pH than at neutral pH. At acidic conditions, histidines become positively charged and more effective in membrane disruption [263].

While there is no agreement in the case of human LL-37 regarding the carpet or pore formation, recent structural determination of dermcidin provides evidence for possible pore formation in bacteria membranes. In the crystal structure [216], the peptide forms a hexamer, where two trimers are connected by zinc (Figure 1C). It is proposed that this structure might be directly inserted into bacterial membranes, serving as an ion channel.

In addition to α-defensins (HD-5 and HD-6), RegIII peptides are expressed to control the microbiota and keep the bacteria away from the epithelial surface of intestine. In particular, specific bacteria (e.g., *Bifidobacterium breve* NCC2950) can effectively induce the expression of RegIIIγ (an ortholog of human RegIIIα) in the intestine of mice via the MyD88-Ticam1 pathway [264]. RegIIIα is a lectin that binds to peptidoglycans of Gram-positive bacteria. However, it adopts a hexametic membrane-permeating pore structure to kill bacteria [246]. Such a pore is reminiscent of other pore structures solved for toxins [265–267]. The structure also provides a basis for selective killing of Gram-positive bacteria such as *L. monocytogenes*, *L. innocua*, and *E. faecalis* but not Gram-negative bacteria. This is because LPS, the major component of the outer membranes of Gram-negative bacteria, inhibits the pore-forming activity of RegIIIα [246].

5.3. *Cell-Penetrating Peptides and Intracellular Targets*

There are other AMPs that may work primarily by binding DNA. Buforin is such an example [83]. This is not surprising because this AMP was derived from DNA-binding histone 2A. In addition, SLPI, a small protein that inhibits elastase and cathepsin G, displayed antibacterial activity against *E. coli* by binding nucleic acids [268]. It is also likely that AMPs kill bacteria by more than one mechanism. For example, human LL-37 may first damage bacterial membranes followed by DNA binding, leading to the shutdown of bacterial machinery [83].

Unlike human LL-37, histatin 5 caused only small membrane damaging effects [269]. To interpret the killing effect of this peptide, two models have been proposed. In the first model, treatment of *C. albicans* with histatin 5 induces the efflux of ATP and increases cell permeability to small molecules, leading to ion imbalance. Thus, *C. albicans* cells respond by activating the osmotic stress responding pathways to minimize ion loss. This model is supported by the fact that knocking out the TRK1 gene that encodes a major K^+ uptake system made histatin 5 ineffective. A second model was also proposed based on the observation that the candida killing ability of histatin 5 is lost using a mitochondrial respiration mutant or after treatment with sodium azide that inhibits cellular metabolism [270]. In addition to the requirement of the mitochondrial respiration machinery [271], cellular internalization of histatins is also facilitated by peptide binding to heat shock protein Ssa2p on the surface of *C. albicans* [272]. This interference with mitochondrial respiration chain may be responsible for the formation of reactive oxygen species (ROS), leading to cell death [273]. Vylkova *et al.* performed a DNA microarray study of the effect of histatin 5 and found that these two models can be unified. This is because the oxidative stress could be produced as a secondary effect of osmotic stress. This proposal is in line with the observation that the killing of histatin 5 is facilitated in the presence of an osmotic agent sorbital but not an oxidant agent H_2O_2 [274]. It should be mentioned that human GAPDH(2–32), an antifungal peptide derived from the highly conserved protein GAPDH, can also enter *C. albicans* to induce apoptosis [275].

As a different mechanism to combat bacterial infection, some AMPs are reported to penetrate immune cells and activate them to boost immune response. For example, chromagranin A-derived peptides can penetrate neutrophils, bind to cytoplasmic calmodulin, and induce Ca^{2+} influx, leading to neutrophil activation and immune system augmentation [276].

Granulysin is an effector molecule in the cytotoxic granules of cytotoxic T lymphocytes and natural killer (NK) cells. It can kill intracellular pathogens in infected cells in the presence of perforin and to induce a cytotoxic effect against tumor cells. Although perforin and granulysin can colocalize [277], it is unclear how they work together in bacterial killing. A recent study reveals that perforin can form pores that preferentially allow the entry of cationic molecules [278]. Thus, granulysin might have entered the cell via the perforin pores, thereby providing yet another mechanism for intracellular bacterial killing by forming a molecular pair.

6. Concluding Remarks and Potential Therapeutic Strategies

Human antimicrobial peptides and proteins occupy an important niche in the current research on human host defense and innate immunity [1–6,279]. Except for antimicrobial protein lysozyme, which was found in 1922, most of short cationic peptides were discovered after 1980 (Table 1). By the time this article was written, over 100 human AMPs have been identified and characterized. They were either isolated from human tissues or predicted from the human genome by bioinformatics. Although genomic prediction constitutes an invaluable method, isolation from natural sources remains important in determining the exact mature form of AMPs. The discovery story of LL-37 nicely illustrates this point (Section 2.3). These peptides have diverse amino acid sequences (Table 1) and physical properties (Table 2), leading to a panel of defense molecules with varying activities (Table 1). While psoriasin and KDAMP primarily inhibit the growth of Gram-negative bacteria, RegIIIα is mainly active against Gram-positive bacteria. In addition, histatins and drosomycin-like defensin are primarily fungicidal. Many human AMPs such as LL-37 and defensins are broad-spectrum peptides against pathogens.

Remarkably, human AMPs are able to hinder bacterial growth by interactions with different targets, ranging from surface molecules (e.g., cell walls), inner membranes, to intracellular molecules (Table 3). Some AMPs can interact with two or more molecules. For example, the binding of RegIIIα to peptidoglycans constitutes only the initial recognition step and subsequent pore formation in bacterial membranes could be the lethal step [246].

Table 3. Select human antimicrobial peptides and their proposed targets.

APD ID	AMP	Structure	Molecular target
181	HD-6	β	Aggregate on bacterial surface
283	hBD-3	αβ	Bacterial cell wall (lipid II)
176	HNP-1	β	Bacterial cell wall (lipid II)
2257	Lysozyme	α	Cell wall carbohydrate
2071	RegIIIα	αβ	Membrane pores
310	LL-37	α	Bacterial membranes and/or DNA
433	Dermcidin	α	Membranes ion channel
2017	hGAPDH(2-32)	Unknown	Intracellular targets of fungi
505	Histatin 5	α	Intracellular mitochondria
2352	Chromagranin A-derived peptides	Unknown	Cytoplasmic calmodulin of neutrophils
1161	Granulysin	α	Perforin generates a pore to allow granulysin to enter the cell and kill intracellular bacteria

For interactions with different molecules, human AMPs are capable of adopting a variety of 3D structures (Figures 1–4). It is clearly important to determine the structure to high quality so that the molecular basis of these interactions can be uncovered accurately (reviewed in ref. [52]). It is also important to correlate the structure with the active state of the peptide. In the case of dermcidin, which oligomerizes on bacterial surface, the helix-bundle structure determined by X-ray crystallography [216] should be more relevant. Likewise, the disulfide-bonded structure of HBD-1 does not explain peptide activity under reduced conditions [226]. Therefore, human AMPs are diverse in terms of amino acid sequence, 3D structure, activity, and mechanism of action.

Many human AMPs are currently under close examination for their functional roles as well as potential applications in detection and diagnosis of human diseases. The type and expression level of human AMPs, if accurately mapped, may have clinical relevance. A clear variation in the expression level of AMPs can serve as biomarkers for human diseases, such as eczema severity and cancer [280–283]. In addition, this remarkable array of molecules may be used for detection, imaging, and diagnosis of bacterial infection. An example of this application is based on the preferential association of Technetium-99m labeled ubiquicidin with bacteria, enabling the physician to differentiate infection from aseptic loosening of hip prostheses in 30 min with high accuracy [284–286].

The collection of human AMPs discussed herein also inspires us in developing novel therapeutics [287]. First, new antimicrobials may be developed using human AMPs as templates. The rationale is that AMPs have remained potent for millions of years and are thus less prone to microbial resistance [1–6]. In particular, peptides with different structural scaffolds may kill the same bacterium by different mechanisms (Table 3). Furthermore, the same peptide sequence can be tailored into various peptides that selectively target pathogens such as Gram-positive, Gram-negative bacteria, or viruses [83]. This is highly desirable for selective bacterial elimination without destroying the probiotic microbial flora. The success of this line depends on whether a selected template will achieve the desired potency *in vivo* against a target pathogen, low cytotoxicity to humans, stability to proteases, and cost-effective production [287]. One can also consider alternative peptide forms. For instance, a pro-drug can be used to reduce the cytotoxicity of AMPs if a mechanism can be found to release it when needed [288]. While portions of antimicrobial proteins are preferred to design novel antimicrobials [222,223,242,289], a whole protein may also be considered. Unlike short peptides, the folded structure of proteins confers stability to the action of proteases. However, the production of such a long polypeptide chain may require recombinant expression in bacteria or cell-free systems [199].

Second, new strategies are actively sought to bring the invading pathogens under control. It is appreciated that different receptors and signal pathways are activated in response to the invasion of different microbes [65]. Of outstanding interest is that non-pathogen factors can also induce AMP expression (Table 4). One of the earliest examples might be the light therapy invented by Niel Finsen [290]. The establishment of a link between light therapy, vitamin D and human cathelicidin LL-37 expression provides a completely different way for infection treatment. Instead of treating patients with traditional antibiotics, doctors may be able to use light or vitamin D [291,292]. Indeed using narrow-band UV B light, the level of vitamin D was increased in psoriasis patients (psoriasis is a common autoimmune disease on skin) [293]. In addition, other small molecules such as butyrate can induce LL-37 expression [294]. Components from Traditional Chinese Medicine may regulate the AMP expression as well [295]. These factors may induce the expression of a single peptide or multiple AMPs [296]. It is also possible that certain factors can work together to induce AMP expression. While cyclic AMP and butyrate synergistically stimulate the expression of chicken β-defensin 9 [297], 4-phenylbutyrate (PBA) and 1,25-dihydroxyvitamin D3 (or lactose) can induce AMP gene expression synergistically [294,298]. It appears that stimulation of LL-37 expression by histone deacetylase (HDAC) inhibitors is cell dependent. Trichostatin and sodium butyrate increased the peptide expression in human NCI-H292 airway epithelial cells but not in the primary cultures of normal nasal epithelial cells [299]. However, the induction of the human LL-37 expression may not be a general approach for bacterial clearance. During *Salmonella enterica* infection of human monocyte-derived macrophages, LL-37 is neither induced nor required for bacterial clearance [300].

Table 4. Some known factors that induce antimicrobial peptide expression

Factor	AMP induced	Cells	Ref
Bacteria/LPS	LL-37, HBD-2	keratinocytes	[296]
TNF-α	LL-37, HBD-2	keratinocytes	[286]
UV Light	LL-37, HBD-2, chemerin	keratinocytes	[286,301]
Vitamin D3	LL-37	neutrophil progenitors and EBV-transformed B cells	[302,303]
Lactose	LL-37	colonic epithelial cells T84, THP-1 monocytes and macrophages	[304]
Short-chain fatty acids	LL-37; pBD-2, pBD-3, pEP2C, and protegrins	human HT-29 colonic epithelial cells and U-937 monocytic cells;	[305,306]
Isoleucine	hBD-1; epithelial defensins	human colon cells, HCT-116; bovine kidney epithelial cells	[307–309]
Arginine	hBD-1	human colon cells, HCT-116	[307]
Ca^{2+}	hBD-2, hBD-3	human keratinocyte monolayers	[310]
Zn^{2+}	LL-37; pBD-1, pBD-2, pBD-3	Caco-2 cell; Intestinal epithelial cells	[311]
Butyrate	LL-37	colon, gastric and hepatocellular cells	[312]
Albumin	hBD-1	human colon cells, HCT-116	[307]
Cyclic AMP/Butyrate	Chicken β-defensin 9	macrophages and primary jejunal explants	[297]
Phenylbutyrate/ 1,25-dihydroxyvitamin D3	cathelicidins	immortalized human bronchial epithelial cell line VA10	[298]

Finally, immune modulation peptides may find therapeutic use because they do not act on microbes directly and thereby are less likely to induce antimicrobial resistance [4,5]. Immune modulation is activated via peptide binding to host cell receptors that initiate various signal transduction pathways. Recently, a natural peptide was found to have immune modulating activity but no antimicrobial activity [313]. Besides engineering peptides with distinct properties, there has been growing interest in elucidating the bacterial mechanisms in generating resistance to AMPs or by subverting host immune systems [314,315]. It can be anticipated that new therapeutic approaches will continue to emerge from our understanding of the host-pathogen interactions. All these strategies will facilitate the development of AMPs into novel antimicrobials to meet the challenge of antibiotics-resistant superbugs, RNA viral infections and difficult-to-treat cancers [287].

Acknowledgments: The author is grateful for the support of the fundings from the NIH (R56AI081975) and the state of Nebraska during this study.

Conflicts of Interest: The author does not declare a conflict of interest.

References

1. Boman, H.G. Antibacterial peptides: Basic facts and emerging concepts. *J. Inter. Med.* **2003**, *254*, 197–215. [CrossRef]
2. Ganz, T.; Lehrer, R.I. Defensins. *Curr. Opin. Immunol.* **1994**, *6*, 584–589. [CrossRef]
3. Zasloff, M. Antimicrobial peptides of multicellullar organisms. *Nature* **2002**, *415*, 359–365. [CrossRef]
4. Hancock, R.E.W.; Sahl, H.G. Antimicrobial and host-defense peptides as new anti-infective therapeutic strategies. *Nat. Biotechnol.* **2006**, *24*, 1551–1557. [CrossRef]
5. Lai, Y.; Gallo, R.L. AMPed up immunity: How antimicrobial peptides have multiple roles in immune defense. *Trends Immunol.* **2009**, *30*, 131–141. [CrossRef]
6. Yount, N.Y.; Yeaman, M.R. Emerging themes and therapeutic prospects for anti-infective peptides. *Annu. Rev. Pharmacol. Toxicol.* **2012**, *52*, 337–360. [CrossRef]
7. Wang, Z.; Wang, G. APD: The antimicrobial peptide database. *Nucleic Acids Res.* **2004**, *32*, D590–D592. [CrossRef]
8. Wang, G.; Li, X.; Wang, Z. The updated antimicrobial peptide database and its application in peptide design. *Nucleic Acids Res.* **2009**, *37*, D933–D937. [CrossRef]
9. Marchini, G.; Lindow, S.; Brismar, H.; Ståbi, B.; Berggren, V.; Ulfgren, A.K.; Lonne-Rahm, S.; Agerberth, B.; Gudmundsson, G.H. The newborn infant is protected by an innate antimicrobial barrier: Peptide antibiotics are present in the skin and vernix caseosa. *Br. J. Dermatol.* **2002**, *147*, 1127–1134. [CrossRef]
10. Gschwandtner, M.; Zhong, S.; Tschachler, A.; Mlitz, V.; Karner, S.; Elbe-Bürger, A.; Mildner, M. Fetal Human Keratinocytes Produce Large Amounts of Antimicrobial Peptides: Involvement of Histone-Methylation Processes. *J. Invest. Dermatol.* **2014**. [CrossRef]
11. Wittersheim, M.; Cordes, J.; Meyer-Hoffert, U.; Harder, J.; Hedderich, J.; Gläser, R. Differential expression and *in vivo* secretion of the antimicrobial peptides psoriasin (S100A7), RNase 7, human beta-defensin-2 and -3 in healthy human skin. *Exp. Dermatol.* **2013**, *22*, 364–366. [CrossRef]
12. Gläser, R.; Meyer-Hoffert, U.; Harder, J.; Cordes, J.; Wittersheim, M.; Kobliakova, J.; Fölster-Holst, R.; Proksch, E.; Schröder, J.M.; Schwarz, T. The antimicrobial protein psoriasin (S100A7) is upregulated in atopic dermatitis and after experimental skin barrier disruption. *J. Invest. Dermatol.* **2009**, *129*, 641–649. [CrossRef]
13. McDermott, A.M. Antimicrobial compounds in tears. *Exp. Eye Res.* **2013**, *117*, 53–61. [CrossRef]
14. Underwood, M.; Bakaletz, L. Innate immunity and the role of defensins in otitis media. *Curr. Allergy Asthma Rep.* **2011**, *11*, 499–507. [CrossRef]
15. Sato, J.; Nishimura, M.; Yamazaki, M.; Yoshida, K.; Kurashige, Y.; Saitoh, M.; Abiko, Y. Expression profile of drosomycin-like defensin in oral epithelium and oral carcinoma cell lines. *Arch. Oral Biol.* **2013**, *58*, 279–285. [CrossRef]
16. Da Silva, B.R.; de Freitas, V.A.; Nascimento-Neto, L.G.; Carneiro, V.A.; Arruda, F.V.; de Aguiar, A.S.; Cavada, B.S.; Teixeira, E.H. Antimicrobial peptide control of pathogenic microorganisms of the oral cavity: A review of the literature. *Peptides* **2012**, *36*, 315–321. [CrossRef]
17. Tollner, T.L.; Bevins, C.L.; Cherr, G.N. Multifunctional glycoprotein DEFB126—A curious story of defensin-clad spermatozoa. *Nat. Rev. Urol.* **2012**, *9*, 365–375. [CrossRef]
18. Yu, H.; Dong, J.; Gu, Y.; Liu, H.; Xin, A.; Shi, H.; Sun, F.; Zhang, Y.; Lin, D.; Diao, H. The novel human β-defensin 114 regulates lipopolysaccharide (LPS)-mediated inflammation and protects sperm from motility loss. *J. Biol. Chem.* **2013**, *288*, 12270–12282.
19. Tollner, T.L.; Yudin, A.I.; Tarantal, A.F.; Treece, C.A.; Overstreet, J.W.; Cherr, G.N. Beta-defensin 126 on the surface of macaque sperm mediates attachment of sperm to oviductal epithelia. *Biol. Reprod.* **2008**, *78*, 400–412. [CrossRef]
20. Fleming, A. On a remarkable bacteriolytic element found in tissues and secretions. *Proc. R. Soc. B* **1922**, *93*, 306–317. [CrossRef]
21. Selsted, M.E.; Harwig, S.S.; Ganz, T.; Schilling, J.W.; Lehrer, R.I. Primary structures of three human neutrophil defensins. *J. Clin. Invest.* **1985**, *76*, 1436–1439. [CrossRef]

22. Oppenheim, F.G.; Xu, T.; McMillian, F.M.; Levitz, S.M.; Diamond, R.D.; Offner, G.D.; Troxler, R.F. Histatins, a novel family of histidine-rich proteins in human parotid secretion. Isolation, characterization, primary structure, and fungistatic effects on *Candida albicans*. *J. Biol. Chem.* **1988**, *263*, 7472–7477.
23. Wilde, C.G.; Griffith, J.E.; Marra, M.N.; Snable, J.L.; Scott, R.W. Purification and characterization of human neutrophil peptide 4, a novel member of the defensin family. *J. Biol. Chem.* **1989**, *264*, 11200–11203.
24. Hamann, K.J.; Gleich, G.J.; Checkel, J.L.; Loegering, D.A.; McCall, J.W.; Barker, R.L. *In vitro* killing of microfilariae of *Brugia pahangi* and *Brugia malayi* by eosinophil granule proteins. *J. Immunol.* **1990**, *144*, 3166–3173.
25. Jones, D.E.; Bevins, C.L. Paneth cells of the human small intestine express an antimicrobial peptide gene. *J. Biol. Chem.* **1992**, *267*, 23216–23225.
26. Jones, D.E.; Bevins, C.L. Defensin-6 mRNA in human Paneth cells: Implications for antimicrobial peptides in host defense of the human bowel. *FEBS Lett.* **1993**, *315*, 187–192. [CrossRef]
27. Bensch, K.W.; Raida, M.; Mägert, H.J.; Schulz-Knappe, P.; Forssmann, W.G. hBD-1: A novel beta-defensin from human plasma. *FEBS Lett.* **1995**, *368*, 331–335. [CrossRef]
28. Agerberth, B.; Gunne, H.; Odeberg, J.; Kogner, P.; Boman, H.G.; Gudmundsson, G.H. FALL-39, a putative human peptide antibiotic, is cysteine-free and expressed in bone marrow and testis. *Proc. Natl. Acad. Sci. USA* **1995**, *92*, 195–199. [CrossRef]
29. Larrick, J.W.; Hirata, M.; Balint, R.F.; Lee, J.; Zhong, J.; Wright, S.C. Human CAP18: A novel antimicrobial lipopolysaccharide-binding protein. *Infect. Immun.* **1995**, *63*, 1291–1297.
30. Cowland, J.B.; Johnsen, A.H.; Borregaard, N. hCAP-18, a cathelin/pro-bactenecin-like protein of human neutrophil specific granules. *FEBS Lett.* **1995**, *368*, 173–176. [CrossRef]
31. Harder, J.; Bartels, J.; Christophers, E.; Schröder, J.M. A peptide antibiotic from human skin. *Nature* **1997**, *387*, 861. [CrossRef]
32. Stenger, S.; Hanson, D.A.; Teitelbaum, R.; Dewan, P.; Niazi, K.R.; Froelich, C.J.; Ganz, T.; Thoma-Uszynski, S.; Melián, A.; Bogdan, C.; *et al.* An antimicrobial activity of cytolytic T cells mediated by granulysin. *Science* **1998**, *282*, 121–125. [CrossRef]
33. Hieshima, K.; Ohtani, H.; Shibano, M.; Izawa, D.; Nakayama, T.; Kawasaki, Y.; Shiba, F.; Shiota, M.; Katou, F.; Saito, T.; *et al.* CCL28 has dual roles in mucosal immunity as a chemokine with broad-spectrum antimicrobial activity. *J. Immunol.* **2003**, *170*, 1452–1461. [CrossRef]
34. Krijgsveld, J.; Zaat, S.A.; Meeldijk, J.; van Veelen, P.A.; Fang, G.; Poolman, B.; Brandt, E.; Ehlert, J.E.; Kuijpers, A.J.; Engbers, G.H.; *et al.* Thrombocidins, microbicidal proteins from human blood platelets, are C-terminal deletion products of CXC chemokines. *J. Biol. Chem.* **2000**, *275*, 20374–20381. [CrossRef]
35. Krause, A.; Neitz, S.; Mägert, H.J.; Schulz, A.; Forssmann, W.G.; Schulz-Knappe, P.; Adermann, K. LEAP-1, a novel highly disulfide-bonded human peptide, exhibits antimicrobial activity. *FEBS Lett.* **2000**, *480*, 147–150. [CrossRef]
36. Cutuli, M.; Cristiani, S.; Lipton, J.M.; Catania, A. Antimicrobial effects of alpha-MSH peptides. *J. Leukoc. Biol.* **2000**, *67*, 233–239.
37. Harder, J.; Bartels, J.; Christophers, E.; Schroeder, J.M. Isolation and characterization of human deta-defensin-3, a novel human inducible peptide antibiotic. *J. Biol. Chem.* **2001**, *276*, 5707–5713. [CrossRef]
38. García, J.R.; Krause, A.; Schulz, S.; Rodríguez-Jiménez, F.J.; Klüver, E.; Adermann, K.; Forssmann, U.; Frimpong-Boateng, A.; Bals, R.; Forssmann, W.G. Human beta-defensin 4: A novel inducible peptide with a specific salt-sensitive spectrum of antimicrobial activity. *FASEB J.* **2001**, *15*, 1819–1821.
39. Schittek, B.; Hipfel, R.; Sauer, B.; Bauer, J.; Kalbacher, H.; Stevanovic, S.; Schirle, M.; Schroeder, K.; Blin, N.; Meier, F.; *et al.* Dermcidin: A novel human antibiotic peptide secreted by sweat glands. *Nat. Immunol.* **2001**, *2*, 1133–1137. [CrossRef]
40. Harder, J.; Schroder, J.M. RNase 7, a novel innate immune defense antimicrobial protein of healthy human skin. *J. Biol. Chem.* **2002**, *277*, 46779–46784. [CrossRef]
41. Hooper, L.V.; Stappenbeck, T.S.; Hong, C.V.; Gordon, J.I. Angiogenins: A new class of microbicidal proteins involved in innate immunity. *Nat. Immunol.* **2003**, *4*, 269–273. [CrossRef]
42. Yang, D.; Chen, Q.; Hoover, D.M.; Staley, P.; Tucker, K.D.; Lubkowski, J.; Oppenheim, J.J. Many chemokines including CCL20/MIP-3alpha display antimicrobial activity. *J. Leukoc. Biol.* **2003**, *74*, 448–455. [CrossRef]
43. Gläser, R.; Harder, J.; Lange, H.; Bartels, J.; Christophers, E.; Schröder, J.M. Antimicrobial psoriasin (S100A7) protects human skin from *Escherichia coli* infection. *Nat. Immunol.* **2005**, *6*, 57–64. [CrossRef]

44. Cash, H.L.; Whitham, C.V.; Behrendt, C.L.; Hooper, L.V. Symbiotic bacteria direct expression of an intestinal bactericidal lectin. *Science* **2006**, *313*, 1126–1130. [CrossRef]
45. El Karim, I.A.; Linden, G.J.; Orr, D.F.; Lundy, F.T. Antimicrobial activity of neuropeptides against a range of micro-organisms from skin, oral, respiratory and gastrointestinal tract sites. *J. Neuroimmunol.* **2008**, *200*, 11–16. [CrossRef]
46. Simon, A.; Kullberg, B.J.; Tripet, B.; Boerman, O.C.; Zeeuwen, P.; van der Ven-Jongekrijg, J.; Verweij, P.; Schalkwijk, J.; Hodges, R.; van der Meer, J.W.; *et al.* Drosomycin-like defensin, a human homologue of Drosophila melanogaster drosomycin with antifungal activity. *Antimicrob. Agents Chemother.* **2008**, *52*, 1407–1412. [CrossRef]
47. Marischen, L.; Wesch, D.; Schröder, J.M.; Wiedow, O.; Kabelitz, D. Human γδ T cells produce the protease inhibitor and antimicrobial peptide elafin. *Scand. J. Immunol.* **2009**, *70*, 547–552. [CrossRef]
48. Soscia, S.J.; Kirby, J.E.; Washicosky, K.J.; Tucker, S.M.; Ingelsson, M.; Hyman, B.; Burton, M.A.; Goldstein, L.E.; Duong, S.; Tanzi, R.E.; *et al.* The Alzheimer's disease-associated amyloid beta-protein is an antimicrobial peptide. *PLoS One* **2010**, *5*, e9505. [CrossRef]
49. Kulig, P.; Kantyka, T.; Zabel, B.A.; Banas, M.; Chyra, A.; Stefanska, A.; Tu, H.; Allen, S.J.; Handel, T.M.; Kozik, A.; *et al.* Regulation of chemerin chemoattractant and antibacterial activity by human cysteine cathepsins. *J. Immunol.* **2011**, *187*, 1403–1410. [CrossRef]
50. Wang, L.; Liu, Q.; Chen, J.C.; Cui, Y.X.; Zhou, B.; Chen, Y.X.; Zhao, Y.F.; Li, Y.M. Antimicrobial activity of human islet amyloid polypeptides: An insight into amyloid peptides' connection with antimicrobial peptides. *Biol. Chem.* **2012**, *393*, 641–646.
51. Tam, C.; Mun, J.J.; Evans, D.J.; Fleiszig, S.M. Cytokeratins mediate epithelial innate defense through their antimicrobial properties. *J. Clin. Invest.* **2012**, *122*, 3665–3677. [CrossRef]
52. Wang, G. Database-guided discovery of potent peptides to combat HIV-1 or superbugs. *Pharmaceuticals* **2013**, *6*, 728–758. [CrossRef]
53. Zhao, C.; Wang, I.; Lehrer, R.I. Widespread expression of beta-defensin hBD-1 in human secretory glands and epithelial cells. *FEBS Lett.* **1996**, *396*, 319–322. [CrossRef]
54. Ouellette, A.J.; Greco, R.M.; James, M.; Frederick, D.; Naftilan, J.; Fallon, J.T. Developmental regulation of cryptdin, a corticostatin/defensin precursor mRNA in mouse small intestinal crypt epithelium. *J. Cell Biol.* **1989**, *108*, 1687–1695. [CrossRef]
55. Ganz, T. Defensins in the urinary tract and other tissues. *J. Infect. Dis.* **2001**, *183* Suppl 1, S41–S42. [CrossRef]
56. Valore, E.V.; Park, C.H.; Quayle, A.J.; Wiles, K.R.; McCray, P.B., Jr.; Ganz, T. Human beta-defensin-1: An antimicrobial peptide of urogenital tissues. *J. Clin. Invest.* **1998**, *101*, 1633–1642. [CrossRef]
57. Goldman, M.J.; Anderson, G.M.; Stolzenberg, E.D.; Kari, U.P.; Zasloff, M.; Wilson, J.M. Human beta-defensin-1 is a salt-sensitive antibiotic in lung that is inactivated in cystic fibrosis. *Cell* **1997**, *88*, 553–560. [CrossRef]
58. Bals, R.; Wang, X.; Wu, Z.; Freeman, T.; Bafna, V.; Zasloff, M.; Wilson, J.M. Human beta-defensin 2 is a salt-sensitive peptide antibiotic expressed in human lung. *J. Clin. Invest.* **1998**, *102*, 874–880. [CrossRef]
59. Jia, H.P.; Schutte, B.C.; Schudy, A.; Linzmeier, R.; Guthmiller, J.M.; Johnson, G.K.; Tack, B.F.; Mitros, J.P.; Rosenthal, A.; Ganz, T.; *et al.* Discovery of new human beta-defensins using a genomics-based approach. *Gene* **2001**, *263*, 211–218. [CrossRef]
60. García, J.R.; Jaumann, F.; Schulz, S.; Krause, A.; Rodríguez-Jiménez, J.; Forssmann, U.; Adermann, K.; Klüver, E.; Vogelmeier, C.; Becker, D.; *et al.* Identification of a novel, multifunctional beta-defensin (human beta-defensin 3) with specific antimicrobial activity. Its interaction with plasma membranes of Xenopus oocytes and the induction of macrophage chemoattraction. *Cell Tissue Res.* **2001**, *306*, 257–264. [CrossRef]
61. Scheetz, T.; Bartlett, J.A.; Walters, J.D.; Schutte, B.C.; Casavant, T.L.; McCray, P.B., Jr. Genomics-based approaches to gene discovery in innate immunity. *Immunol. Rev.* **2002**, *190*, 137–145. [CrossRef]
62. Huang, L.; Leong, S.S.; Jiang, R. Soluble fusion expression and characterization of bioactive human beta-defensin 26 and 27. *Appl. Microbiol. Biotechnol.* **2009**, *84*, 301–308. [CrossRef]
63. Schulz, A.; Klüver, E.; Schulz-Maronde, S.; Adermann, K. Engineering disulfide bonds of the novel human beta-defensins hBD-27 and hBD-28: Differences in disulfide formation and biological activity among human beta-defensins. *Biopolymers* **2005**, *80*, 34–49. [CrossRef]
64. Xin, A.; Zhao, Y.; Yu, H.; Shi, H.; Liu, H.; Diao, H.; Zhang, Y. Soluble fusion expression, characterization and localization of human β-defensin 6. *Mol. Med. Rep.* **2014**, *9*, 149–155.

65. Lemaitre, B.; Reichhart, J.M.; Hoffmann, J.A. Drosophila host defense: Differential induction of antimicrobial peptide genes after infection by various classes of microorganisms. *Proc. Natl. Acad. Sci. USA* **1997**, *94*, 14614–14619. [CrossRef]
66. Selsted, M.E. Theta-defensins: cyclic antimicrobial peptides produced by binary ligation of truncated alpha-defensins. *Curr Protein Pept Sci.* **2004**, *5*, 365–371. [CrossRef]
67. Tang, Y.Q.; Yuan, J.; Osapay, G.; Osapay, K.; Tran, D.; Miller, C.J.; Ouellette, A.J.; Selsted, M.E. A cyclic antimicrobial peptide produced in primate leukocytes by the ligation of two truncated alpha-defensins. *Science* **1999**, *286*, 498–502. [CrossRef]
68. Cole, A.M.; Wang, W.; Waring, A.J.; Lehrer, R.I. Retrocyclins: Using past as prologue. *Curr. Protein Pept. Sci.* **2004**, *5*, 373–381. [CrossRef]
69. Yang, C.; Boone, L.; Nguyen, T.X.; Rudolph, D.; Limpakarnjanarat, K.; Mastro, T.D.; Tappero, J.; Cole, A.M.; Lal, R.B. Theta-Defensin pseudogenes in HIV-1-exposed, persistently seronegative female sex-workers from Thailand. *Infect Genet Evol.* **2005**, *5*, 11–15. [CrossRef]
70. Lehrer, R.I.; Cole, A.M.; Selsted, M.E. θ-Defensins: Cyclic peptides with endless potential. *J. Biol. Chem.* **2012**, *287*, 27014–27019. [CrossRef]
71. Troxler, R.F.; Offner, G.D.; Xu, T.; Vanderspek, J.C.; Oppenheim, F.G. Structural relationship between human salivary histatins. *J. Dent. Res.* **1990**, *69*, 2–6. [CrossRef]
72. Sabatini, L.M.; Azen, E.A. Histatins, a family of salivary histidine-rich proteins, are encoded by at least two loci (HIS1 and HIS2). *Biochem. Biophys. Res. Commun.* **1989**, *160*, 495–502. [CrossRef]
73. vanderSpek, J.C.; Wyandt, H.E.; Skare, J.C.; Milunsky, A.; Oppenheim, F.G.; Troxler, R.F. Localization of the genes for histatins to human chromosome 4q13 and tissue distribution of the mRNAs. *Am. J. Hum. Genet.* **1989**, *45*, 381–387.
74. Nizet, V.; Ohtake, T.; Lauth, X.; Trowbridge, J.; Rudisill, J.; Dorschner, R.A.; Pestonjamasp, V.; Piraino, J.; Huttner, K.; Gallo, R.L. Innate antimicrobial peptide protects the skin from invasive bacterial infection. *Nature* **2001**, *414*, 454–457. [CrossRef]
75. Braff, M.H.; Zaiou, M.; Fierer, J.; Nizet, V.; Gallo, R.L. Keratinocyte production of cathelicidin provides direct activity against bacterial skin pathogens. *Infect. Immun.* **2005**, *73*, 6771–6781. [CrossRef]
76. Lee, P.H.; Ohtake, T.; Zaiou, M.; Murakami, M.; Rudisill, J.A.; Lin, K.H.; Gallo, R.L. Expression of an additional cathelicidin antimicrobial peptide protects against bacterial skin infection. *Proc. Natl. Acad. Sci. USA* **2005**, *102*, 3750–3755.
77. Romeo, D.; Skerlavaj, B.; Bolognesi, M.; Gennaro, R. Structure and bactericidal activity of an antibiotic dodecapeptide purified from bovine neutrophils. *J. Biol. Chem.* **1988**, *263*, 9573–9575.
78. Zanetti, M. Cathelicidins, multifunctional peptides of the innate immunity. *J. Leukoc. Biol.* **2004**, *75*, 39–48. [CrossRef]
79. Gudmundsson, G.H.; Agerberth, B.; Odeberg, J.; Bergman, T.; Olsson, B.; Salcedo, R. The human gene FALL-39 and processing of the cathelin precursor to the antibacterial peptide LL-37 in granulocytes. *Eur. J. Biochem.* **1996**, *238*, 325–332.
80. Sørensen, O.E.; Gram, L.; Johnsen, A.H.; Andersson, E.; Bangsbøll, S.; Tjabringa, G.S.; Hiemstra, P.S.; Malm, J.; Egesten, A.; Borregaard, N. Processing of seminal plasma hCAP-18 to ALL-38 by gastricsin: A novel mechanism of generating antimicrobial peptides in vagina. *J. Biol. Chem.* **2003**, *278*, 28540–28546. [CrossRef]
81. Zhao, H.; Lee, W.H.; Shen, J.H.; Li, H.; Zhang, Y. Identification of novel semenogelin I-derived antimicrobial peptide from liquefied human seminal plasma. *Peptides* **2008**, *29*, 505–511. [CrossRef]
82. Yamasaki, K.; Schauber, J.; Coda, A.; Lin, H.; Dorschner, R.A.; Schechter, N.M.; Bonnart, C.; Descargues, P.; Hovnanian, A.; Gallo, R.L. Kallikrein-mediated proteolysis regulates the antimicrobial effects of cathelicidins in skin. *FASEB J.* **2006**, *20*, 2068–2080. [CrossRef]
83. Wang, G.; Mishra, B.; Epand, R.F.; Epand, R.M. High-quality 3D structures shine light on antibacterial, anti-biofilm and antiviral activities of human cathelicidin LL-37 and its fragments. *Biochim. Biophys. Acta* **2014**. [CrossRef]
84. Tailor, R.H.; Acland, D.P.; Attenborough, S.; Cammue, B.P.; Evans, I.J.; Osborn, R.W.; Ray, J.A.; Rees, S.B.; Broekaert, W.F. A novel family of small cysteine-rich antimicrobial peptides from seed of Impatiens balsamina is derived from a single precursor protein. *J. Biol. Chem.* **1997**, *272*, 24480–24487. [CrossRef]
85. Scocchi, M.; Bontempo, D.; Boscolo, S.; Tomasinsig, L.; Giulotto, E.; Zanetti, M. Novel cathelicidins in horse leukocytes. *FEBS Lett.* **1999**, *457*, 459–464. [CrossRef]

86. Anderson, R.C.; Yu, P.L. Isolation and characterisation of proline/arginine-rich cathelicidin peptides from ovine neutrophils. *Biochem. Biophys. Res. Commun.* **2003**, *312*, 1139–1146. [CrossRef]
87. Skerlavaj, B.; Benincasa, M.; Risso, A.; Zanetti, M.; Gennaro, R. SMAP-29: A potent antibacterial and antifungal peptide from sheep leukocytes. *FEBS Lett.* **1999**, *463*, 58–62. [CrossRef]
88. Castiglioni, B.; Scocchi, M.; Zanetti, M.; Ferretti, L. Six antimicrobial peptide genes of the cathelicidin family map to bovine chromosome 22q24 by fluorescence in situ hybridization. *Cytogenet. Cell Genet.* **1996**, *75*, 240–242. [CrossRef]
89. Murakami, M.; Ohtake, T.; Dorschner, R.A.; Schittek, B.; Garbe, C.; Gallo, R.L. Cathelicidin anti-microbial peptide expression in sweat, an innate defense system for the skin. *J. Invest. Dermatol.* **2002**, *119*, 1090–1095. [CrossRef]
90. Rieg, S.; Garbe, C.; Sauer, B.; Kalbacher, H.; Schittek, B. Dermcidinis constitutively produced by eccrine sweat glands and is not induced in epidermal cells under inflammatory skin conditions. *Br. J. Dermatol.* **2004**, *151*, 534–539. [CrossRef]
91. Rieg, S.; Saborowski, V.; Kern, W.V.; Jonas, D.; Bruckner-Tuderman, L.; Hofmann, S.C. Expression of the sweat-derived innate defence antimicrobial peptide dermcidin is not impaired in *Staphylococcus aureus* colonization or recurrent skin infections. *Clin. Exp. Dermatol.* **2013**. [CrossRef]
92. Schittek, B. The multiple facets of dermcidin in cell survival and host defense. *J. Innate Immun.* **2012**, *4*, 349–360.
93. Ghosh, R.; Maji, U.K.; Bhattacharya, R.; Sinha, A.K. The role of dermcidin isoform 2: A two-faceted atherosclerotic risk factor for coronary artery disease and the effect of acetyl salicylic acid on it. *Thrombosis* **2012**, *2012*, 987932.
94. Park, C.H.; Valore, E.V.; Waring, A.J.; Ganz, T. Hepcidin, a urinary antimicrobial peptide synthesized in the liver. *J. Biol. Chem.* **2001**, *276*, 7806–7801. [CrossRef]
95. Jordan, J.B.; Poppe, L.; Haniu, M.; Arvedson, T.; Syed, R.; Li, V.; Kohno, H.; Kim, H.; Schnier, P.D.; Harvey, T.S.; *et al.* Hepcidin revisited, disulfide connectivity, dynamics, and structure. *J. Biol. Chem.* **2009**, *284*, 24155–24167. [CrossRef]
96. Pigeon, C.; Ilyin, G.; Courselaud, B.; Leroyer, P.; Turlin, B.; Brissot, P.; Loréal, O. A new mouse liver-specific gene, encoding a protein homologous to human antimicrobial peptide hepcidin, is overexpressed during iron overload. *J. Biol. Chem.* **2001**, *276*, 7811–7819.
97. Roetto, A.; Papanikolaou, G.; Politou, M.; Alberti, F.; Girelli, D.; Christakis, J.; Loukopoulos, D.; Camaschella, C. Mutant antimicrobial peptide hepcidin is associated with severe juvenile hemochromatosis. *Nat. Genet.* **2003**, *33*, 21–22.
98. Krause, A.; Sillard, R.; Kleemeier, B.; Klüver, E.; Maronde, E.; Conejo-García, J.R.; Forssmann, W.G.; Schulz-Knappe, P.; Nehls, M.C.; Wattler, F.; *et al.* Isolation and biochemical characterization of LEAP-2, a novel blood peptide expressed in the liver. *Protein Sci.* **2003**, *12*, 143–152.
99. Park, C.B.; Kim, M.S.; Kim, S.C. A novel antimicrobial peptide from Bufo bufo gargarizans. *Biochem. Biophys. Res. Commun.* **1996**, *218*, 408–413. [CrossRef]
100. Minn, I.; Kim, H.S.; Kim, S.C. Antimicrobial peptides derived from pepsinogens in the stomach of the bullfrog, Rana catesbeiana. *Biochim. Biophys. Acta* **1998**, *1407*, 31–39. [CrossRef]
101. Cole, A.M.; Kim, Y.H.; Tahk, S.; Hong, T.; Weis, P.; Waring, A.J.; Ganz, T. Calcitermin, a novel antimicrobial peptide isolated from human airway secretions. *FEBS Lett.* **2001**, *504*, 5–10. [CrossRef]
102. Park, C.J.; Park, C.B.; Hong, S.S.; Lee, H.S.; Lee, S.Y.; Kim, S.C. Characterization and cDNA cloning of two glycine- and histidine-rich antimicrobial peptides from the roots of shepherd's purse, *Capsella. bursa*-pastoris. *Plant. Mol. Biol.* **2000**, *44*, 187–197. [CrossRef]
103. Chang, C.I.; Pleguezuelos, O.; Zhang, Y.A.; Zou, J.; Secombes, C.J. Identification of a novel cathelicidin gene in the rainbow trout, *Oncorhynchus. mykiss*. *Infect. Immun.* **2005**, *73*, 5053–5064. [CrossRef]
104. Bayer, A.; Freund, S.; Jung, G. Post-translational heterocyclic backbone modifications in the 43-peptide antibiotic microcin B17. Structure elucidation and NMR study of a ^{13}C,^{15}N-labelled gyrase inhibitor. *Eur. J. Biochem.* **1995**, *234*, 414–426.
105. Sousa1, J.C.; Berto1, R.F.; Gois, E.A.; Fontenele-Cardi, N.C.; Honório-Júnior, J.E.; Konno, K.; Richardson, M.; Rocha, M.F.; Camargo, A.A.; Pimenta, D.C.; *et al.* Leptoglycin: A new Glycine/Leucine-rich antimicrobial peptide isolated from the skin secretion of the South American frog *Leptodactylus. pentadactylus* (Leptodactylidae). *Toxicon* **2009**, *54*, 23–32. [CrossRef]

106. Couillault, C.; Pujol, N.; Reboul, J.; Sabatier, L.; Guichou, J.F.; Kohara, Y.; Ewbank, J.J. TLR-independent control of innate immunity in Caenorhabditis elegans by the TIR domain adaptor protein TIR-1, an ortholog of human SARM. *Nat. Immunol.* **2004**, *5*, 488–494. [CrossRef]
107. Hao, X.; Yang, H.; Wei, L.; Yang, S.; Zhu, W.; Ma, D.; Yu, H.; Lai, R. Amphibian cathelicidin fills the evolutionary gap of cathelicidin in vertebrate. *Amino Acids* **2012**, *43*, 677–685. [CrossRef]
108. Lorenzini, D.M.; da Silva, P.I., Jr.; Fogaça, A.C.; Bulet, P.; Daffre, S. Acanthoscurrin: A novel glycine-rich antimicrobial peptide constitutively expressed in the hemocytes of the spider *Acanthoscurria. gomesiana. Dev. Comp. Immunol.* **2003**, *27*, 781–791. [CrossRef]
109. Zeng, Y. Procambarin: A glycine-rich peptide found in the haemocytes of red swamp crayfish Procambarus clarkii and its response to white spot syndrome virus challenge. *Fish. Shellfish Immunol.* **2013**, *35*, 407–412. [CrossRef]
110. Lee, S.Y.; Moon, H.J.; Kurata, S.; Natori, S.; Lee, B.L. Purification and cDNA cloning of an antifungal protein from the hemolymph of *Holotrichia. diomphalia* larvae. *Biol. Pharm. Bull.* **1995**, *18*, 1049–1052. [CrossRef]
111. Hiemstra, P.S.; van den Barselaar, M.T.; Roest, M.; Nibbering, P.H.; van Furth, R. Ubiquicidin, a novel murine microbicidal protein present in the cytosolic fraction of macrophages. *J. Leukoc. Biol.* **1999**, *66*, 423–428.
112. Linde, C.M.; Grundström, S.; Nordling, E.; Refai, E.; Brennan, P.J.; Andersson, M. Conserved structure and function in the granulysin and NK-lysin peptide family. *Infect. Immun.* **2005**, *73*, 6332–6339. [CrossRef]
113. Drannik, A.G.; Nag, K.; Sallenave, J.M.; Rosenthal, K.L. *Antiviral activity of trappin-2 and elafin in vitro* and *in vivo* against genital herpes. *J. Virol.* **2013**, *87*, 7526–7538. [CrossRef]
114. Strub, J.M.; Garcia-Sablone, P.; Lonning, K.; Taupenot, L.; Hubert, P.; van Dorsselaer, A.; Aunis, D.; Metz-Boutigue, M.H. Processing of chromogranin B in bovine adrenal medulla. Identification of secretolytin, the endogenous C-terminal fragment of residues 614–626 with antibacterial activity. *Eur. J. Biochem.* **1995**, *229*, 356–368. [CrossRef]
115. Lugardon, K.; Raffner, R.; Goumon, Y.; Corti, A.; Delmas, A.; Bulet, P.; Aunis, D.; Metz-Boutigue, M.H. Antibacterial and antifungal activities of vasostatin-1, the N-terminal fragment of chromogranin A. *J. Biol. Chem.* **2000**, *275*, 10745–10753.
116. Briolat, J.; Wu, S.D.; Mahata, S.K.; Gonthier, B.; Bagnard, D.; Chasserot-Golaz, S.; Helle, K.B.; Aunis, D.; Metz-Boutigue, M.H. New antimicrobial activity for the catecholamine release-inhibitory peptide from chromogranin A. *Cell. Mol. Life Sci.* **2005**, *62*, 377–385. [CrossRef]
117. Goumon, Y.; Strub, J.M.; Moniatte, M.; Nullans, G.; Poteur, L.; Hubert, P.; van Dorsselaer, A.; Aunis, D.; Metz-Boutigue, M.H. The C-terminal bisphosphorylated proenkephalin-A-(209-237)-peptide from adrenal medullary chromaffin granules possesses antibacterial activity. *Eur. J. Biochem.* **1996**, *235*, 516–525.
118. Vindrola, O.; Padrós, M.R.; Sterin-Prync, A.; Ase, A.; Finkielman, S.; Nahmod, V. Proenkephalin system in human polymorphonuclear cells. Production and release of a novel 1.0-kD peptide derived from synenkephalin. *J. Clin. Invest.* **1990**, *86*, 531–537. [CrossRef]
119. Metz-Boutigue, M.H.; Goumon, Y.; Strub, J.M.; Lugardon, K.; Aunis, D. Antimicrobial chromogranins and proenkephalin-A-derived peptides. *Ann. N. Y. Acad. Sci.* **2003**, *992*, 168–178.
120. Shimizu, M.; Shigeri, Y.; Tatsu, Y.; Yoshikawa, S.; Yumoto, N. Enhancement of antimicrobial activity of neuropeptide Y by N-terminal truncation. *Antimicrob. Agents Chemother.* **1998**, *42*, 2745–2746.
121. Hansen, C.J.; Burnell, K.K.; Brogden, K.A. Antimicrobial activity of Substance P and Neuropeptide Y against laboratory strains of bacteria and oral microorganisms. *J. Neuroimmunol.* **2006**, *177*, 215–218. [CrossRef]
122. Allaker, R.P.; Zihni, C.; Kapas, S. An investigation into the antimicrobial effects of adrenomedullin on members of the skin, oral, respiratory tract and gut microflora. *FEMS Immunol. Med. Microbiol.* **1999**, *23*, 289–293. [CrossRef]
123. Chu, H.; Pazgier, M.; Jung, G.; Nuccio, S.P.; Castillo, P.A.; de Jong, M.F.; Winter, M.G.; Winter, S.E.; Wehkamp, J.; Shen, B.; *et al.* Human α-defensin 6 promotes mucosal innate immunity through self-assembled peptide nanonets. *Science* **2012**, *337*, 477–481. [CrossRef]
124. Wada, A.; Wong, P.F.; Hojo, H.; Hasegawa, M.; Ichinose, A.; Llanes, R.; Kubo, Y.; Senba, M.; Ichinose, Y. Alarin but not its alternative-splicing form, GALP (Galanin-like peptide) has antimicrobial activity. *Biochem. Biophys. Res. Commun.* **2013**, *434*, 223–227. [CrossRef]
125. Brogden, K.A.; Guthmiller, J.M.; Salzet, M.; Zasloff, M. The nervous system and innate immunity: The neuropeptide connection. *Nat. Immunol.* **2005**, *6*, 558–564.

126. Khemtémourian, L.; Killian, J.A.; Höppener, J.W.; Engel, M.F. Recent insights in islet amyloid polypeptide-induced membrane disruption and its role in beta-cell death in type 2 diabetes mellitus. *Exp. Diabetes Res.* **2008**, *2008*, 421287.
127. Shahnawaz, M.; Soto, C. Microcin amyloid fibrils A are reservoir of toxic oligomeric species. *J. Biol. Chem.* **2012**, *287*, 11665–11676. [CrossRef]
128. Domachowske, J.B.; Bonville, C.A.; Dyer, K.D.; Rosenberg, H.F. Evolution of antiviral activity in the ribonuclease A gene superfamily: Evidence for a specific interaction between eosinophil-derived neurotoxin (EDN/RNase 2) and respiratory syncytial virus. *Nucleic Acids Res.* **1998**, *26*, 5327–5332. [CrossRef]
129. Pulido, D.; Torrent, M.; Andreu, D.; Nogués, M.V.; Boix, E. Two human host defense ribonucleases against mycobacteria, the eosinophil cationic protein (RNase 3) and RNase 7. *Antimicrob. Agents Chemother.* **2013**, *57*, 3797–3805. [CrossRef]
130. Huang, Y.C.; Lin, Y.M.; Chang, T.W.; Wu, S.J.; Lee, Y.S.; Chang, M.D.; Chen, C.; Wu, S.H.; Liao, Y.D. The flexible and clustered lysine residues of human ribonuclease 7 are critical for membrane permeability and antimicrobial activity. *J. Biol. Chem.* **2007**, *282*, 4626–4633. [CrossRef]
131. Spencer, J.D.; Schwaderer, A.L.; Dirosario, J.D.; McHugh, K.M.; McGillivary, G.; Justice, S.S.; Carpenter, A.R.; Baker, P.B.; Harder, J.; Hains, D.S. Ribonuclease 7 is a potent antimicrobial peptide within the human urinary tract. *Kidney Int.* **2011**, *80*, 174–180. [CrossRef]
132. Spencer, J.D.; Schwaderer, A.L.; Wang, H.; Bartz, J.; Kline, J.; Eichler, T.; DeSouza, K.R.; Sims-Lucas, S.; Baker, P.; Hains, D.S. Ribonuclease 7, an antimicrobial peptide upregulated during infection, contributes to microbial defense of the human urinary tract. *Kidney Int.* **2013**, *83*, 615–625.
133. Nielsen, K.L.; Dynesen, P.; Larsen, P.; Jakobsen, L.; Andersen, P.S.; Frimodt-Møller, N. Role of urinary cathelicidin LL-37 and human β-defensin 1 in uncomplicated *Escherichia coli* urinary tractinfections. *Infect Immun.* **2014**, *82*, 1572–1578. [CrossRef]
134. Chromek, M.; Slamová, Z.; Bergman, P.; Kovács, L.; Podracká, L.; Ehrén, I.; Hökfelt, T.; Gudmundsson, G.H.; Gallo, R.L.; Agerberth, B.; *et al.* The antimicrobial peptide cathelicidin protects the urinary tract against invasive bacterial infection. *Nat. Med.* **2006**, *12*, 636–641. [CrossRef]
135. Becknell, B.; Spencer, J.D.; Carpenter, A.R.; Chen, X.; Singh, A.; Ploeger, S.; Kline, J.; Ellsworth, P.; Li, B.; Proksch, E.; *et al.* Expression and antimicrobial function of beta-defensin 1 in the lower urinary tract. *PLoS One.* **2013**, *8*, e77714.
136. Wiedłocha, A. Following angiogenin during angiogenesis: A journey from the cell surface to the nucleolus. *Arch. Immunol. Ther. Exp. (Warsz)* **1999**, *47*, 299–305.
137. Avdeeva, S.V.; Chernukha, M.U.; Shaginyan, I.A.; Tarantul, V.Z.; Naroditsky, B.S. Human angiogenin lacks specific antimicrobial activity. *Curr. Microbiol.* **2006**, *53*, 477–478. [CrossRef]
138. Rudolph, B.; Podschun, R.; Sahly, H.; Schubert, S.; Schröder, J.M.; Harder, J. Identification of RNase 8 as a novel human antimicrobial protein. *Antimicrob. Agents Chemother.* **2006**, *50*, 3194–3196. [CrossRef]
139. Boix, E.; Torrent, M.; Sánchez, D.; Nogués, M.V. The antipathogen activities of eosinophil cationic protein. *Curr. Pharm. Biotechnol.* **2008**, *9*, 141–152. [CrossRef]
140. Hoffmann, H.J.; Olsen, E.; Etzerodt, M.; Madsen, P.; Thøgersen, H.C.; Kruse, T.; Celis, J.E. Psoriasin binds calcium and is upregulated by calcium to levels that resemble those observed in normal skin. *J. Invest. Dermatol.* **1994**, *103*, 370–375.
141. Porre, S.; Heinonen, S.; Mäntyjärvi, R.; Rytkönen-Nissinen, M.; Perola, O.; Rautiainen, J.; Virtanen, T. Psoriasin, a calcium-binding protein with chemotactic properties is present in the third trimester amniotic fluid. *Mol. Hum. Reprod.* **2005**, *11*, 87–92. [CrossRef]
142. Ostergaard, M.; Rasmussen, H.H.; Nielsen, H.V.; Vorum, H.; Orntoft, T.F.; Wolf, H.; Celis, J.E. Proteome profiling of bladder squamous cell carcinomas: Identification of markers that define their degree of differentiation. *Cancer Res.* **1997**, *57*, 4111–4117.
143. Narushima, Y.; Unno, M.; Nakagawara, K.; Mori, M.; Miyashita, H.; Suzuki, Y.; Noguchi, N.; Takasawa, S.; Kumagai, T.; Yonekura, H.; *et al.* Structure, chromosomal localization and expression of mouse genes encoding type III Reg, RegIII α, RegIII β, RegIII γ. *Gene* **1997**, *185*, 159–168. [CrossRef]
144. Feng, Y.; Huang, N.; Wu, Q.; Wang, B. HMGN2: A novel antimicrobial effector molecule of human mononuclear leukocytes? *J. Leukoc. Biol.* **2005**, *78*, 1136–1141. [CrossRef]

145. Domachowske, J.B.; Dyer, K.D.; Bonville, C.A.; Rosenberg, H.F. Recombinant human eosinophil-derived neurotoxin/RNase 2 functions as an effective antiviral agent against respiratory syncytial virus. *J. Infect. Dis.* **1998**, *177*, 1458–64. [CrossRef]
146. Domachowske, J.B.; Dyer, K.D.; Adams, A.G.; Leto, T.L.; Rosenberg, H.F. Eosinophil cationic protein/RNase 3 is another RNase A-family ribonuclease with direct antiviral activity. *Nucleic Acids Res.* **1998**, *26*, 3358–63. [CrossRef]
147. Shugars, D.C. Endogenous mucosal antiviral factors of the oral cavity. *J. Infect. Dis.* **1999**, *179*, S431–S435. [CrossRef]
148. Wang, W.; Owen, S.M.; Rudolph, D.L.; Cole, A.M.; Hong, T.; Waring, A.J.; Lal, R.B.; Lehrer, R.I. Activity of alpha- and theta-defensins against primary isolates of HIV-1. *J. Immunol.* **2004**, *173*, 515–520. [CrossRef]
149. Dugan, A.S.; Maginnis, M.S.; Jordan, J.A.; Gasparovic, M.L.; Manley, K.; Page, R.; Williams, G.; Porter, E.; O'Hara, B.A.; Atwood, W.J. Human alpha-defensins inhibit BK virus infection by aggregating virions and blocking binding to host cells. *J. Biol. Chem.* **2008**, *283*, 31125–31132. [CrossRef]
150. Quiñones-Mateu, M.E.; Lederman, M.M.; Feng, Z.; Chakraborty, B.; Weber, J.; Rangel, H.R.; Marotta, M.L.; Mirza, M.; Jiang, B.; Kiser, P.; *et al.* Human epithelial beta-defensins 2 and 3 inhibit HIV-1 replication. *AIDS* **2003**, *17*, F39–F48.
151. Bergman, P.; Walter-Jallow, L.; Broliden, K.; Agerberth, B.; Söderlund, J. The antimicrobial peptide LL-37 inhibits HIV-1 replication. *Curr. HIV Res.* **2007**, *5*, 410–415. [CrossRef]
152. Wang, G.; Watson, K.M.; Buckheit, R.W., Jr. Anti-human immunodeficiency virus type 1 activities of antimicrobial peptides derived from human and bovine cathelicidins. *Antimicrob. Agents Chemother.* **2008**, *52*, 3438–3440. [CrossRef]
153. Groot, F.; Sanders, R.W.; ter Brake, O.; Nazmi, K.; Veerman, E.C.; Bolscher, J.G.; Berkhout, B. Histatin 5-derived peptide with improved fungicidal properties enhances human immunodeficiency virus type 1 replication by promoting viral entry. *J. Virol.* **2006**, *80*, 9236–9243. [CrossRef]
154. Wang, G. Natural antimicrobial peptides as promising anti-HIV candidates. *Curr. Topics Peptide Protein Res.* **2012**, *13*, 93–110.
155. López-García, B.; Lee, P.H.; Yamasaki, K.; Gallo, R.L. Anti-fungal activity of cathelicidins and their potential role in Candida albicans skin infection. *J. Invest. Dermatol.* **2005**, *125*, 108–115. [CrossRef]
156. Den Hertog, A.L.; van Marle, J.; Veerman, E.C.; Valentijn-Benz, M.; Nazmi, K.; Kalay, H.; Grün, C.H.; Van't Hof, W.; Bolscher, J.G.; Nieuw Amerongen, A.V. The human cathelicidin peptide LL-37 and truncated variants induce segregation of lipids and proteins in the plasma membrane of *Candida albicans*. *Biol. Chem.* **2006**, *387*, 1495–1502.
157. Dabirian, S.; Taslimi, Y.; Zahedifard, F.; Gholami, E.; Doustdari, F.; Motamedirad, M.; Khatami, S.; Azadmanesh, K.; Nylen, S.; Rafati, S. Human neutrophil peptide-1 (HNP-1): A new anti-leishmanial drug candidate. *PLoS Negl. Trop. Dis.* **2013**, *7*, e2491. [CrossRef]
158. Söbirk, S.K.; Mörgelin, M.; Egesten, A.; Bates, P.; Shannon, O.; Collin, M. Human chemokines as antimicrobial peptides with direct parasiticidal effect on Leishmania mexicana *in vitro*. *PLoS One* **2013**, *8*, e58129.
159. Rico-Mata, R.; De Leon-Rodriguez, L.M.; Avila, E.E. Effect of antimicrobial peptides derived from human cathelicidin LL-37 on Entamoeba histolytica trophozoites. *Exp. Parasitol.* **2013**, *133*, 300–306. [CrossRef]
160. Love, M.S.; Millholland, M.G.; Mishra, S.; Kulkarni, S.; Freeman, K.B.; Pan, W.; Kavash, R.W.; Costanzo, M.J.; Jo, H.; Daly, T.M.; *et al.* Platelet factor 4 activity against P. falciparum and its translation to nonpeptidic mimics as antimalarials. *Cell Host Microbe.* **2012**, *12*, 815–823. [CrossRef]
161. Baker, M.A.; Maloy, W.L.; Zasloff, M.; Jacob, L.S. Anticancer efficacy of Magainin2 and analogue peptides. *Cancer Res.* **1993**, *53*, 3052–3057.
162. Winder, D.; Günzburg, W.H.; Erfle, V.; Salmons, B. Expression of antimicrobial peptides has an antitumour effect in human cells. *Biochem. Biophys. Res. Commun.* **1998**, *242*, 608–612. [CrossRef]
163. Lichtenstein, A.; Ganz, T.; Selsted, M.E.; Lehrer, R.I. *In vitro* tumor cell cytolysis mediated by peptide defensins of human and rabbit granulocytes. *Blood* **1986**, *68*, 1407–1410.
164. Gaspar, D.; Veiga, A.S.; Castanho, M.A. From antimicrobial to anticancer peptides. A review. *Front. Microbiol.* **2013**, *4*, 294.
165. Riedl, S.; Zweytick, D.; Lohner, K. Membrane-active host defense peptides—Challenges and perspectives for the development of novel anticancer drugs. *Chem. Phys. Lipids* **2011**, *164*, 766–781. [CrossRef]

166. Hoskin, D.W.; Ramamoorthy, A. Studies on anticancer activities of antimicrobial peptides. *Biochim. Biophys. Acta* **2008**, *1778*, 357–375.
167. Kishi, A.; Takamori, Y.; Ogawa, K.; Takano, S.; Tomita, S.; Tanigawa, M.; Niman, M.; Kishida, T.; Fujita, S. Differential expression of granulysin and perforin by NK cells in cancer patients and correlation of impaired granulysin expression with progression of cancer. *Cancer Immunol. Immunother.* **2002**, *50*, 604–614. [CrossRef]
168. Sekiguchi, N.; Asano, N.; Ito, T.; Momose, K.; Momose, M.; Ishida, F. Elevated serum granulysin and its clinical relevance in mature NK-cell neoplasms. *Int. J. Hematol.* **2012**, *96*, 461–468. [CrossRef]
169. Xu, N.; Wang, Y.S.; Pan, W.B.; Xiao, B.; Wen, Y.J.; Chen, X.C.; Chen, L.J.; Deng, H.X.; You, J.; Kan, B.; *et al.* Human alpha-defensin-1 inhibits growth of human lung adenocarcinoma xenograft in nude mice. *Mol. Cancer Ther.* **2008**, *7*, 1588–1597. [CrossRef]
170. Mizukawa, N.; Sugiyama, K.; Fukunaga, J.; Ueno, T.; Mishima, K.; Takagi, S.; Sugahara, T. Defensin-1, a peptide detected in the saliva of oral squamous cell carcinoma patients. *Anticancer Res.* **1998**, *18*, 4645–4649.
171. Müller, C.A.; Markovic-Lipkovski, J.; Klatt, T.; Gamper, J.; Schwarz, G.; Beck, H.; Deeg, M.; Kalbacher, H.; Widmann, S.; Wessels, J.T.; *et al.* Human alpha-defensins HNPs-1, -2, and -3 in renal cell carcinoma: Influences on tumor cell proliferation. *Am. J. Pathol.* **2002**, *160*, 1311–1324. [CrossRef]
172. Sun, C.Q.; Arnold, R.; Fernandez-Golarz, C.; Parrish, A.B.; Almekinder, T.; He, J.; Ho, S.M.; Svoboda, P.; Pohl, J.; Marshall, F.F.; *et al.* Human beta-defensin-1, a potential chromosome 8p tumor suppressor: Control of transcription and induction of apoptosis in renal cell carcinoma. *Cancer Res.* **2006**, *66*, 8542–8549.
173. Bullard, R.S.; Gibson, W.; Bose, S.K.; Belgrave, J.K.; Eaddy, A.C.; Wright, C.J.; Hazen-Martin, D.J.; Lage, J.M.; Keane, T.E.; Ganz, T.A.; *et al.* Functional analysis of the host defense peptide Human Beta Defensin-1: New insight into its potential role in cancer. *Mol. Immunol.* **2008**, *45*, 839–848. [CrossRef]
174. Winter, J.; Pantelis, A.; Reich, R.; Martini, M.; Kraus, D.; Jepsen, S.; Allam, J.P.; Novak, N.; Wenghoefer, M. Human beta-defensin-1, -2, and -3 exhibit opposite effects on oral squamous cell carcinoma cell proliferation. *Cancer Invest.* **2011**, *29*, 196–201.
175. Wu, W.K.; Wang, G.; Coffelt, S.B.; Betancourt, A.M.; Lee, C.W.; Fan, D.; Wu, K.; Yu, J.; Sung, J.J.; Cho, C.H. Emerging roles of the host defense peptide LL-37 in human cancer and its potential therapeutic applications. *Int. J. Cancer.* **2010**, *127*, 1741–1747. [CrossRef]
176. van den Broek, I.; Sparidans, R.W.; Engwegen, J.Y.; Cats, A.; Depla, A.C.; Schellens, J.H.; Beijnen, J.H. Evaluation of human neutrophil peptide-1, -2 and -3 as serum markers for colorectal cancer. *Cancer Biomark.* **2010**, *7*, 109–115.
177. Albrethsen, J.; Bøgebo, R.; Gammeltoft, S.; Olsen, J.; Winther, B.; Raskov, H. Upregulated expression of human neutrophil peptides 1, 2 and 3 (HNP 1–3) in colon cancer serum and tumours: A biomarker study. *BMC Cancer* **2005**, *5*, 8. [CrossRef]
178. Albrethsen, J.; Møller, C.H.; Olsen, J.; Raskov, H.; Gammeltoft, S. Human neutrophil peptides 1, 2 and 3 are biochemical markers for metastatic colorectal cancer. *Eur. J. Cancer* **2006**, *42*, 3057–3064. [CrossRef]
179. Li, X.; Li, Y.; Han, H.; Miller, D.W.; Wang, G. Solution structures of human LL-37 fragments and NMR-based identification of a minimal membrane-targeting antimicrobial and anticancer region. *J. Am. Chem. Soc.* **2006**, *128*, 5776–5785. [CrossRef]
180. Ren, S.X.; Shen, J.; Cheng, A.S.; Lu, L.; Chan, R.L.; Li, Z.J.; Wang, X.J.; Wong, C.C.; Zhang, L.; Ng, S.S.; *et al.* FK-16 derived from the anticancer peptide LL-37 induces caspase-independent apoptosis and autophagic cell death in colon cancer cells. *PLoS One* **2013**, *8*, e63641. [CrossRef]
181. Zhou, J.; Shi, J.; Hou, J.; Cao, F.; Zhang, Y.; Rasmussen, J.T.; Heegaard, C.W.; Gilbert, G.E. Phosphatidylserine exposure and procoagulant activity in acute promyelocytic leukemia. *J. Thromb. Haemost.* **2010**, *8*, 773–782. [CrossRef]
182. Wang, G. Structures of human host defense cathelicidin LL-37 and its smallest antimicrobial peptide KR-12 in lipid micelles. *J. Biol. Chem.* **2008**, *283*, 32637–32643.
183. Svensson, D.; Westman, J.; Wickström, C.; Jönsson, D.; Herwald, H.; Nilsson, B.O. Human endogenous peptide p33 inhibits detrimental effects of LL-37 on osteoblast viability. *J. Periodontal Res.* **2014**. [CrossRef]
184. Hiemstra, T.F.; Charles, P.D.; Gracia, T.; Hester, S.S.; Gatto, L.; Al-Lamki, R.; Floto, R.A.; Su, Y.; Skepper, J.N.; Lilley, K.S.; *et al.* Human Urinary Exosomes as Innate Immune Effectors. *J. Am. Soc. Nephrol.* **2014**, in press.
185. Yung, S.C.; Murphy, P.M. Antimicrobial chemokines. *Front Immunol.* **2012**, *3*, 276.

186. Yang, D.; Chen, Q.; Schmidt, A.P.; Anderson, G.M.; Wang, J.M.; Wooters, J.; Oppenheim, J.J.; Chertov, O. LL-37, the neutrophil granule- and epithelial cell-derived cathelicidin, utilizes formyl peptide receptor-like 1 (FPRL1) as a receptor to chemoattract human peripheral blood neutrophils, monocytes, and T cells. *J. Exp. Med.* **2000**, *192*, 1069–1074. [CrossRef]
187. Ciornei, C.D.; Tapper, H.; Bjartell, A.; Sternby, N.H.; Bodelsson, M. Human antimicrobial peptide LL-37 is present in atherosclerotic plaques and induces death of vascular smooth muscle cells: A laboratory study. *BMC Cardiovasc. Disord.* **2006**, *6*, 49. [CrossRef]
188. Barlow, P.G.; Li, Y.; Wilkinson, T.S.; Bowdish, D.M.; Lau, Y.E.; Cosseau, C.; Haslett, C.; Simpson, A.J.; Hancock, R.E.; Davidson, D.J. The human cationic host defense peptide LL-37 mediates contrasting effects on apoptotic pathways in different primary cells of the innate immune system. *J. Leukoc. Biol.* **2006**, *80*, 509–520. [CrossRef]
189. Aarbiou, J.; Tjabringa, G.S.; Verhoosel, R.M.; Ninaber, D.K.; White, S.R.; Peltenburg, L.T.; Rabe, K.F.; Hiemstra, P.S. Mechanisms of cell death induced by the neutrophil antimicrobial peptides alpha-defensins and LL-37. *Inflamm. Res.* **2006**, *55*, 119–127. [CrossRef]
190. Okumura, K.; Itoh, A.; Isogai, E.; Hirose, K.; Hosokawa, Y.; Abiko, Y.; Shibata, T.; Hirata, M.; Isogai, H. C-terminal domain of human CAP18 antimicrobial peptide induces apoptosis in oral squamous cell carcinoma SAS-H1 cells. *Cancer Lett.* **2004**, *212*, 185–194. [CrossRef]
191. Ciornei, C.D.; Egesten, A.; Bodelsson, M. Effects of human cathelicidin antimicrobial peptide LL-37 on lipopolysaccharide-induced nitric oxide release from rat aorta *in vitro*. *Acta Anaesthesiol. Scand.* **2003**, *47*, 213–220. [CrossRef]
192. Chamorro, C.I.; Weber, G.; Grönberg, A.; Pivarcsi, A.; Ståhle, M. The human antimicrobial peptide LL-37 suppresses apoptosis *in* keratinocytes. *J. Invest. Dermatol.* **2009**, *129*, 937–944. [CrossRef]
193. Nagaoka, I.; Tamura, H.; Hirata, M. An antimicrobial cathelicidin peptide, human CAP18/LL-37, suppresses neutrophil apoptosis via the activation of formyl-peptide receptor-like 1 and P2X7. *J. Immunol.* **2006**, *176*, 3044–3052. [CrossRef]
194. Lee, W.Y.; Savage, J.R.; Zhang, J.; Jia, W.; Oottamasathien, S.; Prestwich, G.D. Prevention of anti-microbial peptide LL-37-induced apoptosis and ATP release in the urinary bladder by a modified glycosaminoglycan. *PLoS One* **2013**, *8*, e77854.
195. Suzuki, K.; Murakami, T.; Kuwahara-Arai, K.; Tamura, H.; Hiramatsu, K.; Nagaoka, I. Human anti-microbial cathelicidin peptide LL-37 suppresses the LPS-induced apoptosis of endothelial cells. *Int. Immunol.* **2011**, *23*, 185–193. [CrossRef]
196. Ren, S.X.; Cheng, A.S.; To, K.F.; Tong, J.H.; Li, M.S.; Shen, J.; Wong, C.C.; Zhang, L.; Chan, R.L.; Wang, X.J.; *et al.* Host immune defense peptide LL-37 activates caspase-independent apoptosis and suppresses colon cancer. *Cancer Res.* **2012**, *72*, 6512–6523. [CrossRef]
197. Oudhoff, M.J.; Blaauboer, M.E.; Nazmi, K.; Scheres, N.; Bolscher, J.G.; Veerman, E.C. The role of salivary histatin and the human cathelicidin LL-37 in wound healing and innate immunity. *Biol. Chem.* **2010**, *391*, 541–548.
198. Wang, G. NMR of membrane-associated peptides and proteins. *Curr. Protein Pept. Sci.* **2008**, *9*, 50–69. [CrossRef]
199. Wang, G. NMR of membrane proteins. In "Advances in Protein and Peptide Sciences" (edited by Dunn BM). *Bentham Sci.* **2013**, *1*, 128–188.
200. Nguyen, L.T.; Haney, E.F.; Vogel, H.J. The expanding scope of antimicrobial peptide structures and their modes of action. *Trends Biotechnol.* **2011**, *29*, 464–472. [CrossRef]
201. Wang, G.; Li, X.; Zasloff, M. A Database View of Natural Antimicrobial Peptides: Nomenclature, Classification and Amino acid Sequence Analysis. In *Antimicrobial Peptides: Discovery, Design and Novel Therapeutic Strategies*; Wang, G., Ed.; CABI: Wallingford, UK, 2010; pp. 1–21.
202. Rose, P.W.; Bi, C.; Bluhm, W.F.; Christie, C.H.; Dimitropoulos, D.; Dutta, S.; Green, R.K.; Goodsell, D.S.; Prlic, A.; Quesada, M.; *et al.* The RCSB Protein Data Bank: New resources for research and education. *Nucleic Acids Res.* **2013**, *41*, D475–D482. [CrossRef]
203. Xu, T.; Levitz, S.M.; Diamond, R.D.; Oppenheim, F.G. Anticandidal activity of major human salivary histatins. *Infect. Immun.* **1991**, *59*, 2549–2554.
204. Raj, P.A.; Edgerton, M.; Levine, M.J. Salivary histatin 5: Dependence of sequence, chain length, and helical conformation for candidacidal activity. *J. Biol. Chem.* **1990**, *265*, 3898–3905.

205. Rothstein, D.M.; Spacciapoli, P.; Tran, L.T.; Xu, T.; Roberts, F.D.; Dalla Serra, M.; Buxton, D.K.; Oppenheim, F.G.; Friden, P. Anticandida activity is retained in P-113, a 12-amino-acid fragment of histatin 5. *Antimicrob. Agents Chemother.* **2001**, *45*, 1367–1373. [CrossRef]
206. Zuo, Y.; Xu, T.; Troxler, R.F.; Li, J.; Driscoll, J.; Oppenheim, F.G. Recombinant histatins: Functional domain duplication enhances candidacidal activity. *Gene* **1995**, *161*, 87–91. [CrossRef]
207. Situ, H.; Tsai, H.; Bobek, L.A. Construction and characterization of human salivary histatin-5 multimers. *J. Dent. Res.* **1999**, *78*, 690–698. [CrossRef]
208. Situ, H.; Balasubramanian, S.V.; Bobek, L.A. Role of alpha-helical conformation of histatin-5 in candidacidal activity examined by proline variants. *Biochim. Biophys. Acta* **2000**, *1475*, 377–382. [CrossRef]
209. Melino, S.; Rufini, S.; Sette, M.; Morero, R.; Grottesi, A.; Paci, M.; Petruzzelli, R. Zn^{2+} ions selectively induce antimicrobial salivary peptide histatin-5 to fuse negatively charged vesicles. Identification and characterization of a zinc-binding motif present in the functional domain. *Biochemistry* **1999**, *38*, 9626–9633. [CrossRef]
210. Rydengård, V.; Andersson Nordahl, E.; Schmidtchen, A. Zinc potentiates the antibacterial effects of histidine-rich peptides against *Enterococcus faecalis*. *FEBS J.* **2006**, *273*, 2399–2406. [CrossRef]
211. Melino, S.; Gallo, M.; Trotta, E.; Mondello, F.; Paci, M.; Petruzzelli, R. Metal-binding and nuclease activity of an antimicrobial peptide analogue of the salivary histatin 5. *Biochemistry* **2006**, *45*, 15373–15383. [CrossRef]
212. Wang, G. Structural studies of antimicrobial peptides provide insight into their mechanisms of action. In *Antimicrobial Peptides: Discovery, Design and Novel Therapeutic Strategies*; Wang, G., Ed.; CABI: Wallingford, UK, 2010; pp. 141–168.
213. Xhindoli, D.; Pacor, S.; Guida, F.; Antcheva, N.; Tossi, A. Native oligomerization determines the mode of action and biological activities of human cathelicidin LL-37. *Biochem. J.* **2014**, *457*, 263–275. [CrossRef]
214. Wang, G.; Elliott, M.; Cogen, A.L.; Ezell, E.L.; Gallo, R.L.; Hancock, R.E.W. Structure, dynamics, antimicrobial and immune modulatory activities of human LL-23 and its single residue variants mutated based on homologous primate cathelicidins. *Biochemistry* **2012**, *51*, 653–664. [CrossRef]
215. Paulmann, M.; Arnold, T.; Linke, D.; Özdirekcan, S.; Kopp, A.; Gutsmann, T.; Kalbacher, H.; Wanke, I.; Schuenemann, V.J.; Habeck, M.; *et al.* Structure-activity analysis of the dermcidin-derived peptide DCD-1L, an anionic antimicrobial peptide present in human sweat. *J. Biol. Chem.* **2012**, *287*, 8434–8443. [CrossRef]
216. Song, C.; Weichbrodt, C.; Salnikov, E.S.; Dynowski, M.; Forsberg, B.O.; Bechinger, B.; Steinem, C.; de Groot, B.L.; Zachariae, U.; Zeth, K. Crystal structure and functional mechanism of a human antimicrobial membrane channel. *Proc. Natl. Acad. Sci. USA* **2013**, *110*, 4586–4591. [CrossRef]
217. Jung, H.H.; Yang, S.T.; Sim, J.Y.; Lee, S.; Lee, J.Y.; Kim, H.H.; Shin, S.Y.; Kim, J.I. Analysis of the solution structure of the human antibiotic peptide dermcidin and its interaction with phospholipid vesicles. *BMB Rep.* **2010**, *43*, 362–368. [CrossRef]
218. Koradi, R.; Billeter, M.; Wüthrich, K. MOLMOL: A program for display and analysis of macromolecular structures. *J. Mol. Graph.* **1996**, *14*, 51–55. [CrossRef]
219. Anderson, D.H.; Sawaya, M.R.; Cascio, D.; Ernst, W.; Modlin, R.; Krensky, A.; Eisenberg, D. Granulysin crystal structure and a structure-derived lytic mechanism. *J. Mol. Biol.* **2003**, *325*, 355–365.
220. Peña, S.V.; Krensky, A.M. Granulysin, a new human cytolytic granule-associated protein with possible involvement in cell-mediated cytotoxicity. *Semin. Immunol.* **1997**, *9*, 117–125. [CrossRef]
221. Bruhn, H. A short guided tour through functional and structural features of saposin-like proteins. *Biochem. J.* **2005**, *389*, (Pt 2). 249–257.
222. da Silva, A.P.; Unks, D.; Lyu, S.C.; Ma, J.; Zbozien-Pacamaj, R.; Chen, X.; Krensky, A.M.; Clayberger, C. *In vitro* and *in vivo* antimicrobial activity of granulysin-derived peptides against Vibrio cholerae. *J. Antimicrob Chemother.* **2008**, *61*, 1103–1109. [CrossRef]
223. McInturff, J.E.; Wang, S.J.; Machleidt, T.; Lin, T.R.; Oren, A.; Hertz, C.J.; Krutzik, S.R.; Hart, S.; Zeh, K.; Anderson, D.H.; *et al.* Granulysin-derived peptides demonstrate antimicrobial and anti-inflammatory effects against *Propionibacterium. acnes*. *J. Invest. Dermatol.* **2005**, *125*, 256–263.
224. Ericksen, B.; Wu, Z.; Lu, W.; Lehrer, R.I. Antibacterial activity and specificity of the six human α-defensins. *Antimicrob. Agents Chemother.* **2005**, *49*, 269–275. [CrossRef]
225. Schibli, D.J.; Hunter, H.N.; Aseyev, V.; Starner, T.D.; Wiencek, J.M.; McCray PB, Jr.; Tack, B.F.; Vogel, H.J. The solution structures of the human beta-defensins lead to a better understanding of the potent bactericidal activity of HBD3 against *Staphylococcus aureus*. *J. Biol. Chem.* **2002**, *277*, 8279–8289. [CrossRef]

226. Schroeder, B.O.; Wu, Z.; Nuding, S.; Groscurth, S.; Marcinowski, M.; Beisner, J.; Buchner, J.; Schaller, M.; Stange, E.F.; Wehkamp, J. Reduction of disulphide bonds unmasks potent antimicrobial activity of human β-defensin 1. *Nature* **2011**, *469*, 419–423. [CrossRef]
227. Keizer, D.W.; Crump, M.P.; Lee, T.W.; Slupsky, C.M.; Clark-Lewis, I.; Sykes, B.D. Human CC chemokine I-309, structural consequences of the additional disulfide bond. *Biochemistry* **2000**, *39*, 6053–6059. [CrossRef]
228. Blaszczyk, J.; Coillie, E.V.; Proost, P.; Damme, J.V.; Opdenakker, G.; Bujacz, G.D.; Wang, J.M.; Ji, X. Complete crystal structure of monocyte chemotactic protein-2, a CC chemokine that interacts with multiple receptors. *Biochemistry* **2000**, *39*, 14075–14081.
229. Crump, M.P.; Rajarathnam, K.; Kim, K.S.; Clark-Lewis, I.; Sykes, B.D. Solution structure of eotaxin, a chemokine that selectively recruits eosinophils in allergic inflammation. *J. Biol. Chem.* **1998**, *273*, 22471–22479.
230. Love, M.; Sandberg, J.L.; Ziarek, J.J.; Gerarden, K.P.; Rode, R.R.; Jensen, D.R.; McCaslin, D.R.; Peterson, F.C.; Veldkamp, C.T. Solution structure of CCL21 and identification of a putative CCR7 binding site. *Biochemistry* **2012**, *51*, 733–735.
231. Jansma, A.L.; Kirkpatrick, J.P.; Hsu, A.R.; Handel, T.M.; Nietlispach, D. NMR analysis of the structure, dynamics, and unique oligomerization properties of the chemokine CCL27. *J. Biol. Chem.* **2010**, *285*, 14424–14437.
232. Veldkamp, C.T.; Ziarek, J.J.; Su, J.; Basnet, H.; Lennertz, R.; Weiner, J.J.; Peterson, F.C.; Baker, J.E.; Volkman, B.F. Monomeric structure of the cardioprotective chemokine SDF-1/CXCL12. *Protein Sci.* **2009**, *18*, 1359–1369.
233. Hoover, D.M.; Boulegue, C.; Yang, D.; Oppenheim, J.J.; Tucker, K.; Lu, W.; Lubkowski, J. The structure of human macrophage inflammatory protein-3alpha/CCL20. Linking antimicrobial and CC chemokine receptor-6-binding activities with human beta-defensins. *J. Biol. Chem.* **2002**, *277*, 37647–37654.
234. Barinka, C.; Prahl, A.; Lubkowski, J. Structure of human monocyte chemoattractant protein 4 (MCP-4/CCL13). *Acta. Crystallogr. D Biol. Crystallogr.* **2008**, *64*, (Pt 3). 273–278. [CrossRef]
235. Kim, K.S.; Clark-Lewis, I.; Sykes, B.D. Solution structure of GRO/melanoma growth stimulatory activity determined by ^{1}H-NMR spectroscopy. *J. Biol. Chem.* **1994**, *269*, 32909–32915.
236. Swaminathan, G.J.; Holloway, D.E.; Colvin, R.A.; Campanella, G.K.; Papageorgiou, A.C.; Luster, A.D.; Acharya, K.R. Crystal structures of oligomeric forms of the IP-10/CXCL-10 chemokine. *Structure* **2003**, *11*, 521–532. [CrossRef]
237. Yung, S.C.; Parenti, D.; Murphy, P.M. Host chemokines bind to *Staphylococcus aureus* and stimulate protein A release. *J. Biol. Chem.* **2011**, *286*, 5069–5077. [CrossRef]
238. Nguyen, L.T.; Kwakman, P.H.; Chan, D.I.; Liu, Z.; de Boer, L.; Zaat, S.A.; Vogel, H.J. Exploring platelet chemokine antimicrobial activity: Nuclear magnetic resonance backbone dynamics of NAP-2 and TC-1. *Antimicrob. Agents Chemother.* **2011**, *55*, 2074–2083. [CrossRef]
239. Wang, G.; Epand, R.F.; Mishra, B.; Lushnikova, T.; Thomas, V.C.; Bayles, K.W.; Epand, R.M. Decoding the functional roles of cationic side chains of the major antimicrobial region of human cathelicidin LL-37. *Antimicrob. Agents Chemother.* **2012**, *56*, 845–856. [CrossRef]
240. Lequin, O.; Thüring, H.; Robin, M.; Lallemand, J.Y. Three-dimensional solution structure of human angiogenin determined by ^{1}H,^{15}N-NMR spectroscopy–characterization of histidine protonation states and pKa values. *Eur. J. Biochem.* **1997**, *250*, 712–726.
241. Wang, H.; Schwaderer, A.L.; Kline, J.; Spencer, J.D.; Kline, D.; Hains, D.S. Contribution of structural domains to the activity of ribonuclease 7 against uropathogenic bacteria. *Antimicrob. Agents Chemother.* **2013**, *57*, 766–774. [CrossRef]
242. Torrent, M.; Pulido, D.; Valle, J.; Nogués, M.V.; Andreu, D.; Boix, E. Ribonucleases as a host-defence family: Evidence of evolutionarily conserved antimicrobial activity at the N-terminus. *Biochem. J.* **2013**, *456*, 99–108. [CrossRef]
243. Boix, E.; Salazar, V.A.; Torrent, M.; Pulido, D.; Nogués, M.V.; Moussaoui, M. Structural determinants of the eosinophil cationic protein antimicrobial activity. *Biol. Chem.* **2012**, *393*, 801–815.
244. Spencer, J.D.; Schwaderer, A.L.; Eichler, T.; Wang, H.; Kline, J.; Justice, S.S.; Cohen, D.M.; Hains, D.S. An endogenous ribonuclease inhibitor regulates the antimicrobial activity of ribonuclease 7 in the human urinary tract. *Kidney Int.* **2013**, *85*, 1179–1191.
245. Lehotzky, R.E.; Partch, C.L.; Mukherjee, S.; Cash, H.L.; Goldman, W.E.; Gardner, K.H.; Hooper, L.V. Molecular basis for peptidoglycan recognition by a bactericidal lectin. *Proc. Natl. Acad. Sci. USA* **2010**, *107*, 7722–7727.

246. Mukherjee, S.; Zheng, H.; Derebe, M.G.; Callenberg, K.M.; Partch, C.L.; Rollins, D.; Propheter, D.C.; Rizo, J.; Grabe, M.; Jiang, Q.X.; *et al.* Antibacterial membrane attack by a pore-forming intestinal C-type lectin. *Nature* **2013**, *505*, 103–107. [CrossRef]
247. De Leeuw, E.; Li, C.; Zeng, P.; Li, C.; Diepeveen-de Buin, M.; Lu, W.Y.; Breukink, E.; Lu, W. Functional interaction of human neutrophil peptide-1 with the cell wall precursor lipid II. *FEBS Lett.* **2010**, *584*, 1543–1548. [CrossRef]
248. Böhling, A.; Hagge, S.O.; Roes, S.; Podschun, R.; Sahly, H.; Harder, J.; Schröder, J.M.; Grötzinger, J.; Seydel, U.; Gutsmann, T. Lipid-specific membrane activity of human beta-defensin-3. *Biochemistry* **2006**, *45*, 5663–5670. [CrossRef]
249. Sass, V.; Schneider, T.; Wilmes, M.; Körner, C.; Tossi, A.; Novikova, N.; Shamova, O.; Sahl, H.G. Human beta-defensin 3 inhibits cell wall biosynthesis in Staphylococci. *Infect. Immun.* **2010**, *78*, 2793–2800. [CrossRef]
250. Schmitt, P.; Wilmes, M.; Pugnière, M.; Aumelas, A.; Bachère, E.; Sahl, H.G.; Schneider, T.; Destoumieux-Garzón, D. Insight into invertebrate defensin mechanism of action: Oyster defensins inhibit peptidoglycan biosynthesis by binding to lipid II. *Biol. Chem.* **2010**, *285*, 29208–29216. [CrossRef]
251. Bierbaum, G.; Sahl, H.G. Lantibiotics: Mode of action, biosynthesis and bioengineering. *Curr. Pharm. Biotechnol.* **2009**, *10*, 2–18. [CrossRef]
252. Schneider, T.; Kruse, T.; Wimmer, R.; Wiedemann, I.; Sass, V.; Pag, U.; Jansen, A.; Nielsen, A.K.; Mygind, P.H.; Raventós, D.S.; *et al.* Plectasin, a fungal defensin, targets the bacterial cell wall precursor Lipid II. *Science* **2010**, *328*, 1168–1172. [CrossRef]
253. Derouaux, A.; Turk, S.; Olrichs, N.K.; Gobec, S.; Breukink, E.; Amoroso, A.; Offant, J.; Bostock, J.; Mariner, K.; Chopra, I.; *et al.* Small molecule inhibitors of peptidoglycan synthesis targeting the lipid II precursor. *Biochem. Pharmacol.* **2011**, *81*, 1098–1105. [CrossRef]
254. Varney, K.M.; Bonvin, A.M.; Pazgier, M.; Malin, J.; Yu, W.; Ateh, E.; Oashi, T.; Lu, W.; Huang, J.; Diepeveen-de Buin, M.; *et al.* Turning Defense into Offense: Defensin Mimetics as Novel Antibiotics Targeting Lipid II. *PLoS Pathog.* **2013**, *9*, e1003732. [CrossRef]
255. Poon, I.K.h.; Baxter, A.A.; Lay, F.T.; Mills, G.D.; Adda, C.G.; Payne, J.A.; Phan, T.K.; Ryan, G.F.; White, J.A.; Veneer, P.K.; *et al.* Phosphoinositide-mediated oligomerization of a defensin induces cell lysis. *Elife* **2014**, *3*, e01808. [CrossRef]
256. Silva, P.M.; Gonçalves, S.; Santos, N.C. Defensins: Antifungal lessons from eukaryotes. *Front. Microbiol.* **2014**, *5*, 97.
257. Sagaram, U.S.; El-Mounadi, K.; Buchko, G.W.; Berg, H.R.; Kaur, J.; Pandurangi, R.S.; Smith, T.J.; Shah, D.M. Structural and functional studies of a phosphatidic acid-binding antifungal plant defensin MtDef4: identification of an RGFRRR motif governing fungal cell entry. *PLoS One.* **2013**, *8*, e82485. [CrossRef]
258. Miki, T.; Holst, O.; Hardt, W.D. The bactericidal activity of the C-type lectin RegIIIβ against Gram-negative bacteria involves binding to lipid A. *J. Biol. Chem.* **2012**, *287*, 34844–34855. [CrossRef]
259. Formanek, H. A three dimensional model of the digestion of peptidoglycan by lysozyme. *Biophys. Struct. Mech.* **1977**, *4*, 1–14. [CrossRef]
260. Ma, G.; Greenwell-Wild, T.; Lei, K.; Jin, W.; Swisher, J.; Hardegen, N.; Wild, C.T.; Wahl, S.M. Secretory leukocyte protease inhibitor binds to annexin II, a cofactor for macrophage HIV-1 infection. *J. Exp. Med.* **2004**, *200*, 1337–1346. [CrossRef]
261. Oren, Z.; Lerman, J.C.; Gudmundsson, G.H.; Agerberth, B.; Shai, Y. Structure and organization of the human antimicrobial peptide LL-37 in phospholipid membranes: Relevance to the molecular basis for its non-cell-selective activity. *Biochem. J.* **1999**, *341*, (Pt. 3). 501–513.
262. Lee, C.C.; Sun, Y.; Qian, S.; Huang, H.W. Transmembrane pores formed by human antimicrobial peptide LL-37. *Biophys. J.* **2011**, *100*, 1688–1696. [CrossRef]
263. Maisetta, G.; Vitali, A.; Scorciapino, M.A.; Rinaldi, A.C.; Petruzzelli, R.; Brancatisano, F.L.; Esin, S.; Stringaro, A.; Colone, M.; Luzi, C.; *et al.* pH-dependent disruption of *Escherichia coli* ATCC 25922 and model membranes by the human antimicrobial peptides hepcidin 20 and 25. *FEBS J.* **2013**, *280*, 2842–2854. [CrossRef]
264. Natividad, J.M.; Hayes, C.L.; Motta, J.P.; Jury, J.; Galipeau, H.J.; Philip, V.; Garcia-Rodenas, C.L.; Kiyama, H.; Bercik, P.; Verdu, E.F. Differential Induction of Antimicrobial REGIII by the Intestinal Microbiota and Bifidobacterium breve NCC2950. *Appl. Environ. Microbiol.* **2013**, *79*, 7745–7754. [CrossRef]

265. Parker, M.W.; Feil, S.C. Pore-forming protein toxins: From structure to function. *Prog. Biophys. Mol. Biol.* **2005**, *88*, 91–142. [CrossRef]
266. Birck, C.; Damian, L.; Marty-Detraves, C.; Lougarre, A.; Schulze-Briese, C.; Koehl, P.; Fournier, D.; Paquereau, L.; Samama, J.P. A new lectin family with structure similarity to actinoporins revealed by the crystal structure of Xerocomus chrysenteron lectin XCL. *J. Mol. Biol.* **2004**, *344*, 1409–1420. [CrossRef]
267. Mechaly, A.E.; Bellomio, A.; Gil-Cartón, D.; Morante, K.; Valle, M.; González-Mañas, J.M.; Guérin, D.M. Structural insights into the oligomerization and architecture of eukaryotic membrane pore-forming toxins. *Structure* **2011**, *19*, 181–191. [CrossRef]
268. Miller, K.W.; Evans, R.J.; Eisenberg, S.P.; Thompson, R.C. Secretory leukocyte protease inhibitor binding to mRNA and DNA as a possible cause of toxicity to Escherichia coli. *J. Bacteriol.* **1989**, *171*, 2166–2172.
269. den Hertog, A.L.; van Marle, J.; van Veen, H.A.; Van't Hof, W.; Bolscher, J.G.; Veerman, E.C.; Nieuw Amerongen, A.V. Candidacidal effects of two antimicrobial peptides: Histatin 5 causes small membrane defects, but LL-37 causes massive disruption of the cell membrane. *Biochem. J.* **2005**, *388*, 689–695. [CrossRef]
270. Gyurko, C.; Lendenmann, U.; Troxler, R.F.; Oppenheim, F.G. *Candida albicans* mutants deficient in respiration are resistant to the small cationic salivary antimicrobial peptide histatin 5. *Antimicrob. Agents Chemother.* **2000**, *44*, 348–354. [CrossRef]
271. Gyurko, C.; Lendenmann, U.; Helmerhorst, E.J.; Troxler, R.F.; Oppenheim, F.G. Killing of *Candida albicans* by histatin 5: Cellular uptake and energy requirement. *Antonie. Van Leeuwenhoek.* **2001**, *79*, 297–309. [CrossRef]
272. Li, X.S.; Sun, J.N.; Okamoto-Shibayama, K.; Edgerton, M. *Candida albicans* cell wall ssa proteins bind and facilitate import of salivary histatin 5 required for toxicity. *J. Biol. Chem.* **2006**, *281*, 22453–22463.
273. Helmerhorst, E.J.; Breeuwer, P.; Van't Hof, W.; Walgreen-Weterings, E.; Amerongen, A.V.; Abee, T. The cellular target of histatin 5 on *Candida albicans* is the energized mitochondrion. *J. Biol. Chem.* **1999**, *274*, 7286–7291.
274. Vylkova, S.; Jang, W.S.; Li, W.; Nayyar, N.; Edgerton, M. Histatin 5 initiates osmotic stress response in *Candida albicans* via activation of the Hog1 mitogen-activated protein kinase pathway. *Eukaryot. Cell* **2007**, *6*, 1876–1888. [CrossRef]
275. Wagener, J.; Schneider, J.J.; Baxmann, S.; Kalbacher, H.; Borelli, C.; Nuding, S.; Küchler, R.; Wehkamp, J.; Kaeser, M.D.; Mailänder-Sanchez, D.; *et al.* A peptide derived from the highly conserved protein Glyceraldehyde-3-phosphate dehydrogenase (GAPDH) is involved in tissue protection by different antifungal strategies and epithelial immunomodulation. *J. Invest. Dermatol.* **2013**, *133*, 144–153. [CrossRef]
276. Aslam, R.; Atindehou, M.; Lavaux, T.; Haïkel, Y.; Schneider, F.; Metz-Boutigue, M.H. Chromogranin A-derived peptides are involved in innate immunity. *Curr. Med. Chem.* **2012**, *19*, 4115–4123. [CrossRef]
277. Ochoa, M.T.; Stenger, S.; Sieling, P.A.; Thoma-Uszynski, S.; Sabet, S.; Cho, S.; Krensky, A.M.; Rollinghoff, M.; Nunes Sarno, E.; Burdick, A.E.; *et al.* T-cell release of granulysin contributes to host defense in leprosy. *Nat. Med.* **2001**, *7*, 174–179. [CrossRef]
278. Stewart, S.E.; Kondos, S.C.; Matthews, A.Y.; D'Angelo, M.E.; Dunstone, M.A.; Whisstock, J.C.; Trapani, J.A.; Bird, P.I. The Perforin Pore Facilitates the Delivery of Cationic Cargos. *J. Biol. Chem.* **2014**, *289*, 9172–9181. [CrossRef]
279. Diamond, G.; Beckloff, N.; Weinberg, A.; Kisich, K.O. The roles of antimicrobial peptides in innate host defense. *Curr. Pharm Des.* **2009**, *15*, 2377–2392. [CrossRef]
280. Leung, T.F.; Ching, K.W.; Kong, A.P.; Wong, G.W.; Chan, J.C.; Hon, K.L. Circulating LL-37 is a biomarker for eczema severity in children. *J. Eur. Acad. Dermatol. Venereol.* **2012**, *26*, 518–522. [CrossRef]
281. Weber, G.; Chamorro, C.I.; Granath, F.; Liljegren, A.; Zreika, S.; Saidak, Z.; Sandstedt, B.; Rotstein, S.; Mentaverri, R.; Sánchez, F.; *et al.* Human antimicrobial protein hCAP18/LL-37 promotes a metastatic phenotype in breast cancer. *Breast Cancer Res.* **2009**, *11*, R6. [CrossRef]
282. Cheng, W.L.; Wang, C.S.; Huang, Y.H.; Liang, Y.; Lin, P.Y.; Hsueh, C.; Wu, Y.C.; Chen, W.J.; Yu, C.J.; Lin, S.R.; *et al.* Overexpression of a secretory leukocyte protease inhibitor in human gastric cancer. *Int. J. Cancer* **2008**, *123*, 1787–1796. [CrossRef]
283. Emson, C.L.; Fitzmaurice, S.; Lindwall, G.; Li, K.W.; Hellerstein, M.K.; Maibach, H.I.; Liao, W.; Turner, S.M. A pilot study demonstrating a non-invasive method for the measurement of protein turnover in skin disorders: Application to psoriasis. *Clin. Transl. Med.* **2013**, *2*, 12. [CrossRef]

284. Welling, M.M.; Paulusma-Annema, A.; Balter, H.S.; Pauwels, E.K.; Nibbering, P.H. Technetium-99m labeled antimicrobial peptides discriminate between bacterial infections and sterile inflammations. *Eur. J. Nucl. Med.* **2000**, *27*, 292–301. [CrossRef]
285. Saeed, S.; Zafar, J.; Khan, B.; Akhtar, A.; Qurieshi, S.; Fatima, S.; Ahmad, N.; Irfanullah, J. Utility of ^{99}mTc-labelled antimicrobial peptide ubiquicidin (29–41) in the diagnosis of diabetic foot infection. *Eur. J. Nucl. Med. Mol. Imaging* **2013**, *40*, 737–743. [CrossRef]
286. Aryana, K.; Hootkani, A.; Sadeghi, R.; Davoudi, Y.; Naderinasab, M.; Erfani, M.; Ayati, N. (99m)Tc-labeled ubiquicidin scintigraphy: A promising method in hip prosthesis infection diagnosis. *Nuklearmedizin* **2012**, *51*, 133–139. [CrossRef]
287. Wang, G. *Antimicrobial Peptides: Discovery, Design and Novel Therapeutic Strategies*; CABI: Wallingford, UK, 2010.
288. Forde, E.; Humphreys, H.; Greene, C.M.; Fitzgerald-Hughes, D.; Devocelle, M. The potential of host defence peptide prodrugs as neutrophil elastase-dependent anti-infective agents for cystic fibrosis. *Antimicrob. Agents. Chemother.* **2013**, *58*, 978–985.
289. Reynolds, N.L.; de Cecco, M.; Taylor, K.; Stanton, C.; Kilanowski, F.; Kalapothakis, J.; Seo, E.; Uhrin, D.; Campopiano, D.; Govan, J.; *et al.* Peptide fragments of a beta-defensin derivative with potent bactericidal activity. *Antimicrob. Agents Chemother.* **2010**, *54*, 1922–1929. [CrossRef]
290. Roelandts, R. The history of phototherapy: Something new under the sun? *J. Am. Acad. Dermatol.* **2002**, *46*, 926–930. [CrossRef]
291. Wang, T.T.; Nestel, F.P.; Bourdeau, V.; Nagai, Y.; Wang, Q.; Liao, J.; Tavera-Mendoza, L.; Lin, R.; Hanrahan, J.W.; Mader, S.; *et al.* Cutting edge: 1,25-dihydroxyvitamin D3 is a direct inducer of antimicrobial peptide gene expression. *J. Immunol.* **2004**, *173*, 2909–2912. [CrossRef]
292. Gombart, A.F.; Borregaard, N.; Koeffler, H.P. Human cathelicidin antimicrobial peptide (CAMP) gene is a direct target of the vitamin D receptor and is strongly up-regulated in myeloid cells by 1,25-dihydroxyvitamin D3. *FASEB J.* **2005**, *19*, 1067–1077. [CrossRef]
293. Ala-Houhala, M.J.; Karppinen, T.; Vähävihu, K.; Kautiainen, H.; Dombrowski, Y.; Snellman, E.; Schauber, J.; Reunala, T. Narrow-band Ultraviolet B Treatment Boosts Serum 25-hydroxyvitamin D in Patients with Psoriasis on Oral Vitamin D Supplementation. *Acta Derm. Venereol.* **2014**, *94*, 146–151.
294. Steinmann, J.; Halldórsson, S.; Agerberth, B.; Gudmundsson, G.H. Phenylbutyrate (PBA) induces antimicrobial peptide expression. *Antimicrob. Agents Chemother.* **2009**, *53*, 5127–5133. [CrossRef]
295. Gan, Y.; Cui, X.; Ma, T.; Liu, Y.; Li, A.; Huang, M. Paeoniflorin Upregulates β-Defensin-2 Expression in Human Bronchial Epithelial Cell Through the p38 MAPK, ERK, and NF-κB Signaling Pathways. *Inflammation.* **2014**, in press.
296. Kim, B.J.; Rho, Y.K.; Lee, H.I.; Jeong, M.S.; Li, K.; Seo, S.J.; Kim, M.N.; Hong, C.K. The effect of calcipotriol on the expression of human beta defensin-2 and LL-37 in cultured human keratinocytes. *Clin. Dev. Immunol.* **2009**, *2009*, 645898.
297. Sunkara, L.T.; Zeng, X.; Curtis, A.R.; Zhang, G. Cyclic AMP synergizes with butyrate in promoting β-defensin9 expression in chickens. *Mol. Immunol.* **2014**, *57*, 171–180. [CrossRef]
298. Cederlund, A.; Nylén, F.; Miraglia, E.; Bergman, P.; Gudmundsson, G.H.; Agerberth, B. Label-Free Quantitative Mass Spectrometry Reveals Novel Pathways Involved in LL-37 Expression. *J. Innate Immun.* **2014**, *6*, 365–376.
299. Liu, Q.; Liu, J.; Roschmann, K.I.; van Egmond, D.; Golebski, K.; Fokkens, W.J.; Wang, D.; van Drunen, C.M. Histone deacetylase inhibitors up-regulate LL-37 expression independent of toll-like receptor mediated signalling in airway epithelial cells. *J. Inflamm. (Lond)* **2013**, *10*, 15. [CrossRef]
300. Strandberg, K.L.; Richards, S.M.; Gunn, J.S. Cathelicidin antimicrobial peptide expression is not induced or required for bacterial clearance during *salmonella enterica* infection of human monocyte-derived macrophages. *Infect. Immun.* **2012**, *80*, 3930–3938. [CrossRef]
301. Yin, Q.; Xu, X.; Lin, Y.; Lv, J.; Zhao, L.; He, R. Ultraviolet B irradiation induces skin accumulation of plasmacytoid dendritic cells: A possible role for chemerin. *Autoimmunity.* **2013**, *47*, 185–192.
302. Karlsson, J.; Carlsson, G.; Larne, O.; Andersson, M.; Pütsep, K. Vitamin D3 induces pro-LL-37 expression in myeloid precursors from patients with severe congenital neutropenia. *J. Leukoc. Biol.* **2008**, *84*, 1279–1286. [CrossRef]

303. Martineau, A.R.; Wilkinson, K.A.; Newton, S.M.; Floto, R.A.; Norman, A.W.; Skolimowska, K.; Davidson, R.N.; Sørensen, O.E.; Kampmann, B.; Griffiths, C.J.; *et al.* IFN-gamma- and TNF-independent vitamin D-inducible human suppression of mycobacteria: The role of cathelicidin LL-37. *J. Immunol.* **2007**, *178*, 7190–7198. [CrossRef]
304. Cederlund, A.; Kai-Larsen, Y.; Printz, G.; Yoshio, H.; Alvelius, G.; Lagercrantz, H.; Strömberg, R.; Jörnvall, H.; Gudmundsson, G.H.; Agerberth, B. Lactose in human breast milk an inducer of innate immunity with implications for a role in intestinal homeostasis. *PLoS One* **2013**, *8*, e53876.
305. Jiang, W.; Sunkara, L.T.; Zeng, X.; Deng, Z.; Myers, S.M.; Zhang, G. Differential regulation of human cathelicidin LL-37 by free fatty acids and their analogs. *Peptides* **2013**, *50C*, 129–138.
306. Zeng, X.; Sunkara, L.T.; Jiang, W.; Bible, M.; Carter, S.; Ma, X.; Qiao, S.; Zhang, G. Inductionof porcine host defense peptidegene expression by short-chain fatty acids and their analogs. *PLoS One* **2013**, *8*, e72922.
307. Sherman, H.; Chapnik, N.; Froy, O. Albumin and amino acids upregulate the expression of human beta-defensin 1. *Mol. Immunol.* **2006**, *43*, 1617–1623. [CrossRef]
308. Fehlbaum, P.; Rao, M.; Zasloff, M.; Anderson, G.M. An essential amino acid induces epithelial beta-defensin expression. *Proc. Natl. Acad. Sci. USA* **2000**, *97*, 12723–12728. [CrossRef]
309. Rivas-Santiago, C.E.; Rivas-Santiago, B.; León, D.A.; Castañeda-Delgado, J.; Hernández Pando, R. Induction of β-defensins by l-isoleucine as novel immunotherapy in experimental murine tuberculosis. *Clin. Exp. Immunol.* **2011**, *164*, 80–89. [CrossRef]
310. Pernet, I.; Reymermier, C.; Guezennec, A.; Branka, J.E.; Guesnet, J.; Perrier, E.; Dezutter-Dambuyant, C.; Schmitt, D.; Viac, J. Calcium triggers beta-defensin (hBD-2 and hBD-3) and chemokine macrophage inflammatory protein-3 alpha (MIP-3alpha/CCL20) expression in monolayers of activated human keratinocytes. *Exp. Dermatol.* **2003**, *12*, 755–760. [CrossRef]
311. Talukder, P.; Satho, T.; Irie, K.; Sharmin, T.; Hamady, D.; Nakashima, Y.; Kashige, N.; Miake, F. Trace metal zinc stimulates secretion of antimicrobial peptide LL-37 from Caco-2 cells through ERK and p38 MAP kinase. *Int. Immunopharmacol.* **2011**, *11*, 141–144. [CrossRef]
312. Schauber, J.; Iffland, K.; Frisch, S.; Kudlich, T.; Schmausser, B.; Eck, M.; Menzel, T.; Gostner, A.; Lührs, H.; Scheppach, W. Histone-deacetylase inhibitors induce the cathelicidin LL-37 in gastrointestinal cells. *Mol. Immunol.* **2004**, *41*, 847–854. [CrossRef]
313. Thivierge, K.; Cotton, S.; Schaefer, D.A.; Riggs, M.W.; To, J.; Lund, M.E.; Robinson, M.W.; Dalton, J.P.; Donnelly, S.M. Cathelicidin-like helminth defence molecules (HDMs): Absence of cytotoxic, anti-microbial and anti-protozoan activities imply a specific adaptation to immune modulation. *PLoS Negl. Trop. Dis.* **2013**, *7*, e2307.
314. Yeaman, M.R.; Yount, N.Y. Mechanisms of antimicrobial peptide action and resistance. *Pharmacol. Rev.* **2003**, *55*, 27–55. [CrossRef]
315. Peschel, A. How do bacteria resist human antimicrobial peptides? *Trends Microbiol.* **2002**, *10*, 179–186. [CrossRef]

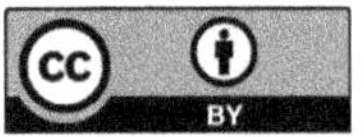

© 2014 by the author. Licensee MDPI, Basel, Switzerland. This article is an open access article distributed under the terms and conditions of the Creative Commons Attribution (CC BY) license (http://creativecommons.org/licenses/by/4.0/).

Part III:
Therapeutic Potential of Antimicrobial Peptides

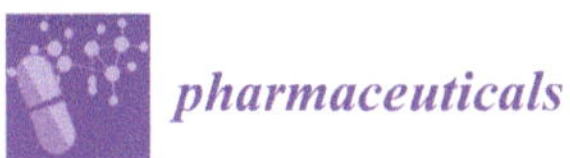

MDPI

Article

Chapter 10:

Therapeutic Potential of Gramicidin S in the Treatment of Root Canal Infections

Marina Berditsch [1], Hannah Lux [1], Oleg Babii [1], Sergii Afonin [2] and Anne S. Ulrich [1,2,*]

[1] Institute of Organic Chemistry, Karlsruhe Institute of Technology (KIT), Fritz-Haber-Weg 6, Karlsruhe 76131, Germany; marina.berditsch@kit.edu (M.B.); luxhannah89@gmail.com (H.L.); oleg.babii@kit.edu (O.B.)

[2] Institute of Biological Interfaces (IBG-2), KIT, P. O. Box 3640, Karlsruhe 76021, Germany; sergii.afonin@kit.edu

* Correspondence: anne.ulrich@kit.edu; Tel.: +49-721-608-43912

Academic Editor: Guangshun Wang
Received: 27 May 2016; Accepted: 23 August 2016; Published: 7 September 2016

Abstract: An intrinsic clindamycin-resistant *Enterococcus faecalis*, the most common single species present in teeth after failed root canal therapy, often possesses acquired tetracycline resistance. In these cases, root canal infections are commonly treated with Ledermix® paste, which contains demeclocycline, or the new alternative endodontic paste Odontopaste, which contains clindamycin; however, these treatments are often ineffective. We studied the killing activity of the cyclic antimicrobial peptide gramicidin S (GS) against planktonic and biofilm cells of tetracycline-resistant clinical isolates of *E. faecalis*. The high therapeutic potential of GS for the topical treatment of problematic teeth is based on the rapid bactericidal effect toward the biofilm-forming, tetracycline-resistant *E. faecalis*. GS reduces the cell number of planktonic cells within 20–40 min at a concentration of 40–80 μg/mL. It kills the cells of pre-grown biofilms at concentrations of 100–200 μg/mL, such that no re-growth is possible. The translocation of the peptide into the cell interior and its complexation with intracellular nucleotides, including the alarmon ppGpp, can explain its anti-biofilm effect. The successful treatment of persistently infected root canals of two volunteers confirms the high effectiveness of GS. The broad GS activity towards resistant, biofilm-forming *E. faecalis* suggests its applications for approval in root canal medication.

Keywords: gramicidin S; *Enterococcus faecalis*; tetracycline resistance; biofilms; root canal infections; alarmone ppGpp; polymyxin B

1. Introduction

Teeth with necrotic pulps and periapical radiolucencies indicate the presence of bacteria in a root canal system. They can cause apical periodontitis, an inflammatory process around the apex of a tooth root accompanied by bone resorption [1,2]. Root canal infections are characterized by a wide variety of combinations of a few oral anaerobic bacteria, such as *Actinomyces* species and peptostreptococci. The non-oral but environmental bacterium *Pseudomonas aeruginosa* is frequently isolated from treatment-resistant cases because of its intrinsic multidrug resistance, including resistance to tetracycline [3]. However, more and more evidence has been provided on the prevalence of *Enterococcus faecalis* in teeth associated with a failed endodontic treatment of root canal infections [2,4–7]. The success rate for the re-treatment of teeth with *E. faecalis* is lower (66%) than the overall success rate of re-treatment (75%) [8]. Previous studies reported about up to 77% prevalence of *E. faecalis* in teeth with failed endodontic treatment [7]. *E. faecalis* can best adapt to and tolerate the conditions in the filled root canal [6]. This facultative anaerobe is able to grow at 6.5% NaCl and temperatures up to 45 °C and is even able to colonize dentine under alkaline pH and glucose starvation [9]. It has a remarkable ability to avoid leukocyte-dependent antibacterial mechanisms and to utilize collagen within dentin, using this property for adhesion within the root canal [2]. A number of other virulence factors in *E. faecalis*, such as a plasmid-encoded surface localized adhesion protein, gelatinase (metalloendopeptidase), a serine protease, hemolysin, which is classified as a type A lantibiotic, and extracellular superoxide, permit adherence and facilitate invasion [6]. The surface adherence of biofilms is significant in persistent endodontic infections because it increases the difficulty of eliminating biofilms by conventional treatment measures [10]. Although the conventional endodontic irrigant sodium hypochlorite (1%–6%) exhibits more efficient elimination of *E. faecalis* biofilms in comparison to chlorhexidine, calcium hydroxide, povidone iodine and ethylendiamintetraacetat [11,12], this intracanal medication was found to have a limited action against bacterial biofilms [13].

Currently, there are no clinically available compounds that disassemble biofilms of *E. faecalis*, although several antimicrobial peptides are in development, such as siamycin I, which affects quorum sensing, as well as protegrin, and oritavancin that can damage the bacterial membrane [14]. Recently, the use of the commercially available Ledermix® paste, which contains demeclocycline, or the new alternative endodontic paste Odontopaste, which contains clindamycin, was reported to be ineffective in the treatment of *E. faecalis* infections due to the natural clindamycin and acquired tetracycline resistance of these bacteria [6,15]. Their dominance in nosocomial infections is based on their ability to develop multidrug resistance via the acquisition of antibiotic resistance genes on plasmids or transposons from other bacteria. Notably, surface aggregation facilitates the contact between the cells, which leads to the exchange of plasmids that carry resistance. Approximately 70% of *E. faecalis* isolates from primary endodontic infections showed a resistance to tetracycline [16]. In genomic analysis, the tetracycline resistance genes *tetM* and *tetL*, as well as gelatinase, aggregation substance and enterococcal surface protein genes, were detected in these *E. faecalis* isolates.

In this paper, we report the antimicrobial and anti-biofilm activity of the cyclic decapeptide gramicidin S (GS) against tetracycline-resistant *E. faecalis* illustrated by two cases of successful treatment of Ledermix®-resistant root canal infections using this peptide.

2. Results

2.1. Susceptibility of Tetracycline-Resistant E. faecalis to GS

According to the data of the Clinical and Laboratory Standards Institute [17], enterococci are defined to be resistant to tetracycline if the minimum inhibitory concentration (MIC) values are $\geq$16 µg/mL and they are called susceptible at MIC $\leq$ 4 µg/mL. Table 1 shows the resistance of the *E. faecalis* DSM 2570, which was isolated from urine and represents a quality control strain for antimicrobial susceptibility testing [18], the WW4 cheese isolate and four tetracycline-resistant clinical isolates, designated TRE1–TRE5. For comparison, the clinical root canal isolate WW6, which is susceptible to tetracycline (MIC < 1 µg/mL) but forms robust biofilms (Figure 1A), was also studied (Table 1). Tetracycline inhibits protein synthesis, and its action is therefore bacteriostatic. GS is a bactericidal antibiotic peptide. As shown in Table 1, its MIC, minimum bactericidal concentration (MBC), and minimum biofilm inhibitory concentration ($MBIC_{90}$) are mostly in the range of 8–16 µg/mL for all studied *E. faecalis* strains. This small difference between inhibitory and bactericidal concentrations as well as the concentrations required for the inhibition of biofilm formation, explains the great bactericidal activity of GS, which gives bacterial cells no chance to remain alive or to respond to the stress caused by GS treatment.

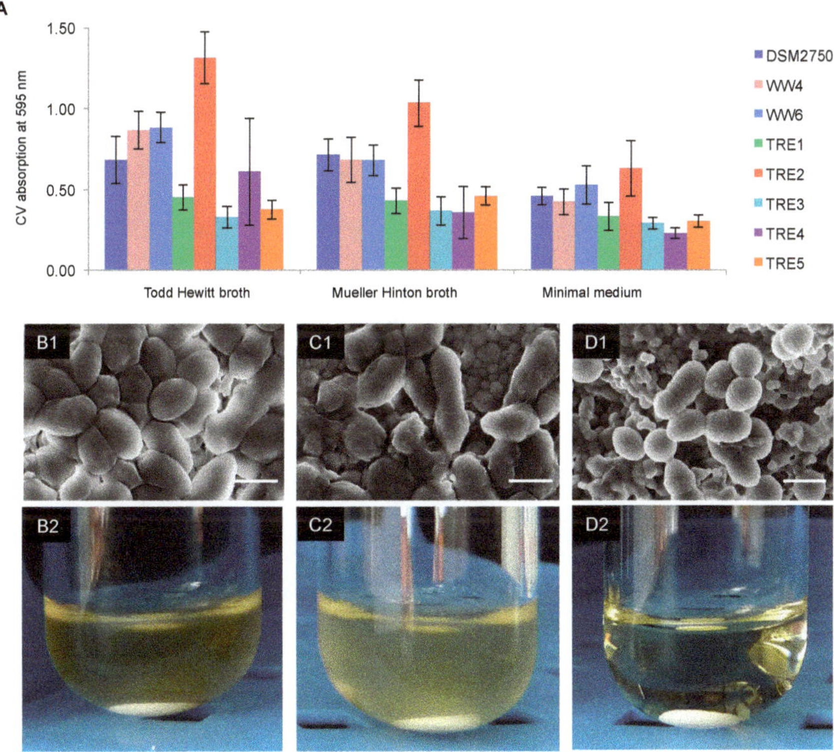

Figure 1. Anti-biofilm activity of GS. (**A**) When eight *E. faecalis* strains were compared using a crystal violet staining assay, the tetracycline-resistant clinical isolate TRE2 exhibited the strongest biofilm formation in all three nutrient media; (**B1**) SEM image of a TRE2 biofilm formed on a hydroxyapatite disk, which served as a control and as a starting point for antibiotic treatment; (**B2**) when B1 was incubated in TH broth, the biofilm is found to re-grow in a suspended form; (**C1**) SEM image of B1 after treatment with 400 μg/mL demeclocycline, and (**C2**) re-growth of a biofilm in suspension; (**D1**) B1 after treatment with 400 μg/mL GS; and (**D2**) no biofilm re-growth was observed after treatment, even when only 200 μg/mL of GS were used in D1. Reproducible results were obtained in two independent experiments. The scale on the SEM images is 1 μm.

Table 1. Minimum inhibitory concentration (MIC), minimum bactericidal concentration (MBC) and minimum biofilm inhibitory concentration (MBIC) of GS against *E. faecalis*.

E. faecalis Strain	Resistance/Susceptibility (μg/mL) to		Antimicrobial Activity of GS (μg/mL)		
	Tetracycline	Demeclocycline			
	MIC [a]	MIC	MIC	MBC	$MBIC_{90}$
DSM 2570	16	8	8	8	4–8
TRE1	16	16	8	16	-
TRE2	16	32	16	16	8–16
TRE4	16	8	8	8	-
TRE5	16	16	8	16	-
WW4	64	16	8	16	-
WW6	<1	<1	8	16	8–16

[a] MICs, MBCs and MBICs were determined in at least in two independent experiments, each performed in triplicate. MBIC was determined only for the three best biofilm-formers (see Figure 1A).

2.2. Time-Dependent Killing Effect of GS

The bactericidal activity of GS against *E. faecalis* strains over time was studied in killing assays. For this experiment, we used stationary cultures, which contained metabolically inactive, slow- or non-dividing dormant cells that tolerate conventional antibiotics and cause persistent infections [19]. At the time points of 20 min and 40 min after the addition of GS, the undiluted 100-μL bacterial aliquots revealed no colonies on agar plates. This indicates a prompt and complete reduction of the cell number in planktonic suspension, which contained 10^8 CFU/mL cells (Figure 2). Notably, the metabolically inactive dormant cells were also killed at the studied concentrations, which corresponded to the 5 × MIC and 10 × MIC values (Table 1). The increase from 5 to 10 × MICs led to a decrease in killing time from 40 to 20 min for the *E. faecalis* DSM 2570 and WW6. The same killing curve was observed at 5 × MIC values of GS for the best biofilm former, the tetracycline-resistant clinical isolate *E. faecalis* TRE2. However, its effective concentration was 80 μg/mL because its MIC value was 16 μg/mL.

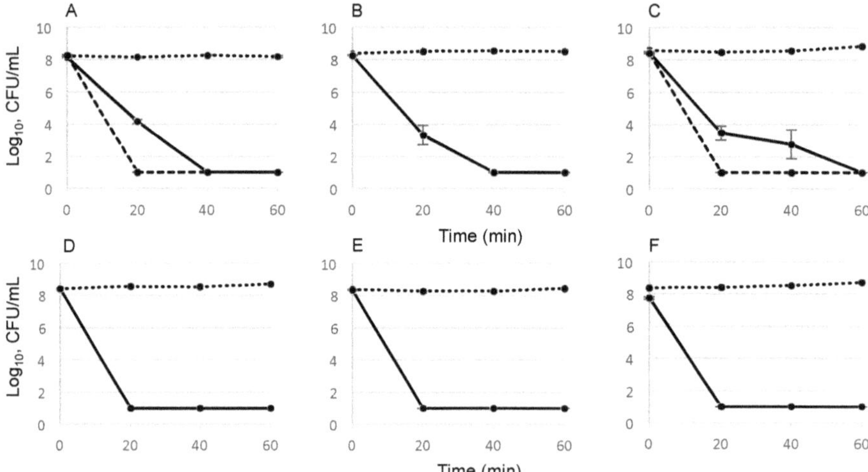

Figure 2. Reduction of the number of *E. faecalis* bacteria during exposure to GS: (**A**) control strain DSM 2570; (**B**) cheese isolate WW4; (**C**) root canal isolate WW6; and (**D–F**) clinical tetracycline-resistant isolates TRE1, TRE2, and TRE4, respectively. The bacterial number remained unchanged in the controls (dotted lines), but decreased drastically during exposure to 5 × MIC of GS (solid lines). The dashed lines show the faster bactericidal effect of 10 × MIC for DSM 2570 and WW6 strains; 10 CFU/mL was taken as the detection limit although no colonies were grown from undiluted sample. The standard deviations were calculated from at least two independent experiments.

2.3. Biofilm-Killing Effect of GS

For these experiments, it was necessary to determine the biofilm forming capacity of all *E. faecalis* isolates to choose the strongest biofilm formers and the most suitable medium. A standard crystal violet staining assay was applied to evaluate the mass of the biofilms that were pre-grown for 24 h in 96-well microtiter plates (Figure 1A).

The strongest biofilm growth was found to occur in the Todd Hewitt (TH) broth, which contains glucose. The Mueller Hinton (MH) broth and minimal medium were less suitable for biofilm formation. The biofilm-forming capacity of the control strain DSM 2570 was comparable with that of the tetracycline-resistant WW4 (cheese isolate) and the tetracycline-susceptible WW6 (root canal isolate) (Table 1). The tetracycline-resistant clinical isolate *E. faecalis* TRE2 was the best biofilm former. Scanning electron microscopy (SEM) showed that the cells in this biofilm completely covered the surface of the hydroxyapatite disc (HAD) and were attached to the HAD nanoparticles (Figure 1B1). After exposure to 400 μg/mL of GS for 18 h, the cell morphology of *E. faecalis* TRE2 was drastically altered (Figure 1D1) in comparison to the control or to the treatment with 400 μg/mL of demeclocycline (Figure 1C1). The GS-treated cells decreased in size from 1 to 0.6–0.8 μm, the cell surface got wrinkled, and the cells detached from the HAD particles (Figure 1D1). Treatment of the pre-grown biofilms with 400 μg/mL of GS led to a disappearance of the matrix layer and to a partial elimination of biofilm cells, so that the nanoparticles of the HAD were clearly exposed underneath the cells. No re-growth of the robust TRE2 biofilm in the fresh TH broth was observed, even when only 200 μg/mL GS has been applied (Figure 1D2). This concentration represents the minimal biofilm bactericidal concentration (MBBC) of GS against *E. faecalis* TRE2, because subsequent plating of this non re-grown culture on nutrient agar did not reveal any viable cells. The control biofilm (Figure 1B2) as well as the biofilm after demeclocycline treatment (Figure 1C2) were clearly found to re-grow in the fresh TH nutrient broth after cultivation at 37 °C for 24 h. The second strongest biofilm former, the tetracycline-susceptible root canal isolate *E. faecalis* WW6 (Figure 1A), did not exhibit re-growth after treatment with 400 μg/mL demeclocycline, as expected due to its high susceptibility (see Table 1). We note, however, that the MBBC of GS against this strain was even lower (100 μg/mL) (data not shown).

2.4. GS Penetration into the Bacterial Cells and Binding Affinity to Nucleotides

Microbiological assays helped to elucidate the complex action of GS at the cellular level. To understand the anti-biofilm activity at the molecular level, we first studied the membrane-penetrating ability of GS, in order to find out whether it has any access to intracellular targets. For comparative fluorescent microscopy, we used the dye 5(6)-carboxy-fluorescein-*N*-hydroxysuccinimide ester (CFSE) as a control, which cannot penetrate the cell membrane. To detect GS by fluorecscence microscopy, the photo-switchable GS analog GS-sw(FP) was used, which possesses an intrinsic green fluorescence upon irradiation with visible light [20]. The fluorescence image of *E. faecalis* TRE2 stained with CFSE showed strong fluorescence of only the cell envelope (Figure 3A). On the other hand, bacteria that were incubated with GS peptide for 30 min (Figure 3B) showed an even fluorescence internally. The same result was obtained by staining the other *E. faecalis* strains (data not shown).

The access of cationic GS to the cytoplasm suggests that it may engage in electrostatic interactions with intracellular anionic targets. A key target could be the alarmon ppGpp, which regulates biofilm formation [21]. Indeed, the addition of ppGpp to GS at different molar ratios led to their co-precipitation as a result of mutual binding. At ppGpp:GS ratios of 2:1, 1:1 and 1:2 (Figure 3C), floating white flakes could be seen, suggesting the presence of large aggregates. A further excess of GS led to the formation of a stable milky opalescent suspension, which contained smaller nano-rods (Figure 3D). ^{31}P-NMR analysis of the intrinsic ppGpp phosphate signals confirmed the binding and aggregation, as sharp signals were observed only in the presence of low concentrations of GS (Figure 3E). The broadening and disappearance of the ^{31}P-NMR signals with excess peptide indicated the precipitation of the alarmone/GS complex. Electron microscopy of the milky suspension at a molar ratio of ppGpp:GS 1:8 (Figure 3D) revealed the assembly of GS with ppGpp into nano-rods with 50 nm width and 200 nm length. The ability of GS to bind to ppGpp and thus to deplete its free cytoplasmic pool may explain the strong inhibition of biofilm formation by GS described above (see $MBIC_{90}$ values in Table 1).

Notably, ppGpp is not the only possible intracellular target of GS. In the literature, complex formation of GS with nucleic acids and adenosine phosphates has already been described [22,23]. Because the triphosphates GTP and ATP are utilized in the biosynthesis of ppGpp, their binding to GS may further enhance the anti-biofilm effect of the peptide. Using the same ^{31}P-NMR approach as described above, we also compared the ability of several other phosphorus-containing nucleotides to bind GS. Judged by the molar ratio at which the ^{31}P-NMR signal disappeared (see Figures in Supplementary Materials), the studied nucleotides exhibited GS binding affinities in the following order: ADP < ppGpp < ATP = GTP < GDP. In particular, this means that the ppGpp precursors represent even stronger complex partners for GS, and their binding to GS should additionally contribute to the overall inhibitory and bactericidal effects in bacterial biofilms.

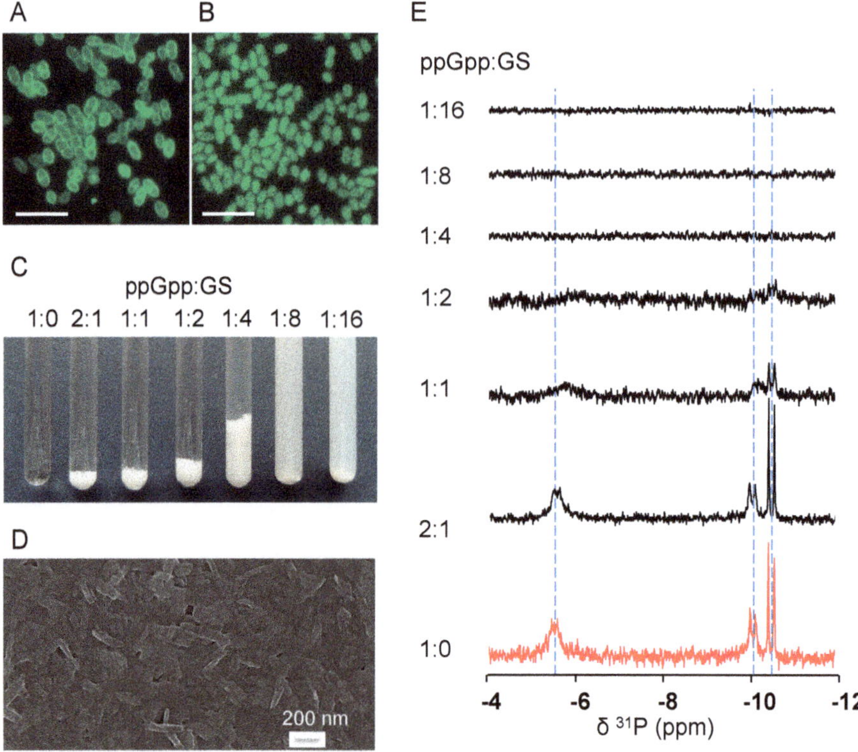

Figure 3. Translocation of GS into the cells and its binding affinity to the bacterial alarmon ppGpp. (**A**) Green fluorescence of the *E. faecalis* cell envelope upon staining with the dye CFSE, which cannot penetrate the cellular membrane. (**B**) Fluorescence throughout the interior of the cells is seen upon staining with a fluorescent GS-sw(FP) analog, confirming that the peptide can translocate across the cell membrane into the cytoplasm. (**C**) Co-precipitation of GS and ppGpp is seen to occur at roughly equimolar ratios, and a stable opalescent suspension is formed when GS is in large (i.e., electrostatic) excess. (**D**) SEM showed that the aggregation ppGpp by GS led to the formation of short nano-rods of about 50 nm width and 200 nm length. (**E**) When GS was added to ppGpp at different molar ratios, the ^{31}P-NMR signals of the latter disappeared successively. The pure ppGpp sample (1:0) is shown in red. The scale on the fluorescent images is 5 μm.

2.5. Medication Reports

Case I of root canal infection: Molar 38 of a 59-year-old female patient (M.B.) was percussion-sensitive and responded negative to cold testing with CO_2 snow. The initial root canal treatment was carried out in a standard way using irrigation with sodium hypochlorite. An intracanal Ledermix® Paste dressing was administered. For the next six weeks, the tooth remained percussion sensitive and painful, so the root canals were again treated in the same way for the next four weeks, but the second treatment with Ledermix® Paste was also unsuccessful. The pain was stronger and radiated into the ear and head. At the patient's request, the tooth was medicated using a mixture of the antimicrobial peptides GS and polymyxin B (PMB) at a molar ratio of 2:1. The powders were co-dissolved in a drop of 50% ethanol and applied as an intracanal dressing with a temporary Cavit™ restoration. Alleviation of pain was experienced after one hour, and a positive healing effect was noted. After a few weeks without symptoms the tooth was sealed, and in the following five years no recurrence was observed.

Case II of root canal infection: Decay in molar 36 of a 25-year-old male patient (M.B.'s son) was observed by X-ray as a radiolucent spot in the pulp region (Figure 4A). Without treatment, an irreversible pulpitis developed within six months. The root canals were treated in a standard way, but a painful root canal infection appeared after two months. After the direct application of ~2 mg GS, which was suspended in sterile isotonic saline, the pain receded within an hour, and the root canals were sealed (Figure 4B). After treatment, no reoccurrence of root canal infection was observed in the following five years.

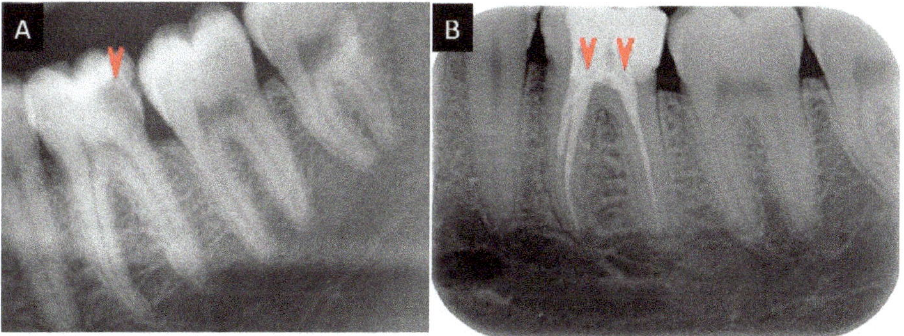

Figure 4. Molar 36 of a 25-year-old male patient before and after treatment. (**A**) The radiolucent area in the X-ray image indicates decay. (**B**) The sealed root canals after treatment with GS. The red arrowheads mark the decayed area and the sealed root canals, respectively.

3. Discussion

The cyclic decapeptide gramicidin S (S = "Soviet") was isolated by Gause and Brazhnikova from soil bacilli and described in *Nature* and *Lancet* in 1944 [24,25]. The symmetric structure of GS is a double-repeated sequence of five amino acids, which are arranged in an antiparallel cyclic manner ($_{cyclo}$[phe-Pro-Val-Orn-Leu]$_2$) [26]. GS has an amphiphilic structure, consisting of the cationic non-canonical amino acid ornithine and the hydrophobic ^{D}phenylalanine, valine and leucine. As pharmaceuticals, antimicrobial peptides generally exhibit some unfavorable properties, such as instability, salt sensitivity, high cost of production, and a rather non-specific spectrum of activity, including hemolytic effects [27]. GS, on the other hand, is a very stable peptide. Its cyclic structure and the presence of the unusual amino acids ornithine and ^{D}phenylalanine avoid the typical proteolytic degradation by common proteases. Overall, GS has a high hemolytic activity, which limits its use to topical applications, though the addition of polyethylene glycol has been shown to prevent its hemolytic effects [28]. The production of GS via the fermentation of producing *Aneurinibacillus migulanus* phenotypes [29] is less costly than the usual chemical synthesis of antimicrobial peptides of non-bacterial origin. GS is approved as the bioactive agent in Grammidin®Neo, a lozenge used against sore throat and mouth ulcers, produced by Russian JSC Valenta Pharmaceuticals. Notably, despite a long treatment history, no clinical cases of bacterial resistance against GS have been reported [30].

The promising observation that GS does not lead to bacterial resistance can be attributed to its ability to attack multiple targets in bacterial cells at the same time. The first target of GS is the prokaryotic plasma membrane; therefore, the peptide possesses enhanced activity against Gram-positive bacteria like *Staphylococcus* spp., *Streptococcus* spp., and *Enterococcus* spp. [31]. In addition to depolarization, presumably via the formation of short-lived pores at sub-MICs [32], it also inhibits the respiratory enzymes NADH dehydrogenase and cytochrome *bd* terminal oxidase in the bacterial membrane [33], and it detaches several vital peripheral membrane proteins, namely the cell-division regulator MinD, the Lipid II biosynthesis protein MurG, and cytochrome c [34]. Here, we have shown that GS does not only interact with the bacterial membrane, which causes structural and functional damage as described above.

In fact, it can also penetrate into the cytoplasm, where it can bind to ppGpp, the intracellular regulator of biofilm growth [35], and to its precursors ATP and GTP, as well as the energy metabolites ADP and GDP (Figures S1–S4 in the Supplementary Materials). These new modes of activity broaden the spectrum of effects known so far for GS. It is especially important to realize that this multifaceted activity profile provides GS with unique bactericidal properties toward Gram-positive bacteria irrespective of their physiological state, virulence, resistance, tolerance and phenotypic variation. Generally, the stationary phase of a liquid bacterial culture contains a population of metabolically inactive non- or slow-growing reversible phenotypes, which are known as persister cells. They are tolerant to conventional antibiotics, even at 100 × MIC [36], because these antibiotics target only growing cells. The ability of GS to disrupt membrane function and to form complexes with intracellular targets after its rapid penetration into the cell interior leads to a complete and rapid killing. This was demonstrated in our killing assays of stationary cells (Figure 2), and in the biofilm re-growth experiments with each of the selected three strongest biofilm forming strains of *E. faecalis* (Table 1 and Figure 1).

The origin of *E. faecalis* in the root canal is unclear, as enterococci do not belong to the normal oral microbial flora [7]. However, 77% of British-produced cheeses [37], 60% of French soft cheeses, and 20% of mozzarella, feta and Swiss Tilsiter cheese [38], contain enterococci. A genetic analysis of saliva, previously treated root canal samples, and of cheeses, using repetitive extragenic palindromic (REP)-PCR, revealed nine *E. faecalis* genotypes in all specimens studied. The transitional colonization of the oral cavity after the consumption of cheese may thus be a possible reason for the prevalence of *E. faecalis* in root canal infections [37,38]. Tetracycline-resistant enterococcal or multispecies infections may provoke treatment failure, requiring tooth extraction, if the therapy using an intracanal Ledermix® paste dressing is applied [16]. Even if several bacteria cause the infection, a GS-containing dressing would be an unsurpassable choice for successful treatment due to the broad-spectrum activity of GS [30]. Although microbiological analysis was not performed in two above described medication cases, a cure using GS alone and in combination with PMB has been successfully achieved. Recently, we also reported that these two peptides exert a synergistic effect against multidrug-resistant strains and against biofilms of *P. aeruginosa* [39]. In the treatment of root canal infections caused by this pathogen, which is frequently isolated from treatment-resistant cases, we expect that the combination of GS/PMB could play a very promising role. Remarkably, the pain-alleviating effect, which we describe here for both medication cases, had been previously observed in Russian clinical trials as a characteristic property only of GS but not of the related tyrothricin complex [40]—a peptide mixture of the lineal gramicidin A and cyclic tyrocidines [41]. This unique property of GS should thus be highly advantageous in the treatment of painful root canal infections.

Biofilm formation is a key virulence factor in the pathogenicity of persistent *E. faecalis* infections [42]. Nutrients such as hemin, vitamin K and glucose enhance biofilm formation. The tetracycline-resistant *E. faecalis* strain TRE2 was the best biofilm former amongst all clinical isolates. The exposure of its pre-grown biofilm to an aqueous solution of GS showed a bactericidal effect (no re-growth of biofilms was observed, and no viable cells were found in this culture upon plating), and some drastic morphological alterations of the biofilm remnants were observed (Figure 3). Our results thus highlight the promising potential of GS in the successful treatment of root canal infections caused by tetracycline-resistant biofilms of *E. faecalis*. In persistent infections, these bacteria can penetrate the cellular and tissue barrier and thereby present an imminent risk to human health, causing further non-oral, life-threatening infections, such as bacteremia or endocarditis [6,43]. Therefore, the successful treatment of root canal infections and their prevention are vital tasks. GS alone or in combination with PMB offers an opportunity to help patients with untreatable root canal infections, to save their natural teeth and to avoid high prosthetic costs.

4. Materials and Methods

4.1. *E. faecalis* Strains, Antibiotics and the Determination of the Minimum Inhibitory Concentrations

The control strain *Enterococcus faecalis* DSM 2570 (ATCC 29212) was purchased from the German Collection of Microorganisms and Cell Cultures (DSMZ). The WW4 isolate from cheese and the root canal isolate WW6 were a kind gift from William G. Wade (Department of Microbiology, King's College London, London, UK). The tetracycline-resistant clinical isolates TRE1-TRE5 were obtained from the medical laboratory of Staber & Kollegen, Heilbronn, Germany.

GS was produced by fermentation, extracted from producer cells and HPLC purified as described earlier [28]. Other antibiotics (tetracycline and demeclocycline hydrochlorides) were purchased form Sigma-Aldrich Chemie GmbH (Taufkirchen, Germany).

The bacterial strains were maintained at −80 °C using a Cryobank™System (Mast Diagnostica, Reinfeld, Germany). To refresh the bacterial cells, single beads were recovered in 10 mL BHI broth (Becton, Dickinson and Co., Sparks, MD, USA) in an overnight incubation at 37 °C and 200 rpm, in the 50 mL culture flasks. Single colonies were obtained by streaking these cultures on BHI agar plates, which were then stored at 4 °C. Subsequently, the colonies were used to inoculate 10 mL MH broth (Becton, Dickinson and Co., Sparks, MD, USA) to an optical density (OD) of 0.02 at 550 nm, and the cultures were grown overnight. The test cultures were prepared by inoculating 10 mL MH broth to an OD_{550} of 0.2 with the overnight cultures and allowing them to grow until the bacteria reached OD_{550} of 1–2 at 37 °C and 200 rpm. For inoculation, the test cultures were diluted immediately prior to the experiment in MH broth to obtain final inoculation doses of 5×10^5 CFU/mL according to the CLSI recommendations [17].

For the determination of the MIC, the standard broth microdilution procedure [18] was modified to obtain the uniform medium concentration after the addition of antibiotic stock solutions dissolved in sterile deionized water (tetracycline and demeclocycline) or in 50% ethanol (GS). Briefly, 50 µL of the double-strength MH broth was added to the upper row of the 96-well microtiter plates (Nunclon™, Nunc GmbH & Co., Wiesbaden, Germany). Next, 50 µL of the standard MH broth was added to the remaining wells, including the columns for the ethanol control and the positive (without peptides) and negative (sterility) controls. Addition of the antibiotic stock solutions (50 µL) to the upper wells provided a standard medium concentration and the antibiotic concentration to establish a concentration gradient. Once the two-fold dilution series of the antibiotic concentration was prepared according to [44], the plates were inoculated with 50 µL of bacterial suspensions from the exponentially growing culture to reach 5×10^5 CFU/mL. The plates were incubated for 22 h at 37 °C and 5% CO_2 without agitation. To examine bacterial growth, 20 µL of an aqueous 80 µM solution of the redox indicator resazurin was added to each well. The plates were incubated for another 2 h at 37 °C. The respiration activity was calculated for each well as the difference in the absorbance of resorufin at 570 nm and resazurin at 600 nm using the microtiter plate reader FlashScan550 (Analytic Jena GmbH, Jena, Germany) and the WinFlash program. Positive values indicated bacterial growth and allowed the determination of the lowest peptide concentrations that inhibit bacterial growth. All results were obtained from several independent experiments, and each was performed in triplicate.

4.2. Determination of the Minimum Bactericidal Concentration (MBC)

Determination of MBC was carried out directly after the MIC assay. The 10-µL samples of all 8 dilution rows of microtiter plates were spotted on the square agar plates and incubated overnight at 37 °C and 5% CO_2. The MBC was determined as the lowest concentration at which no bacterial growth was observed on the two parallel spotted plates in several independent experiments.

4.3. Determination of the Minimum Biofilm Inhibitory Concentration (MBIC)

The MBIC leading to a 90% decrease in biofilm growth ($MBIC_{90}$) was obtained using the microdilution procedure in the same way as for the determination of MIC, but the inoculation of the wells was performed with bacterial cells from stationary cultures to reach 5×10^7 CFU/mL. In contrast to the determination of MBIC for the peptide IDR-1018 in [21], we used TH broth as a medium, which facilitated maximum biofilm growth (Figure 1A). After incubation at 37 °C and 5% CO_2 without agitation for 24 h, the planktonic cells were washed and the crystal violet staining method was applied to evaluate the biofilm growth [45] under the different peptide concentrations. The results were obtained from two independent experiments, and each was performed in triplicate.

4.4. Determination of the Biofilm-Forming Capacity of the *E. faecalis* Strains

Three nutrition media—TH broth, MH broth and minimal medium [21], containing 62 mM potassium phosphate (pH 7.0), 7 mM ammonium sulfate, 2 mM $MgSO_4$, 10 µM $FeSO_4$, 0.4% glucose and 0.5% casamino acids—were used to determine the best biofilm formers and the medium that supported the best biofilm growth. The central 6 × 3 wells separated by the empty columns in the 96-well microtiter plates were filled with overnight bacterial suspensions of OD_{550} = 0.2 in three different media and incubated at 37 °C and 5% CO_2 without agitation for 24 h. The adherent biofilms were washed, dried, fixed in methanol and dried again. The staining was carried out according to previously described methods [45] in 100 µL of the 0.1% crystal violet solution for 20 min. The excess dye was removed with water, and the wells were thoroughly dried. The dye absorbed by biofilms was dissolved in absolute ethanol, and its absorption was evaluated in a microtiter plate reader at 595 nm.

4.5. Determination of GS Killing Activity

The killing activity of GS was monitored during the 60 min after exposure to GS concentrations of 5 × MIC and 10 × MIC if needed. The stationary cultures were diluted up to OD_{550} = 0.2 calculated for 1.5 mL culture in MH broth, including the addition of GS stock solution. The 200-µL aliquots were removed from the cultures, which were incubated in 4 mL culture tubes at 37 °C with agitation of about 220 rpm, at 0 min, 20 min, 40 min and 60 min. For each time point, the culture samples were diluted 1:10 in 900 µL MH broth and 100 µL of undiluted culture, and each dilution was spotted as ten 10 µL on the agar plates according to the drop plate method [46]. After the incubation of the plates, the bacterial growth was evaluated by the enumeration of colonies. The decrease in bacterial number indicated the killing activity for the each time point.

4.6. Biofilms on HAD: Scanning Electron Microscopy and Re-Growth

The three best biofilm formers were grown on HAD (3D Biotek, NJ, USA), which served as a tooth-like material. The discs were placed into the 24-well microtiter plates (Nunc GmbH & Co., Wiesbaden, Germany) and inoculated with a cell suspension from the overnight stationary cultures, which were grown in TH broth and diluted to OD_{550} = 0.2. After 30 h growth at 37 °C without agitation, biofilms on HAD were placed into solutions containing 50 µg/mL, 100 µg/mL, 200 µg/mL and 400 µg/mL of GS, 400 µg/mL of demeclocycline, or 150 mM sodium phosphate buffer (SPB, pH 7.2) for 18 h. After that, the biofilms on the HAD were washed in SPB and placed into 1 mL of fresh TH broth to examine their re-growth. Cultures were incubated at 37 °C with agitation at 200 rpm for 24 h. To determine the number of viable cells after exposure to GS, the 100 µL of TH culture after re-growth experiment were spotted as described in 4.5. The second series of biofilms on HAD after the treatment were washed in SPB, fixed for 1 h in 2% glutaraldehyde dissolved in SPB, washed twice in distilled water and dried in the sample box. The samples were sputtered to obtain a 1-nm platinum layer using the high vacuum coating system Leica EM MED020 (Leica Microsystems, Wetzlar, Germany). The biofilm images were obtained with a Supra 55 VP scanning electron microscope (Carl Zeiss, Ostfildern, Germany).

4.7. Fluorescence Microscopy

The fluorescence of the photo-switchable analog GS-sw(FP), described previously [20], was used to study GS translocation into the bacterial cytoplasm. Approximately 1 mL of the *E. faecalis* cell suspension adjusted to OD_{550} = 1.0 was co-incubated with 100 µg/mL of GS-sw(FP) in less active closed-ring form and incubated at 37 °C for 30 min without agitation. To observe the fluorescence this form was converted to the fluorescent open-ring form upon the irradiation with visible light directly under the microscope for 5 min. The CFSE dye (Sigma-Aldrich, St. Louis, MO, USA), which cannot penetrate the cell membrane, was applied for comparison. The bacterial suspension for this staining was resuspended in the fresh 150 mM $NaHCO_3$ buffer (pH 8.3). This was necessary because at this pH, the amino groups of membrane proteins remain deprotonated and can better bind to CFSE. The dye concentration used for the cell staining was 1 µL/mL (stock solution 10 mg/mL in DMSO). The staining procedure was carried out at the same conditions (37 °C, 30 min, without agitation). The fluorescence was observed using a Axioskop 40 light microscope (Carl Zeiss Light Microscopy, Göttingen, Germany) equipped with an "A-Plan" objective (100x/1.25 Ph3), a fluorescence filter (type 09, λ_{ex} 450–490, λ_{em} 515) and a digital camera (PowerShot G5, Canon, Tokyo, Japan). The sensitivity setting ISO 50 was used in experiments with the highly fluorescent CFSE dye. Due to the low fluorescence quantum yield of GS-sw(FP), the sensitivity setting was increased to the ISO 400.

4.8. ^{31}P-NMR Spectroscopy of GS with Nucleotides in An Aqueous Environment

The ppGpp solution was purchased from TriLink BioTechnologies (San Diego, CA, USA), and the nucleotides ATP, ADP, GTP, and GDP were purchased from Sigma-Aldrich (Munich, Germany). 600 µL of 1 mM or 0.5 mM ppGpp solution in D_2O (pH 7.2) were added to lyophilized aliquots of GS, yielding 0.5 mM, 1.0 mM, 2.0 mM, 4.0 mM and 8.0 mM for the end volume of 600 µL and thoroughly vortexed. Each NMR sample was then allowed to remain without any perturbation at ambient temperature for at least 2 h to allow precipitate formation. Proton-decoupled ^{31}P-NMR spectra were acquired on a Bruker AVANCE 400 MHz spectrometer (Bruker-Biospin, Rheinstetten, Germany), operating at a ^{31}P frequency of 161.974 MHz. The experiments were performed without temperature control (room temperature) using a Bruker 5 mm BB-PABBO probe. A single pulse (30 degrees, 15 µs) using a standard pulse sequence zgpg30 (Bruker library) was used. For ^{1}H decoupling, a waltz16 decoupling sequence (Bruker library) was used. A total of 3500 scans were accumulated for each spectrum with an interpulse delay of 2 s. Spectra were processed with TopSpin 3.1 software (Bruker) using line broadening of 5 Hz.

4.9. Medication of the Root Canal Infections

In Case I, lyophilized powders of 9.0 mg GS (1141.4 g/mol) and 5.5 mg PMB-sulfate (1385.6 g/mol) were placed onto a glass slide, mechanically mixed with a spatula, and suspended by addition a 50 µL droplet of 50% ethanol. In Case II, about 4 mg of GS powder were suspended by addition a 50 µL droplet of sterile isotonic saline. A fraction of the resulting slurry was applied to the open root canal as an intracanal dressing, employing standard filling instruments. The tooth was temporarily restored by Cavit™. When a few weeks without pain had passed, both teeth were permanently sealed. Both individual cases studies (of the first author and a family member) were carried out privately and with full responsibility and awareness of the risks, as the only alternative would have been to have the decayed tooth extracted. Both the participants in medication signed a "Note of patient consent".

5. Conclusions

In this study, we have demonstrated the considerable therapeutic potential of GS, which can be used for the treatment of root canal infections caused by tetracycline-resistant *E. faecalis* and by any of its tenacious biofilm-forming strains. The rapid killing by GS is based not only on its membrane-perturbing activity but also on further intracellular effects. The latter seem to involve the ability of the peptide to cross the lipid bilayer and bind to anionic intracellular targets (e.g., the alarmone ppGpp, and energetic nucleotides), as demonstrated here. The persistently infected root canals of two patients have been successfully treated, exhibiting rapid pain-alleviating effects. The broad activity spectrum of GS should thus be especially beneficial if the taxonomic status of the bacterial burden in root canals cannot be rapidly identified. For multispecies infections containing multidrug-resistant *P. aeruginosa*, the combination with PMB can significantly promote the curing effect further. Therefore, we recommend the approval of GS alone and/or as a complex with PMB for the treatment of persistent tetracycline-resistant root canal infections.

Supplementary Materials: The following are available online at http://www.mdpi.com/1424-8247/9/3/56/s1, Figure S1. Binding of ATP by GS; Figure S2. Binding of ADP by GS; Figure S3. Binding of GTP by GS; Figure S4. Binding of GDP by GS.

Acknowledgments: We thank Thomas Wittgens, Kristina Schkolin (Labor Staber & Kollegen, Heilbronn, Germany) and William G. Wade (Department of Microbiology, King's College London, London, UK) for providing the clinical *E. faecalis* isolates. We are grateful to Christian Engel (Zahnaerzte Engel, Karlsruhe, Germany) for the root canal therapy, and Stefan Kuhn (Laboratory of Electron Microscopy, Karlsruhe Institute of Technology, Germany) for the technical assistance with SEM.

Author Contributions: M.B. conceived the study, designed the experiments, performed biofilm studies on hydroxyapatite discs, prepared ^{31}P-NMR experiments, was the first patient, and wrote the paper; H.L. determined the biofilm-forming capacity and performed the time-killing assay, fluorescence microscopy, and MIC, MBC and MBIC experiments; O.B. performed the chemical synthesis of the fluorescent GS-Sw(FP) derivate and its application for bacterial staining; S.A. performed and analyzed the ^{31}P-NMR spectra and wrote the paper; and A.S.U. discussed the results, supervised the entire study and wrote the paper.

Conflicts of Interest: The authors declare no conflict of interest.

Abbreviations

The following abbreviations are used in this manuscript:

GS	gramicidin S
PMB	polymyxin B
MIC	minimum inhibitory concentration
MBC	minimum bactericidal concentration
$MBIC_{90}$	minimum biofilm inhibitory concentration, 90% inhibition
MBBC	minimal biofilm bactericidal concentration
TRE	tetracycline resistant enterococci
CFU/mL	colony forming units per mL
OD	optical density
SEM	scanning electron microscopy
CFSE	5(6)-carboxy-fluorescein-*N*-hydroxysuccinimide ester
HAD	hydroxyapatite disc
NMR	nuclear magnet resonance analysis
MH	Mueller Hinton broth
TH	Todd Hewitt broth
BHI	brain heart infusion broth
MM	minimal medium
SPB	sodium phosphate buffer

References

1. Tronstad, L. Recent development in endodontic research. *Eur. J. Oral Sci.* **1992**, *100*, 52–59. [CrossRef]
2. Figdor, D.; Sundqvist, G. A big role for the very small—understanding the endodontic microbial flora. *Aust. Dent. J.* **2007**, *52*, S38–S51. [CrossRef] [PubMed]
3. Li, X.Z.; Livermore, D.M.; Nikaido, H. Role of efflux pump(s) in intrinsic resistance of *Pseudomonas aeruginosa*: Resistance to tetracycline, chloramphenicol, and norfloxacin. *Antimicrob. Agents Chemother.* **1994**, *38*, 1732–1741. [CrossRef] [PubMed]
4. Wang, Q.Q.; Zhang, C.F.; Chu, C.H.; Zhu, X.F. Prevalence of *Enterococcus faecalis* in saliva and filled root canals of teeth associated with apical periodontitis. *Int. J. Oral Sci.* **2012**, *4*, 19–23. [CrossRef] [PubMed]
5. Stuart, C.H.; Schwartz, S.A.; Beeson, T.J.; Owatz, C.B. *Enterococcus faecalis*: Its role in root canal treatment failure and current concepts in retreatment. *J. Endod.* **2006**, *32*, 93–98. [CrossRef] [PubMed]

6. Portenier, I.; Waltimo, T.M.T.; Haapasalo, M. *Enterococcus faecalis*—The root canal survivor and "star" in post-treatment disease. *Endod. Topics* **2003**, *6*, 135–159. [CrossRef]
7. Vidana, R.; Sullivan, A.; Billstrom, H.; Ahlquist, M.; Lund, B. *Enterococcus faecalis* infection in root canals—Host-derived or exogenous source? *Lett. Appl. Microbiol.* **2011**, *52*, 109–115. [CrossRef] [PubMed]
8. Molander, A.; Warfvinge, J.; Reit, C.; Kvist, T. Clinical and radiographic evaluation of one- and two-visit endodontic treatment of asymptomatic necrotic teeth with apical periodontitis: a randomized clinical trial. *J. Endod.* **2007**, *33*, 1145–1148. [CrossRef] [PubMed]
9. Ran, S.; Wang, J.; Jiang, W.; Zhu, C.; Liang, J. Assessment of dentinal tubule invasion capacity of *Enterococcus faecalis* under stress conditions ex vivo. *Int. Endontic. J.* **2015**, *48*, 362–372. [CrossRef] [PubMed]
10. De Paz, L.C. Redefining the persistent infection in root canals: Possible role of biofilm communities. *J. Endod.* **2007**, *33*, 652–662. [CrossRef] [PubMed]
11. Abdullah, M.; Ng, Y.L.; Gulabivala, K.; Moles, D.R.; Spratt, D.A. Susceptibilties of two *Enterococcus faecalis* phenotypes to root canal medications. *J. Endod.* **2005**, *31*, 30–36. [CrossRef] [PubMed]
12. Dunavant, T.R.; Regan, J.D.; Glickman, G.N.; Solomon, E.S.; Honeyman, A.L. Comparative evaluation of endodontic irrigants against *Enterococcus faecalis* biofilms. *J. Endod.* **2006**, *32*, 527–531. [CrossRef] [PubMed]
13. Estrela, C.; Sydney, G.B.; Figueiredo, J.A.; Estrela, C.R. Antibacterial efficacy of intracanal medicaments on bacterial biofilm: A critical review. *J. Appl. Oral Sci.* **2009**, *17*, 1–7. [CrossRef] [PubMed]
14. Paganelli, F.L.; Willems, R.J.; Leavis, H.L. Optimizing future treatment of enterococcal infections: Attacking the biofilm? *Trends Microbiol.* **2012**, *20*, 40–49. [CrossRef] [PubMed]
15. Hollenbeck, B.L.; Rice, L.B. Intrinsic and acquired resistance mechanisms in enterococcus. *Virulence* **2012**, *3*, 421–433. [CrossRef] [PubMed]
16. Lins, R.X.; de Oliveira Andrade, A.; Junior, R.H.; Lewis, M.A.O.; Wilson, M.J.; Fidel, R.A.S. Antimicrobial resistance and virulence traits of *Enterococcus faecalis* from primary endodontic infections. *J. Dent.* **2013**, *41*, 779–786. [CrossRef] [PubMed]
17. Clinical and Laboratory Standards Institute. Performance Standards for Antimicrobial Susceptibility Testing. Twenty-Fourth Informational Supplement; Wayne, PA, USA, 2014; PP. 76–79.
18. Wiegand, I.; Hilpert, K.; Hancock, R.E. Agar and broth dilution methods to determine the minimal inhibitory concentration (MIC) of antimicrobial substances. *Nat. Protoc.* **2008**, *3*, 163–175. [CrossRef] [PubMed]
19. Maisonneuve, E.; Gerdes, K. Molecular mechanisms underlying bacterial persisters. *Cell* **2014**, *157*, 539–548. [CrossRef] [PubMed]
20. Babii, O.; Afonin, S.; Berditsch, M.; Reibetaer, S.; Mykhailiuk, P.K.; Kubyshkin, V.S.; Steinbrecher, T.; Ulrich, A.S.; Komarov, I.V. Controlling biological activity with light: Diarylethene-containing cyclic peptidomimetics. *Angew. Chem. Int. Ed. Engl.* **2014**, *53*, 3392–3395. [CrossRef] [PubMed]
21. de la Fuente-Nunez, C.; Reffuveille, F.; Haney, E.F.; Straus, S.K.; Hancock, R.E. Broad-spectrum anti-biofilm peptide that targets a cellular stress response. *PLoS Pathog.* **2014**, *10*, e1004152. [CrossRef] [PubMed]
22. Krauss, E.M.; Chan, S.I. Complexation and phase transfer of nucleotides by gramicidin S. *Biochemistry* **1983**, *22*, 4280–4291. [CrossRef] [PubMed]
23. Krauss, E.M.; Chan, S.I. Complexation and phase transfer of nucleic acids by gramicidin S. *Biochemistry* **1984**, *23*, 73–77. [CrossRef] [PubMed]
24. Gause, G.F.; Brazhnikova, M.G. Gramicidin S and its use in the treatment of infected wounds. *Nature* **1944**, *154*, 703. [CrossRef]
25. Gause, G.F.; Brazhnikova, M.G. Gramicidin S Origin and mode of action. *Lancet* **1944**, *244*, 715–716.
26. Hoyer, K.M.; Mahlert, C.; Marahiel, M.A. The iterative gramicidin s thioesterase catalyzes peptide ligation and cyclization. *Chem. Biol.* **2007**, *14*, 13–22. [CrossRef] [PubMed]
27. Aoki, W.; Ueda, M. Characterization of Antimicrobial Peptides toward the Development of Novel Antibiotics. *Pharmaceuticals* **2013**, *6*, 1055–1081. [CrossRef] [PubMed]
28. Katsu, T.; Ninomiya, C.; Kuroko, M.; Kobayashi, H.; Hirota, T.; Fujita, Y. Action mechanism of amphipathic peptides gramicidin S and melittin on erythrocyte membrane. *Biochim. Biophys. Acta* **1988**, *939*, 57–63. [CrossRef]
29. Berditsch, M.; Afonin, S.; Ulrich, A.S. The ability of *Aneurinibacillus migulanus* (*Bacillus brevis*) to produce the antibiotic gramicidin S is correlated with phenotype variation. *Appl. Environ. Microbiol.* **2007**, *73*, 6620–6628. [CrossRef] [PubMed]

30. Polin, A.N.; Egorov, N.S. Structural and functional characteristics of gramicidin S in connection with its antibiotic activity. *Antibiot. Khimioter.* **2003**, *48*, 29–32. [PubMed]
31. Salgado, J.; Grage, S.L.; Kondejewski, L.H.; Hodges, R.S.; McElhaney, R.N.; Ulrich, A.S. Membrane-bound structure and alignment of the antimicrobial β-sheet peptide gramicidin S derived from angular and distance constraints by solid state ^{19}F-NMR. *J. Biomol. NMR* **2001**, *21*, 191–208. [CrossRef] [PubMed]
32. Zhang, L.; Rozek, A.; Hancock, R.E. Interaction of cationic antimicrobial peptides with model membranes. *J. Biol. Chem.* **2001**, *276*, 35714–35722. [CrossRef] [PubMed]
33. Mogi, T.; Kita, K. Gramicidin S and polymyxins: the revival of cationic cyclic peptide antibiotics. *Cell. Mol. Life Sci.* **2009**, *66*, 3821–3826. [CrossRef] [PubMed]
34. Wenzel, M.; Chiriac, A.I.; Otto, A.; Zweytick, D.; May, C.; Schumacher, C.; Gust, R.; Albada, H.B.; Penkova, M.; Krämer, U.; et al. Small cationic antimicrobial peptides delocalize peripheral membrane proteins. *Proc. Natl. Acad. Sci. USA* **2014**, *111*, E1409–E1418. [CrossRef] [PubMed]
35. de la Fuente-Nunez, C.; Korolik, V.; Bains, M.; Nguyen, U.; Breidenstein, E.B.; Horsman, S.; Lewenza, S.; Burrows, L.; Hancock, R.E. Inhibition of bacterial biofilm formation and swarming motility by a small synthetic cationic peptide. *Antimicrob. Agents Chemother.* **2012**, *56*, 2696–2704. [CrossRef] [PubMed]
36. Lechner, S; Lewis, K.; Bertram, R. *Staphylococcus aureus* persisters tolerant to bactericidal antibiotics. *J. Mol. Microbiol. Biotechnol.* **2012**, *22*, 235–244. [CrossRef] [PubMed]
37. Williams, S.C.; Wade, W.G. A comparison of enterococcal genotypes from the human mouth and cheese. *Int. Endontic. J.* **2010**, *43*, 352–353. [CrossRef]
38. Razavi, A.; Gmur, R.; Imfeld, T.; Zehnder, M. Recovery of *Enterococcus faecalis* from cheese in the oral cavity of healthy subjects. *Oral Microbiol. Immunol.* **2007**, *22*, 248–251. [CrossRef] [PubMed]
39. Berditsch, M.; Jager, T.; Strempel, N.; Schwartz, T.; Overhage, J.; Ulrich, A.S. Synergistic effect of membrane-active peptides polymyxin B and gramicidin S on multidrug-resistant strains and biofilms of *Pseudomonas aeruginosa*. *Antimicrob. Agents Chemother.* **2015**, *59*, 5288–5296. [CrossRef] [PubMed]
40. Sergiev, P.G. Clinical use of Gramicidin S. *Lancet* **1944**, *244*, 717–718. [CrossRef]
41. Lapage, G. Gramicidin-S. *Nature* **1945**, *155*, 246–246. [CrossRef]
42. Seneviratne, C.J.; Yip, J.W.; Chang, J.W.; Zhang, C.F.; Samaranayake, L.P. Effect of culture media and nutrients on biofilm growth kinetics of laboratory and clinical strains of *Enterococcus faecalis*. *Arch. Oral Biol.* **2013**, *58*, 1327–1334. [CrossRef] [PubMed]
43. Murray, C.A.; Saunders, W.P. Root canal treatment and general health: A review of the literature. *Int. Endontic. J.* **2000**, *33*, 1–18. [CrossRef]
44. Amsterdam, D. Susceptibility testing of antimicrobials in liquid media. *Antibiot. Laboratory Med.* **1996**, *4*, 61–143.
45. Stepanovic, S.; Vukovic, D.; Dakic, I.; Savic, B.; Svabic-Vlahovic, M. A modified microtiter-plate test for quantification of staphylococcal biofilm formation. *J. Microbiol. Methods* **2000**, *40*, 175–179. [CrossRef]
46. Herigstad, B.; Hamilton, M.; Heersink, J. How to optimize the drop plate method for enumerating bacteria. *J. Microbiol. Methods* **2001**, *44*, 121–129. [CrossRef]

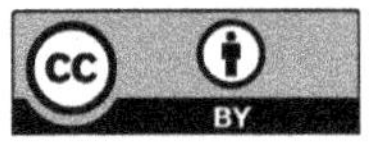

© 2016 by the authors. Licensee MDPI, Basel, Switzerland. This article is an open access article distributed under the terms and conditions of the Creative Commons Attribution (CC BY) license (http://creativecommons.org/licenses/by/4.0/).

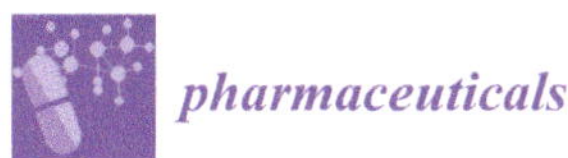

MDPI

Review

Chapter 10:

The Role of Antimicrobial Peptides in Influenza Virus Infection and Their Potential as Antiviral and Immunomodulatory Therapy

I-Ni Hsieh and Kevan L. Hartshorn *

Department of Medicine, Boston University School of Medicine, Boston, MA 02118, USA; inhsieh@bu.edu
* Correspondence: khartsho@bu.edu; Tel.: +1-617-638-5638; Fax: +1-617-638-7530

Academic Editor: Guangshun Wang
Received: 28 June 2016; Accepted: 31 August 2016; Published: 6 September 2016

Abstract: Influenza A virus (IAV) remains a major threat that can cause severe morbidity and mortality due to rapid genomic variation. Resistance of IAVs to current anti-IAV drugs has been emerging, and antimicrobial peptides (AMPs) have been considered to be potential candidates for novel treatment against IAV infection. AMPs are endogenous proteins playing important roles in host defense through direct antimicrobial and antiviral activities and through immunomodulatory effects. In this review, we will discuss the anti-IAV and immunomodulatory effects of classical AMPs (defensins and cathelicidins), and proteins more recently discovered to have AMP-like activity (histones and Alzheimer's associated β-amyloid). We will discuss the interactions between AMPs and other host defense proteins. Major emphasis will be placed on novel synthetic AMPs derived from modification of natural proteins, and on potential methods of increasing expression of endogenous AMPs, since these approaches may lead to novel antiviral therapeutics.

Keywords: cathelicidin; defensin; LL-37; histone; amyloid

---

1. Introduction

IAV presents an ongoing major threat to human health and there is much yet to be learned about the role of innate immunity during IAV infection [1]. Although IAV elicits strong adaptive immune responses, it is prone to rapid genomic variation either through small incremental mutations or major changes resulting from exchange of genome segments with those of animal strains (reassortment). These genomic changes allow IAV to escape immune responses generated against prior strains. Generally, the small incremental changes lead to seasonal epidemics, whereas reassortment leads to pandemics. The presence of animal reservoirs allows introduction of avian or pig strains (or genes from these strains) into humans resulting in pandemics, as in 2009 [2]. Seasonal epidemics of influenza virus still contribute tremendous morbidity and mortality including annual mortality in the USA of ~40,000 [3]. Certain groups of individuals are more susceptible to severe outcomes of seasonal IAV: those at extremes of age, smokers, individuals with COPD, cystic fibrosis or asthma, diabetes mellitus, cardiovascular disease, or immune compromise. Some otherwise healthy young people die during seasonal epidemics, sometimes due to bacterial super-infection (e.g., note recent association of IAV with MRSA pneumonia) [4]. Pandemics cause more indiscriminate mortality in young healthy adults than seasonal IAV [5]. There is a period of 5–7 days prior to arrival of CD8+ T cells in the lung after exposure to a new IAV strain and innate defense is critical at this time.

There is clearly a need for more therapies for IAV infection. Currently there are only two classes of antiviral drugs active against IAV: inhibitors of the viral proton channel (M protein) and neuraminidase inhibitors. High level of resistance to amantadines and emerging resistance to neuraminidase inhibitors have been reported. In this review, we evaluate the potential of antimicrobial peptides (AMPs) as therapies for IAV through summarizing in vitro and in vivo antiviral and immunomodulatory activity of natural and modified forms these peptides.

2. Antiviral Activity of Various AMPs in Vitro and in Vivo vs. IAV

IAV is a respiratory tract infection that rarely causes viremia or direct infection of organs outside the lung. Despite this it can induce severe systemic illness largely through the production of pro-inflammatory cytokines. Mortality is most often linked to respiratory failure due to acute lung injury and/or bacterial super-infection. In addition, some deaths occur due to cardiovascular events likely triggered by the profound inflammatory state resulting from IAV infection in some vulnerable subjects. There has been extensive interest in development of antivirals for IAV, but also in designing therapies to dampen inflammatory injury induced by the virus. AMPs are attractive as potential therapies for IAV since they have antiviral and antibacterial activity and also exert immunomodulatory effects.

There are two major classes of amphipathic AMPs present in human respiratory lining fluids: defensins and cathelicidins. There is evidence that both of these classes of AMPs play a role during IAV infection. We will review the antiviral and immune modulatory activities of defensins, cathelicidins, and also other peptides that have other important functions but also act as AMPs (e.g., histones and Alzheimer's associated amyloid beta). We will then discuss novel modified versions of AMPs synthesized with the aim of increasing antiviral activity. Finally, we will review potential means of inducing increased production of endogenous AMPs as an approach to antiviral treatment.

2.1. Defensins and Influenza

There are two major classes of defensins: α- and β-defensins. One group of α-defensins are packaged in neutrophil granules and these are termed human neutrophil peptides (HNPs) 1–4. The HNPs are very likely to interact with IAV in vivo since neutrophils predominate in the early infiltrate in the IAV infected airway and play a pivotal role in initiation of the immune response to the virus. HNPs are also displayed on neutrophil extracellular traps (NETs), which are formed in response to IAV infection in vitro [6] and in vivo [7]. Another group of α-defensins is expressed by epithelial cells, predominantly in the gut and genitourinary tracts. These are termed human defensins (HDs) 5 and 6. There is less reason to believe that HDs play a role in vivo during IAV infection, although they are of interest for their strong antiviral activity [8]. β-defensins are expressed predominantly by epithelial cells and are relevant in particular to IAV since they are expressed by the respiratory epithelium.

2.1.1. HNPs and IAV

These have strong neutralizing activity for many IAV strains [8–10]. The mechanisms of antiviral activity of HNPs have not been fully elucidated. We have found that HNPs induce viral aggregation and inhibit infectivity mainly through direct interactions with the virus [8,10–12]. In our studies, incubating epithelial cells with defensins pre- or post-infection had minimal inhibitory activity and direct incubation of HNPs with the virus was needed. In contrast, Salvatore et al. have found that HNPs also inhibit IAV through binding to epithelial cells and inhibition of protein kinase C [9]. In addition, the viral binding activity of defensins is potentiated by formation of multimolecular assemblies of defensins [8,13,14]. This may help to account for viral aggregating activity of defensins. Unlike the collectins and other proteins that bind the viral hemagglutinin (HA), HNPs do not inhibit HA activity of IAV [10]. Mice do not have neutrophil α-defensins but have other antimicrobial peptides that may play a similar role; hence, it has not been possible to use mouse models to test the role of neutrophil α-defensins.

2.1.2. β-Defensins and IAV

Human β-defensins (HBDs), are produced by respiratory epithelial cells either constitutively or in response to inflammatory stimuli and also inhibit IAV [8,15,16]. The HBDs are less potent as direct inhibitors of IAV than the HNPs; however, they may have important immunomodulatory roles during IAV infection as well. Ryan et al. have demonstrated that mice lacking mouse β defensin 1 (mBD1) have more severe lung inflammation when infected with IAV although viral titers were not different compared to control mice [16]. This paper also demonstrated that IAV infection increases production of mBD1 by plasmacytoid dendritic cells. Further studies of the in vivo contributions of this and other β-defensins during IAV infection will be of great interest.

2.1.3. Retrocyclins

Of interest, there is a third class of defensins called θ-defensins or retrocylins (because of their cyclic nature) that are expressed in primates but not humans and have very strong anti-IAV activity [8,17]. The retrocyclins, like HNPs, can induce aggregation of IAV and they appear to have stronger intrinsic antiviral activity than HNPs [8]. As with HNPs, it was necessary to directly incubate the virus with the retrocyclins to achieve optimal inhibition of infectivity in our studies. There is evidence that retrocyclins and other defensins can act as lectins binding to viral carbohydrates [18,19], and this may be an important contributor to their activity against viruses.

2.1.4. Potential for Paradoxical Activity of Defensins

HD5 and HD6 have been found to promote infection by human immunodeficiency virus (HIV) in vitro by increasing viral entry [20]. These defensins also counteract anti-HIV effects of polyanion microbicides [21]. HNP1 was also reported to increase HIV infectivity by facilitating transfer of the virus across epithelial barriers [22]. Note that other studies show an ability of these defensins to inhibit HIV [23–25]. No studies have indicated promotion of infection of IAV by defensins.

2.2. LL-37 and Influenza

A distinct group of antimicrobial peptides is called the cathelicidins and the one representative of this class in humans is LL-37. Recent reviews have discussed the extraordinary range of activities of LL-37, which include direct antimicrobial and antiviral activities, chemotactic activities for various immune cells, modulation of macrophage responses to inflammatory stimuli, and modulation of dendritic cell responses [26,27]. It is very likely that LL-37 participates in the host response to IAV. LL-37 resembles HNPs in that it is packaged in neutrophil granules and released upon cellular activation. LL-37 is also displayed on NETs where it can interact with IAV, which binds to NETs [6]. Like HBDs, LL-37 is produced by respiratory (and other) epithelial cells in response to various stimuli [26]. Leukotriene B4 (LTB4) has been shown to promote defense against IAV probably through its ability to stimulate release of LL-37 and β-defensins from respiratory epithelial cells [28].

As with other AMPs there is considerably more literature about the anti-bacterial activity than there is about the antiviral activity of LL-37. Recently, however, LL-37 has been found to inhibit several viruses including IAV, adenovirus, respiratory syncytial virus and HIV [29–32]. Several studies have recently established a role of LL-37 during IAV infection. Barlow et al. first demonstrated that LL-37 has direct antiviral activity against IAV and contributes to host defense against the virus in vivo both by limiting viral replication and virus-induced inflammation [33]. There is also a single murine cathelicidin, called CRAMP, which also inhibits IAV in vitro and in vivo [33,34]. Our laboratory then reported on the mechanism of antiviral activity of LL-37 that is distinct from that of collectins or defensins [34]. As with the defensins, direct incubation of the virus with LL-37 was needed to cause optimal inhibition of viral replication. Adding LL-37 to cells before or after infection was less effective.

In contrast to the HNPs, LL-37 did not induce viral aggregation. In addition, LL-37 did not alter viral uptake by epithelial cells, although it markedly limited subsequent viral replication in the cells. Using electron microscopy, there was evidence of viral membrane degradation that could alter infectivity after viral internalization. This is consistent with the known membrane perturbing activities of LL-37. A similar finding was obtained by Currie et al. with respect to neutralization of RSV by LL-37 [35].

2.3. Other Peptides with Antiviral Activity for IAV

Fragments of other host defense molecules or peptides not commonly known to serve host defense functions have been showed to have AMP like activity with regard to bacteria and viruses.

2.3.1. Histones

Histones are cationic peptides that resemble AMPs in some regards. There is increasing evidence that histones serve a host defense role vs. various organisms [36]. Histones are mainly known for their ability to bind to and regulate expression of DNA. However, histones are also found in cytosol and extracellular fluids where they appear to serve other functions, including antimicrobial activity. There are several reasons to believe histones may participate in the immune response during IAV infection. Like defensins and LL-37, histones are a major component of NETs [37]. In addition, histones are released into respiratory lining fluids during a variety of lung inflammatory states [38].

The bulk of studies of the antimicrobial activity of histones have focused on antibacterial activity. The lysine rich histones, H2A and H2B, have generally been found to have stronger anti-bacterial activity than the arginine rich histones H3 and H4 [39]. Several studies have demonstrated antiviral activity for histones as well [36,40]. We have recently reported that histones are able to neutralize influenza A viruses, with H3 and H4 having greater antiviral activity than H1, H2A and H2B [40]. The antiviral effect of the H4 was mediated by direct interaction with the virus rather than the host cells. In addition, H4 did not cause cell injury in a wide range of concentrations that reduced viral infectivity. H4 was able to strongly aggregate viral particles and this was associated with reduced uptake of the virus by target cells. Further studies of antiviral mechanisms of histones are warranted.

2.3.2. Amyloid Beta (Aβ) Peptides

Aβ peptides are mainly known for their key role in the development of Alzheimer's disease. However, Aβ peptides resemble some anti-microbial peptides or AMPs in their structure [41,42]. Aβ peptides are similar to the porcine AMP, protegrin, in ability to form channels in membrane structures, which is believed to be one of the anti-bacterial and anti-fungal mechanisms of AMPs. Soscia et al. demonstrated antibacterial and antifungal activity for Aβ peptides [43]. In addition, this study showed that Aβ isolated from the brain of AD patients had antimicrobial activity and that incubation of these brain derived samples with antibodies to Aβ ablated the antimicrobial activity. We recently reported that Aβ peptides also have antiviral activity against IAV [44]. A study by Bourgade et al. also showed inhibition of herpes simplex virus by Aβ peptides [45]. In our study and that of Soscia et al., Aβ1-42 was found to have greater antimicrobial or antiviral activity than Aβ1-40. We demonstrated that Aβ1-42, but not Aβ1-40, caused viral aggregation which appears to contribute to its antiviral effects. This implies a possible connection between the ability of Aβ1-42 to assemble into oligomers and its antiviral activity, since this peptide has a greater propensity to form oligomers and fibrils than Aβ1-40. An important recent study showed that Aβ peptides exert protective effects in mouse and worm models in vivo [46]. This study demonstrated that the antimicrobial mechanism of the peptides involved direct binding and then agglutination of the bacteria and fungi.

3. Immunomodulatory Effects of AMPs

In addition to their direct antimicrobial and antiviral effects, AMPs have important modulatory effects on responses of many immune cells (see Table 1).

Table 1. Antiviral and immunomodulatory activity of AMPs with respect to IAV.

AMP	Principle Human Lung Source	Antiviral Activity [a]	Immune Modulation [b]
α Defensin	Neutrophil	Seasonal strains: 3+ Pandemic strains: 1+	*Neutrophils:* increased viral uptake, reduced H_2O_2 response *Monocytes:* cytokines reduced
β Defensin	Epithelial Cells	Seasonal strains: 2+ Pandemic strains: ND	*Neutrophils:* increased viral uptake *Monocytes:* cytokines reduced
θ Defensin	Not present in humans	Seasonal strains: 4+ Pandemic strains: ND	*Neutrophils:* increased viral uptake *Monocytes:* cytokines reduced
LL-37	Neutrophils, macrophages, epithelial cells	Seasonal strains: 3+ Pandemic strains: +/−	*Neutrophils:* increased H_2O_2 and NETs, reduced IL-8 *Monocytes:* cytokines reduced
Amyloid Beta (Aβ)	Unknown	Seasonal strains: 2+ Pandemic strains: 2+	*Neutrophils:* increased viral uptake, increased H_2O_2 and NET response *Monocytes:* cytokines reduced
Histones H3 and H4	NETs and necrotic cells	Seasonal strains: 3+ Pandemic strains: +/−	*Neutrophils:* increased viral uptake, increased H_2O_2 response
Lactoferrin peptides	Neutrophils	Seasonal strains: 4+ Pandemic strains: ND	ND

[a] Antiviral activity for seasonal and pandemic IAV strains are indicated by a scale of 0 to 4+ to give a general idea of the relative potency of the different peptides. In some instances activity against pandemic strains were not determined (ND). [b] Results for immune modulation are not comprehensive.

3.1. Effects on Viral Uptake, Respiratory Burst and NET Formation by Neutrophils

We have studied extensively the ability of AMPs to modulate viral interactions with neutrophils. HNPs, retrocyclins, histones and Aβ1-42 increase viral uptake by human neutrophils ([8,12,44] and unpublished data). We obtained similar results with human monocytes ([11,44], and unpublished data). It appears likely that the ability of these AMPs to increase viral uptake is linked to their viral aggregating activity. Consistent with this interpretation, LL-37 did not alter viral uptake by neutrophils [6]. The AMPs have varied effects on respiratory burst responses of neutrophils. IAV itself stimulates a respiratory burst response characterized by H_2O_2 production. Pre-incubation of IAV with HNPs reduced this H_2O_2 response, whereas histones, Aβ1-42, and LL-37 potentiated the response. LL-37 and Aβ1-42 also increased NET formation in response to IAV [47]. LL-37 has several known receptors on phagocytes, including formyl peptide receptor 2 (FPR2), CXCR2, the epidermal growth factor receptor and the P2X7 receptor [48]. By use of a specific inhibitor for FPR2 and other means we were able to show that the enhanced H_2O_2 and NET response to IAV caused by LL-37 is mediated by FPR2 [6].

3.2. Effects on Cytokine Responses to IAV

IAV is a potent stimulator of neutrophil IL-8 production and monocyte or macrophage pro-inflammatory cytokine production (e.g., TNF or IL-6). Pro-inflammatory cytokine production in vivo correlates with symptomatology and with lung injury caused by IAV. A major goal of current IAV research has been to reduce inflammatory effects of the virus to reduce lung injury [49]. In mouse models, lung injury can be reduced even when viral loads are unaffected in some cases [49]. LL-37 has been reported to reduce cytokine responses to various stimuli [50–54], and, indeed we found that it reduced neutrophil IL-8 responses to IAV and LPS [6]. We are in the process of studying the effects of the various AMPs on monocyte and macrophage cytokine responses to IAV. As noted, LL-37 treatment of mice infected with IAV reduces cytokine responses [33]. This effect appeared be in part independent of reduction of viral load by LL-37 in vivo.

HNPs released from dying neutrophils have been shown to mediate anti-inflammatory effects [55]. In addition, HNPs can be taken up by macrophages during bacterial infection where they inhibit macrophage inflammatory cytokine production by restricting protein translation [56]. The relevance of these findings to IAV infection has not been evaluated thus far. As noted also, deletion of HBD-1 resulted in greater inflammatory reaction to IAV, despite no change in viral titers. HBD 3 has been shown to have strong anti-inflammatory effects as well in an LPS model [57,58]. It will be of interest to test this peptide in the context of IAV infection. Even though Aβ1-42 has been extensively studied as a pro-inflammatory stimulus [59], we found that it reduced inflammatory cytokine production triggered by IAV in monocytes in vitro [44].

Overall, these results indicate that maximizing anti-inflammatory effects as well as antiviral activity should be considered when designing novel AMPs for treatment of IAV. A contrasting perspective has arisen from several studies in which increasing inflammation prior to IAV or SARS-CoV infection was protective [60–62]. In the study by Wohlford-Lenane et al. intranasal instillation of retrocyclin 1 alone induced lung inflammation and this was associated with protection vs. SARS-CoV. In another study, direct instillation of HNPs into the airway of mice had pro-inflammatory effects independent of infection [63]. Note that in other models listed above HNPs had anti-inflammatory effects. Hence, further study is needed to determine how to best administer AMPs in vivo and whether possible pro-inflammatory effects would be harmful or beneficial with respect to infection.

Although histones have antimicrobial and antiviral activities, they have been considered to instigate several systemic inflammatory diseases and tissue injuries, including sepsis, peritonitis, pancreatitis, stroke, acute lung injury, liver injury and kidney injury [36]. The injection of histones into mice can stimulate pro-inflammatory cytokine/chemokine release (e.g., IL-6, IL-8 and TNF) and leukocyte infiltration, resulting in sepsis-like pathology [64–67]. In these cases histones function as damage-associated molecular pattern molecules, and possible mechanisms for them to induce cytokine storm may be through the interactions with toll-like receptors (TLR), especially TLR2, -4 and -9, and the NLRP3 inflammasome [68]. Knowing the possible detrimental pro-inflammatory effects of histones, further study is needed to investigate the roles of histones during severe IAV and IAV-related lung injury.

3.3. Effects of AMPs on Adaptive Immune Responses

AMPs have been termed "alarmins", in that they are able to trigger recruitment and activation of immune cells. AMPs modulate adaptive immune responses in various ways. This topic is beyond the scope of this paper; however, we refer the reader to other reviews [48,69]. As examples, HBDs and other defensins bind to receptors on lymphocytes and act as chemoattractants [70,71] and LL-37 facilitates presentation of antigens to by DCs to T cells [48,72]. α-defensins have been shown to potentiate neutralizing antibody responses to enteric viral infection [73]. The contribution of these activities to IAV infection have not been studied but certainly are valuable areas for future research.

3.4. Effects on Bacterial Superinfection

Bacterial superinfections are a major contributor to mortality during pandemics and seasonal epidemics of IAV [4]. These bacterial superinfections are difficult to treat with antibiotics. As a result there is great interest in identifying the cause of bacterial superinfection and how to intervene to prevent or treat these infections. The role of AMPs in bacterial superinfection, or for possible treatment of bacterial superinfection, has not been studied. However, given the combined antiviral and antibacterial activity of many AMPs they are attractive candidates for treatment of combined IAV and bacterial infection.

3.5. Interactions of AMPs with Other Host Defense Proteins

It is likely that the activity of AMPs in vivo reflects complex interactions among various AMPs and other host defense molecules [74,75]. We found that HNPs 1-3 bind to the lung host defense and surfactant regulatory protein, surfactant protein D (SP-D) [10,74]. The importance of this binding in vivo is not clear; however, HNPs inhibited antiviral activity of SP-D and caused precipitation of SP-D out of human BAL fluid. Since SP-D has anti-inflammatory properties in the uninfected and infected lung, this property of HNPs could account for inflammatory responses seen upon instillation of HNPs in the lung [63]. On the other hand, SP-D might aid in clearance of HNPs after neutrophil infiltration. Of note, we found that LL-37 and HBDs do not bind to SP-D [8], which may be advantageous when considering use of these peptides for therapy in the lung. Retrocyclins and LL-37 had additive antiviral effects when combined with SP-D [8,34].

Histones have been considered to augment inflammatory responses and promote thrombosis and thus can be responsible for IAV-related acute lung injury as noted above. There is evidence that other host defense proteins can bind histones and modulate their potential adverse effects. Little is known about the relationship between histones and SP-D. Evidence suggests that SP-D can simultaneously bind to both pathogens and NETs [64], and we recently found that SP-D can bind to histones and inhibit histone-induced respiratory burst in neutrophils (unpublished data). C-reactive protein (CRP), an acute phase reactant, is another host defense protein that is usually elevated during infections or inflammation, and CRP treatment in mice has been found to alleviate histone-induced toxicity, including endothelial damage, thrombosis and lung edema [76]. Other proteins like thrombomodulin have similar effects [77]. These findings suggest some possible modulators for histones, but further studies are needed [76].

4. Production of Modified Synthetic AMPs with Increased Antiviral Activity

4.1. Novel Cyclic or Alpha Defensins

There has been extensive research into ways to modify or mimic the structure of defensins in order to improve anti-bacterial or antiviral activity. Results of some of these studies are summarized in Table 2. Even single amino acid substitutions can potentiate antiviral activity. For instance, replacement of a single arginine with a lysine in retrocyclin 1 resulted in increased binding to, and inhibition of, HIV [14]. This modified retrocyclin also had increased IAV neutralizing activity [27]. Similarly, replacement of a single amino acid in HD5 resulted in increased activity vs. HSV [78]. The strong activity of retrocyclins also inspired construction of a panel of cyclic peptides by Ruchala and Lehrer [11]. The intent was to retain or improve on antiviral activities of naturally occurring retrocyclins with cyclic peptides that are easier to synthesize. These peptides were termed hapivirins and diprovirins and they incorporated systematic substitutions of key cationic or hydrophobic residues and also incorporated several synthetic amino acids. Several of the hapivirins and diprovirins had markedly increased neutralizing activity for IAV [11]. In addition, the peptides retained the properties of viral aggregation and increasing viral uptake by neutrophils. Like the retrocyclins, they did not interfere with the viral neutralizing activity of SP-D. In the case of the hapivirins, substitutions that increased hydrophobicity caused clear increase in antiviral activity, indicating that hydrophobicity is as important a feature as cationic charge for antiviral activity. The most active hapivirins and diprovirins also had strong ability to suppress TNF generation by human monocytes.

Table 2. Therapeutic Directions: Creation of Novel AMPs.

Prototype Peptide	Antiviral Activity	Immune modulation
β Defensin	Novel p9 peptide has increased antiviral activity against human and avian IAV strains	Mediate anti-inflammatory effects
Cyclic defensins	Hapivirins and Diprovirins have increased antiviral activity against seasonal IAV	Cause increased neutrophil uptake compared with HNPs and suppress TNF generation by monocytes
LL-37	GI-20 gains activity against pandemic strain	Have similar immunomodulatory effects to LL-37
Lactoferrin	Shorter peptide fragments show increased anti-IAV activity for seasonal and mouse adapted strains	Not tested
BPI	27 amino acid N-terminal fragment of human BPI inhibits infectivity of various IAV strains	Inhibit monocyte cytokine production in response to IAV

4.2. Novel β-Defensins

A recent paper by Zhao et al. took the approach of preparing a series of fragments of mouse beta defensin 4 and testing their activity against a panel of clinically important respiratory viruses, including human and avian IAV strains, SARS-CoV and MERS-CoV [79]. A 30 amino acid fragment of mBD4 (termed P9 by the authors) was found to have activity exceeding that of the full 40 amino acid protein both in vitro and in vivo in mice. In fact, 100% of mice survived lethal challenge with a mouse adapted H1N1 viral strain when they were pretreated with 50 μg/mouse of P9 intranasally. The P9 peptide also reduced lung inflammation and viral loads in the mice. P9 also increased survival of mice infected with a lethal dose of avian H5N1 or H7N9 and had in vitro antiviral activity against SARS-CoV and MERS-CoV. All of these respiratory viral strains are of great concern due to pandemic potential and severe outcomes of infection in humans. The mechanism of action of P9 was found to include binding to H1N1 IAV, entering the cell along with the virus and impairing endosomal acidification and hence viral escape from endosomes. This study provides and interesting example of a shortened fragment of a naturally occurring defensin having greater activity than the parent peptide.

4.3. LL-37 Derived Peptides

In a similar vein, shortened or subtly modified version of LL-37 have been tested for antiviral and antibacterial activity. A 20 amino acid fragment, termed GI-20, was found to have retained the antiviral activity of the full molecule against seasonal IAV [80] and against HIV [81]. Another fragment called K-13 had no activity for IAV, despite the fact that it inhibits HIV and has anti-bacterial activity as well [82,83]. Two N-terminal fragments (LL-23 and LL-23V9) that have anti-bacterial activity [84] failed to inhibit IAV [85]. The GI-20 fragment incorporates the central helix of LL-37 and differs by one amino acid from the LL-37 sequence (isoleucine 13 is changed to glycine). Of note, pandemic H1N1 of 2009 was inhibited in vitro by GI-20, but not by LL-37 or the other peptides [85]. This provides another example of a shortened version of a natural AMP with increased antiviral activity compared to the parent peptide. GI-20 also retained the ability of LL-37 to increase neutrophil respiratory burst and NET responses to IAV, while also suppressing neutrophil IL-8 response to the virus [80]. The ability of GI-20 to increase virus induced respiratory burst and NET responses was also mediated through binding to FPR2. Using molecular modeling GI-20 was found to incorporate the domain of the protein predicted to bind to the FPR2 receptor.

4.4. Lactoferrin and Bacterial/Permeability Increasing Protein (BPI) Based Peptides

Lactoferrin is an evolutionarily conserved innate immune protein present in breast milk and other mucosal secretions that is cationic and has activity against bacteria and several viruses, including IAV [86]. Lactoferrin has two lobes (the N and C lobes) both of which contain an iron binding site. Although the N and C lobes have similar structures they have distinct sequences within them. The two lobes can be separated by proteolytic cleavage and shown to have distinct functional activities [87]. A recent study by Ammendolia et al. showed that all of the anti-influenza activity of bovine lactoferrin is in the C lobe and that shorter peptide domains within the C lobe have picomolar activity against IAV [88]. These peptides had greater antiviral activity in vitro and greater selectivity indices (a measure that combines antiviral activity and cellular cytotoxicity) than the whole lactoferrin protein. The antiviral activity of lactoferrin was related to binding to the HA_2 subunit of the viral hemagglutinin (which contains the fusion domain).

A 27 amino acid N-terminal fragment of human BPI was recently shown to inhibit various IAV strains (including H1N1, H3N2 and H5N1 strains) in vitro through a direct action on the virus [89]. Of interest, the murine homolog of this peptide lacked anti-IAV activity. In addition, the human peptide inhibited IL-6 and TNF responses of monocytes triggered by IAV.

5. Potential for Resistance of IAV to AMPs

Mechanisms of resistance to AMPs have been well described in bacteria; however, there are no similar data for viruses. As noted above we found that pandemic IAV was not inhibited by LL-37 (although the GI-20 fragment was inhibitory). Similarly we found that the murine cathelicidin CRAMP [85] and human histone H4 did not inhibit pandemic H1N1 of 2009 [40]. HNP-1 had reduced activity for the pandemic strain as well. The mechanism of resistance of the pandemic strain is not clear since all of these AMP have activity against seasonal or mouse adapted strains of IAV. Using reverse genetics a viral strain was prepared having only the HA of the pandemic strain but all other gene segments from a seasonal H1N1 strain and this re-assorted strain was sensitive to LL-37, CRAMP and histone H4. This indicates that resistance is not mediated by the hemagglutinin of the pandemic strain. Further studies will be important to determine which components of the pandemic strain confer resistance to several AMPs.

6. Induction of Endogenous AMPs

One of the challenging features of developing AMPs as therapeutics is determining how to administer them. As noted above, there is evidence that direct administration into the airway may induce inflammatory responses. Another approach under exploration is increasing endogenous production of AMPs through various means [90]. Results of these studies are summarized in Table 3. As noted, LTB-4 can potentiate generation of both LL-37 and HBD in the respiratory tract [28,91]. LL-37 generation by epithelial cells is regulated by vitamin D; hence, repletion of vitamin D may have host defense benefits. LL-37 generation is also enhanced by histone deacetylase inhibitors (e.g., phenylbutyrate) [92]. This approach was found to improve outcomes when added to standard antibiotic treatment of mycobacterium tuberculosis infection in humans [93]. An interesting report also showed that supplementation with the amino acid isoleucine can increase HBD expression [94]. Further studies of this phenomenon will be of special interest given the low toxicity of this approach. IL-17 and IL-22 have been shown to induce expression of HBD and S100 peptides (another group of AMPs) in human keratinocytes [95]. One paper reported on endogenous generation of retrocyclins in human cells after exposure to aminoglycoside antibiotics [96]. Human cells actually contain the gene for retrocyclins but they are not expressed due to a premature stop codon in the signal sequence [97]. Clearly the study of AMP induction is in its infancy. However, there are several tantalizing findings that certainly support further exploration of this approach.

Table 3. Therapeutic Directions: Increase endogenous AMP generation.

Mediator	AMPs Effected
LTB4	Increase LL-37 and β Defensin generation
HDAC inhibitors	Increase LL-37 generation
Vitamin D	Increase LL-37 generation
Isoleucine	Increase HBD expression
IL-22, IL-17	Increase AMP expression

7. Conclusions

IAV causes many deaths or severe illness every year in seasonal outbreaks and has the potential to cause massive morbidity and mortality during pandemics. Resistance to two classes of drugs that are currently used for IAV treatment has been emerging, so there has been extensive interest in developing new antiviral treatment for this virus. Deaths caused by IAV infection mostly resulted from acute lung injury, systemic inflammation or bacterial superinfection, suggesting that new treatments with anti-viral, anti-bacterial and anti-inflammation effects would be ideal. AMPs are antimicrobial peptides that not only play important roles as host defense against pathogens but also modulate inflammatory responses, and thus they are potential candidates for IAV treatment. We discussed the interactions of two classes of classical AMPs (defensins and cathelicidins) and two non-classical AMPs (histones and Aβ) with IAVs in this paper. For the most part, these AMPs possess anti-IAV activity by direct interacting with the virus, although in some instances direct interactions with mammalian cells may contribute to antiviral effects. All of AMPs we discussed also have immunomodulatory effects, with some up-regulating and others down-regulating inflammation. We provide some examples (e.g., hapivirins and diprovirins or GI-20) in which novel synthetic AMPs or AMP fragments have improved anti-IAV or immunomodulatory activities, suggesting that modification of AMPs is an attractive strategy. Further studies are required to determine the interactions between AMPs and other host defense proteins in the lung, the best methods to administer or induce generation of AMPs, and to explain instances of resistance of pandemic IAV strains to AMPs.

Acknowledgments: This work was supported by NIH R01 HL069031 (KH).

Conflicts of Interest: The authors declare no conflict of interest.

References

1. Tripathi, S.; White, M.R.; Hartshorn, K.L. The amazing innate immune response to influenza a virus infection. *Innate Immun.* **2013**, *96*, 931–938. [CrossRef] [PubMed]
2. Dawood, F.S.; Jain, S.; Finelli, L.; Shaw, M.W.; Lindstrom, S.; Garten, R.J.; Gubareva, L.V.; Xu, X.; Bridges, C.B.; Uyeki, T.M. Emergence of a novel swine-origin influenza a (H1N1) virus in humans. *N. Engl. J. Med.* **2009**, *360*, 2605–2615. [PubMed]
3. Morens, D. Influenza-related mortality: Considerations for practice and public health. *J. Am. Med. Assoc.* **2003**, *289*, 227–229. [CrossRef]
4. Hartshorn, K.L. New look at an old problem: Bacterial superinfection after influenza. *Am. J. Pathol.* **2010**, *176*, 536–539. [CrossRef] [PubMed]
5. Hartshorn, K.L. Why does pandemic influenza virus kill? *Am. J. Pathol.* **2013**, *183*, 1125–1127. [CrossRef] [PubMed]
6. Tripathi, S.; Verma, A.; Kim, E.J.; White, M.R.; Hartshorn, K.L. LL-37 modulates human neutrophil responses to influenza a virus. *J. Leukoc. Biol.* **2014**. [CrossRef] [PubMed]
7. Narasaraju, T.; Yang, E.; Samy, R.P.; Ng, H.H.; Poh, W.P.; Liew, A.A.; Phoon, M.C.; Van Rooijen, N.; Chow, V.T. Excessive neutrophils and neutrophil extracellular traps contribute to acute lung injury of influenza pneumonitis. *Am. J. Pathol.* **2011**, *179*, 199–210. [CrossRef] [PubMed]
8. Doss, M.; White, M.R.; Tecle, T.; Gantz, D.; Crouch, E.C.; Jung, G.; Ruchala, P.; Waring, A.J.; Lehrer, R.I.; Hartshorn, K.L. Interactions of alpha-, beta-, and theta-defensins with influenza a virus and surfactant protein D. *J. Immunol.* **2009**, *182*, 7878–7887. [CrossRef] [PubMed]
9. Salvatore, M.; Garcia-Sastre, A.; Ruchala, P.; Lehrer, R.I.; Chang, T.; Klotman, M.E. β-defensin inhibits influenza virus replication by cell-mediated mechanism(s). *J. Infect. Dis.* **2007**, *196*, 835–843. [CrossRef] [PubMed]
10. Hartshorn, K.L.; White, M.R.; Tecle, T.; Holmskov, U.; Crouch, E.C. Innate defense against influenza a virus: Activity of human neutrophil defensins and interactions of defensins with surfactant protein d. *J. Immunol.* **2006**, *176*, 6962–6972. [CrossRef] [PubMed]

11. Doss, M.; Ruchala, P.; Tecle, T.; Gantz, D.; Verma, A.; Hartshorn, A.; Crouch, E.C.; Luong, H.; Micewicz, E.D.; Lehrer, R.I. Hapivirins and diprovirins: Novel theta-defensin analogs with potent activity against influenza a virus. *J. Immunol.* **2012**, *188*, 2759–2768. [CrossRef] [PubMed]
12. Tecle, T.; White, M.R.; Gantz, D.; Crouch, E.C.; Hartshorn, K.L. Human neutrophil defensins increase neutrophil uptake of influenza a virus and bacteria and modify virus-induced respiratory burst responses. *J. Immunol.* **2007**, *178*, 8046–8052. [CrossRef] [PubMed]
13. Hoover, D.M.; Rajashankar, K.R.; Blumenthal, R.; Puri, A.; Oppenheim, J.J.; Chertov, O.; Lubkowski, J. The structure of human β-defensin-2 shows evidence of higher order oligomerization. *J. Biol. Chem.* **2000**, *275*, 32911–32918. [CrossRef] [PubMed]
14. Owen, S.M.; Rudolph, D.L.; Wang, W.; Cole, A.M.; Waring, A.J.; Lal, R.B.; Lehrer, R.I. RC-101, a retrocyclin-1 analogue with enhanced activity against primary HIV type 1 isolates. *AIDS Res. Hum. Retrovir.* **2004**, *20*, 1157–1165. [CrossRef] [PubMed]
15. Jiang, Y.; Wang, Y.; Kuang, Y.; Wang, B.; Li, W.; Gong, T.; Jiang, Z.; Yang, D.; Li, M. Expression of mouse beta-defensin-3 in mdck cells and its anti-influenza-virus activity. *Arch. Virol.* **2009**, *154*, 639–647. [CrossRef] [PubMed]
16. Ryan, L.K.; Dai, J.; Yin, Z.; Megjugorac, N.; Uhlhorn, V.; Yim, S.; Schwartz, K.D.; Abrahams, J.M.; Diamond, G.; Fitzgerald-Bocarsly, P. Modulation of human beta-defensin-1 (hBD-1) in plasmacytoid dendritic cells (PDC), monocytes, and epithelial cells by influenza virus, herpes simplex virus, and sendai virus and its possible role in innate immunity. *J. Leukoc. Biol.* **2011**, *90*, 343–356. [CrossRef] [PubMed]
17. Liang, Q.L.; Zhou, K.; He, H.X. Retrocyclin 2: A new therapy against avian influenza H5N1 virus in vivo and vitro. *Biotechnol. Lett.* **2009**, *32*, 387–392. [CrossRef] [PubMed]
18. Leikina, E.; Delanoe-Ayari, H.; Melikov, K.; Cho, M.S.; Chen, A.; Waring, A.J.; Wang, W.; Xie, Y.; Loo, J.A.; Lehrer, R.I. Carbohydrate-binding molecules inhibit viral fusion and entry by crosslinking membrane glycoproteins. *Nat. Immunol.* **2005**, *6*, 995–1001. [CrossRef] [PubMed]
19. Wang, W.; Cole, A.M.; Hong, T.; Waring, A.J.; Liang, Q.L.; Zhou, K.; He, H.X. Retrocyclin 2: A new therapy against avian influenza h5n1 virus in vivo and vitro. *Biotechnol. Lett.* **2009**, *32*, 387–392. [CrossRef] [PubMed]
20. Klotman, M.E.; Rapista, A.; Teleshova, N.; Micsenyi, A.; Jarvis, G.A.; Lu, W.; Porter, E.; Chang, T.L. Neisseria gonorrhoeae-induced human defensins 5 and 6 increase HIV infectivity: Role in enhanced transmission. *J. Immunol.* **2008**, *180*, 6176–6185. [CrossRef] [PubMed]
21. Ding, J.; Rapista, A.; Teleshova, N.; Lu, W.; Klotman, M.E.; Chang, T.L. Mucosal human defensins 5 and 6 antagonize the anti-HIV activity of candidate polyanion microbicides. *J. Innate. Immun.* **2011**, *3*, 208–212. [CrossRef] [PubMed]
22. Valere, K.; Rapista, A.; Eugenin, E.; Lu, W.; Chang, T.L. Human alpha-defensin hnp1 increases hiv traversal of the epithelial barrier: A potential role in sti-mediated enhancement of HIV transmission. *Viral Immunol.* **2015**, *28*, 609–615. [CrossRef] [PubMed]
23. Furci, L.; Tolazzi, M.; Sironi, F.; Vassena, L.; Lusso, P. Inhibition of HIV-1 infection by human α-defensin-5, a natural antimicrobial peptide expressed in the genital and intestinal mucosae. *PLoS ONE* **2012**, *7*, e45208. [CrossRef] [PubMed]
24. Wang, W.; Owen, S.M.; Rudolph, D.L.; Cole, A.M.; Hong, T.; Waring, A.J.; Lal, R.B.; Lehrer, R.I. Activity of alpha- and theta-defensins against primary isolates of HIV-1. *J. Immunol.* **2004**, *173*, 515–520. [CrossRef] [PubMed]
25. Wilson, S.S.; Wiens, M.E.; Holly, M.K.; Smith, J.G. Defensins at the mucosal surface: Latest insights into defensin-virus interactions. *J. Virol.* **2016**, *90*, 5216–5218. [CrossRef] [PubMed]
26. Tecle, T.; Tripathi, S.; Hartshorn, K.L. Review: Defensins and cathelicidins in lung immunity. *Innate. Immun.* **2010**, *16*, 151–159. [CrossRef] [PubMed]
27. Doss, M.; White, M.R.; Tecle, T.; Hartshorn, K.L. Human defensins and LL-37 in mucosal immunity. *J. Leukoc. Biol.* **2010**, *87*, 79–92. [CrossRef] [PubMed]
28. Gaudreault, E.; Gosselin, J. Leukotriene B4 induces release of antimicrobial peptides in lungs of virally infected mice. *J. Immunol.* **2008**, *180*, 6211–6221. [CrossRef] [PubMed]
29. Currie, S.M.; Findlay, E.G.; McHugh, B.J.; Mackellar, A.; Man, T.; Macmillan, D.; Wang, H.; Fitch, P.M.; Schwarze, J.; Davidson, D.J. The human cathelicidin LL-37 has antiviral activity against respiratory syncytial virus. *PLoS ONE* **2013**, *8*, e73659. [CrossRef] [PubMed]

30. Uchio, E.; Inoue, H.; Kadonosono, K. Anti-adenoviral effects of human cationic antimicrobial protein-18/LL-37, an antimicrobial peptide, by quantitative polymerase chain reaction. *Korean J. Ophthalmol.* **2013**, *27*, 199–203. [CrossRef] [PubMed]
31. Wang, G.; Watson, K.M.; Buckheit, R.W., Jr. Anti-human immunodeficiency virus type 1 activities of antimicrobial peptides derived from human and bovine cathelicidins. *Antimicrob. Agents Chemother.* **2008**, *52*, 3438–3440. [CrossRef] [PubMed]
32. Bergman, P.; Walter-Jallow, L.; Broliden, K.; Agerberth, B.; Soderlund, J. The antimicrobial peptide LL-37 inhibits HIV-1 replication. *Curr. HIV Res.* **2007**, *5*, 410–415. [CrossRef] [PubMed]
33. Barlow, P.G.; Svoboda, P.; Mackellar, A.; Nash, A.A.; York, I.A.; Pohl, J.; Davidson, D.J.; Donis, R.O. Antiviral activity and increased host defense against influenza infection elicited by the human cathelicidin LL-37. *PLoS ONE* **2011**, *6*, e25333. [CrossRef] [PubMed]
34. Tripathi, S.; Tecle, T.; Verma, A.; Crouch, E.; White, M.; Hartshorn, K.L. The human cathelicidin LL-37 inhibits influenza a viruses through a mechanism distinct from that of surfactant protein D or defensins. *J. Gen. Virol.* **2013**, *94*, 40–49. [CrossRef] [PubMed]
35. Currie, S.M.; Gwyer Findlay, E.; McFarlane, A.J.; Fitch, P.M.; Bottcher, B.; Colegrave, N.; Paras, A.; Jozwik, A.; Chiu, C.; Schwarze, J. Cathelicidins have direct antiviral activity against respiratory syncytial virus in vitro and protective function in vivo in mice and humans. *J. Immunol.* **2016**, *196*, 2699–2710. [CrossRef] [PubMed]
36. Hoeksema, M.; Van Eijk, M.; Haagsman, H.P.; Hartshorn, K.L. Histones as mediators of host defense, inflammation and thrombosis. *Future Microbiol.* **2016**, *11*, 441–453. [CrossRef] [PubMed]
37. Lewis, H.D.; Liddle, J.; Coote, J.E.; Atkinson, S.J.; Barker, M.D.; Bax, B.D.; Bicker, K.L.; Bingham, R.P.; Campbell, M.; Chen, Y.H. Inhibition of PAD4 activity is sufficient to disrupt mouse and human net formation. *Nat. Chem. Biol.* **2015**, *11*, 189–191. [CrossRef] [PubMed]
38. Cheng, O.Z.; Palaniyar, N. Net balancing: A problem in inflammatory lung diseases. In *NETosis: At the Intersection of Cell Biology, Microbiology, and Immunology*; Frontiers Media SA: Lausanne, Switzerland, 2013; Volume 4, p. 1.
39. Morita, S.; Tagai, C.; Shiraishi, T.; Miyaji, K.; Iwamuro, S. Differential mode of antimicrobial actions of arginine-rich and lysine-rich histones against gram-positive staphylococcus aureus. *Peptides* **2013**, *48*, 75–82. [CrossRef] [PubMed]
40. Hoeksema, M.; Tripathi, S.; White, M.; Qi, L.; Taubenberger, J.; van Eijk, M.; Haagsman, H.; Hartshorn, K.L. Arginine-rich histones have strong antiviral activity for influenza a viruses. *Innate Immun.* **2015**. [CrossRef] [PubMed]
41. Kagan, B.L.; Jang, H.; Capone, R.; Teran Arce, F.; Ramachandran, S.; Lal, R.; Nussinov, R. Antimicrobial properties of amyloid peptides. *Mol. Pharm.* **2012**, *9*, 708–717. [CrossRef] [PubMed]
42. Jang, H.; Ma, B.; Lal, R.; Nussinov, R. Models of toxic beta-sheet channels of protegrin-1 suggest a common subunit organization motif shared with toxic alzheimer β-amyloid ion channels. *Biophys. J.* **2008**, *95*, 4631–4642. [CrossRef] [PubMed]
43. Soscia, S.J.; Kirby, J.E.; Washicosky, K.J.; Tucker, S.M.; Ingelsson, M.; Hyman, B.; Burton, M.A.; Goldstein, L.E.; Duong, S.; Tanzi, R.E. The alzheimer's disease-associated amyloid beta-protein is an antimicrobial peptide. *PLoS ONE* **2010**, *5*, e9505. [CrossRef] [PubMed]
44. White, M.R.; Kandel, R.; Tripathi, S.; Condon, D.; Qi, L.; Taubenberger, J.; Hartshorn, K.L. Alzheimer's associated beta-amyloid protein inhibits influenza a virus and modulates viral interactions with phagocytes. *PLoS ONE* **2014**, *9*, e101364. [CrossRef] [PubMed]
45. Bourgade, K.; Garneau, H.; Giroux, G.; Le Page, A.Y.; Bocti, C.; Dupuis, G.; Frost, E.H.; Fulop, T., Jr. Beta-amyloid peptides display protective activity against the human alzheimer's disease-associated herpes simplex virus-1. *Biogerontology* **2015**, *16*, 85–98. [CrossRef] [PubMed]
46. Kumar, D.; Choi, S.; Washicosky, K.; Eimer, W.; Tucker, S.; Ghofrani, J.; Lefkowitz, A.; McColl, G.; Goldstein, L.; Tanzi, R. Amyloid-β peptide protects against microbial infection in mouse and worm models of alzheimer's disease. *Sci. Transl. Med.* **2016**, *8*, 340ra372. [CrossRef] [PubMed]
47. Hartshorn, K.L.; Collamer, M.; White, M.R.; Schwartz, J.H.; Tauber, A.I. Characterization of influenza a virus activation of the human neutrophil. *Blood* **1990**, *75*, 218–226. [PubMed]
48. Kahlenberg, J.M.; Kaplan, M.J. Little peptide, big effects: The role of LL-37 in inflammation and autoimmune disease. *J. Immunol.* **2013**, *191*, 4895–4901. [CrossRef] [PubMed]

49. Tripathi, S.; White, M.R.; Hartshorn, K.L. The amazing innate immune response to influenza a virus infection. *Innate Immun.* **2015**, *21*, 73–98. [CrossRef] [PubMed]
50. Hu, Z.; Murakami, T.; Suzuki, K.; Tamura, H.; Kuwahara-Arai, K.; Iba, T.; Nagaoka, I. Antimicrobial cathelicidin peptide LL-37 inhibits the LSP/ATP-induced pyroptosis of macrophages by dual mechanism. *PLoS ONE* **2014**, *9*, e85765. [CrossRef] [PubMed]
51. Chen, X.; Takai, T.; Xie, Y.; Niyonsaba, F.; Okumura, K.; Ogawa, H. Human antimicrobial peptide LL-37 modulates proinflammatory responses induced by cytokine milieus and double-stranded rna in human keratinocytes. *Biochem. Biophys. Res. Commun.* **2013**, *433*, 532–537. [CrossRef] [PubMed]
52. Ruan, Y.; Shen, T.; Wang, Y.; Hou, M.; Li, J.; Sun, T. Antimicrobial peptide LL-37 attenuates lta induced inflammatory effect in macrophages. *Int. Immunopharmacol.* **2013**, *15*, 575–580. [CrossRef] [PubMed]
53. Brown, K.L.; Poon, G.F.; Birkenhead, D.; Pena, O.M.; Falsafi, R.; Dahlgren, C.; Karlsson, A.; Bylund, J.; Hancock, R.E.; Johnson, P. Host defense peptide LL-37 selectively reduces proinflammatory macrophage responses. *J. Immunol.* **2011**, *186*, 5497–5505. [CrossRef] [PubMed]
54. Braff, M.H.; Hawkins, M.A.; Di Nardo, A.; Lopez-Garcia, B.; Howell, M.D.; Wong, C.; Lin, K.; Streib, J.E.; Dorschner, R.; Leung, D.Y. Structure-function relationships among human cathelicidin peptides: Dissociation of antimicrobial properties from host immunostimulatory activities. *J. Immunol.* **2005**, *174*, 4271–4278. [CrossRef] [PubMed]
55. Miles, K.; Clarke, D.J.; Lu, W.; Sibinska, Z.; Beaumont, P.E.; Davidson, D.J.; Barr, T.A.; Campopiano, D.J.; Gray, M. Dying and necrotic neutrophils are anti-inflammatory secondary to the release of alpha-defensins. *J. Immunol.* **2009**, *183*, 2122–2132. [CrossRef] [PubMed]
56. Brook, M.; Tomlinson, G.H.; Miles, K.; Smith, R.W.; Rossi, A.G.; Hiemstra, P.S.; van't Wout, E.F.; Dean, J.L.; Gray, N.K.; Lu, W. Neutrophil-derived alpha defensins control inflammation by inhibiting macrophage mrna translation. *Proc. Natl. Acad. Sci. USA* **2016**, *113*, 4350–4355. [CrossRef] [PubMed]
57. Semple, F.; MacPherson, H.; Webb, S.; Cox, S.L.; Mallin, L.J.; Tyrrell, C.; Grimes, G.R.; Semple, C.A.; Nix, M.A.; Millhauser, G.L. Human beta-defensin 3 affects the activity of pro-inflammatory pathways associated with MyD88 and TRIF. *Eur. J. Immunol.* **2011**, *41*, 3291–3300. [CrossRef] [PubMed]
58. Semple, F.; Webb, S.; Li, H.N.; Patel, H.B.; Perretti, M.; Jackson, I.J.; Gray, M.; Davidson, D.J.; Dorin, J.R. Human β-defensin 3 has immunosuppressive activity in vitro and in vivo. *Eur. J. Immunol.* **2010**, *40*, 1073–1078. [CrossRef] [PubMed]
59. Gold, M.; El Khoury, J. Beta-amyloid, microglia, and the inflammasome in alzheimer's disease. *Semin. Immunopathol.* **2015**, *37*, 607–611. [CrossRef] [PubMed]
60. Tuvim, M.J.; Gilbert, B.E.; Dickey, B.F.; Evans, S.E. Synergistic TLR2/6 and TLR9 activation protects mice against lethal influenza pneumonia. *PLoS ONE* **2012**, *7*, e30596. [CrossRef] [PubMed]
61. Tuvim, M.J.; Evans, S.E.; Clement, C.G.; Dickey, B.F.; Gilbert, B.E. Augmented lung inflammation protects against influenza a pneumonia. *PLoS ONE* **2009**, *4*, e4176. [CrossRef] [PubMed]
62. Wohlford-Lenane, C.L.; Meyerholz, D.K.; Perlman, S.; Zhou, H.; Tran, D.; Selsted, M.E.; McCray, P.B., Jr. Rhesus theta-defensin prevents death in a mouse model of sars coronavirus pulmonary disease. *J. Virol.* **2009**, *83*. [CrossRef] [PubMed]
63. Zhang, H.; Porro, G.; Orzech, N.; Mullen, B.; Liu, M.; Slutsky, A.S. Neutrophil defensins mediate acute inflammatory response and lung dysfunction in dose-related fashion. *Am. J. Physiol. Lung Cell. Mol. Physiol.* **2001**, *280*, 947–954.
64. Xu, J.; Zhang, X.; Monestier, M.; Esmon, N.L.; Esmon, C.T. Extracellular histones are mediators of death through TLR2 and TLR4 in mouse fatal liver injury. *J. Immunol.* **2011**, *187*, 2626–2631. [CrossRef] [PubMed]
65. Xu, J.; Zhang, X.; Pelayo, R.; Monestier, M.; Ammollo, C.T.; Semeraro, F.; Taylor, F.B.; Esmon, N.L.; Lupu, F.; Esmon, C.T. Extracellular histones are major mediators of death in sepsis. *Nat. Med.* **2009**, *15*, 1318–1321. [CrossRef] [PubMed]
66. Chen, R.; Kang, R.; Fan, X.G.; Tang, D. Release and activity of histone in diseases. *Cell Death Dis.* **2014**, *5*, e1370. [CrossRef] [PubMed]
67. Westman, J.; Papareddy, P.; Dahlgren, M.W.; Chakrakodi, B.; Norrby-Teglund, A.; Smeds, E.; Linder, A.; Morgelin, M.; Johansson-Lindbom, B.; Egesten, A. Extracellular histones induce chemokine production in whole blood ex vivo and leukocyte recruitment in vivo. *PLoS Pathog.* **2015**, *11*, e1005319. [CrossRef] [PubMed]

68. Huang, H.; Chen, H.W.; Evankovich, J.; Yan, W.; Rosborough, B.R.; Nace, G.W.; Ding, Q.; Loughran, P.; Beer-Stolz, D.; Billiar, T.R. Histones activate the NLRP3 inflammasome in kupffer cells during sterile inflammatory liver injury. *J. Immunol.* **2013**, *191*, 2665–2679. [CrossRef] [PubMed]
69. Oppenheim, J.J.; Yang, D. Alarmins: Chemotactic activators of immune responses. *Curr. Opin. Immunol.* **2005**, *17*, 359–365. [CrossRef] [PubMed]
70. Grigat, J.; Soruri, A.; Forssmann, U.; Riggert, J.; Zwirner, J. Chemoattraction of macrophages, T lymphocytes, and mast cells is evolutionarily conserved within the human alpha-defensin family. *J. Immunol.* **2007**, *179*, 3958–3965. [CrossRef] [PubMed]
71. Chertov, O.; Michiel, D.F.; Xu, L.; Wang, J.M.; Tani, K.; Murphy, W.J.; Longo, D.L.; Taub, D.D.; Oppenheim, J.J. Identification of defensin-1, defensin-2, and CAP37/azurocidin as T-cell chemoattractant proteins released from interleukin-8-stimulated neutrophils. *J. Biol. Chem.* **1996**, *271*, 2935–2940. [CrossRef] [PubMed]
72. Davidson, D.J.; Currie, A.J.; Reid, G.S.; Bowdish, D.M.; MacDonald, K.L.; Ma, R.C.; Hancock, R.E.; Speert, D.P. The cationic antimicrobial peptide LL-37 modulates dendritic cell differentiation and dendritic cell-induced T cell polarization. *J. Immunol.* **2004**, *172*, 1146–1156. [CrossRef] [PubMed]
73. Gounder, A.P.; Myers, N.D.; Treuting, P.M.; Bromme, B.A.; Wilson, S.S.; Wiens, M.E.; Lu, W.; Ouellette, A.J.; Spindler, K.R.; Parks, W.C. Defensins potentiate a neutralizing antibody response to enteric viral infection. *PLoS Pathog.* **2016**, *12*, e1005474. [CrossRef] [PubMed]
74. White, M.R.; Tecle, T.; Crouch, E.C.; Hartshorn, K.L. Impact of neutrophils on antiviral activity of human bronchoalveolar lavage fluid. *Am. J. Physiol. Lung Cell. Mol. Physiol.* **2007**, *293*, 1293–1299. [CrossRef] [PubMed]
75. Bals, R.; Hiemstra, P.S. Innate immunity in the lung: How epithelial cells fight against respiratory pathogens. *Eur. Respir. J.* **2004**, *23*, 327–333. [CrossRef] [PubMed]
76. Abrams, S.T.; Zhang, N.; Dart, C.; Wang, S.S.; Thachil, J.; Guan, Y.; Wang, G.; Toh, C.H. Human CRP defends against the toxicity of circulating histones. *J. Immunol.* **2013**, *191*, 2495–2502. [CrossRef] [PubMed]
77. Nakahara, M.; Ito, T.; Kawahara, K.; Yamamoto, M.; Nagasato, T.; Shrestha, B.; Yamada, S.; Miyauchi, T.; Higuchi, K.; Takenaka, T. Recombinant thrombomodulin protects mice against histone-induced lethal thromboembolism. *PLoS ONE* **2013**, *8*, e75961. [CrossRef] [PubMed]
78. Wang, A.; Chen, F.; Wang, Y.; Shen, M.; Xu, Y.; Hu, J.; Wang, S.; Geng, F.; Wang, C.; Ran, X. Enhancement of antiviral activity of human alpha-defensin 5 against herpes simplex virus 2 by arginine mutagenesis at adaptive evolution sites. *J. Virol.* **2013**, *87*, 2835–2845. [CrossRef] [PubMed]
79. Zhao, H.; Zhou, J.; Zhang, K.; Chu, H.; Liu, D.; Poon, V.K.; Chan, C.C.; Leung, H.C.; Fai, N.; Lin, Y.P. A novel peptide with potent and broad-spectrum antiviral activities against multiple respiratory viruses. *Sci. Rep.* **2016**, *6*, 22008. [CrossRef] [PubMed]
80. Tripathi, S.; Wang, G.; White, M.; Rynkiewicz, M.; Seaton, B.; Hartshorn, K. Identifying the critical domain of LL-37 involved in mediating neutrophil activation in the presence of influenza virus: Functional and structural analysis. *PLoS ONE* **2015**, *10*, e0133454. [CrossRef] [PubMed]
81. Wang, G. Database-guided discovery of potent peptides to combat HIV-1 or superbugs. *Pharmaceuticals* **2013**, *6*, 728–758. [CrossRef] [PubMed]
82. Wang, G.; Mishra, B.; Epand, R.F.; Epand, R.M. High-quality 3D structures shine light on antibacterial, anti-biofilm and antiviral activities of human cathelicidin LL-37 and its fragments. *Biochim. Biophys. Acta* **2014**, *1838*, 2160–2172. [CrossRef] [PubMed]
83. Jacob, B.; Park, I.S.; Bang, J.K.; Shin, S.Y. Short KR-12 analogs designed from human cathelicidin LL-37 possessing both antimicrobial and antiendotoxic activities without mammalian cell toxicity. *J. Pept. Sci.* **2013**, *19*, 700–707. [CrossRef] [PubMed]
84. Wang, G.; Elliott, M.; Cogen, A.L.; Ezell, E.L.; Gallo, R.L.; Hancock, R.E. Structure, dynamics, and antimicrobial and immune modulatory activities of human LL-23 and its single-residue variants mutated on the basis of homologous primate cathelicidins. *Biochemistry* **2012**, *51*, 653–664. [CrossRef] [PubMed]
85. Tripathi, S.; Wang, G.; White, M.; Qi, L.; Taubenberger, J.; Hartshorn, K.L. Antiviral activity of the human cathelicidin, LL-37, and derived peptides on seasonal and pandemic influenza a viruses. *PLoS ONE* **2015**, *10*, e0124706. [CrossRef] [PubMed]
86. Wakabayashi, H.; Oda, H.; Yamauchi, K.; Abe, F. Lactoferrin for prevention of common viral infections. *J. Infect. Chemother.* **2014**, *20*, 666–671. [CrossRef] [PubMed]

87. Sharma, S.; Sinha, M.; Kaushik, S.; Kaur, P.; Singh, T.P. C-lobe of lactoferrin: The whole story of the half-molecule. *Biochem. Res. Int.* **2013**, *2013*, 271641. [CrossRef] [PubMed]
88. Ammendolia, M.G.; Agamennone, M.; Pietrantoni, A.; Lannutti, F.; Siciliano, R.A.; De Giulio, B.; Amici, C.; Superti, F. Bovine lactoferrin-derived peptides as novel broad-spectrum inhibitors of influenza virus. *Pathog. Glob. Health* **2012**, *106*, 12–19. [CrossRef] [PubMed]
89. Pinkenburg, O.; Meyer, T.; Bannert, N.; Norley, S.; Bolte, K.; Czudai-Matwich, V.; Herold, S.; Gessner, A.; Schnare, M. The human antimicrobial protein bactericidal/permeability-increasing protein (BPI) inhibits the infectivity of influenza a virus. *PLoS ONE* **2016**, *11*, e0156929. [CrossRef] [PubMed]
90. Zasloff, M. Inducing endogenous antimicrobial peptides to battle infections. *Proc. Natl. Acad. Sci. USA* **2006**, *103*, 8913–8914. [CrossRef] [PubMed]
91. Flamand, L.; Tremblay, M.J.; Borgeat, P. Leukotriene B4 triggers the in vitro and in vivo release of potent antimicrobial agents. *J. Immunol.* **2007**, *178*, 8036–8045. [CrossRef] [PubMed]
92. Mily, A.; Rekha, R.S.; Kamal, S.M.; Akhtar, E.; Sarker, P.; Rahim, Z.; Gudmundsson, G.H.; Agerberth, B.; Raqib, R. Oral intake of phenylbutyrate with or without vitamin D3 upregulates the cathelicidin LL-37 in human macrophages: A dose finding study for treatment of tuberculosis. *BMC Pulm. Med.* **2013**, *13*, 23.
93. Mily, A.; Rekha, R.S.; Kamal, S.M.; Arifuzzaman, A.S.; Rahim, Z.; Khan, L.; Haq, M.A.; Zaman, K.; Bergman, P.; Brighenti, S. Significant effects of oral phenylbutyrate and vitamin D3 adjunctive therapy in pulmonary tuberculosis: A randomized controlled trial. *PLoS ONE* **2015**, *10*, e0138340.
94. Fehlbaum, P.; Rao, M.; Zasloff, M.; Anderson, G.M. An essential amino acid induces epithelial beta-defensin expression. *Proc. Natl. Acad. Sci. USA* **2000**, *97*, 12723–12728. [CrossRef] [PubMed]
95. Liang, S.C.; Tan, X.Y.; Luxenberg, D.P.; Karim, R.; Dunussi-Joannopoulos, K.; Collins, M.; Fouser, L.A. Interleukin (IL)-22 and IL17 are coexpressed by TH17 cells and cooperatively enhance expression of antimicrobial peptides. *J. Exp. Med.* **2006**, *203*, 2271–2279. [CrossRef] [PubMed]
96. Venkataraman, N.; Cole, A.L.; Ruchala, P.; Waring, A.J.; Lehrer, R.I.; Stuchlik, O.; Pohl, J.; Cole, A.M. Reawakening retrocyclins: Ancestral human defensins active against HIV-1. *PLoS Biol.* **2009**, *7*, e95.
97. Lehrer, R.I.; Cole, A.M.; Selsted, M.E. Theta-defensins: Cyclic peptides with endless potential. *J. Biol. Chem.* **2012**, *287*, 27014–27019. [CrossRef] [PubMed]

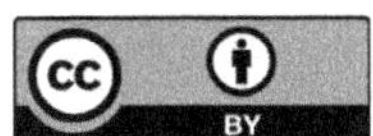

© 2016 by the authors. Licensee MDPI, Basel, Switzerland. This article is an open access article distributed under the terms and conditions of the Creative Commons Attribution (CC BY) license (http://creativecommons.org/licenses/by/4.0/).

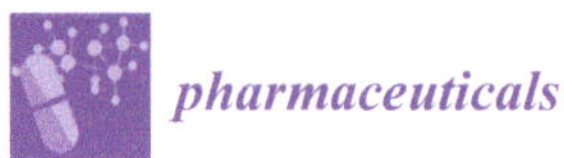

MDPI

Review

Chapter 12:

Potential Use of Antimicrobial Peptides as Vaginal Spermicides/Microbicides

Nongnuj Tanphaichitr [1,2,3,*], Nopparat Srakaew [1,4], Rhea Alonzi [1,3,†], Wongsakorn Kiattiburut [1,†], Kessiri Kongmanas [1,5], Ruina Zhi [1,6], Weihua Li [6], Mark Baker [7], Guanshun Wang [8] and Duane Hickling [1,9]

1 Chronic Disease Program, Ottawa Hospital Research Institute, Ottawa, ON K1H 8L6, Canada; fscinrsr@ku.ac.th (N.S.); ralonzi@ohri.ca (R.A.); wkiattiburut@ohri.ca (W.K.); kessiri.kon@mahidol.ac.th (K.K.); ruina.zhi@gmail.com (R.Z.); dhickling@toh.ca (D.H.)
2 Department of Obstetrics and Gynecology, Faculty of Medicine, University of Ottawa, Ottawa, ON K1H 8L6, Canada
3 Department of Biochemistry, Microbiology, Immunology, Faculty of Medicine, University of Ottawa, Ottawa, ON K1H 8M5, Canada
4 Department of Zoology, Faculty of Science, Kasetsart University, Bangkok 10900, Thailand
5 Division of Dengue Hemorrhagic Fever Research Unit, Office of Research and Development, Faculty of Medicine Siriraj Hospital, Mahidol University, Bangkok 10700, Thailand
6 Key Laboratory of Reproduction Regulation of NPFPC, Shanghai Institute of Planned Parenthood Research, and School of Public Health, Fudan University, Shanghai 200032, China; iamliweihua@foxmail.com
7 Reproductive Proteomics, Department of Science and Information technology, University of Newcastle, Callaghan Drive, Newcastle, NSW 2308 Australia; mark.baker@newcastle.edu.au
8 Department of Pathology and Microbiology, College of Medicine, University of Nebraska Medical Center, 986495 Nebraska Medical Center, Omaha, NE 68198-6495, USA; gwang@unmc.edu
9 Division of Urology, Department of Surgery, Faculty of Medicine, University of Ottawa, Ottawa, ON K1Y 4E9 , Canada
* Correspondence: ntanphaichitr@ohri.ca; Tel.: +1-737-8899 (ext. 72793)
† These authors contributed equally to this work.

Academic Editor: Jean Jacques Vanden Eynde
Received: 25 January 2016; Accepted: 3 March 2016; Published: 11 March 2016

Abstract: The concurrent increases in global population and sexually transmitted infection (STI) demand a search for agents with dual spermicidal and microbicidal properties for topical vaginal application. Previous attempts to develop the surfactant spermicide, nonoxynol-9 (N-9), into a vaginal microbicide were unsuccessful largely due to its inefficiency to kill microbes. Furthermore, N-9 causes damage to the vaginal epithelium, thus accelerating microbes to enter the women's body. For this reason, antimicrobial peptides (AMPs), naturally secreted by all forms of life as part of innate immunity, deserve evaluation for their potential spermicidal effects. To date, twelve spermicidal AMPs have been described including LL-37, magainin 2 and nisin A. Human cathelicidin LL-37 is the most promising spermicidal AMP to be further developed for vaginal use for the following reasons. First, it is a human AMP naturally produced in the vagina after intercourse. Second, LL-37 exerts microbicidal effects to numerous microbes including those that cause STI. Third, its cytotoxicity is selective to sperm and not to the female reproductive tract. Furthermore, the spermicidal effects of LL-37 have been demonstrated *in vivo* in mice. Therefore, the availability of LL-37 as a vaginal spermicide/microbicide will empower women for self-protection against unwanted pregnancies and STI.

Keywords: antimicrobial peptide; spermicide; spermicidal antimicrobial peptide; vaginal microbicide; vaginal contraceptive; sexually transmitted infection; vaginitis; LL-37; cathelicidin; hCAP-18

---

1. The Need for New Types of Contraceptives

As the world population continues to grow at an exponential rate, so does the need for novel contraceptives. Oral contraceptive pills (OC), formulated with a balanced combination of estrogen and progestin, are praised for their highest contraceptive efficacy and reversibility. The high, non-physiological dosages of estrogen and progestin in OCs induce an imbalance of reproductive hormones in the hypothalamus-pituitary-ovary axis, and subsequently a failure in ovulation. Progestin also thickens the cervical mucus, thus impeding sperm from swimming into the uterus and oviduct. These features empower women to protect themselves from unwanted pregnancies and therefore have become the most widely used form of contraception. However, these sex steroid based pills are not without risks, as estrogen and progestin are also involved in other physiological processes outside of ovulation and pregnancy. Excess circulating amounts of either hormone can lead to undesirable side effects. The most common minor side effects include nausea, weight gain and acne formation, whereas major side effects can include thromboembolism, hypertension, hyperlipidemia, cardiovascular disease, and breast and cervical malignancies. Long-term exposure to these hormones has also been shown to cause vaginal atrophy, which can lead to local symptoms and predisposition to infection. Women with a personal or family history of the aforementioned medical abnormalities or those who engage in high-risk behaviours such as smoking are medically advised against the use of OCs [1]. Estrogen and/or progestin can also be systemically administered via transdermal patch, subdermal implant, intradermal injection, vaginal ring, or intrauterine device (IUD). Regardless of the administration route, the side effects associated with estrogen/progestin are similar. Recent studies further suggest that the intradermally injected progestin, depo-medroxyprogesterone acetate (DMPA), may induce the thinning of the vaginal epithelium, and therefore increase the infection risk of microbes [2,3]. What is more, there is now growing concern about bioaccumulation of these hormonally based contraceptives and their associated negative impact on ecologic systems of all scales [4,5]. Therefore, development of reversible, locally acting and non-hormonal contraceptives should be considered.

As the global population increases, so does the rate of sexually transmitted infection (STI). HIV/AIDS continues to be a prevalent condition, affecting approximately 37 million people worldwide (http://www.who.int/hiv/data/epi_core_july2015.png?ua=1). The vaginal mucosa is the portal by which HIV from semen of seropositive men infects women following intercourse [6]. Many other viruses, bacteria, yeasts and protozoa also cause sexually transmitted infection (Table 1) via this route. Physical barriers such as male and female condoms prevent transmission of potential pathogens between both sexes. STI-induced microorganisms, as well as sperm, cannot penetrate through the condom layer, made from polyurethane or polyisoprene [1]. Therefore, the use of condoms is considered part of a safe sex practice for both men and women, as they are protected against unwanted pregnancies and STIs. However, the main drawback of condom use is decreased sensation and sensual pleasure during intercourse. Also, improper use and breakage during intercourse are concerns of the contraceptive efficacy of condoms [1]. Development for chemical spermicides and microbicides for vaginal use is therefore much needed.

Table 1. Common microorganisms that cause sexually transmitted infection and genitourinary tract infection.

Sexually Transmitted Infection	Vaginitis	Urinary Tract Infection
Viral Infection	**Yeast Infection**	**Yeast Infection**
• Human immunodeficiency virus (HIV) • Herpes simplex virus 1 & 2 (HSV-1 & HSV-2) • Human papillomavirus (HPV) • Hepatitis B and C	• *Candida albicans*	• *Candida albicans*
Protozoal Infection	**Protozoal Infection**	**Bacterial infection**
• *Trichomonas vaginalis*	• *Trichomonas vaginalis*	• *Escherichia coli* • *Klebsiella pneumoniae* • *Enterococcus* spp. • *Streptococcus agalactiae* • *Proteus mirabilis* • *Staphylococcus saprophyticus* • *Viridans streptococci* • *Klebsiella oxytoca* • *Staphylococcus aureus*
Bacterial infection	**Bacterial Vaginosis**	
• *Chlamydia trachomatis* • *Neisseria gonorrhoeae* • *Treponema pallidum*	• *Gardnerella vaginalis* • *Prevotella* spp. • *Porphyromonas* spp. • *Bacteroides* spp. • *Peptostreptococcus* spp. • *Mycoplasma hominis* • *Ureaplasma urealyticum* • *Mobiluncus* spp.	

2. Vaginally Administered Compounds with Dual Actions as Spermicides and Microbicides

Clearly, compounds with dual spermicide/microbicide action need to be developed. Various approaches to this can be considered, including microbicide screening against compounds with known spermicidal activity. Indeed, this was the approach taken for the spermicide, nonoxynol-9 (N-9). However, the final development of N-9 into a vaginal microbicide was not successful due to its deleterious effects on the vaginal epithelium as well as its microbicide inefficacy. Apparently, the development of N-9 into a spermicide over 50 years ago did not take into account the physiology of sperm function, the knowledge of which has been slowly unfolding over the past decades. Details of the current knowledge on sperm physiology/biochemistry are therefore given herein for consideration of the development of the next generation of vaginal contraceptive/microbicide compounds.

2.1. Mechanisms on How Mammalian Sperm Gain Fertilizing Ability

The fertilizing potential of sperm in the ejaculate correlates with a number of basic parameters including motility, concentration, total sperm number, and sperm morphology [7]. However, sperm can fertilize eggs only after they undergo the capacitation process. This occurs naturally in the female reproductive tract, and can be mimicked *in vitro* by incubating isolated sperm relatively free of seminal plasma in a medium containing calcium, bicarbonate and albumin. "Capacitation" defines the overall biochemical and physiological changes that allow sperm to bind to the egg and then enter into its cytoplasm. During capacitation significant changes occur on the sperm plasma membrane [8]. This is partly attributed to a cholesterol efflux [8,9], which subsequently increases overall sperm plasma membrane fluidity, preparing sperm for the two membrane fusion events essential for completing the fertilization process. The first event is part of the onset of the acrosome reaction. The acrosome is a membrane enveloped cap-like structure that is underneath the plasma membrane of the sperm head anterior. Upon exposure to stimulators such as zona pellucida (ZP) glycoproteins and progesterone, calcium is rapidly transported into sperm, and the acrosome reaction is initiated with the multi-site fusion between the sperm anterior head plasma membrane and the outer acrosomal membrane. This membrane fusion results in the pore formation in the sperm head anterior and finally exocytosis of the acrosomal content, mainly composed of hydrolytic enzymes, into the surrounding. These hydrolytic enzymes digest the egg vestments (networks of cumulus cell layers composed of proteo-glycosaminoglycans and the egg extracellular matrix-the ZP), thus facilitating sperm to swim towards the egg plasma membrane [8]. Without the completion of the acrosome reaction, fertilization cannot take place [8,10]. On the other hand, if the acrosome reaction is completed prematurely, sperm will have problems penetrating the egg vestments and also binding to the egg ZP.

Once acrosome reacted sperm penetrate through the ZP, they reach and bind to the egg plasma membrane. At this time the second membrane fusion event occurs between the plasma membrane of the head (post-acrosomal) region of an acrosome reacted sperm and the egg plasma membrane. This fusion is immediately followed by incorporation of the whole sperm into the egg proper and this signifies that fertilization has occurred.

The increase of the membrane fluidity due to cholesterol efflux also leads to a change in the sperm movement patterns. Sperm swim with a progressive forward pattern before capacitation. Capacitated sperm, however, swim with "hyperactivated motility" patterns, which are whiplash like with a high amplitude of lateral head (ALH) displacement. These swimming patterns endow sperm with a high thrusting force, facilitating them to penetrate through the egg vestments [8,11]. CatSper calcium cation channels play an integral role in sperm acquisition of hyperactivated motility patterns [12]. Male mice genetically deleted of *CatSperδ* are infertile; despite normal sperm production, sperm of these knockout mice cannot move with hyperactivated motility patterns [13]. Changes in the sperm plasma membrane composition during capacitation also lead to the exposure of sperm head surface molecules that are responsible for binding to the egg ZP in a species specific manner [8]. These ZP binding molecules are localized to the sperm anterior head plasma membrane overlying the acrosome. To date, more than 15 proteins, as well as a male germ cell specific sulfoglycolipid, sulfogalactosylglycerolipid (SGG, aka seminolipid) [14–16], have been shown for their affinity for the egg ZP. Results from knockout mouse studies indicate that most of these proteins and SGG are not essential for sperm fertilizing ability, since the knockout male mice remain fertile [17]. These results can be interpreted by the possibility that these proteins/SGG have backups for one another, as the fertilization process is of utmost importance for the maintenance of life in the next generation within a species [18]. Supporting this concept is the fact that sperm head surface proteins with ZP affinity exist together as high molecular weight complexes, which have direct ZP binding ability [19,20].

With sperm physiological events described above, it is logical to search for compounds that disable sperm fertilizing ability through the following processes: forward motility in non-capacitated sperm, and hyperactivated motility, acrosome reaction and sperm-ZP binding in capacitated sperm. However, targeting each individual event may be a complicated task, especially at the step of sperm-ZP binding in which numerous sperm surface molecules are engaged. Hypothetically, inhibiting sperm capacitation would result in inability of sperm to fertilize eggs. However, there are several challenges towards this approach. First, compounds used to inhibit sperm capacitation should be specific to only this sperm event, so as to minimize unrelated side effects. Second, sperm swim out from the seminal plasma in the vagina through the cervix and into the uterine cavity to undergo capacitation at different rates. Therefore, it is important that the tested compounds administered in the vagina can travel through the cervix into the upper part of the uterine cavity.

2.2. Unsuccessful Attempts to Develop the Spermicide, Nonoxynol-9, as a Microbicide

Since the search for spermicides started over 50 years ago before the significant unfolding of the molecular mechanisms on how sperm gain fertilizing ability, a simple Sander-Cramer assay based on sperm immotility was implemented at the time for spermicide screening. Compounds are considered as spermicides if they can completely inhibit motility of sperm in the diluted semen suspension within 20 s. However, these criteria are unlikely to represent the physiological events occurring during conception. First, motile sperm swim out from the liquefied semen in the vagina to enter the cervix and then the uterine cavity, while most of the seminal plasma is left in the vagina along with sperm that have much less progressive motility. Given this scenario, a spermicide needs to target those motile sperm with only residual amounts of the seminal plasma. In contrast, in the Sander-Cramer assay, semen is diluted three to four-fold with medium, leaving 20%–25% of seminal plasma in the sperm suspension. The seminal plasma contains high amounts of amyloid peptide complexes, which surround sperm in the ejaculate [21]. In general, this makes it hard for compounds added exogenously to reach the surface of sperm in the seminal plasma. As such, only compounds that have the strength to immediately disaggregate the amyloid complexes, such as harsh surfactants, can accomplish the task. Thus, the major compound identified by the Sander-Cramer assay for its spermicidal effects is nonoxynol-9 (N-9), which is a non-ionic detergent with a very similar structure to Triton X-100 (Figure 1). At 0.0075% to 0.012%, N-9 can irreversibly immobilize human sperm in a saline/medium diluted semen suspension (3-4 fold dilution) within 20 s [22–24], and therefore it has been used for more than 50 years as a spermicide in condom coating and in various vaginal contraceptive devices (*i.e.*, foams, suppositories, creams, gels and films). As a detergent, it is not surprising that N-9 exerts microbicidal effects *in vitro* against various types of STI-induced microbes as well as HIV [25–29]. N-9 formulated foam was further shown to prevent rhesus macaques from SIV and SHIV infection, albeit in a very small cohort of monkeys (<10) [30,31]. Nonetheless, these results paved the way to clinical trials on the anti-STI activity of N-9 in women. However, a systematic review using meta-analyses of 10 respectable clinical trials, including 5909 participating women, failed to demonstrate significant protective effects of N-9 against a wide range of STI-induced microbes including *Neisseria gonorrhoeae*, *Chlamydia trachomatis*, HIV, *Candida albicans* and *Trichomonas vaginalis* [32]. In fact, in one clinical trial, the HIV infection rate was shown to increase twofold in women using N-9 gel, compared with those without any application [33] and in another clinical trial, the gonorrhoea infection rate was shown to be higher in N-9 vaginal gel users [34]. These increased rates of STI are likely due to the "detergent" action of N-9 on cervicovaginal surface membranes. In most of the clinical trials, vaginal toxicity including irritation, ulcerations, histological inflammation as well as vulvitis was observed in women who were vaginally exposed to N-9 in various forms (e.g., N-9 formulated gels, films, sponges and suppositories, and N-9 coated condoms) [35–40]. Vaginal epithelial disruption was in fact observed by colposcopy in women frequently using N-9 vaginal suppositories [41]. Similar results were observed in mice intravaginally inoculated with N-9 [42]. These cervicovaginal epithelial disruptions likely facilitate the entry of HIV and possibly also other microbes through the genital mucosa. In addition, specific cytokines are produced in N-9 using women with cervicovaginal inflammation, resulting in recruitment of immune cells, which are typical HIV host cells, to the vaginal lumen. Essentially, this enhances HIV replication [43]. Currently, N-9 is not promoted for its use as a microbicide and most established pharmaceutical companies have stopped coating condoms with N-9. However, all vaginal products, such as foam and cream, which contain N-9 (can be up to 28%), are still available over the counter for contraceptive use, although the products contain a warning message against their use in women who are prone to HIV and other microbe exposure. Scientifically, it is hard to understand why N-9, a detergent, was even developed as a spermicide with a false hope that its disruption effect would be specific to sperm membranes, and not cervicovaginal epithelial cell membranes. Nonetheless, the adverse outcomes of the attempts to develop N-9 as vaginal microbicides provide a valuable lesson to the scientific/medical community. Namely, the integrity of the female reproductive tract must be considered for all future microbicide/spermicide development.

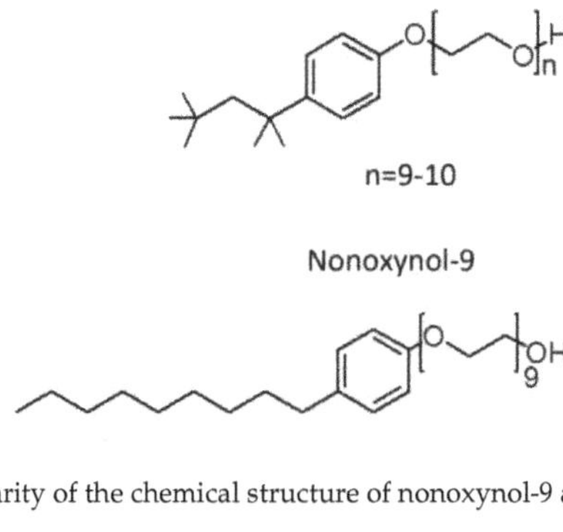

Triton X-100

n=9-10

Nonoxynol-9

Figure 1. Similarity of the chemical structure of nonoxynol-9 and Triton X-100.

3. Antimicrobial Peptides as Spermicides

An alternative approach to search for compounds with both spermicidal and microbicidal actions can be taken by screening for spermicidal properties of known microbicidal agents. However, conventional antibiotics must be excluded in this pursuit due to the growing antibiotic resistance [44,45]. In this regard, antimicrobial peptides (AMPs) have been appropriately considered, as they are small peptides (<10 kDa) produced by all domains of life as part of innate immunity. In humans and eutherian mammals, AMPs are produced by neutrophils and other immune cells as well as epithelial cells of various tissues especially those that are connected or exposed to an external environment (e.g., genitourinary tract, lung, skin) [46,47]. As natural compounds, resistance against the microbicidal activities of AMPs is less anticipated and AMPs are considered to be the next generation of anti-infectives [45]. The broad spectrum activity against Gram positive and Gram negative bacteria, fungi, viruses and certain protozoa is another attractive property of AMPs [46–48]. In addition to the direct microbicidal properties, AMPs can abrogate the action of lipopolysaccharides (LPS), a pathogen associated molecular pattern (PAMP) from Gram negative bacteria [47], through their affinity for LPS [49–51]. Therefore, the binding of LPS to the host cell surface Toll-like receptor 4 and subsequent cell signalling events that lead to inflammatory responses cannot occur [52]. AMPs can also act as immune modulators with various positive consequences to the target cells (reviews [53–55]). For this reason, AMPs are also referred to as host defence peptides [46,55]. Immunomodulatory effects of AMPs, which are relevant to the health of the lower female genital tract tissues include wound repair, angiogenesis and cell proliferation [46,48,52,56–59], as these processes would be beneficial to the vaginal mucosa after intercourse that often induces abrasion to the mucosal surface.

Most of AMPs are cationic and amphipathic peptides. To date, over 2500 natural AMPs with diverse sequence, structure and property have been archived in the APD3 database (http://aps.unmc.edu/AP/ [60]). Based on the types of secondary structures, AMPs are categorized into four classes (α, β, $\alpha\beta$, and non-$\alpha\beta$) [61]. Because less than 12% of the AMPs in the APD3 database have a 3D structure, covalent bonding patterns of polypeptide chains are also used to categorize AMPs into four classes: linear (UCLL, with no covalent bonds between different amino acids in the polypeptide chain, e.g., human cathelicidin LL-37 and frog magainins), side-chain linked (UCSS, covalent bonds between different amino acid side chains, e.g., disulfide bonded defensins and lanthionine ether bonded lantibiotics), sidechain-backbone linked (UCSB, such as those present in bacterial lasso peptides), and backbone-backbone connected circular peptides (UCBB, such as those present in plant cyclotides) [62]. In addition, specific properties have been used to define AMP families. For example, cathelicidins are AMPs, where their precursors contain a conserved cathelin domain in the N-terminal region [46]. Examples include LL-37 in humans, CRAMP in mice, indolicidin in cows. Another family of AMPs containing disulfide bonds is called "defensins", which are sub-classified to the α, β and θ groups. The α- and β-defensins are differentiated from each other based on the positions of the disulfide bonds (α having C^{I}–C^{VI}, C^{II}–C^{IV} and C^{III}–C^{V}, whereas β having C^{I}–C^{V}, C^{II}–C^{IV} and C^{III}–C^{VI}). So are θ-defensins, which possess three different disulfide bonds (C^{I}–C^{VI}, C^{II}–C^{V} and C^{III}–C^{IV}). Interestingly, most of defensins with known 3-D structure (α: HNP-1, HNP-2, HNP-3, HNP-4, HD-5 and HD-6; β: hBD-3; θ: RTD-1) have β-sheet secondary structure, while hBD-1 (human β-defensin-1) contains both α-helix and β-sheet structures. In addition, "bacteriocins" is used to define AMPs produced by bacteria. Notably, a number of bacteriocins contain intramolecular lanthionine or methyl lanthionine ethers (formed through thioether linkages between serine/threonine and cysteine); such bacteriocins are referred to as lantibiotics and lantipeptides depending on whether they have antibacterial activity [63]. In addition, some bacteriocins such as gramicidin A contain D-amino acids [64]. Both lanthionines and D-amino acids contribute to the 3-D structure of bacteriocins [65]. It is notable that a number of bacteriocins differ substantially from cationic cathelicidins and defensins. For example, gramicidin A has a net charge of zero and consists of essentially all hydrophobic amino acids, allowing it to insert into bacterial membranes as an ion channel. In addition to structural categorization, APD3 classifies AMPs according to their functions (e.g., antimicrobial (as expected), anti-HIV, antimalarial, wound healing). Relevant to this review is the spermicidal activity of certain AMPs, at least *in vitro*. These AMPs are referred to as spermicidal AMPs.

Being positively charged, AMPs first bind to anionic molecular components of the cell wall of Gram positive bacteria (*i.e.*, lipoteichoic acid) and outer membrane of Gram negative bacteria (*i.e.*, LPS) [66]. This initial binding results in destabilization of these outer surfaces, thus allowing AMPs to reach and bind to anionic molecules of the bacterial cell membrane (*i.e.*, phosphatidylglycerol (PG) and cardiolipin (CL)). Initially, AMPs may lie horizontally through their affinity for PG and CL on the bacterial cell membrane. Since AMPs are amphiphathic, clusters of their hydrophobic amino acids would then interact with the hydrocarbon chains of lipids in the membrane bilayers. This may result in the vertical insertion of AMP peptides into the lipid bilayer. AMPs adjacent to each other also tend to polymerize through the interaction of their hydrophobic domains. Alternatively, these peptides may intersperse in the membranes by preferentially interacting with anionic lipids. All of these could lead to pore formation in the bacterial cell membrane and the eventual loss of cellular homeostasis, and finally death [46,48,67]. In addition, some AMPs can inhibit bacterial cell wall synthesis [67], while others can enter the bacteria to bind to their ribosomes, resulting in inhibition of protein translation [60]. The fungicidal, virucidal and protozoacidal mechanisms, however, are less understood [48].

The desire to use AMPs as spermicides has been in place for decades, although in the early phase of work, the selective action of AMPs on sperm and not on epithelial cells of the vagina (the most logical site for their administration) may not have been well considered. Mammalian sperm are known to have a negatively charged surface [68,69] in the head region. This is due to the specific presence of SGG in the outer leaflet of the plasma membrane. The level of SGG is at 10 mole% of total sperm lipids with the main molecular species having C16:0 in both its *sn-1* alkyl chain and *sn-2* acyl chain [70,71] (Figure 2). SGG is a structural analog of sulfogalactosylceramide (SGC, aka sulfatide) (Figure 2), which is known to be an integral component of membrane lipid rafts. Likewise, SGG is a major lipid in sperm lipid rafts; it exists together with its lipid binding partner, cholesterol [72,73]. Our lab has shown that lipid rafts in capacitated sperm, housing a number of ZP binding proteins [19,20,74], are surface platforms on sperm for the ZP binding [72]. SGG itself also has a direct affinity for the ZP, contributing to the ZP binding ability of sperm lipid rafts [15,16]. It is expected that positively charged molecules, including AMPs, would interact electrostatically with SGG on the sperm head surface and thus reduce the sperm-ZP binding process. In addition to SGG, polysialyated glycoproteins found in the sperm plasma membrane endow negative charges to the sperm surface [75,76].

Sulfogalactosylglycerolipid (SGG)

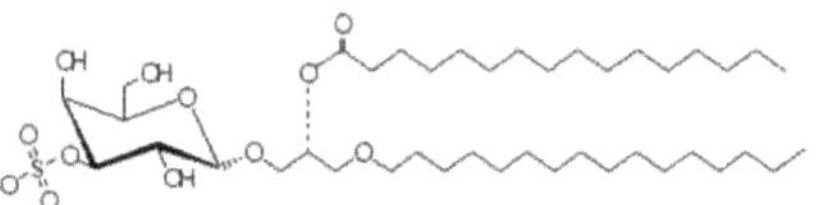

Sulfogalactosylceramide (SGC)

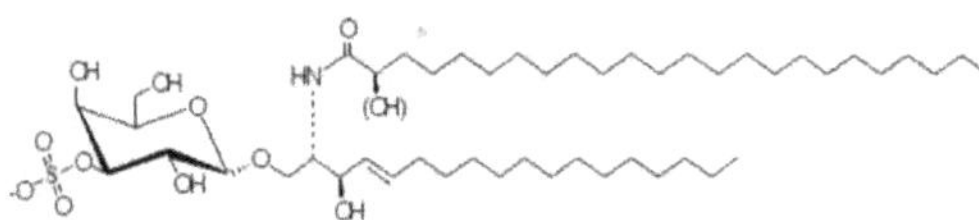

Figure 2. Chemical structure of sulfogalactosylglycerolipid (SGG) and sulfogalactosylceramide (SGC).

Table 2 lists all spermicidal AMPs described in the literature and the antimicrobial peptide database (http://aps.unmc.edu/AP/ [60]), with their sequences and relevant biochemical properties described in Table 3.

Table 2. Spermicidal antimicrobial peptides: microbicidal, structural and spermicidal properties.

Peptide Name APD [1] ID UniProt ID PDB ID	Source	Microbicidal/Biological/ Biochemical Properties	References for Spermicidal Effects	Remarks
LL-37 APD: AP00310 UniProt: P49913 PDB: 2K6O	Neutrophils, monocytes, lymphocytes, keratinocytes, epithelial cells of the lung, nasal cavity, genitourinary tract, gastrointestinal tract, ocular surface, and gingiva of *Homo sapiens*, Expression of LL-37 in *Pan troglodytes* (chimpanzee), *Macaca mulatta* (rhesus macaque) have also been described.	LL-37 exerts microbicidal effects on Gram positive and Gram negative bacteria, yeasts, *Candida albicans*, and HIV and other viruses, including those that cause STIs (see Table 4). In an aqueous solution, the structure of LL-37 is disordered. However, when it interacts with lipid membranes such as SDS and dodecylphosphocholine micelles, LL-37 adopts an alpha helical amphipathic structure, as revealed by NMR analysis with one side of the helix enriched in hydrophilic amino acids and the other side hydrophobic residues [77,78].	[79]	LL-37 completely inhibits human and mouse sperm motility within 5 min at 10.8 μM and 3.7 μM, respectively. This inhibition is likely due to the specific disruptive effects of LL-37 on sperm surface membranes, as shown by electron microscopy and Sytox Green (a membrane impermeable DNA dye) staining. In addition, LL-37 treated sperm become prematurely acrosome reacted, thus hindering them to effectively bind to the egg. These specific adverse effects of LL-37 on sperm are likely due to its affinity for the negatively charged sulfogalactosylglycerolipid (SGG) present selectively on the sperm surface. The contraceptive effect of LL-37 is further demonstrated in female mice. Females, naturally cycling to the estrous phase and transcervically injected with sperm + LL-37, fail to become pregnant, whereas pregnancy occurs in 92% of females injected with sperm alone. The reproductive tract tissues of the females administered with LL-37 appears to be normal like that observed in females unexposed to LL-37 [79].
Maximin 1 APD:AP00058 UniProt: P83080 PDB:None and Maximin 3 APD:AP00060 UniProt: P83082 PDB:None	Skin: Chinese red belly toad *Bombina maxima*	Lai *et al.* [80] have shown that maximin 1 and maximin 3 have microbicidal activities against both Gram positive and Gram negative bacteria and yeasts, *Candida albicans*. Both also have anti-cancer and anti-HIV activities. Although both maximin 1 and maximin 4 have no PDB ID, they are close homologs of maximin 4 (PDB: 2MHW). The 3D structure of maximin 4, as revealed by NMR analyses, is a linear cationic amphipathic peptide in solution, but forms a kinked alpha helix with lipid micelles [81].	[80]	The spermicidal work is based only on sperm immotility. At 100 μg/mL (37 μM) of maximin 1 or maximin 3, ~80% of human sperm become immotile.
Magainin 2 APD:AP00144 UniProt: P11006 for magainins; magainin 2 is one of the five cleaved products of magainins. PDB: 2MAG	Skin and stomach: African clawed frog, *Xenopus laevis*	Magainin 2 has microbicidal effects on Gram positive and Gram negative bacteria, yeasts and viruses. It also acts against certain protozoa including malaria causing *Plasmodium falciparum*. However, magainin 2 does not have an anti-HIV activity [82]. NMR analysis indicates that magainin 2 adopts an alpha helical structure in the presence of SDS and other lipid micelles [83].	[84–87]	Magainin A, a synthetic derivatives of magainin 2 [88] possess sperm immobilizing activity, as shown in rat, rabbit, monkey and human sperm. At ~50 μg/mL (20 μM), magainin A completely inhibit human/monkey sperm motility within 7–10 min of treatment, although it takes ~300 μg/mL (120 μM) of the peptide for the immediate immobilization of human sperm. Lower doses are required for rat and rabbit sperm for the same results [82,85,86]. These spermistatic effects are likely due to the ability of magainin A to disrupt the sperm surface membranes [85]. Magainin 2-amide (250 μg/mL (101 μM)) also exerts spermistatic effects on human sperm, although it is at 50% efficacy. Only when sperm are treated with both cyclodextrin and magainin 2-amide, sperm immotility is enhanced to 80%. Reddy's group have demonstrated vaginal contraceptive effects of magainin A in rabbits and monkeys. Females each administered with 1 mg magainin A did not become pregnant upon natural mating. Side effects of magainin A on the female reproductive tract appeared to be minimum [82,84].
Dermaseptin S1 APD:AP00157 UniProt: 80277 PDB:None	Skin: Sauvage's leaf frog, *Phyllomedusa sauvagii*	Dermaseptin S1 has microbicidal activities against Gram positive and Gram negative bacteria and herpes simplex virus. It also kills the protozoa, Leishmania. Dermaseptin S1 has an alpha helix structure as revealed by circular dichroism analyses [89].	[90]	The spermicidal work is based only on sperm immotility. Human sperm become completely immotile immediately after treatment with 200 μg/mL (58 μM) of dermaseptin S1.

Table 2. *Cont.*

Peptide Name APD [1] ID UniProt ID PDB ID	Source	Microbicidal/Biological/ Biochemical Properties	References for Spermicidal Effects	Remarks
Dermaseptin S4 APD:AP00160 UniProt: P80280 PDB: 2DD6 for a close analog of truncated dermaseptin-S4 (aa1-13).	Skin:Sauvage's leaf frog, *Phyllomedusa sauvagii*	Dermaseptin S4 has microbicidal activities against Gram positive and Gram negative bacteria and viruses (herpes simplex virus and HIV). It also kills *P falciparum* protozoa. NMR analyses of a close analog of truncated dermaseptin S4 (aa1-13) indicates its alpha helix structure when interacting with lipid micelles [91].	[90,92,93]	Despite a similar structure to dermaseptin S1, only 100 μg/mL (36 μM) of dermaseptin S4 is required to induce complete human sperm motility, indicating a twice spermistatic potency of dermaseptin S4 [90]. A higher spermistatic effect is further observed in a dermaseptin S4 derivative with one amino acid replacement with lysine to increase the positive charge. Only 20 μg/mL (7.2 μM) of this derivative is required to induce complete sperm immotility effects. The native dermaseptin S4 (100 μg/mL (36 μM)) and its derivative (20 μg/mL (7.2 μM)) cause 100% and 50% cytotoxicity to HeLa cells, respectively [92].
Sarcotoxin Pd APD:AP02212 UniProt: None for this sarcotoxin but available for other sarcotoxin isoforms. PDB:None	Insects: rove beetles, *Paederus dermatitis*	Sarcotoxin Pd has microbicidal effects on Gram positive and Gram negative bacteria. Although there is no PDB information on sarcotoxin Pd, in the publication of Zare-Zardini *et al.* [94], a 3D structure of sarcotoxin Pd was shown to consist of two alpha helices. This structural information was obtained from computational modeling, although no details were given on how this modeling was performed.	[94]	The spermicidal work is based only on sperm immotility. The concentration of sarcotoxin Pd to immobilize human sperm is 80 μg/mL (22 μM). Cytotoxicity MTT assay was done on HeLa cells; at 80 μg/mL of sarcotoxin Pd, close to 100% of cells show cytotoxicity.
Nisin A APD:AP00205 UniProt:P13068 PDB: 1WCO	Bacteriocin from lactic acid bacteria (LAB), *Lactococcus lactis* (formerly called *Streptococcus lactis*)	The microbicidal effects of nisin A are more preferential to Gram positive bacteria; this may be attributed to its ability to bind to lipid II, a structural component of Gram positive bacterial peptidoglycans. The interaction between nisin A and lipid II leads to inhibition of the bacterial cell wall synthesis [95]. It is a cationic amphipathic lantipeptide (i.e., containing a lanthionine ether linkage between S3-C7 and 4 methyllanthionines: T8-C11, T13-C19, T23-C26 and T25-C28) (see Table 3). These thioether linkages create a constraint polycyclic feature to the peptide. However, NMR analysis revealed that nisin A is still flexible enough to interact with SDS micelles, first via ionic interaction and then through hydrophobic interaction. It was therefore proposed that nisin A can create pores in lipid bilayers following its tran-bilayer insertion [96,97].	[98–103]	The sperm immobilizing effects of nisin A have been shown in various species, *i.e.*, rats, rabbits, bulls, horses/ponies, boars, monkeys and humans [98,99,101]. The instantaneous spermistatic concentration of nisin A is 300–400 μg/mL (86–114 μM) for human/monkey sperm, 200 μg/mL (57 μM) for rabbit sperm and 50 μg/mL (14 μM) for rat sperm. Scanning electron microscopy revealed obvious disruption of the human sperm plasma membrane following treatment with 360 μg/mL (103 μM) of nisin A. This disruption was similar to what observed on the surface of *Staphylococcus aureus* bacteria, which were treated with a similar nisin A concentration. In contrast, human red blood cells were not affected by treatment with equivalent concentrations of nisin A. The preferential effects of nisin A on sperm plasma membrane permeabilization was also confirmed by propidium iodide nuclear staining of the treated sperm [102] Reddy *et al.* have further demonstrated that nisin A is an effective vaginal contraceptive in rats and rabbits. Female rats naturally cycling in the proestrous/estrous phase and vaginally administered with nisin A (200 μg each) did not become pregnant following natural mating [98]. Successful contraceptive results were likewise obtained in female rabbits intravaginally injected with nisin A (1 mg each), provided that mating took place within 30 min of the peptide administration [99]. In both animal species, the authors claimed that there were no changes to the anatomy of the female reproductive tract tissues or cytokine production profile in the females vaginally administered with nisin A at the contraceptive dose or even higher and repeated doses of nisin A [98–100]. By MTT assay, HeLa cells appeared to be less susceptible to cytotoxic effects of nisin A, as compared with sperm.
Pediocin CP2 APD:AP00634 UniProt: Q8RL96 PDB:None	Bacteriocin from LAB, *Pediococcus acidilactici*	Pediocin CP2 exerts microbicidal effects on both Gram positive and Gram negative bacteria as well as yeasts, *Candida albicans* [104] No PDB ID is available. However, the 3-D structure of its homolog, sakacin P (PDB: 1OG7, 68% identical peptide sequence to pediocin CP), reveals the presence of an alpha helix in the middle region of the peptide.	[104]	The spermicidal work is based only on sperm immotility. The concentration of pediocin CP2 to immobilize human sperm is >250 μg/mL (54 μM). There is no reported work on the cytoxicity concentration of pediocin CP2 on female reproductive tract tissues/cells.

Table 2. *Cont.*

Peptide Name APD [1] ID UniProt ID PDB ID	Source	Microbicidal/Biological/ Biochemical Properties	References for Spermicidal Effects	Remarks
Gramicidin A APD:AP00499 UniProt: None PDB: 1MAG	Bacteriocin from soil bacterium, *Bacillus brevis*	Gramicidin A exerts microbicidal effects on both Gram positive and Gram negative bacteria as well as viruses (including HIV) [105]. Gramicidin A has a special β-helix structure because of its possession of D-amino acids. Gramicidin A dimerizes with the N-terminus of each peptide being adjacent to each other. As a result, the dimer forms a cation channel in lipid bilayers with the two C-termini exposed [64].	[105–107]	Gramicidin has been used for a long time in Russia as a spermicide as referred to in Bourinbaiar *et al.* [105], although detailed data of its efficacy is not available. Experimentally, the spermicidal effects of gramicidin A are based on human sperm immotility and consequently the inability of sperm to penetrate lamb cervical mucus [106]. Only 5 μg/mL (2.8 μM) of gramicidin A could completely immobilize sperm. Gramicidin D (mixture of gramicidin A, B and C) has similar sperm immobilizing effects but at a higher concentration than gramicidin A.
Subtilosin A APD:AP00928 UniProt:007623 PDB: 1PXQ	Bacteriocin from *Bacillus subtilis, Bacillus amyloliquefaciens, Bacillus atrophaeus*	Subtilosin A has microbicidal effects on both Gram positive and Gram negative bacteria as well as herpes simplex viruses. It is a lantipeptide, containing a high percentage of hydrophobic residues (60%) with an overall negative charge of -2. Lanthionines between C13 and F22, C7 andT28, and C4 and F31 make the N-terminus and C-terminus fold towards each other, giving an overall boat conformation, as revealed by NMR analysis. There is an alpha helix in the C-terminus starting from G29 to W34 [108].	[101,109]	The spermicidal test is based only on sperm immotility. At a single concentration tested, 800 μg/mL (233 μM), subtilosin A instantaneously immobilized bull and horse/pony sperm. The same spermicidal effects were observed in boar and rat sperm at 200 μg/mL (58 μM) of subtilosin A [101]. Human sperm treated with subtilosin also became immotile in a dose-dependent manner with complete immobilization at 110 μg/mL (32 μM). Notably, subtilosin at this concentration does not reduce cell viability in the human EpiVaginal ectocervical tissue model [109].
Lacticin 3147 APD:AP01194 UniProt: 087236 PDB:None	Bacteriocin from LAB *Lactococcus lactis DPC3147*	Lacticin 3147 is composed of two lantipeptide components, LtnA1 and LtnA2. Microbicidal activity of lacticin 3147 is preferential on Gram positive bacteria and is stronger with LtnA1 and LtnA2 combined, compared with each lacticin 3147 chain alone. There are four lanthionines in LtnA1 and two in LtnA2, which generate a polycyclic structure to both peptides. NMR analyses also reveal a helical structure in LtnA2 [110]. Note that there are a few D-Ala residues in both lantipeptide chains, and their existence is important for the microbicidal activity of lacticin [110].	[101]	The spermicidal test is based only on sperm immotility. LtnA1 chain had much less spermicidal effects than LtnA2. The combination of LtnA1 + LtnA2 at 200 μg/mL (31 μM) could effectively immobilize rat, bull, and horse/pony sperm. But only 50 μg/mL (7.8 μM) of LtnA1 + LtnA2 was required to induce immotility of bull sperm [101].

[1] The listing of spermicidal AMPs is essentially from the antimicrobial peptide database (APD) (http://aps.unmc.edu/AP/ [60]).

Table 3. Sequences and biochemical properites of spermicidal antimicrobial.

Name	Sequence	Net Charge, % Hydrophobicity	Theoretical pI/MW
LL-37	LLGDFFRKSKEKIGKEFKRIVQRIKDFLRNLVPRTES [1]	+6, 43.2%	10.61/4493.3
Maximin 1	GIGTKILGGVKTALKGALKELASTYAN	+3, 59.3%	9.83/2675.2
Maximin 3	GIGGKILSGLKTALKGAAGELASTYLH	+3, 59.3%	9.83/2698.3
Maximin 4 [2]	GIGGVLLSAGKAALKGLAKVLAEKYAN	+3, 70.4%	9.83/2613.1
Magainin 2	GIGKFLHSAKKFGKAFVGEIMNS	+3, 60.9%	10.00/2466.9
Dermaseptin S1	ALWKTMLKKLGTMALHAGKAALGAAADTISQGTQ	+3, 61.8%	10.00/3455.1
Dermaseptin S4	ALWMTLLKKVLKAAAKALNAVLVGANA	+4, 74.1%	10.48/2779.5
Sarcotoxin Pd	GWLKKIGKKIERVGQHTRGLGIAQIAANVAATAR	+6, 58.8%	11.74/3613.3
Nisin A	ITSISLCTPGCKTGALMGCNMKTATCHCSIHVSK [3]	+3, 41.2%	8.78/3498.2
Pediocin CP2	KYYGNGVTCGKHSCSVDWGKATTCIINNGAMAWATGGHQGNHKC	+6, 43.0%	8.85/4628.2
Gramicidin A	VGA*L*A*V*V*V*W*L*W*L*W*L*W [4]	0, 100%	5.49/1811.3
Subtilosin A	NKGCATCSIGAACLVDGPIPDFEIAGATGLFGLWG	−2, 68.6%	4.03/3425.9
Lacticin 3147 chain A1	CSTNTF*A*LSDYWGNNGAWCTLTHECMAWCK	−1, 40.0%	5.32/3430.8
Lacticin 3147 chain A2	TPATPAI*A*IL*A*AYISTNTCPTTKCTRAC	+2, 46.4%	8.65/2886.4

[1] Amino acids are color coded according to their charges, hydrophilicity and hydrophobicity. Positively charged amino acids (K, R and H) are in red, whereas negatively charged residues (D, E) are in green. Uncharged hydrophilic amino acids (S, T, Y, N, Q, C) are in purple. Hydrophobic amino acids are in different shades of blue, with strong blue indicating the highest hydrophobicity level (L, F, I, V, A), followed by light blue (G), and very light blue (W, M, P) with the least hydrophobicity. [2] Although maximin 4 has not been shown to be spermicidal, its sequence is shown here because of its high similarity to maximin 1 and maximin 3 and its 3D structure is shown in Figure 3. [3] Brackets denote lanthionine ethers. [4] Italic letters denote D-amino acids.

In addition to these 12 AMPs, cecropin D2A21 was mentioned but without any data on its spermicidal effects in the publication describing its chlamydiacidal property [111]. Seven of these AMPs are produced in humans and animals, *i.e.*, LL-37-humans; maximin 1, maximin 3, magainin 2, dermaseptin S1 and dermaseptin S4-lower vertebrate animals (frogs and toads); and sarcotoxin Pd-invertebrates (insects). The other five AMPs (nisin A, pediocin CP2, gramicidin A, subtilosin A and lacticin 3147) are bacteriocins produced by various bacteria species. Interestingly, gramicidin A has been used for decades in humans in Russia [105], although the scientific and medical details of this use are not available in the literature. Except for our work on LL-37, the screening for the spermicidal action of AMPs listed in Table 1 was based primarily on their ability to immobilize sperm in the suspension that still contained 20%–25% of seminal plasma within 20 s of treatment (Sander-Cramer test). As discussed above, this approach is likely an "overkill", since motile sperm swim out of the seminal plasma and carry only residual amounts of seminal plasma into the cervix and uterine cavity. Rather "swim-up" sperm and "Percoll-gradient centrifuged", prepared in a laboratory, would be more representative of motile sperm that swim through the cervix into the uterine cavity [23]. Swim-up sperm are simply prepared by overlaying semen placed in a tube with appropriate medium. Swim-up sperm are motile sperm that have swum up into the medium layer that still carry a small amount of seminal plasma [112]. Percoll-gradient centrifuged sperm are prepared by loading semen onto a discontinuous gradient of Percoll solutions (usually 45% and 90%) followed by centrifugation at ~600 g. Motile sperm have "clean" morphology (devoid of membranous vesicles and having compact chromatin) with a higher specific density than immotile/morphologically abnormal sperm, and therefore they sediment as a pellet, which can then be resuspended in a medium for experimental use. Percoll-gradient centrifuged sperm have the highest fertilizing ability [113] and therefore they should be used for the screening of a candidate spermicide. However, an assay for human sperm motility that is more physiologically representative is to observe the rate of sperm to swim through cervical mucus collected from women in the middle of their menstrual cycle (ovulation time) and placed in a capillary tube [7,114]. The cervical mucus fluid is viscoelastic due to the abundance of proteo-glycosaminoglycans. Sperm must have sufficient motility force as well as biochemical components to digest the proteo-glycosaminoglycan networks in order to swim through the cervical mucus column, a situation that does not exist in sperm resuspended in medium [11,115]. This sperm-cervical mucus assay was performed with gramicidin A treated human sperm. This assay, however, is impractical to be used for screening of spermicide compounds due to the restriction in obtaining sufficient quantities of mid-menstrual cycle cervical mucus from women.

Among all spermicidal AMPs listed in Table 2, LL-37, magainin 2 and nisin A are the only AMPs with confirmed *in vivo* contraceptive effects in experimental animals. The outcome of zero pregnancies is considered the gold standard indicator of contraceptive effects of these AMPs. Our group performed this *in vivo* work on LL-37 in mice [79], whereas Reddy & Aranha's group examined the effects of nisin A in rats and rabbits [98,99], and magainin 2 in rabbits and monkeys [82,84]. Experimentation in animal models is essential in the screening of vaginal spermicides and/or microbicides, since it is a means not only to confirm the spermicidal/microbicidal effects *in vivo* but also to determine whether there are any adverse effects of the compounds on the female reproductive tract. Selection of appropriate animals for these *in vivo* studies is also critical for the next clinical trials in humans. Monkeys are animals with reproductive physiology closest to the human system. However, one may only use a restricted number of monkeys for each trial. In addition, it is important to preserve the female monkey lives after the experiment. Therefore, the examination of any adverse effects on the reproductive system in female monkeys can only be done in an indirect manner (e.g., assessing types and quality of cells from vaginal smears). Such is the case for the study on *in vivo* spermicidal effects of magainin 2 in monkeys [82]. In contrast, histology of the female reproductive tract can be evaluated directly in smaller animals including rabbits, rats and mice following their sacrifice and tissue removal for fixing and processing. Histology images should be explicitly shown such as those described in the studies for LL-37 in mice [79] and nisin A in rabbits [100]. However, interpretation of results from spermicidal and microbicidal studies in female rabbits, rats and mice must be made with caution that the reproductive systems in these animals differ from that of humans in a number of aspects. While insemination in rabbits occurs in the vagina like the situation in humans, rabbit females do not have a reproductive cycle (estrus or menstrual cycle) with peaked estrogen, which enriches the vaginal/cervical secretion and microflora [116]. Therefore, rabbit vaginal microflora are rather simple and in fact contain only residual amounts of lactobacilli [116], which are found abundantly in the human vagina and responsible for acidifying the vaginal luminal milieu due to lactate production [117]. The pH in the rabbit vagina is in the neutral range [118] in contrast to the pH 4 in the human vagina [119,120]. With no defined reproductive cycle, ovulation in rabbits is not hormonally regulated but rather induced by coitus [121], a process so markedly different from human ovulation. The reproductive processes in rats and mice, as well, differ from those in humans in a number of aspects despite the fact that rodents do have a reproductive estrus cycle. Although rodent semen is first deposited in the vagina, sperm together with seminal plasma are swept into the uterus within minutes [11]. In addition, the mouse vaginal pH is at ~6.5, more basic than that of the human vagina. This is due to lower numbers of lactobacilli colonies in the rodent vagina [122]. Regardless, rodents are less expensive to purchase and maintain and the *in vitro* fertilization procedures in rodents are well described, allowing the assessment of candidate spermicides for their direct inhibitory effects on fertilization *in vitro*. While it is logical that various animal models should be used to validate spermicidal and microbicidal effects of the candidate compounds, human vaginal and cervical cell lines as well as reconstructed human vagina models should also be employed in the spermicide and microbicide *ex vivo* studies. The former include immortalized cell lines derived from human vaginal epithelia (Vk2/E6E7), human ectocervical epithelia (Ect1/E6E7) and human endocervical epithelia (End1/E6E7), all established by Deborah Anderson, Brighams and Women's Hospital, Inc. [123], and available from ATCC. For the latter, MatTek Inc. has produced various types of organotypic vaginal-ectocervical tissue models through reconstruction of human vagina and cervix tissues [124]. Vk2/E6E7, Ect1/E6E7 and End1/E6E7 cell lines have been widely used for the studies of candidate microbicides [125–127]. Likewise, MatTek human vaginal-ectocervical tissue models have recently been used for studies on the properties of potential vaginal anti-HIV agents [128–130]. To date, there are no publications on the use of immortalized Vk2/E6E7, Ect1/E6E7 and End1/E6E7 cells for studies of spermicidal AMPs. MatTek organotypic vaginal-ectocervical tissue models were used only in subtilosin A study (Table 2). On the other hand, HeLa cell lines (derived from cervical cancer cells obtained from Henrietta Black over 60 years ago [131]) were used for evaluating cytotoxicity of dermaseptin S4, sarcotoxin Pd and nisin A (see Table 2). However, HeLa cells are highly transformed and may not have the expected properties of human cervical epithelial cells [131].

As discussed above, the acidic pH in the healthy human vagina is attributed to the presence of commensal lactobacilli. The vaginal acidity is essential in inhibition of unwanted proliferation as well as infection of pathogenic microbes such as *Gardnerella vaginalis*, *Prevotella bivia* and HIV [132]. Depletion of lactobacilli in the vagina leads to bacterial vaginosis. In this regard, caution must be taken in the selection of AMPs with no microbicidal effects on lactobacilli for further development into vaginal microbicides. This is the case for nisin A, which has been used as a food preservative for human consumption and shown to be an effective contraceptive in rabbits and monkeys ([98,99], Table 2). However, nisin A is not a good candidate to be developed into a vaginal microbicide, since it exerts microbicidal activity on vaginal *Lactobacillus spp* [132,133].

While the microbicidal effects of AMPs in general are of a broad spectrum, it is most desirable to search for spermicidal AMPs that also have anti-HIV properties. Among spermicidal AMPs listed in Table 2, LL-37 [134–136], maximin 1 [80], maximin 3 [80], dermaseptin S1, dermaseptin S4 [137] and gramicidin A [105] have been shown to possess anti-HIV properties. Therefore, they should be considered for further research studies and development into vaginal contraceptives/microbicides. Most of these HIV infection studies were performed using HIV lab strains in $CD4^+$ T cells, T-cell leukemia cell lines or T4 lymphoblastoid cell lines, and in some cases monocyte derived dendritic cells.

In order to validate the physiological significance of the anti-HIV properties of these AMPs, work should be comprehensively repeated using dual tropic clinical isolates of HIV at sufficiently high titers. In addition, the inhibitory effects of the candidate AMPs on HIV infection in the human cervicovaginal epithelium should be directly assessed using MatTek human vaginal-ectocervical tissue models. On the other hand, since gramicidin A has been used as a spermicide in Russia [105], a population study should be carried out to determine whether women who have been using gramicidin A vaginally and are more prone to exposure to HIV have a lower rate of HIV infection.

The 3D structures of a number of spermicidal AMPs or their close homologs have been determined by NMR spectroscopy. These include human LL-37 [77], frog maximin 4 (homolog of maximin 1) [81], magainin 2 [83], dermaseptin S4 [91], bacterial nisin A [138], gramicidin A [64], subtilosin A [108] and lacticin 3147 (chain A1 and A2) [110].

Figure 3A shows the 3D structures of these AMPs. Interestingly, LL-37, maximin 4, magainin 2, dermaseptin S4 and lacticin 3147 chain A2 contain an alpha helical structure in a significant length of their sequences. A short helix also exists in subtilosin A and nisin A (Figure 3A). However, lacticin 3147 chain A1 (which has a minimal spermicidal activity) does not have an alpha helical structure [110] and is therefore not displayed in Figure 3A. On the other hand, gramicidin A has a β-helical structure (Figure 3A). The helical wheel projections of LL-37 (both the whole peptide and the sequence from amino acids 10-37), maximin 1, maximin 3, maximin 4, magainin 2, dermaseptin S1 and dermaseptin S4 (all from humans and animals) reveal an amphipathic feature of the helix, with hydrophobic amino acids enriched in approximately one half of the top view helical circle and hydrophilic amino acids in the other half (Figure 3B). Such an amphipathic feature can also be seen in Figure 3A, especially for LL-37, magainin 2, and dermaseptin S4 peptide analog. It is remarkable that both LL-37 and magainin 2 possess 3-4 aromatic phenylalanines on the hydrophobic surfaces. NMR studies have demonstrated that the four phenylalanines all interact with acyl chains of anionic PGs [77]. This amphipathic helical structure of AMPs may be required for spermicidal activity. If this is proven, this requirement would be analogous to that needed for AMPs for full exertion of microbicidal activity [135,139,140].

Bacteriocins utilize specific features to maintain their 3D structure. Lacticin chain A1 does not have any helical structure but its 3D confined structure is attributed to the existence of both D-amino acids and lanthionine ethers in its sequence [110]. These two structural components also exist in lacticin 3147 chain A2 with an apparent alpha helical structure [110]. Nisin A and subtilosin A also contain lanthionine ethers [46,141], which contribute to their 3D structure (Table 3). On the other hand, gramicidin A does not contain any lanthionines but it possesses five D-amino acids in its 15-mer sequence (Table 3). This unique feature endows gramicidin A a β-helical structure, which is further stabilized by dimerization, and this allows gramicidin A dimer to form a cation channel in lipid bilayers [64]. The channel and pore formation in the membranes by gramicidin A and other spermicidal bacteriocins like subtilosin A and lacticin 3147 chain A1 is unlikely to be initiated with the electrostatic binding between these AMPs and the negatively charged surface molecules of the microbes, since these AMPs have a net charge of zero or even minus values (Table 3). A close look at the helical regions in these bacteriocins (Figure 3E, G, and H) reveals a lack of amphipathic nature observed with human LL-37, magainin 2 and dermaseptin S4 (Figure 3A,B).

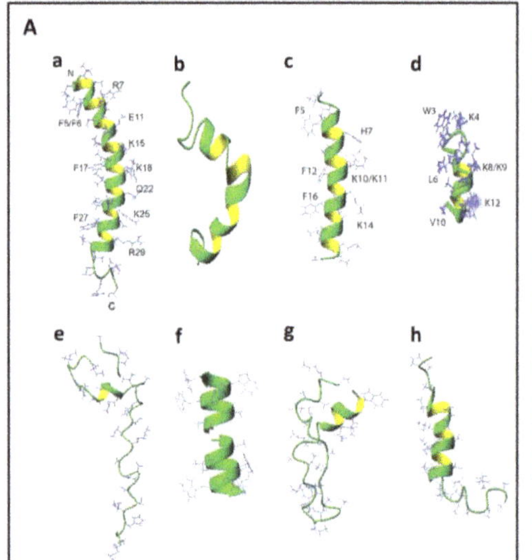

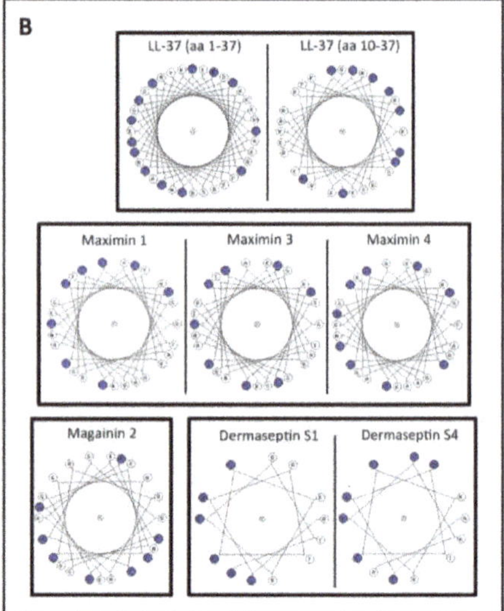

Figure 3. Structures of selected antimicrobial peptides with spermicidal activity annotated in the APD3 [142]. (**A**) 3D structures shown as ribbon diagrams of (**a**) human LL-37 (PDB ID: 2K6O); (**b**) frog maximin 4 (PDB ID: 2MHW); (**c**) magainin 2 (PDB ID: 1MAG); (**d**) a close analog of truncated dermaseptin S4 (amino acids 1-13; PDB ID: 2DD6); (**e**) bacterial nisin A complexed with lipid II (PDB ID: 1WCO); (**f**) gramicidin A (PDB ID: 1MAG); (**g**) subtilosin A (PDB ID: 1PXQ); and (**h**) lacticin 3147 (structural co-ordinates were provided by Dr. John Vedaras, University of Alberta, according to his published work [110]). Except for gramicidin A, the N-terminus of the peptide is positioned at the top. In the case of gramicidin A (**f**), its dimer is shown. The two N-termini of each dimer are positioned next to each other in the middle, whereas the C-termini are exposed and their four tryptophans approximate the lipid head group regions of the lipid bilayers for membrane positioning and ion channel conductance (**f**). Note that the C and N-termini of subtilosin A approximate in the structure (**g**). The side chains of human LL-37, magainin 2, and the dermaseptin S4 analog are selectively labeled to illustrate the amphipathic nature of these AMPs. Images were generated using MOLMOL [143]. (**B**) Helical wheel projections of selected spermicidal AMPs expressed in eukaryotes: LL-37, maximin 1, maximin 3, maximin 4, magainin 2, truncated dermaseptin S1 and dermaseptin S4. All of these AMPs show an amphipathic structure, with hydrophobic amino acids (blue circles) organized in approximately one half of the wheel and the hydrophilic residues in the other half. For LL-37, the wheel projections are shown for both the whole LL-37 sequence (amino acids 1–37) and the sequence from amino acids 10–37. This is because the helical structure of the whole LL-37 sequence has a kink at Ser^9. The LL-37 peptide (amino acids 10-37) actually shows a better distribution of hydrophobic amino acids in one half of the helical wheel. Although maximin 4 has not been shown for the direct microbicidal effects, as demonstrated for maximin 1 and maximin 3, its helical wheel projection is shown herein to corroborate its 3D structure shown in (**A**) and also for a comparison with the wheel projections of maximin 1 and maximin 3. The wheel projections of truncated dermaseptin S1 and dermaseptin S4 are both for their truncated sequence (amino acids 1-13). Again, this is to corroborate the 3D structure of the close analog of the truncated dermaseptin S4 peptide shown in (**A**).

4. LL-37, the Most Promising Spermicidal AMP

Cationic antimicrobial peptide LL-37 is coded by the only human cathelicidin gene [46,47,144]. LL-37 or its very close homologs are also present in non-human primates. Chimpanzees possess LL-37 identical to the human sequence, whereas in Gorillas and orangutans, two and three spots in the human LL-37 sequence are replaced by other amino acids [145]. The name "LL-37" denotes a peptide that contains 37 amino acids with the Leu-Leu sequence at the N-terminus. LL-37 is produced as a propeptide, hCAP-18, by neutrophils [50,146], other immune cells [147,148], normal and inflammatory skin cells [149–151], and epithelial cells of various tissues, especially those that connect with the external (male reproductive tract [152,153], urinary tract [154,155], gastrointestinal tract [156], lung [157,158], gingiva [159], eye [160], nasal cavity [161,162]) (for reviews see [149,163,164]). Of significance to this review is the expression of hCAP-18 by the human epididymal epithelial cells followed by its secretion into the epididymal lumen. This makes hCAP-18 a component of seminal plasma with a physiological concentration range of 2 to 10 μM [152,153,165]. hCAP-18 (MW:16442) is expressed by neutrophils and released during degranulation together with proteinase 3, which immediately processes hCAP-18 at physiological pH into LL-37 (MW:4493) with full microbicidal activity [166]. In skin, LL-37 is generated from hCAP-18 through the proteolytic activity of kallikrein 5 also at the neutral pH. Both kallikrein 5 and kallikrein 7 (also present in the skin surface) then further cleave LL-37 into smaller fragments (*i.e.*, RK-31, KS-30, KS-22, KR-20, LL-29), which have higher antimicrobial activity than LL-37 [151]. However, the processing of hCAP-18 is more complicated. It does not occur in the male reproductive tract or in the ejaculate. Sorensen *et al.* [153] identified gastricsin, secreted from the prostate gland and thus also a component of seminal plasma, to be the enzyme responsible for processing hCAP-18 in seminal plasma into ALL-38 (LL-37 + Ala at the N-terminus) at a pH optimum of approximately 4. Therefore, gastricsin cannot function in seminal plasma, which has a high buffering capacity at neutral pH. Following ejaculation in the vagina, seminal plasma changes the normally acidic pH of the vagina (pH 4) into the neutral range. It takes 2-6 h post-ejaculation for the vaginal lumen to resume its acidic pH and it is only at this time that gastricsin becomes active to process hCAP-18 into ALL-38, with microbicidal activity [153].

However, immediately after semen liquefaction, typically 30 min post-ejaculation, sperm instantaneously swim out from seminal plasma through the cervix into the uterine cavity. Only feeble sperm are left behind together with seminal plasma in the vagina. Therefore, motile sperm with fertilizing ability are never exposed to ALL-38, which is generated long after their movement from the vagina (Figure 4). It is likely that the production of ALL-38 is meant for protection of the vaginal epithelium against microbes introduced during intercourse [167]. As a very close analog of LL-37, ALL-38 should possess all properties described for LL-37. For example, they have identical antibacterial activity against all the organisms tested [153]. LL-37 has been shown for its direct microbicidal effects against numerous Gram negative and Gram positive bacteria, yeast and viruses (including HIV) (Table 4), but not on lactobacilli [168–170], which are essential for maintaining acidic pH and thus health of the vagina (see Section 3).

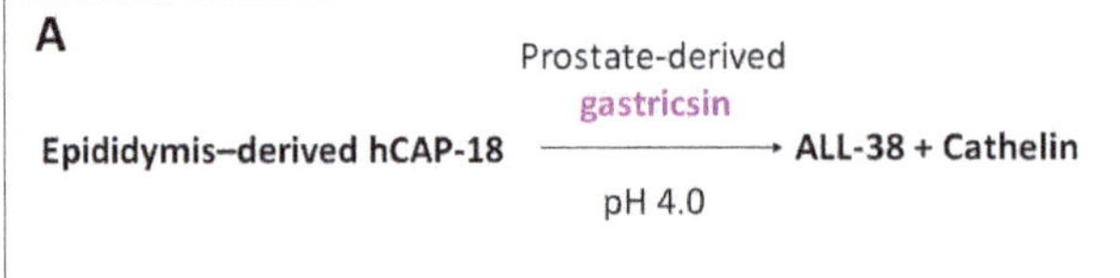

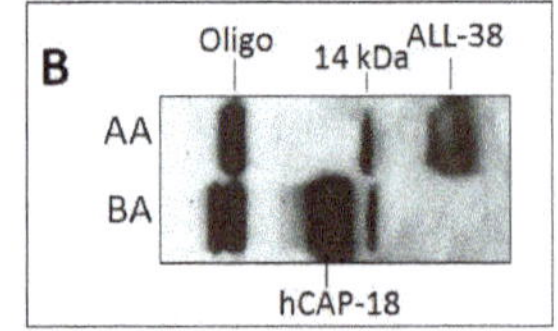

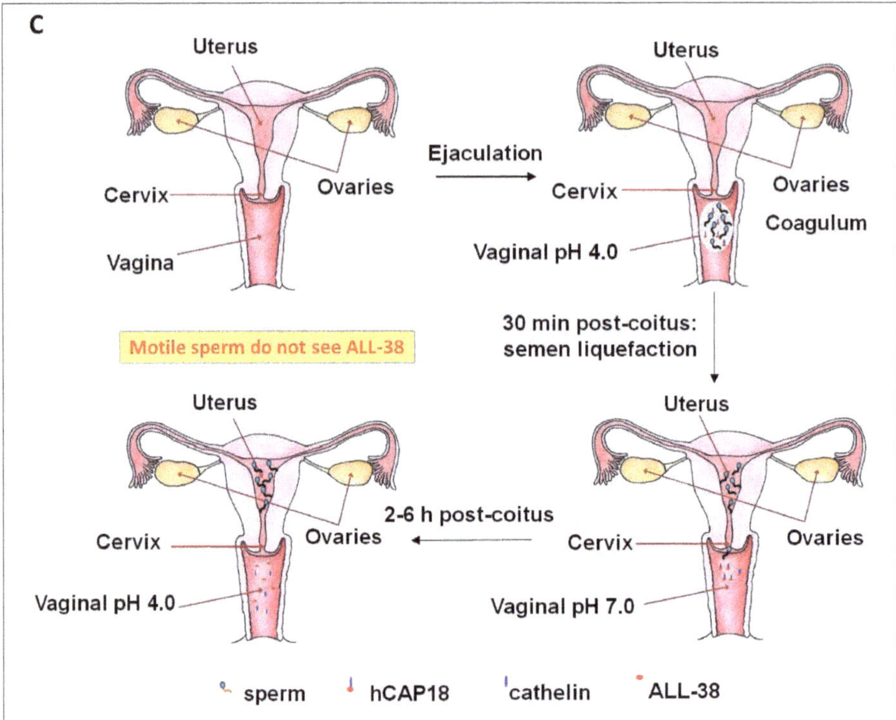

Figure 4. ALL-38 is processed from hCAP-18 post-ejaculation. (**A**) Processing of hCAP-18 to ALL-38 by gastricsin occurs at the optimum pH of 4. Although both hCAP-18 and gastricsin are seminal plasma components, this processing does not occur in the seminal plasma due to its high buffering capacity at neutral pH. (**B**) Immunoblotting showing that processing of hCAP-18 to ALL-38 can occur in acidified seminal plasma. Anti-LL-37 antibody used in immunoblotting was produced against the whole LL-37 sequence [79] and therefore, it recognized only ALL-38 and hCAP-18, but not cathelin. Before acid treatment (BA), seminal plasma contains hCAP-18 and its oligomers (Oligo; ~60 kDa), as well as a 14 kDa band (presumably a cleaved product of hCAP-18). Upon acidification of seminal plasma with HCl to pH 4, hCAP-18 is processed to ALL-38; this is due to the activation of gastricsin. AA = after acid extraction. (**C**) ALL-38 is produced 2–6 h post-ejaculation. Upon ejaculation, seminal plasma neutralizes the vaginal pH, and it takes 2–6 h post-ejaculation for the vagina lumen to resume its acidity. Only at this time, ALL-38 is produced from hCAP-18 via gastricsin activity. However, immediately after semen liquefaction (30 min post-coitus), motile sperm in the ejaculate swim into the uterine cavity. Therefore, motile sperm are never exposed to ALL-38. The drawing is based on Sørensen *et al.* [153].

Table 4. Microbicidal effects of LL-37.

Microbes [1]	Bacteria Gram +/− (B+/−) Virus (V) Yeast (Y)	References: Concentration [2]
Adenovirus (Ad)	V	Gordon *et al.* [160]: 111 μM
Acinetobacter baumannii	B−	Moffatt *et al.* [171]: 1.1 μM Garcia-Quintanilla *et al.* [172]: 0.67 μM
Actinobacillus	B−	Ouhara *et al.* [173]: ~0.26–0.52 μM
Actinobacillus actinomycetemcomitans	B−	Tanaka *et al.* [174]: ~2.2–2.7
Actinobacillus actinomycetemcomitans	B−	Ouhara *et al.* [173]: 2.2 μM
Bacillus anthracis	B−	Thwaite *et al.* [175]: 22 μM
Borrelia burgdorferi	Not applicable [3]	Lusitani *et al.* [176]: 8.8 μM
Borrelia spp	Not applicable [3]	Sambri *et al.* [169]: 100 μM
Burkholderia pseudomallei	B−	Kanthawong *et al.* [177]: 100 μM
Burkholderia thailandensis	B−	Kanthawong *et al.* [178]: 100 μM
Candida albicans	Y	Tsai *et al.* [179,180]: 8.9 μM
Capnocytophaga gingivalis	B−	Tanaka *et al.* [174]: 2.0 μM
Capnocytophaga ochracea	B−	Tanaka *et al.* [174]: 2.4 μM
Chlamydia trachomatis	B−	Tang *et al.* [181]: 20 μM
Clostridium difficile	B+	McQuade *et al.* [182]: 10.7 μM
Enterococcus faecalis	B+	Leszczynska *et al.* [183]: 12.5 μM
Escherichia coli	B−	Benincasa *et al.* [184]: 5 μM Smeianov *et al.* [168]: 25 μM Leszczynska *et al.* [185]: 5.6 μM Chen *et al.* [186]: 0.07 μM Kai-Larsen *et al.* [187]: 20 μM Nagaoka *et al.* [188]: ~1-2 μM
Fusobacterium nucleatum	B−	Ouhara *et al.* [173]: 0.22 μM Leszczynska *et al.* [183]: 49.8 μM
Haemophilus influenzae	B−	Leszczynska *et al.* [183]: 12.5 μM Lysenko *et al.* [189]: 2.2 μM
Helicobacter pylori	B−	Leszczynska *et al.* [183]: 6.2 μM Leszczynska *et al.* [185]: 2.2 μM
Herpes simplex virus type 1	V	Gordon *et al.* [160]: 111 μM
HIV-1	V	Wang *et al.* [135]: 1.6 μM Bergman *et al.* [134]: 11.1 μM
Influenza A virus (IAV)	V	Tripathi *et al.* [190]: 13 μM Barlow *et al.* [191]: 11.1 μM Tripathi *et al.* [192]: 6.7 μM
Klebsiella pneumoniae	B−	De Majumdar *et al.* [193]: >11.1 μM
Moraxella catarrhalis	B−	Leszczynska *et al.* [183]: 6.2 μM
Neisseria gonorrhoeae	B−	Bergman *et al.* [194]: 0.8 μM
Neisseria meningitidis	B−	Leszczynska *et al.* [183]: 12.5 μM for strain B Leszczynska *et al.* [183]: 24.9 μM for strain C Jones *et al.* [195]: 10 μM
Peptostreptococcus anaerobius	B+	Leszczynska *et al.* [183]: 49.8 μM

Table 4. *Cont.*

Microbes [1]	Bacteria Gram +/− (B+/−) Virus (V) Yeast (Y)	References: Concentration [2]
Porphyromonas gingivalis	B−	Leszczynska *et al.* [183]: 49.8 μM Ouhara *et al.* [173]: 11.1 μM
Prevotella intermedia	B−	Ouhara *et al.* [173]: 1.1 μM
Pseudomonas aeruginosa	B−	Bergsson *et al.* [196]: 5.6 μM Dean *et al.* [197]: 0.22 μM Dosler and Karaaslan [198]: ~14.2–28.4 μM Gordon *et al.* [160]: ~11.1–22.2 μM Leszczynska *et al.* [183]: 99.7 μM
Respiratory syncytial virus	V	Currie *et al.* [199]: 5.6 μM
Staphylococcus aureus	B+	Leszczynska *et al.* [183]: 6.2 μM Noore *et al.* [200]: 2 μM Chen *et al.* [186]: 0.67 μM Senyurek *et al.* [201]: 11.1 μM Nagaoka *et al.* [188]: 1 μM Gordon *et al.* [160]: ~11.1–22.2 μM
Staphylococcus epidermidis	B+	Leszczynska *et al.* [183]: 12.5 μM Gordon *et al.* [160]: ~11.1–22.2 μM
Streptococcus mitis	B+	Ouhara *et al.* [173]: 2.2 μM
Streptococcus mutans	B+	Ouhara *et al.* [173]: 0.22 μM Leszczynska *et al.* [183]: 6.2 μM
Streptococcus pneumoniae	B+	Nagaoka *et al.* [188]: 1 μM Leszczynska *et al.* [183]: 3.1 μM
Streptococcus pyogenes	B+	Leszczynska *et al.* [183]: 3.1 μM
Streptococcus salivarius	B+	Ouhara *et al.* [173]: 1.1 μM Leszczynska *et al.* [183]: 6.2 μM
Streptococcus sanguis	B+	Ouhara *et al.* [173]: 0.22 μM Leszczynska *et al.* [183]: 6.2 μM
Streptococcus sobrinus	B+	Ouhara *et al.* [173]: 1.1 μM
Tannerella forsythensis	B+	Leszczynska *et al.* [183]: 49.8 μM
Treponema pallidum	B-	Sambri *et al.* [169]: 100.1 μM
Ureaplasma parvum	NA [3]	Xiao *et al.* [202]: 22.2 μM
Ureaplasma urealyticum	NA [3]	Xiao *et al.* [202]: 22.2 μM
Vaccinia virus	V	Howell *et al.* [203]: 20 μM
Varicella zoster virus (VZV)	V	Crack *et al.* [204]: 0.1 μM

[1] Highlighted microbes: blue causing STI; green causing vaginitis; Red causing UTI; Pink causing vaginitis and UTI. [2] Concentrations of LL-37 given are those that exert microbicidal effects on ⩾90% of the microbes. In some cases where this information is not clearly described in the publication, estimated concentrations are given. [3] NA = not applicable; *Borrelia* spp. and *Ureaplasma* spp. do not react well with the Gram stain.

Besides the direct microbicidal activity, LL-37 possesses other properties including anti-endotoxin activity [49–51], immunomodulation (reviews [53–55]), angiogenesis [59] and wound healing [56–58]. If the anti-endotoxin and immunomodulatory properties are confirmed in the female reproductive tract system, it will strengthen the possibility that LL-37/ALL-38 can be used as vaginal microbicides that can clear infection and minimize infection-associated inflammation. Angiogenesis and wound healing properties would also aid in the repair of minor vaginal tissue damages occurring during intercourse. Further studies on LL-37's direct microbicidal effects must also be carried out in all microbes that are causes of STIs and vaginitis, as well as urinary tract infection (UTI). The vagina and its normal microbiota represent an important barrier against uropathogenic bacteria (Table 1). Perturbations of the normal vaginal microbiota, such as depletion of lactobacilli, can promote colonization of uropathogens, such as uropathogenic *E. coli* (UPEC), within the vagina [205]. The vagina can then become an extra-urinary uropathogen reservoir and in turn increase the risk of UTI [206].LL-37 exerts microbicidal effects on most of the STI-inducing microorganisms including HIV (causing life threatening AIDS with no cure), HSV-1 (causing genital herpes with no cure), *Neisseria gonorrhoeae* (causing gonorrhoea, curable), *Treponema pallidum* (causing syphilis, curable) and *Chlamydia trachomatis* (causing cervicitis, salpingitis and endometriosis, curable) (Table 4). Although gonorrhoea, syphilis and chlamydia infection are curable, a number of complications are associated with these three STIs. They all increase the risk of infertility. A higher susceptibility to HIV transmission is also associated with gonorrhoea and syphilis. Salpingitis and oviductal tubal blockade caused by chlamydia infection can also lead to ovarian cancer. For gonorrhoea, resistance to antibiotics used for the treatment has increasingly become a problem. As listed in Table 1, LL-37 needs to be tested for its microbicidal activity against a number of additional microorganisms that cause STI (viruses:HPV, hepatitis A and C; protozoon, *Trichomonas vaginalis*) and bacterial vaginosis (*Gardnerella vaginalis, Bacteroides* spp., *Mycoplasma hominis* and *Mobiluncus* spp.), prior to its development as a vaginal microbicide. Further testing against uropathogenic microorganisms (Table 1) will also allow LL-37 to be developed for therapeutic and prophylactic uses for urinary tract infection in this system. LL-37 formulated gel administered into the vagina would exert microbicidal action on uropathogenic microbes that opportunistically form a reservoir in the vagina. The vaginal secretion, which can travel upwards into the urinary tract, would also likely contain LL-37 released from the gel, which then can fight against microbes in this tract (see the list in Table 4).

The majority of sperm co-existing with seminal plasma, which contains 2-10 μM of hCAP-18 [153], remain motile in ejaculated semen of fertile donors. Interestingly, despite the negatively charged surface of sperm and the overall positive charge of hCAP-18 (+6, pI = 9.25), hCAP-18 is present at a residual amount on human sperm [79]. However, since motile sperm with fertilizing ability are never exposed to ALL-38 produced from seminal plasma (Figure 4), it raises a possibility that ALL-38/LL-37 may have a deleterious effect on sperm, possibly after the deposition of ALL-38/LL-37 onto the sperm surface. Although hCAP-18/LL-37 is also produced by cervicovaginal epithelial cells, its amount is 1000x less than ALL-38 originated from seminal plasma (i.e., 1.3 nM [136] *versus* 2–10 μM [153], respectively). Therefore, we asked the question of whether LL-37 when added exogenously to a sperm suspension could bind to sperm with a deleterious consequence on their fertilizing ability. Also, if sperm-LL-37 binding did occur, was it dependent on the interaction of LL-37 with a negatively–charged SGG existing specifically on the mammalian sperm head surface? The latter question is relevant in terms of possible development of LL-37 into a spermicide with specificity to sperm and not to other somatic cells such as cervicovaginal epithelial cells. Our results revealed that LL-37 bound to SGG and its anionic lipid analog, sulfogalactosylceramide (SGC), as well as phosphatidylserine (also negatively charged), all immobilized separately in a well of a microtiter plate, in a specific manner. K_d values of the binding of LL-37 to these three anionic lipids were 456, 157 and 24 nM, respectively. In contrast, LL-37 did not bind to neutral lipids, phosphatidylcholine and galactosylglycerolipid (GG—the desulfated form of SGG) [79]. Direct binding of LL-37 to Percoll-gradient centrifuged mouse and human sperm resuspended in medium was further demonstrated. For the reason described in Section 3, Percoll-gradient centrifuged sperm were first used in all studies, and in the case of human sperm replicate experiments were performed with swim-up sperm. The partial dependence of LL-37-sperm interaction on SGG on the sperm surface was then demonstrated by a decrease in LL-37 binding to sperm that were pre-incubated with anti-SGG antibody [79]. Pretreatment of capacitated mouse sperm with 3.6 μM LL-37 resulted in a complete loss of sperm ability to fertilize eggs *in vitro*. This 3.6 μM of LL-37 is equivalent to the concentration of SGG in the mouse sperm suspension used for the treatment [71,79], further corroborating the concept that SGG was involved in LL-37 binding. Notably, 100% of mouse sperm treated with 3.6 μM LL-37 became immotile within 5 min of treatment, and this result would be one of explanations for the inability of these LL-37 treated sperm to fertilize eggs *in vitro*. Likewise, human sperm lost their motility when treated with LL-37, although 10.8 μM of LL-37 was needed for the majority of sperm to become immotile. Furthermore, when non-capacitated sperm and partially capacitated sperm, both human and mouse, were treated with the same LL-37 concentrations as used for fully capacitated sperm, the inhibition of their motility was similarly observed [79]. Non-capacitated sperm, partially capacitated sperm and fully capacitated sperm were prepared in the lab by resuspending sperm in the medium without bicarbonate, calcium and albumin, with bicarbonate and calcium but no albumin, and with all of these three components, respectively. The prepared non-capacitated sperm represent sperm that have just swum out from the seminal plasma *in vivo*, whereas partially capacitated sperm resemble those that are swimming through the cervix. Finally, the prepared capacitated sperm are equivalent to sperm that have swum into the uterine cavity and their cholesterol is induced to release by albumin and HDL present in the uterus [8,207].

The loss of sperm motility upon LL-37 treatment can be from the direct interaction of LL-37 with the axoneme, the motility apparatus, in the sperm tail [8]. However, this possibility is discounted by the lack of binding of LL-37, added exogenously to the sperm suspension, to the sperm tail [79]. It is also unlikely that the mechanism of the effects of LL-37 on sperm motility is through its direct effect on CatSper, the cation channel responsible for sperm hyperactivated motility [12], since LL-37 also induces immotility in non-capacitated sperm, which normally do not have hyperactivated motility patterns. Rather, immotility of LL-37 treated sperm may come from the loss of intracellular homeostasis due to the LL-37 induced damage on the sperm surface, a situation that is parallel to that observed on the microbial membrane [46,67]. This postulation was confirmed by the observation that LL-37 treated sperm became positively stained with Sytox Green (a membrane impermeable DNA fluorescent dye), an indication that the surface membranes of these treated sperm were compromised. Pharmacokinetic studies further indicated that the sperm plasma membrane damage induced by LL-37 occurred prior to the loss of sperm motility. Finally, LL-37 treated sperm became acrosome-reacted, thus markedly lowering their ability to bind to the egg. Transmission electron microscopy confirmed that the damages on the sperm plasma membrane and the outer acrosomal membrane as well as the loss of the acrosome and in some cases the inner acrosomal membrane were the adverse effects of LL-37 on sperm [79]. In contrast, our unpublished results reveal that LL-37 at the spermicidal concentration range did not have any adverse effects to mouse eggs and embryos. Mouse eggs treated with 3.6 μM LL-37 were normally fertilized by sperm collected from a fertile animal, and mouse two-cell embryos treated with the same LL-37 concentration developed into blastocysts at the same rate as untreated two-cell embryos.

We have further demonstrated the loss of sperm fertilizing ability *in vivo*. Mouse sperm treated with LL-37 were transcervically injected into female mice naturally cycling to the estrous phase in the reproductive cycle. None of these female mice (n = 26) became pregnant, whereas pregnancy was observed in 92% of female mice (n = 26) injected with untreated sperm. Significantly, the female reproductive system of mice injected with LL-37 + sperm did not show any apparent changes, as compared with that of control females (injected with medium + sperm) (Figure 5A). In females that were exposed to LL-37, the histology of their vagina and uterus as well as the dimension, shape and color of their reproductive tissues did not differ from those of control females (unexposed to LL-37) (Figure 5A). There were no signs of immune cell recruitment (implicating inflammation) to the vaginal/uterine tissues of these LL-37 exposed females (Figure 5B). This was in contrast to female mice transcervically injected with 2% N-9, whereas numerous neutrophils were apparent in the vaginal epithelium (Figure 5B). In fact, female mice transcervically injected with sperm + LL-37 for three estrus cycles with no pregnancy outcomes could resume their fecundity as shown by pups delivered by these females following their natural mating with fertile males two weeks after the last transcervical injection with LL-37.

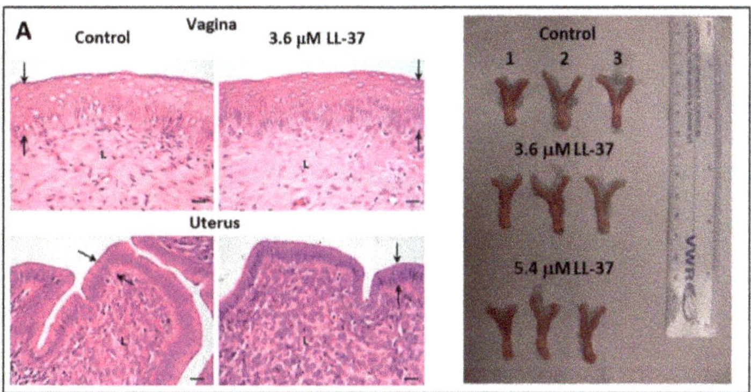

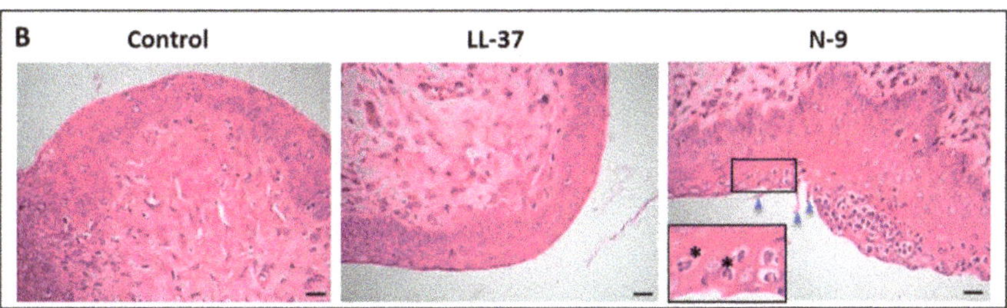

Figure 5. (**A**) Left panel: Normal histology of the vagina and uterus of female mice transcervically injected with LL-37 + sperm. The female reproductive tract tissues were collected for fixing and paraffin embedding one day after the transcervical injection of LL-37 + sperm, or sperm alone (control). Sections of the vagina and uterus revealed that the vaginal stratified epithelial cell layers and the uterine single epithelial cell layer (denoted as the area between the two arrows) as well as the corresponding lamina propria of the LL-37 treated and control animals did not differ from each other. Bar = 20 μm. This image was taken from our published article [79]. Right panel: The anatomy (shape, dimension and color) of the vagina/cervix and uterus, dissected from females injected with LL-37 (3.7or 5.4 μM) + sperm (n = 3 each) or sperm alone (control) (n = 3) one day after the injection, was the same among the three groups of the animals. (**B**) Absence of immune cell recruitment to the vaginal epithelium of mice transcervically injected with LL-37 + sperm. Sections of the vagina were prepared as in (**A**). The vaginal epithelium and lamina propria of both the control and LL-37 treated mice similarly show minimal numbers of immune cells, indicating no recruitment of these cells to the vagina as a consequence of LL-37 injection. In contrast, when females were transcervically injected with 2% nonoxynol-9 (N-9), numerous neutrophils were recruited into the vaginal epithelium. The polymorphonuclear structure of neutrophils is apparent in the close-up image (denoted by asterisks). Triangles point to the N-9 induced rupture of the vaginal epithelial surface. Bar = 20 μm.

We have further confirmed that LL-37 had minimal adverse effects on the immortalized human cervicovaginal epithelial cell lines, *i.e.*, Vk2/E6E7 (vaginal), Ect1/E6E7 (ectocervical) and End1/E6E7 (endocervical) cells. Cytotoxicity MTT (3-(4,5-dimethylthiazol-2-yl)-2,5-diphenyltetrazolium bromide) assays showed no significant differences of percent viable cells of these three cell lines upon treatment with LL-37 at concentrations up to 3.6 μM (Figure 6A). Sytox Green incorporation assays for the membrane intactness of these cell lines revealed similar results. In all of these three cell lines, less than 10% of cells incorporated Sytox Green into their nuclei upon treatment with 3.6 μM. However, these percentages increased to 20, 25 and 40% in Ect1/E6E7, End1/E6E7 and Vk2/E6E7 cells, respectively, following treatment with 10.8 μM of LL-37 (Figure 6B).

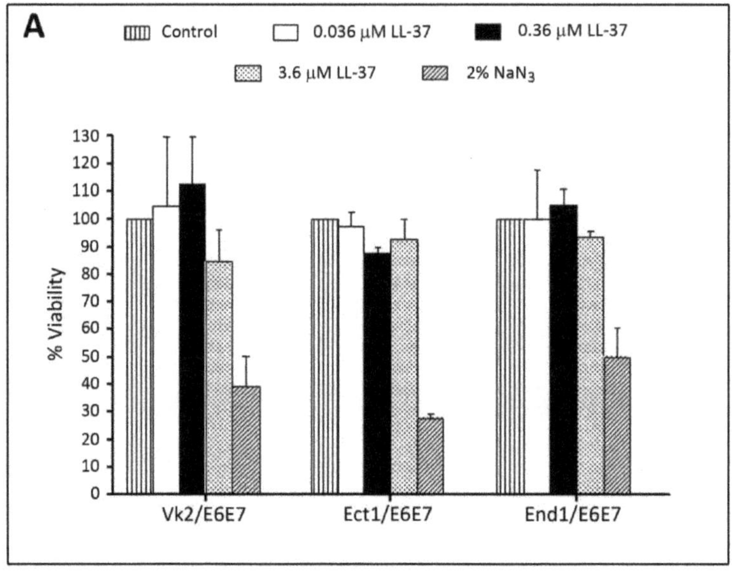

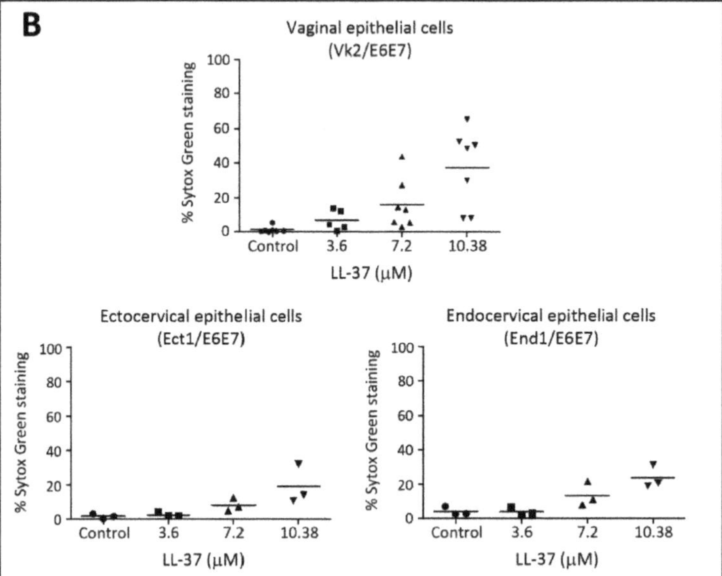

Figure 6. Low adverse effects of LL-37 on human vaginal and cervical cell lines. Vk2/E6E7 (vaginal), Ect1/E6E7 (ectocervical) and End1/E6E7 (endocervical) cells cultured as previously described [123] were treated with various concentrations of LL-37 (24 h, 37 °C, 5% CO_2) and subjected to a cytotoxicity MTT assay (**A**) or a membrane intactness assay using Sytox (**B**). (**A**) Treatment of all three cell lines with LL-37 up to 3.7 μM did not change percentages of viable cells. In contrast, the percentages of viable cells were only 50% or less upon treatment with 2% NaN_3. (**B**) Sytox Green staining was observed in less than 20% of all three cell lines upon treatment with LL-37 up to 3.7 μM. When the LL-37 concentration was increased to 10.8 μM, the numbers of Sytox Green stained cells became higher, although for both End1/E6E7 and Ect1/E6E7 cells, the percentages were still <20%. For Vk2/E6E7 cells, this percentage was 40%.

While the higher susceptibility to LL-37 in the vaginal epithelial cell line should be a matter of concern, the situation *in vivo* may not be as unfavourable as that observed *in vitro*. Cells of the upper layer of the vaginal epithelium continue to slough off into the lumen and it is possible that those cells with compromised membrane intactness due to LL-37 exposure may undergo this sloughing at a higher rate than normal cells.

In summary, we have shown that LL-37 possesses spermicidal effects in both human and mouse sperm with minimal adverse effects on the female reproductive tract epithelia. This spermicidal property with molecular mechanisms described above appears to be unique to LL-37. A number of defensin AMPs are secreted by epididymal epithelial cells (examples-human: HE2β1 (aka SPAG11D) [208], DEFB126 [209–211], DEFB118 [212,213], DEFB114 [214], DEFB1 [215]; -rodents: Bin1b (aka SPAG11E) [216,217], β -defensin 22 [218]) and some of them deposit onto the surface of transit sperm to endow fertilizing ability (e.g., HE2 β 1, DEFB126, DEFB118 and HBD1 in humans, and Bin1b in rodents). We have shown that both HE2 β 1 and Bin1b could bind to SGG/SGC *in vitro*, but sperm incubated with excess amounts (18 μM) of these two defensins were still motile with intact acrosome and in the case of mouse sperm that were treated with these β-defensins, they could still fertilize eggs at 50% control values (our unpublished results).

The physiological significance of LL-37 as a microbicide and an immunomodulatory and wound healing peptide is well documented. In particular, LL-37 exerts microbicidal effects on a number of microbes responsible for STI, vaginitis and UTI (Table 4). With these microbicidal and spermicidal properties, LL-37 warrants further attempts to be developed as a vaginal contraceptive/microbicide. As a natural peptide, its repeated and long-term use will likely create minimal side effects and microbicidal resistance. Further studies, however, are needed in a number of aspects in potential application of LL-37 in the vagina. First, an effective method to deliver LL-37 into the vaginal lumen has to be established. Careful studies on any adverse effects of LL-37, following its repeated/long-term administration, must also be performed at both topical and systemic levels. Regardless, the cost of chemical synthesis of LL-37 for this use is a challenge, and the shortest truncated LL-37 peptide or its mimetic, which still bears spermicidal and microbicidal activity, has to be discovered. In a separate avenue, ultrashort cationic lipopeptides with high antibiotic activity [219–221] may be screened for spermicidal effects. However, the selectivity of the deleterious effects of these lipopeptides to sperm and not to the female reproductive tract epithelial cells must be considered. Nonetheless, success in finding the most cost-effective form of LL-37 as a vaginal contraceptive/microbicide will undoubtedly provide women with empowerment in having a healthy and safe sex practice—the ability to protect themselves from unwanted pregnancies and microbial infections.

Acknowledgments: Our work on LL-37 described in this review is supported by a grant from Canadian Institutes of Health Research and previously by Bill & Melinda Gates Foundation (Grand Challenges Exploration Project) both awarded to NT. GW is supported by the NIH grant R01AI105147 during this study. We thank Ryan Jarratt, RPh, Westboro Pharmasave, Ottawa, ON, Canada for the insightful information on the nonoxynol-9 formulation used in vaginal contraceptives. Help in manuscript preparation from Terri Van Gulik is highly appreciated.

Author Contributions: N.T. conceived and designed the scheme of this review and wrote about 90% of it. N.S. significantly contributed to the results indicating the spermicidal effects of LL-37. As well, he gathered information from databases for the content of Table 4, helped with Table 3 preparation, and drew Figure 4A,C. R.A. contributed to the data shown in Figure 4B and helped in the preparation of Table 4. W.K. helped in all aspects of the writing, including reference citation and checking, and table/figure preparation. K.K. prepared Figure 3B and the first draft of Figure 3A. R.Z. and W.L. contributed to the information on contraceptives. M.B. contributed to information related to sperm physiology and the biochemistry of hCAP-18/LL-37. G.W. prepared Figure 3A and contributed significantly to the up-to-date knowledge of antimicrobial peptides. D.H. prepared Table 1 and contributed to information on the clinical relevance of antimicrobial peptides in the genitourinary system. All authors proofread and edited the manuscript.

Conflicts of Interest: The authors declare no conflicts of interest.

References

1. Shoupe, D.; Mishell, D.R. Contraception. *Women and Health*, 2nd ed.; Goldman, M.B., Troisi, R., Rexrode, K.M., Eds.; Academic Press: London, UK, 2013.
2. Wadman, M. Contraceptive risk of HIV long suspected. *Nature News* **2011**. [CrossRef]
3. Spevack, E. The long-term health implications of depo-provera. *Int. Med.* **2013**, *12*, 27–34.
4. Filby, A.L.; Neuparth, T.; Thorpe, K.L.; Owen, R.; Galloway, T.S.; Tyler, C.R. Health impacts of estrogens in the environment, considering complex mixture effects. *Environ. Health Perspect.* **2007**, *115*, 1704–1710. [CrossRef] [PubMed]
5. Wise, A.; O'Brien, K.; Woodruff, T. Are oral contraceptives a significant contributor to the estrogenicity of drinking water? *Environ. Sci. Technol.* **2011**, *45*, 51–60. [CrossRef] [PubMed]
6. Haase, A.T. Early events in sexual transmission of HIV and SIV and opportunities for interventions. *Annu. Rev. Med.* **2011**, *62*, 127–139. [CrossRef] [PubMed]
7. WHO. Annual technical report. Department of Reproductive Health and Research **2013**.
8. Florman, H.; Fissore, R. Fertilization in mammals. In *Knobil and Neill's Physiology of Reproduction*, 4th ed.; Plant, T.M., Zeleznik, A., Eds.; Elsevier Inc.: New York, NY, USA, 2015; pp. 149–195.
9. Travis, A.J.; Kopf, G.S. The role of cholesterol efflux in regulating the fertilization potential of mammalian spermatozoa. *J. Clin. Investig.* **2002**, *110*, 731–736. [CrossRef] [PubMed]
10. Okabe, M. The cell biology of mammalian fertilization. *Development.* **2013**, *140*, 4471–4479. [CrossRef] [PubMed]
11. Suarez, S.S.; Pacey, A.A. Sperm transport in the female reproductive tract. *Hum. Reprod. Update.* **2006**, *12*, 23–37. [CrossRef] [PubMed]
12. Lishko, P.V.; Kirichok, Y.; Ren, D.; Navarro, B.; Chung, J.J.; Clapham, D.E. The control of male fertility by spermatozoan ion channels. *Annu. Rev. Physiol.* **2012**, *74*, 453–475. [CrossRef] [PubMed]
13. Chung, J.J.; Navarro, B.; Krapivinsky, G.; Krapivinsky, L.; Clapham, D.E. A novel gene required for male fertility and functional *Catsper* channel formation in spermatozoa. *Nature Commun.* **2011**, *2*, 1–12. [CrossRef] [PubMed]
14. Tanphaichitr, N.; Carmona, E.; Bou Khalil, M.; Xu, H.; Berger, T.; Gerton, G.L. New insights into sperm-zona pellucida interaction: Involvement of sperm lipid rafts. *Front. Biosci.* **2007**, *12*, 1748–1766. [CrossRef] [PubMed]
15. White, D.; Weerachatyanukul, W.; Gadella, B.; Kamolvarin, N.; Attar, M.; Tanphaichitr, N. Role of sperm sulfogalactosylglycerolipid in mouse sperm-zona pellucida binding. *Biol. Reprod.* **2000**, *63*, 147–155. [CrossRef] [PubMed]
16. Weerachatyanukul, W.; Rattanachaiyanont, M.; Carmona, E.; Furimsky, A.; Mai, A.; Shoushtarian, A.; Sirichotiyakul, S.; Ballakier, H.; Leader, A.; Tanphaichitr, N. Sulfogalactosylglycerolipid is involved in human gamete interaction. *Mol. Reprod. Dev.* **2001**, *60*, 569–578. [CrossRef] [PubMed]
17. Ikawa, M.; Inoue, N.; Benham, A.M.; Okabe, M. Fertilization: A sperm's journey to and interaction with the oocyte. *J. Clin. Investig.* **2010**, *120*, 984–994. [CrossRef] [PubMed]
18. Lyng, R.; Shur, B.D. Sperm-egg binding requires a multiplicity of receptor-ligand interactions: New insights into the nature of gamete receptors derived from reproductive tract secretions. *Soc. Reprod. Fertil. Suppl.* **2007**, *65*, 335–351. [PubMed]
19. Kongmanas, K.; Kruevaisayawan, H.; Saewu, A.; Sugeng, C.; Fernandes, J.; Souda, P.; Angel, J.B.; Faull, K.F.; Aitken, R.J.; Whitelegge, J.; *et al.* Proteomic characterization of pig sperm anterior head plasma membrane reveals roles of acrosomal proteins in ZP3 binding. *J. Cell Physiol.* **2015**, *230*, 449–463. [CrossRef] [PubMed]
20. Tanphaichitr, N.; Kongmanas, K.; Kruevaisayawan, H.; Saewu, A.; Sugeng, C.; Fernandes, J.; Souda, P.; Angel, J.B.; Faull, K.F.; Aitken, R.J.; *et al.* Remodeling of the plasma membrane in preparation for sperm-egg recognition: Roles of acrosomal proteins. *Asian J. Androl.* **2015**, *17*, 574–582. [CrossRef] [PubMed]
21. Munch, J.; Rucker, E.; Standker, L.; Adermann, K.; Goffinet, C.; Schindler, M.; Wildum, S.; Chinnadurai, R.; Rajan, D.; Specht, A.; *et al.* Semen-derived amyloid fibrils drastically enhance HIV infection. *Cell* **2007**, *131*, 1059–1071. [CrossRef] [PubMed]
22. Chijioke, P.C.; Zaman, S.; Pearson, R.M. Comparison of the potency of d-propanolol, chlorhexidine and nonoxynol-9 in the sander cramer test. *Contraception* **1986**, *34*, 207–211. [CrossRef]

23. Dunmire, E.N.; Katz, D.F. Kinematic response of human spermatozoa to nonoxynol-9. *Biol. Reprod.* **1994**, *50*, 903–911. [CrossRef] [PubMed]
24. Thompson, K.A.; Malamud, D.; Storey, B.T. Assessment of the anti-microbial agent c31g as a spermicide: Comparison with nonoxynol-9. *Contraception* **1996**, *53*, 313–318. [CrossRef]
25. Asculai, S.S.; Weis, M.T.; Rancourt, M.W.; Kupferberg, A.B. Inactivation of herpes simplex viruses by nonionic surfactants. *Antimicrob. Agents Chemother.* **1978**, *13*, 686–690. [CrossRef] [PubMed]
26. Moench, T.R.; Whaley, K.J.; Mandrell, T.D.; Bishop, B.D.; Witt, C.J.; Cone, R.A. The cat/feline immunodeficiency virus model for transmucosal transmission of aids: Nonoxynol-9 contraceptive jelly blocks transmission by an infected cell inoculum. *AIDS* **1993**, *7*, 797–802. [CrossRef] [PubMed]
27. Benes, S.; McCormack, W.M. Inhibition of growth of *Chlamydia trachomatis* by nonoxynol-9 *in vivo*. *Antimicrob. Agents Chemother.* **1985**, *27*, 724–726. [CrossRef] [PubMed]
28. Malkovsky, M.; Newell, A.; Dalgleish, A.G. Inactivation of HIV by nonoxynol-9. *Lancet* **1988**, *1*, 645. [CrossRef]
29. Doncel, G.F. Exploiting common targets in human fertilization and HIV infection: Development of novel contraceptive microbicides. *Hum. Reprod. Update* **2006**, *12*, 103–117. [CrossRef] [PubMed]
30. Miller, C.J.; Alexander, N.J.; Gettie, A.; Hendrickx, A.G.; Marx, P.A. The effect of contraceptives containing nonoxynol-9 on the genital transmission of simian immunodeficiency virus in *Rhesus macaques*. *Fertil. Steril.* **1992**, *57*, 1126–1128. [PubMed]
31. Weber, J.; Nunn, A.; O'Connor, T.; Jeffries, D.; Kitchen, V.; McCormack, S.; Stott, J.; Almond, N.; Stone, A.; Darbyshire, J. Chemical condoms' for the prevention of HIV infection: Evaluation of novel agents against SHIV(89.6PD) *in vitro* and *in vivo*. *AIDS* **2001**, *15*, 1563–1568. [CrossRef] [PubMed]
32. Wilkinson, D.; Tholandi, M.; Ramjee, G.; Rutherford, G.W. Nonoxynol-9 spermicide for prevention of vaginally acquired HIV and other sexually transmitted infections: Systematic review and meta-analysis of randomised controlled trials including more than 5000 women. *Lancet Infect. Dis.* **2002**, *2*, 613–617. [CrossRef]
33. Van Damme, L.; Ramjee, G.; Alary, M.; Vuylsteke, B.; Chandeying, V.; Rees, H.; Sirivongrangson, P.; Mukenge-Tshibaka, L.; Ettiegne-Traore, V.; Uaheowitchai, C.; *et al.* Effectiveness of col-1492, a nonoxynol-9 vaginal gel, on HIV-1 transmission in female sex workers: A randomised controlled trial. *Lancet* **2002**, *360*, 971–977. [CrossRef]
34. Richardson, B.A.; Lavreys, L.; Martin, H.L., Jr.; Stevens, C.E.; Ngugi, E.; Mandaliya, K.; Bwayo, J.; Ndinya-Achola, J.; Kreiss, J.K. Evaluation of a low-dose nonoxynol-9 gel for the prevention of sexually transmitted diseases: A randomized clinical trial. *Sex. Transm. Dis.* **2001**, *28*, 394–400. [CrossRef] [PubMed]
35. Stafford, M.K.; Ward, H.; Flanagan, A.; Rosenstein, I.J.; Taylor-Robinson, D.; Smith, J.R.; Weber, J.; Kitchen, V.S. Safety study of nonoxynol-9 as a vaginal microbicide: Evidence of adverse effects. *J. Acquir. Immune Defic. Syndr.* **1998**, *17*, 327–331. [CrossRef]
36. Schreiber, C.A.; Meyn, L.A.; Creinin, M.D.; Barnhart, K.T.; Hillier, S.L. Effects of long-term use of nonoxynol-9 on vaginal flora. *Obstet. Gynecol.* **2006**, *107*, 136–143. [CrossRef] [PubMed]
37. Klebanoff, S.J. Effects of the spermicidal agent nonoxynol-9 on vaginal microbial flora. *J. Infect. Dis.* **1992**, *165*, 19–25. [CrossRef] [PubMed]
38. Martin, H.L., Jr.; Stevens, C.E.; Richardson, B.A.; Rugamba, D.; Nyange, P.M.; Mandaliya, K.; Ndinya-Achola, J.; Kreiss, J.K. Safety of a nonoxynol-9 vaginal gel in Kenyan prostitutes. A randomized clinical trial. *Sex. Transm. Dis.* **1997**, *24*, 279–283. [CrossRef] [PubMed]
39. Kreiss, J.; Ngugi, E.; Holmes, K.; Ndinya-Achola, J.; Waiyaki, P.; Roberts, P.L.; Ruminjo, I.; Sajabi, R.; Kimata, J.; Fleming, T.R.; *et al.* Efficacy of nonoxynol 9 contraceptive sponge use in preventing heterosexual acquisition of HIV in Nairobi prostitutes. *JAMA* **1992**, *268*, 477–482. [CrossRef] [PubMed]
40. Weber, J.; Desai, K.; Darbyshire, J.; Microbicides Development Program. The development of vaginal microbicides for the prevention of HIV transmission. *PLoS Med* **2005**, *2*, e142. [CrossRef] [PubMed]
41. Niruthisard, S.; Roddy, R.E.; Chutivongse, S. The effects of frequent nonoxynol-9 use on the vaginal and cervical mucosa. *Sex. Transm. Dis.* **1991**, *18*, 176–179. [CrossRef] [PubMed]
42. Lozenski, K.; Ownbey, R.; Wigdahl, B.; Kish-Catalone, T.; Krebs, F.C. Decreased cervical epithelial sensitivity to nonoxynol-9 (N-9) after four daily applications in a murine model of topical vaginal microbicide safety. *BMC Pharmacol. Toxicol.* **2012**, *13*, 1–11. [CrossRef] [PubMed]

43. Fichorova, R.N.; Tucker, L.D.; Anderson, D.J. The molecular basis of nonoxynol-9-induced vaginal inflammation and its possible relevance to human immunodeficiency virus type 1 transmission. *J. Infect. Dis.* **2001**, *184*, 418–428. [CrossRef] [PubMed]
44. Ventola, C.L. The antibiotic resistance crisis: Part 1: Causes and threats. *Pharm. Ther.* **2015**, *40*, 277–283.
45. Reardon, S. Bacterial arms race revs up. *Nature* **2015**, *521*, 402–403. [CrossRef] [PubMed]
46. Kindrachuk, J.; Nijnik, A.; Hancock, R.E.W. Host defense peptides: Bridging antimicrobial and immunomodulatory activities. In *Comprehensive Natural Products II: Chemistry and Biology*; Mander, L., Lui, H.W., Eds.; Elsevier Science: Oxford, UK, 2010; Volume 5, pp. 175–216.
47. Wang, G. Human antimicrobial peptides and proteins. *Pharmaceuticals* **2014**, *7*, 545–594. [CrossRef] [PubMed]
48. Yarbrough, V.L.; Winkle, S.; Herbst-Kralovetz, M.M. Antimicrobial peptides in the female reproductive tract: A critical component of the mucosal immune barrier with physiological and clinical implications. *Hum. Reprod. Update* **2015**, *21*, 353–377. [CrossRef] [PubMed]
49. Lee, S.H.; Jun, H.K.; Lee, H.R.; Chung, C.P.; Choi, B.K. Antibacterial and lipopolysaccharide (LPS)-neutralising activity of human cationic antimicrobial peptides against periodontopathogens. *Int. J. Antimicrob Agents* **2010**, *35*, 138–145. [CrossRef] [PubMed]
50. Larrick, J.W.; Hirata, M.; Balint, R.F.; Lee, J.; Zhong, J.; Wright, S.C. Human CAP18: A novel antimicrobial lipopolysaccharide-binding protein. *Infect. Immun.* **1995**, *63*, 1291–1297. [PubMed]
51. Molhoek, E.M.; den Hertog, A.L.; de Vries, A.M.; Nazmi, K.; Veerman, E.C.; Hartgers, F.C.; Yazdanbakhsh, M.; Bikker, F.J.; van der Kleij, D. Structure-function relationship of the human antimicrobial peptide LL-37 and LL-37 fragments in the modulation of TLR responses. *Biol. Chem.* **2009**, *390*, 295–303. [CrossRef] [PubMed]
52. Bowdish, D.M.; Davidson, D.J.; Lau, Y.E.; Lee, K.; Scott, M.G.; Hancock, R.E. Impact of LL-37 on anti-infective immunity. *J. Leukoc. Biol.* **2005**, *77*, 451–459. [CrossRef] [PubMed]
53. Choi, K.Y.; Mookherjee, N. Multiple immune-modulatory functions of cathelicidin host defense peptides. *Front. Immunol.* **2012**, *3*. [CrossRef] [PubMed]
54. Steinstraesser, L.; Kraneburg, U.; Jacobsen, F.; Al Benna, S. Host defense peptides and their antimicrobial-immunomodulatory duality. *Immunobiology* **2011**, *216*, 322–333. [CrossRef] [PubMed]
55. Hilchie, A.L.; Wuerth, K.; Hancock, R.E. Immune modulation by multifaceted cationic host defense (antimicrobial) peptides. *Nat. Chem Biol.* **2013**, *9*, 761–768. [CrossRef] [PubMed]
56. Carretero, M.; Escamez, M.J.; Garcia, M.; Duarte, B.; Holguin, A.; Retamosa, L.; Jorcano, J.L.; Rio, M.D.; Larcher, F. *In vitro* and *in vivo* wound healing-promoting activities of human cathelicidin LL-37. *J. Investig. Dermatol.* **2008**, *128*, 223–236. [CrossRef] [PubMed]
57. Tokumaru, S.; Sayama, K.; Shirakata, Y.; Komatsuzawa, H.; Ouhara, K.; Hanakawa, Y.; Yahata, Y.; Dai, X.; Tohyama, M.; Nagai, H.; *et al.* Induction of keratinocyte migration via transactivation of the epidermal growth factor receptor by the antimicrobial peptide LL-37. *J. Immunol.* **2005**, *175*, 4662–4668. [CrossRef] [PubMed]
58. Steinstraesser, L.; Hirsch, T.; Schulte, M.; Kueckelhaus, M.; Jacobsen, F.; Mersch, E.A.; Stricker, I.; Afacan, N.; Jenssen, H.; Hancock, R.E.; *et al.* Innate defense regulator peptide 1018 in wound healing and wound infection. *PLoS ONE* **2012**, *7*, e39373. [CrossRef] [PubMed]
59. Koczulla, R.; von Degenfeld, G.; Kupatt, C.; Krotz, F.; Zahler, S.; Gloe, T.; Issbrucker, K.; Unterberger, P.; Zaiou, M.; Lebherz, C.; *et al.* An angiogenic role for the human peptide antibiotic LL-37/hCAP-18. *J. Clin. Investig.* **2003**, *111*, 1665–1672. [CrossRef] [PubMed]
60. Wang, G.; Mishra, B.; Lau, K.; Lushnikova, T.; Golla, R.; Wang, X. Antimicrobial peptides in 2014. *Pharmaceuticals* **2015**, *8*, 123–150. [CrossRef] [PubMed]
61. Wang, G.; Li, X.; Zasloff, M. Part 1: Natural antimicrobial peptides: Nomenclature, classification and interesting templates for peptide engineering. In *Antimicrobial peptides, Discovery, Design and Novel Therapeutic Strategies*, 1st ed.; Wang, G., Ed.; CABI: Oxfordshire, UK, 2010; pp. 1–21.
62. Wang, G. Improved methods for classification, prediction, and design of antimicrobial peptides. *Methods Mol. Biol.* **2015**, *1268*, 43–66. [PubMed]
63. Chatterjee, C.; Paul, M.; Xie, L.; van der Donk, W.A. Biosynthesis and mode of action of lantibiotics. *Chem. Rev.* **2005**, *105*, 633–684. [CrossRef] [PubMed]
64. Ketchem, R.R.; Lee, K.C.; Huo, S.; Cross, T.A. Macromolecular structural elucidation with solid-state NMR-derived orientational constraints. *J. Biomol. NMR* **1996**, *8*, 1–14. [CrossRef] [PubMed]

65. Lohans, C.T.; Li, J.L.; Vederas, J.C. Structure and biosynthesis of carnolysin, a homologue of enterococcal cytolysin with d-amino acids. *J. Am. Chem. Soc.* **2014**, *136*, 13150–13153. [CrossRef] [PubMed]
66. Wang, G.; Mishra, B.; Epand, R.F.; Epand, R.M. High-quality 3D structures shine light on antibacterial, anti-biofilm and antiviral activities of human cathelicidin LL-37 and its fragments. *Biochim. Biophys. Acta* **2014**, *1838*, 2160–2172. [CrossRef] [PubMed]
67. Brogden, K.A. Antimicrobial peptides: Pore formers or metabolic inhibitors in bacteria? *Nat. Rev. Microbiol.* **2005**, *3*, 238–250. [CrossRef] [PubMed]
68. Yanagimachi, R.; Noda, Y.D.; Fujimoto, M.; Nicolson, G.L. The distribution of negative surface charges on mammalian spermatozoa. *Am. J. Anat.* **1972**, *135*, 497–519. [CrossRef] [PubMed]
69. Ainsworth, C.; Nixon, B.; Aitken, R.J. Development of a novel electrophoretic system for the isolation of human spermatozoa. *Hum. Reprod.* **2005**, *20*, 2261–2270. [CrossRef] [PubMed]
70. Tanphaichitr, N.; Bou Khalil, M.; Weerachatyanukul, W.; Kates, M.; Xu, H.; Carmona, E.; Attar, M.; Carrier, D. Physiological and biophysical properties of male germ cell sulfogalactosylglycerolipid. In *Lipid Metabolism and Male Fertility*; De Vriese, S., Ed.; AOCS Press: Champaign, IL, USA, 2003; Volume 11, pp. 125–148.
71. Kongmanas, K.; Xu, H.; Yaghoubian, A.; Franchini, L.; Panza, L.; Ronchetti, F.; Faull, K.; Tanphaichitr, N. Quantification of seminolipid by LC-ESI-MS/MS-multiple reaction monitoring: Compensatory levels in Cgt(+/−) mice. *J. Lipid Res.* **2010**, *51*, 3548–3558. [CrossRef] [PubMed]
72. Bou Khalil, M.; Chakrabandhu, K.; Xu, H.; Weerachatyanukul, W.; Buhr, M.; Berger, T.; Carmona, E.; Vuong, N.; Kumarathasan, P.; Wong, P.T.; *et al.* Sperm capacitation induces an increase in lipid rafts having zona pellucida binding ability and containing sulfogalactosylglycerolipid. *Dev. Biol.* **2006**, *290*, 220–235. [CrossRef] [PubMed]
73. Attar, M.; Kates, M.; Bou Khalil, M.; Carrier, D.; Wong, P.T.T.; Tanphaichitr, N. A fourier-transform infrared study of the interaction between germ-cell specific sulfogalactosylglycerolipid and dimyristoylglycerophosphocholine. *Chem. Phys. Lipids* **2000**, *106*, 101–114. [CrossRef]
74. Tanphaichitr, N.; Faull, K.F.; Yaghoubian, A.; Xu, H. Lipid rafts and sulfogalactosylglycerolipid (SGG) in sperm functions: Consensus and controversy. *Trends Glycosci. Glycotech.* **2007**, *19*, 67–83. [CrossRef]
75. Simon, P.; Baumner, S.; Busch, O.; Rohrich, R.; Kaese, M.; Richterich, P.; Wehrend, A.; Muller, K.; Gerardy-Schahn, R.; Muhlenhoff, M.; *et al.* Polysialic acid is present in mammalian semen as a post-translational modification of the neural cell adhesion molecule NCAM and the polysialyltransferase ST8SiaII. *J. Biol. Chem.* **2013**, *288*, 18825–18833. [CrossRef] [PubMed]
76. Kirchhoff, C.; Schroter, S. New insights into the origin, structure and role of CD52: A major component of the mammalian sperm glycocalyx. *Cells Tiss. Organs* **2001**, *168*, 93–104. [CrossRef]
77. Wang, G. Structures of human host defense cathelicidin LL-37 and its smallest antimicrobial peptide KR-12 in lipid micelles. *J. Biol. Chem.* **2008**, *283*, 32637–32643. [CrossRef] [PubMed]
78. Porcelli, F.; Verardi, R.; Shi, L.; Henzler-Wildman, K.A.; Ramamoorthy, A.; Veglia, G. NMR structure of the cathelicidin-derived human antimicrobial peptide LL-37 in dodecylphosphocholine micelles. *Biochemistry* **2008**, *47*, 5565–5572. [CrossRef] [PubMed]
79. Srakaew, N.; Young, C.D.; Sae-wu, A.; Xu, H.; Quesnel, K.L.; di Brisco, R.; Kongmanas, K.; Fongmoon, D.; Hommalai, G.; Weerachatyanukul, W.; *et al.* Antimicrobial host defence peptide, LL-37, as a potential vaginal contraceptive. *Hum. Reprod.* **2014**, *29*, 683–696. [CrossRef] [PubMed]
80. Lai, R.; Zheng, Y.T.; Shen, J.H.; Liu, G.J.; Liu, H.; Lee, W.H.; Tang, S.Z.; Zhang, Y. Antimicrobial peptides from skin secretions of chinese red belly toad *Bombina maxima*. *Peptides* **2002**, *23*, 427–435. [CrossRef]
81. Toke, O.; Banoczi, Z.; Kiraly, P.; Heinzmann, R.; Burck, J.; Ulrich, A.S.; Hudecz, F. A kinked antimicrobial peptide from *Bombina maxima*. I. Three-dimensional structure determined by NMR in membrane-mimicking environments. *Eur. Biophys. J.* **2011**, *40*, 447–462. [CrossRef] [PubMed]
82. Clara, A.; Manjramkar, D.D.; Reddy, V.K. Preclinical evaluation of magainin-a as a contraceptive antimicrobial agent. *Fertil. Steril.* **2004**, *81*, 1357–1365. [CrossRef] [PubMed]
83. Gesell, J.; Zasloff, M.; Opella, S.J. Two-dimensional 1h nmr experiments show that the 23-residue magainin antibiotic peptide is an alpha-helix in dodecylphosphocholine micelles, sodium dodecylsulfate micelles, and trifluoroethanol/water solution. *J. Biomol. NMR* **1997**, *9*, 127–135. [CrossRef] [PubMed]
84. Reddy, V.R.; Manjramkar, D.D. Evaluation of the antifertility effect of magainin-a in rabbits: *In vitro* and *in vivo* studies. *Fertil. Steril.* **2000**, *73*, 353–358. [CrossRef]

85. Edelstein, M.C.; Gretz, J.E.; Bauer, T.J.; Fulgham, D.L.; Alexander, N.J.; Archer, D.F. Studies on the *in vivo* spermicidal activity of synthetic magainins. *Fertil. Steril.* **1991**, *55*, 647–649. [PubMed]
86. Reddy, K.V.; Shahani, S.K.; Meherji, P.K. Spermicidal activity of magainins: *In vitro* and *in vivo* studies. *Contraception* **1996**, *53*, 205–210. [CrossRef]
87. Wojcik, C.; Sawicki, W.; Marianowski, P.; Benchaib, M.; Czyba, J.C.; Guerin, J.F. Cyclodextrin enhances spermicidal effects of magainin-2-amide. *Contraception* **2000**, *62*, 99–103. [CrossRef]
88. Chen, H.C.; Brown, J.H.; Morell, J.L.; Huang, C.M. Synthetic magainin analogues with improved antimicrobial activity. *FEBS Lett.* **1988**, *236*, 462–466. [CrossRef]
89. Mor, A.; Nicolas, P. The NH2-terminal alpha-helical domain 1-18 of dermaseptin is responsible for antimicrobial activity. *J. Biol. Chem.* **1994**, *269*, 1934–1939. [PubMed]
90. Zairi, A.; Belaid, A.; Gahbiche, A.; Hani, K. Spermicidal activity of dermaseptins. *Contraception* **2005**, *72*, 447–453. [CrossRef] [PubMed]
91. Shalev, D.E.; Rotem, S.; Fish, A.; Mor, A. Consequences of N-acylation on structure and membrane binding properties of dermaseptin derivative K4-S4-(1-13). *J. Biol Chem.* **2006**, *281*, 9432–9438. [CrossRef] [PubMed]
92. Zairi, A.; Serres, C.; Tangy, F.; Jouannet, P.; Hani, K. *In vivo* spermicidal activity of peptides from amphibian skin: Dermaseptin S4 and derivatives. *Bioorg. Med. Chem.* **2008**, *16*, 266–275. [CrossRef] [PubMed]
93. Zairi, A.; Tangy, F.; Bouassida, K.; Hani, K. Dermaseptins and magainins: Antimicrobial peptides from frogs' skin-new sources for a promising spermicides microbicides-a mini review. *J. Biomed. Biotechnol.* **2009**. [CrossRef] [PubMed]
94. Zare-Zardini, H.; Fesahat, F.; Anbari, F.; Halvaei, I.; Ebrahimi, L. Assessment of spermicidal activity of the antimicrobial peptide sarcotoxin Pd: A potent contraceptive agent. *Eur. J. Contracept. Reprod. Health Care* **2015**, *21*, 15–21. [CrossRef] [PubMed]
95. Hasper, H.E.; Kramer, N.E.; Smith, J.L.; Hillman, J.D.; Zachariah, C.; Kuipers, O.P.; de Kruijff, B.; Breukink, E. An alternative bactericidal mechanism of action for lantibiotic peptides that target lipid II. *Science* **2006**, *313*, 1636–1637. [CrossRef] [PubMed]
96. Van Den Hooven, H.W.; Doeland, C.C.; Van De Kamp, M.; Konings, R.N.; Hilbers, C.W.; Van De Ven, F.J. Three-dimensional structure of the lantibiotic nisin in the presence of membrane-mimetic micelles of dodecylphosphocholine and of sodium dodecylsulphate. *Eur. J. Biochem.* **1996**, *235*, 382–393. [CrossRef] [PubMed]
97. Van Den Hooven, H.W.; Spronk, C.A.; Van De Kamp, M.; Konings, R.N.; Hilbers, C.W.; Van De Van, F.J. Surface location and orientation of the lantibiotic nisin bound to membrane-mimicking micelles of dodecylphosphocholine and of sodium dodecylsulphate. *Eur. J. Biochem.* **1996**, *235*, 394–403. [CrossRef] [PubMed]
98. Aranha, C.; Gupta, S.; Reddy, K.V. Contraceptive efficacy of antimicrobial peptide Nisin: *In vitro* and *in vivo* studies. *Contraception* **2004**, *69*, 333–338. [CrossRef] [PubMed]
99. Reddy, K.V.; Aranha, C.; Gupta, S.M.; Yedery, R.D. Evaluation of antimicrobial peptide nisin as a safe vaginal contraceptive agent in rabbits: *In vitro* and *in vivo* studies. *Reproduction* **2004**, *128*, 117–126. [CrossRef] [PubMed]
100. Aranha, C.C.; Gupta, S.M.; Reddy, K.V. Assessment of cervicovaginal cytokine levels following exposure to microbicide nisin gel in rabbits. *Cytokine* **2008**, *43*, 63–70. [CrossRef] [PubMed]
101. Silkin, L.; Hamza, S.; Kaufman, S.; Cobb, S.L.; Vederas, J.C. Spermicidal bacteriocins: Lacticin 3147 and subtilosin a. *Bioorg. Med. Chem. Lett.* **2008**, *18*, 3103–3106. [CrossRef] [PubMed]
102. Gupta, S.M.; Aranha, C.C.; Bellare, J.R.; Reddy, K.V. Interaction of contraceptive antimicrobial peptide nisin with target cell membranes: Implications for use as vaginal microbicide. *Contraception* **2009**, *80*, 299–307. [CrossRef] [PubMed]
103. Reddy, K.V.; Gupta, S.M.; Aranha, C.C. Effect of antimicrobial peptide, nisin, on the reproductive functions of rats. *ISRN Vet. Sci.* **2011**, *2011*. [CrossRef] [PubMed]
104. Kumar, B.; Balgir, P.P.; Kaur, B.; Mittu, B.; Garg, N. Antimicrobial and spermicidal activity of native and recombinant pediocin CP2: A camparative evaluation. *Arch. Clin. Microbiol.* **2012**, *3*, 1–12.
105. Bourinbaiar, A.S.; Krasinski, K.; Borkowsky, W. Anti-HIV effect of gramicidin *in vivo*: Potential for spermicide use. *Life Sci.* **1994**, *54*, 5–9. [CrossRef]

106. Lee, C.H.; Bagdon, R.; Chien, Y.W. Comparative *in vivo* spermicidal activity of chelating agents and synergistic effect with nonoxynol-9 on human sperm functionality. *J. Pharm. Sci.* **1996**, *85*, 91–95. [CrossRef] [PubMed]
107. Centola, G.M. Dose-response effects of gramicidin-D, EDTA, and nonoxynol-9 on sperm motion parameters and acrosome status. *Contraception* **1998**, *58*, 35–38. [CrossRef]
108. Kawulka, K.E.; Sprules, T.; Diaper, C.M.; Whittal, R.M.; McKay, R.T.; Mercier, P.; Zuber, P.; Vederas, J.C. Structure of subtilosin A, a cyclic antimicrobial peptide from *Bacillus subtilis* with unusual sulfur to alpha-carbon cross-links: Formation and reduction of alpha-thio-alpha-amino acid derivatives. *Biochemistry* **2004**, *43*, 3385–3395. [CrossRef] [PubMed]
109. Sutyak, K.E.; Anderson, R.A.; Dover, S.E.; Feathergill, K.A.; Aroutcheva, A.A.; Faro, S.; Chikindas, M.L. Spermicidal activity of the safe natural antimicrobial peptide subtilosin. *Infect. Dis. Obstet. Gynecol.* **2008**, *2008*. [CrossRef] [PubMed]
110. Martin, N.I.; Sprules, T.; Carpenter, M.R.; Cotter, P.D.; Hill, C.; Ross, R.P.; Vederas, J.C. Structural characterization of lacticin 3147, a two-peptide lantibiotic with synergistic activity. *Biochemistry* **2004**, *43*, 3049–3056. [CrossRef] [PubMed]
111. Ballweber, L.M.; Jaynes, J.E.; Stamm, W.E.; Lampe, M.F. *In vivo* microbicidal activities of cecropin peptides D2A21 and D4E1 and gel formulations containing 0.1 to 2% D2A21 against *Chlamydia trachomatis*. *Antimicrob. Agents Chemother.* **2002**, *46*, 34–41. [CrossRef] [PubMed]
112. Tanphaichitr, N.; Randall, M.; Fitzgerald, L.; Lee, G.; Seibel, M.; Taymor, M. An increase in *in vivo* fertilization ability of low-density human sperm capacitated by multiple-tube swim up. *Fert. Steril.* **1987**, *48*, 821–827.
113. Tanphaichitr, N.; Millette, C.F.; Agulnick, A.; Fitzgerald, L.M. Egg-penetration ability and structural properties of human sperm prepared by percoll-gradient centrifugation. *Gamete Res.* **1988**, *20*, 67–81. [CrossRef] [PubMed]
114. Katz, D.F.; Drobnis, E.Z.; Overstreet, J.W. Factors regulating mammalian sperm migration through the female reproductive tract and oocyte vestments. *Gamete Res.* **1989**, *22*, 443–469. [CrossRef] [PubMed]
115. Suarez, S.S. Gamete and zygote transport. In *Knobil and Neill's Physiology of Reproduction*, 4th ed.; Plant, T.M., Zeleznik, A., Eds.; Elsevier Inc.: New York, NY, USA, 2015; pp. 113–145.
116. Noguchi, K.; Tsukumi, K.; Urano, T. Qualitative and quantitative differences in normal vaginal flora of conventionally reared mice, rats, hamsters, rabbits, and dogs. *Comp. Med.* **2003**, *53*, 404–412. [PubMed]
117. Ronnqvist, P.D.; Forsgren-Brusk, U.B.; Grahn-Hakansson, E.E. Lactobacilli in the female genital tract in relation to other genital microbes and vaginal pH. *Acta Obstet. Gynecol. Scand.* **2006**, *85*, 726–735. [CrossRef] [PubMed]
118. Jacques, M.; Olson, M.E.; Crichlow, A.M.; Osborne, A.D.; Costerton, J.W. The normal microflora of the female rabbit's genital tract. *Can. J. Vet. Res.* **1986**, *50*, 272–274. [PubMed]
119. Cohen, L. Influence of pH on vaginal discharges. *Br. J. Vener. Dis.* **1969**, *45*, 241–247. [CrossRef] [PubMed]
120. Tevi-Benissan, C.; Belec, L.; Levy, M.; Schneider-Fauveau, V.; Si Mohamed, A.; Hallouin, M.C.; Matta, M.; Gresenguet, G. *In vivo* semen-associated pH neutralization of cervicovaginal secretions. *Clin. Diagn. Lab. Immunol.* **1997**, *4*, 367–374. [PubMed]
121. Castle, P.E.; Hoen, T.E.; Whaley, K.J.; Cone, R.A. Contraceptive testing of vaginal agents in rabbits. *Contraception* **1998**, *58*, 51–60. [CrossRef]
122. Meysick, K.C.; Garber, G.E. Interactions between *Trichomonas vaginalis* and vaginal flora in a mouse model. *J. Parasitol.* **1992**, *78*, 157–160. [CrossRef] [PubMed]
123. Fichorova, R.N.; Rheinwald, J.G.; Anderson, D.J. Generation of papillomavirus-immortalized cell lines from normal human ectocervical, endocervical, and vaginal epithelium that maintain expression of tissue-specific differentiation proteins. *Biol. Reprod.* **1997**, *57*, 847–855. [CrossRef] [PubMed]
124. Ayehunie, S.; Cannon, C.; Lamore, S.; Kubilus, J.; Anderson, D.J.; Pudney, J.; Klausner, M. Organotypic human vaginal-ectocervical tissue model for irritation studies of spermicides, microbicides, and feminine-care products. *Toxicol. In Vitro* **2006**, *20*, 689–698. [CrossRef] [PubMed]
125. Zalenskaya, I.A.; Joseph, T.; Bavarva, J.; Yousefieh, N.; Jackson, S.S.; Fashemi, T.; Yamamoto, H.S.; Settlage, R.; Fichorova, R.N.; Doncel, G.F. Gene expression profiling of human vaginal cells *in vivo* discriminates compounds with pro-inflammatory and mucosa-altering properties: Novel biomarkers for preclinical testing of HIV microbicide candidates. *PLoS ONE* **2015**, *10*, e0128557. [CrossRef] [PubMed]

126. Krebs, F.C.; Miller, S.R.; Catalone, B.J.; Fichorova, R.; Anderson, D.; Malamud, D.; Howett, M.K.; Wigdahl, B. Comparative *in vivo* sensitivities of human immune cell lines, vaginal and cervical epithelial cell lines, and primary cells to candidate microbicides nonoxynol 9, C31G, and sodium dodecyl sulfate. *Antimicrob. Agents Chemother.* **2002**, *46*, 2292–2298. [CrossRef] [PubMed]
127. Catalone, B.J.; Kish-Catalone, T.M.; Budgeon, L.R.; Neely, E.B.; Ferguson, M.; Krebs, F.C.; Howett, M.K.; Labib, M.; Rando, R.; Wigdahl, B. Mouse model of cervicovaginal toxicity and inflammation for preclinical evaluation of topical vaginal microbicides. *Antimicrob. Agents Chemother.* **2004**, *48*, 1837–1847. [CrossRef] [PubMed]
128. Bon, I.; Lembo, D.; Rusnati, M.; Clo, A.; Morini, S.; Miserocchi, A.; Bugatti, A.; Grigolon, S.; Musumeci, G.; Landolfo, S.; *et al.* Peptide-derivatized SB105-A10 dendrimer inhibits the infectivity of R5 and X4 HIV-1 strains in primary pbmcs and cervicovaginal histocultures. *PLoS ONE* **2013**, *8*, e76482. [CrossRef] [PubMed]
129. Lagenaur, L.A.; Sanders-Beer, B.E.; Brichacek, B.; Pal, R.; Liu, X.; Liu, Y.; Yu, R.; Venzon, D.; Lee, P.P.; Hamer, D.H. Prevention of vaginal SHIV transmission in macaques by a live recombinant lactobacillus. *Mucosal Immunol.* **2011**, *4*, 648–657. [CrossRef] [PubMed]
130. Mahalingam, A.; Simmons, A.P.; Ugaonkar, S.R.; Watson, K.M.; Dezzutti, C.S.; Rohan, L.C.; Buckheit, R.W., Jr.; Kiser, P.F. Vaginal microbicide gel for delivery of IQP-0528, a pyrimidinedione analog with a dual mechanism of action against HIV-1. *Antimicrob. Agents Chemother.* **2011**, *55*, 1650–1660. [CrossRef] [PubMed]
131. Masters, J.R. Hela cells 50 years on: The good, the bad and the ugly. *Nat. Rev. Cancer* **2002**, *2*, 315–319. [CrossRef] [PubMed]
132. Dover, S.E.; Aroutcheva, A.A.; Faro, S.; Chikindas, M.L. Natural antimicrobials and their role in vaginal health: A short review. *Int. J. Probiotics Prebiotics* **2008**, *3*, 219–230. [PubMed]
133. Aroutcheva, A.; Gariti, D.; Simon, M.; Shott, S.; Faro, J.; Simoes, J.A.; Gurguis, A.; Faro, S. Defense factors of vaginal lactobacilli. *Am. J. Obstet. Gynecol.* **2001**, *185*, 375–379. [CrossRef] [PubMed]
134. Bergman, P.; Walter-Jallow, L.; Broliden, K.; Agerberth, B.; Soderlund, J. The antimicrobial peptide LL-37 inhibits HIV-1 replication. *Curr. HIV Res.* **2007**, *5*, 410–415. [CrossRef] [PubMed]
135. Wang, G.; Watson, K.M.; Buckheit, R.W., Jr. Anti-human immunodeficiency virus type 1 activities of antimicrobial peptides derived from human and bovine cathelicidins. *Antimicrob. Agents Chemother.* **2008**, *52*, 3438–3440. [CrossRef] [PubMed]
136. Levinson, P.; Choi, R.Y.; Cole, A.L.; Hirbod, T.; Rhedin, S.; Payne, B.; Guthrie, B.L.; Bosire, R.; Cole, A.M.; Farquhar, C.; *et al.* HIV-neutralizing activity of cationic polypeptides in cervicovaginal secretions of women in HIV-serodiscordant relationships. *PLoS ONE* **2012**, *7*, e31996. [CrossRef] [PubMed]
137. Lorin, C.; Saidi, H.; Belaid, A.; Zairi, A.; Baleux, F.; Hocini, H.; Belec, L.; Hani, K.; Tangy, F. The antimicrobial peptide dermaseptin S4 inhibits HIV-1 infectivity *in vivo*. *Virology* **2005**, *334*, 264–275. [CrossRef] [PubMed]
138. Hsu, S.T.; Breukink, E.; Tischenko, E.; Lutters, M.A.; de Kruijff, B.; Kaptein, R.; Bonvin, A.M.; van Nuland, N.A. The nisin-lipid II complex reveals a pyrophosphate cage that provides a blueprint for novel antibiotics. *Nat. Struct. Mol. Biol.* **2004**, *11*, 963–967. [CrossRef] [PubMed]
139. Li, X.; Li, Y.; Han, H.; Miller, D.W.; Wang, G. Solution structures of human LL-37 fragments and nmr-based identification of a minimal membrane-targeting antimicrobial and anticancer region. *J. Am. Chem. Soc.* **2006**, *128*, 5776–5785. [CrossRef] [PubMed]
140. Epand, R.F.; Wang, G.; Berno, B.; Epand, R.M. Lipid segregation explains selective toxicity of a series of fragments derived from the human cathelicidin LL-37. *Antimicrob. Agents Chemother.* **2009**, *53*, 3705–3714. [CrossRef] [PubMed]
141. Paiva, A.; Breukink, E. Antimicrobial peptides produced by microorganisms. In *Antimicrobial Peptides and Innate Immunity*; Hiemstra, P.S., Zaat, S.A.J., Eds.; Springer: Basel, Switzerland, 2013; pp. 53–95.
142. Wang, G.; Li, X.; Wang, Z. Apd3: The antimicrobial peptide database as a tool for research and education. *Nucleic Acids Res.* **2016**, *44*, D1087–D1093. [CrossRef] [PubMed]
143. Koradi, R.; Billeter, M.; Wuthrich, K. Molmol: A program for display and analysis of macromolecular structures. *J. Mol. Graph.* **1996**, *14*, 51–55. [CrossRef]
144. Durr, U.H.; Sudheendra, U.S.; Ramamoorthy, A. LL-37, the only human member of the cathelicidin family of antimicrobial peptides. *Biochim. Biophys. Acta* **2006**, *1758*, 1408–1425. [CrossRef] [PubMed]
145. Zelezetsky, I.; Pontillo, A.; Puzzi, L.; Antcheva, N.; Segat, L.; Pacor, S.; Crovella, S.; Tossi, A. Evolution of the primate cathelicidin. Correlation between structural variations and antimicrobial activity. *J. Biol. Chem.* **2006**, *281*, 19861–19871. [CrossRef] [PubMed]

146. Cowland, J.B.; Johnsen, A.H.; Borregaard, N. hCAP-18, a cathelin/pro-bactenecin-like protein of human neutrophil specific granules. *FEBS Lett.* **1995**, *368*, 173–176. [CrossRef]
147. Agerberth, B.; Charo, J.; Werr, J.; Olsson, B.; Idali, F.; Lindbom, L.; Kiessling, R.; Jornvall, H.; Wigzell, H.; Gudmundsson, G.H. The human antimicrobial and chemotactic peptides LL-37 and alpha-defensins are expressed by specific lymphocyte and monocyte populations. *Blood* **2000**, *96*, 3086–3093. [PubMed]
148. Di Nardo, A.; Vitiello, A.; Gallo, R.L. Cutting edge: Mast cell antimicrobial activity is mediated by expression of cathelicidin antimicrobial peptide. *J. Immunol.* **2003**, *170*, 2274–2278. [CrossRef] [PubMed]
149. Frohm Nilsson, M.; Sandstedt, B.; Sorensen, O.; Weber, G.; Borregaard, N.; Stahle-Backdahl, M. The human cationic antimicrobial protein (hCAP-18), a peptide antibiotic, is widely expressed in human squamous epithelia and colocalizes with interleukin-6. *Infect. Immun.* **1999**, *67*, 2561–2566. [PubMed]
150. Reinholz, M.; Ruzicka, T.; Schauber, J. Cathelicidin LL-37: An antimicrobial peptide with a role in inflammatory skin disease. *Ann. Dermatol.* **2012**, *24*, 126–135. [CrossRef] [PubMed]
151. Yamasaki, K.; Schauber, J.; Coda, A.; Lin, H.; Dorschner, R.A.; Schechter, N.M.; Bonnart, C.; Descargues, P.; Hovnanian, A.; Gallo, R.L. Kallikrein-mediated proteolysis regulates the antimicrobial effects of cathelicidins in skin. *FASEB J.* **2006**, *20*, 2068–2080. [CrossRef] [PubMed]
152. Malm, J.; Sorensen, O.; Persson, T.; Frohm-Nilsson, M.; Johansson, B.; Bjartell, A.; Lilja, H.; Stahle-Backdahl, M.; Borregaard, N.; Egesten, A. The human cationic antimicrobial protein (hCAP-18) is expressed in the epithelium of human epididymis, is present in seminal plasma at high concentrations, and is attached to spermatozoa. *Infect. Immun.* **2000**, *68*, 4297–4302. [CrossRef] [PubMed]
153. Sorensen, O.E.; Gram, L.; Johnsen, A.H.; Andersson, E.; Bangsboll, S.; Tjabringa, G.S.; Hiemstra, P.S.; Malm, J.; Egesten, A.; Borregaard, N. Processing of seminal plasma hCAP-18 to ALL-38 by gastricsin: A novel mechanism of generating antimicrobial peptides in vagina. *J. Biol. Chem.* **2003**, *278*, 28540–28546. [CrossRef] [PubMed]
154. Chromek, M.; Slamova, Z.; Bergman, P.; Kovacs, L.; Podracka, L.; Ehren, I.; Hokfelt, T.; Gudmundsson, G.H.; Gallo, R.L.; Agerberth, B.; *et al.* The antimicrobial peptide cathelicidin protects the urinary tract against invasive bacterial infection. *Nat. Med.* **2006**, *12*, 636–641. [CrossRef] [PubMed]
155. Nielsen, K.L.; Dynesen, P.; Larsen, P.; Jakobsen, L.; Andersen, P.S.; Frimodt-Moller, N. Role of urinary cathelicidin LL-37 and human β-defensin 1 in uncomplicated *Escherichia coli* urinary tract infections. *Infect. Immun.* **2014**, *82*, 1572–1578. [CrossRef] [PubMed]
156. Hase, K.; Eckmann, L.; Leopard, J.D.; Varki, N.; Kagnoff, M.F. Cell differentiation is a key determinant of cathelicidin LL-37/human cationic antimicrobial protein 18 expression by human colon epithelium. *Infect. Immun.* **2002**, *70*, 953–963. [CrossRef] [PubMed]
157. Bals, R.; Wang, X.; Zasloff, M.; Wilson, J.M. The peptide antibiotic LL-37/hCAP-18 is expressed in epithelia of the human lung where it has broad antimicrobial activity at the airway surface. *Proc. Natl. Acad. Sci. USA* **1998**, *95*, 9541–9546. [CrossRef] [PubMed]
158. Tjabringa, G.S.; Rabe, K.F.; Hiemstra, P.S. The human cathelicidin LL-37: A multifunctional peptide involved in infection and inflammation in the lung. *Pulm. Pharmacol. Ther.* **2005**, *18*, 321–327. [CrossRef] [PubMed]
159. Greer, A.; Zenobia, C.; Darveau, R.P. Defensins and LL-37: A review of function in the gingival epithelium. *Periodontology 2000* **2013**, *63*, 67–79. [CrossRef] [PubMed]
160. Gordon, Y.J.; Huang, L.C.; Romanowski, E.G.; Yates, K.A.; Proske, R.J.; McDermott, A.M. Human cathelicidin (LL-37), a multifunctional peptide, is expressed by ocular surface epithelia and has potent antibacterial and antiviral activity. *Curr. Eye Res.* **2005**, *30*, 385–394. [CrossRef] [PubMed]
161. Cederlund, A.; Olliver, M.; Rekha, R.S.; Lindh, M.; Lindbom, L.; Normark, S.; Henriques-Normark, B.; Andersson, J.; Agerberth, B.; Bergman, P. Impaired release of antimicrobial peptides into nasal fluid of hyper-IgE and CVID patients. *PLoS ONE* **2011**, *6*, e29316. [CrossRef] [PubMed]
162. Nell, M.J.; Tjabringa, G.S.; Vonk, M.J.; Hiemstra, P.S.; Grote, J.J. Bacterial products increase expression of the human cathelicidin hCap-18/LL-37 in cultured human sinus epithelial cells. *FEMS Immunol Med. Microbiol.* **2004**, *42*, 225–231. [CrossRef] [PubMed]
163. Doss, M.; White, M.R.; Tecle, T.; Hartshorn, K.L. Human defensins and LL-37 in mucosal immunity. *J. Leukoc. Biol.* **2010**, *87*, 79–92. [CrossRef] [PubMed]
164. Yang, H.; Reinherz, E.L. Dynamic recruitment of human CD2 into lipid rafts. Linkage to T cell signal transduction. *J. Biol. Chem.* **2001**, *276*, 18775–18785. [CrossRef] [PubMed]

165. Andersson, E.; Sorensen, O.E.; Frohm, B.; Borregaard, N.; Egesten, A.; Malm, J. Isolation of human cationic antimicrobial protein-18 from seminal plasma and its association with prostasomes. *Hum Reprod.* **2002**, *17*, 2529–2534. [CrossRef] [PubMed]
166. Sorensen, O.E.; Follin, P.; Johnsen, A.H.; Calafat, J.; Tjabringa, G.S.; Hiemstra, P.S.; Borregaard, N. Human cathelicidin, hCAP-18, is processed to the antimicrobial peptide LL-37 by extracellular cleavage with proteinase 3. *Blood* **2001**, *97*, 3951–3959. [CrossRef] [PubMed]
167. Cottell, E.; Harrison, R.F.; McCaffrey, M.; Walsh, T.; Mallon, E.; Barry-Kinsella, C. Are seminal fluid microorganisms of significance or merely contaminants? *Fertil. Steril.* **2000**, *74*, 465–470. [CrossRef]
168. Smeianov, V.; Scott, K.; Reid, G. Activity of cecropin p1 and FA-LL-37 against urogenital microflora. *Microbes Infect.* **2000**, *2*, 773–777. [CrossRef]
169. Sambri, V.; Marangoni, A.; Giacani, L.; Gennaro, R.; Murgia, R.; Cevenini, R.; Cinco, M. Comparative *in vivo* activity of five cathelicidin-derived synthetic peptides against leptospira, borrelia and *Treponema pallidum*. *J. Antimicrob. Chemother.* **2002**, *50*, 895–902. [CrossRef] [PubMed]
170. Bai, L.; Takagi, S.; Guo, Y.; Kuroda, K.; Ando, T.; Yoneyama, H.; Ito, K.; Isogai, E. Inhibition of *Streptococcus mutans* biofilm by LL-37. *Int. J. Med. Sci. Biotechnol.* **2013**, *1*, 56–64.
171. Moffatt, J.H.; Harper, M.; Mansell, A.; Crane, B.; Fitzsimons, T.C.; Nation, R.L.; Li, J.; Adler, B.; Boyce, J.D. Lipopolysaccharide-deficient *Acinetobacter baumannii* shows altered signaling through host toll-like receptors and increased susceptibility to the host antimicrobial peptide LL-37. *Infect. Immun.* **2013**, *81*, 684–689.
172. Garcia-Quintanilla, M.; Pulido, M.R.; Moreno-Martinez, P.; Martin-Pena, R.; Lopez-Rojas, R.; Pachon, J.; McConnell, M.J. Activity of host antimicrobials against multidrug-resistant *Acinetobacter baumannii* acquiring colistin resistance through loss of lipopolysaccharide. *Antimicrob. Agents Chemother.* **2014**, *58*, 2972–2975.
173. Ouhara, K.; Komatsuzawa, H.; Yamada, S.; Shiba, H.; Fujiwara, T.; Ohara, M.; Sayama, K.; Hashimoto, K.; Kurihara, H.; Sugai, M. Susceptibilities of periodontopathogenic and cariogenic bacteria to antibacterial peptides, beta-defensins and LL-37, produced by human epithelial cells. *J. Antimicrob. Chemother.* **2005**, *55*, 888–896. [CrossRef] [PubMed]
174. Tanaka, D.; Miyasaki, K.T.; Lehrer, R.I. Sensitivity of actinobacillus actinomycetemcomitans and *Capnocytophaga* spp. To the bactericidal action of LL-37: A cathelicidin found in human leukocytes and epithelium. *Oral Microbiol. Immunol.* **2000**, *15*, 226–231. [CrossRef] [PubMed]
175. Thwaite, J.E.; Hibbs, S.; Titball, R.W.; Atkins, T.P. Proteolytic degradation of human antimicrobial peptide LL-37 by *Bacillus anthracis* may contribute to virulence. *Antimicrob. Agents Chemother.* **2006**, *50*, 2316–2322.
176. Lusitani, D.; Malawista, S.E.; Montgomery, R.R. *Borrelia burgdorferi* are susceptible to killing by a variety of human polymorphonuclear leukocyte components. *J. Infect. Dis.* **2002**, *185*, 797–804. [CrossRef] [PubMed]
177. Kanthawong, S.; Nazmi, K.; Wongratanacheewin, S.; Bolscher, J.G.; Wuthiekanun, V.; Taweechaisupapong, S. *In vitro* susceptibility of *Burkholderia pseudomallei* to antimicrobial peptides. *Int. J. Antimicrob. Agents* **2009**, *34*, 309–314. [CrossRef] [PubMed]
178. Kanthawong, S.; Bolscher, J.G.; Veerman, E.C.; van Marle, J.; Nazmi, K.; Wongratanacheewin, S.; Taweechaisupapong, S. Antimicrobial activities of LL-37 and its truncated variants against *Burkholderia thailandensis*. *Int. J. Antimicrob. Agents* **2010**, *36*, 447–452. [CrossRef] [PubMed]
179. Tsai, P.W.; Yang, C.Y.; Chang, H.T.; Lan, C.Y. Human antimicrobial peptide LL-37 inhibits adhesion of *Candida albicans* by interacting with yeast cell-wall carbohydrates. *PLoS ONE* **2011**, *6*, e17755. [CrossRef] [PubMed]
180. Tsai, P.W.; Cheng, Y.L.; Hsieh, W.P.; Lan, C.Y. Responses of *Candida albicans* to the human antimicrobial peptide LL-37. *J. Microbiol.* **2014**, *52*, 581–589. [CrossRef]
181. Tang, L.; Chen, J.; Zhou, Z.; Yu, P.; Yang, Z.; Zhong, G. Chlamydia-secreted protease CPAF degrades host antimicrobial peptides. *Microbes Infect.* **2015**, *17*, 402–408. [CrossRef] [PubMed]
182. McQuade, R.; Roxas, B.; Viswanathan, V.K.; Vedantam, G. *Clostridium difficile* clinical isolates exhibit variable susceptibility and proteome alterations upon exposure to mammalian cationic antimicrobial peptides. *Anaerobe* **2012**, *18*, 614–620. [CrossRef] [PubMed]
183. Leszczynska, K.; Namiot, D.; Byfield, F.J.; Cruz, K.; Zendzian-Piotrowska, M.; Fein, D.E.; Savage, P.B.; Diamond, S.; McCulloch, C.A.; Janmey, P.A.; *et al.* Antibacterial activity of the human host defence peptide LL-37 and selected synthetic cationic lipids against bacteria associated with oral and upper respiratory tract infections. *J. Antimicrob. Chemother.* **2013**, *68*, 610–618. [CrossRef] [PubMed]
184. Benincasa, M.; Mattiuzzo, M.; Herasimenka, Y.; Cescutti, P.; Rizzo, R.; Gennaro, R. Activity of antimicrobial peptides in the presence of polysaccharides produced by pulmonary pathogens. *J. Peptide Sci.* **2009**, *15*, 595–600. [CrossRef] [PubMed]

185. Leszczynska, K.; Namiot, A.; Fein, D.E.; Wen, Q.; Namiot, Z.; Savage, P.B.; Diamond, S.; Janmey, P.A.; Bucki, R. Bactericidal activities of the cationic steroid CSA-13 and the cathelicidin peptide LL-37 against *Helicobacter pylori* in simulated gastric juice. *BMC Microbiol.* **2009**, *9*. [CrossRef] [PubMed]
186. Chen, X.; Niyonsaba, F.; Ushio, H.; Okuda, D.; Nagaoka, I.; Ikeda, S.; Okumura, K.; Ogawa, H. Synergistic effect of antibacterial agents human beta-defensins, cathelicidin LL-37 and lysozyme against *Staphylococcus aureus* and *Escherichia coli*. *J. Dermatol. Sci.* **2005**, *40*, 123–132. [CrossRef] [PubMed]
187. Kai-Larsen, Y.; Luthje, P.; Chromek, M.; Peters, V.; Wang, X.; Holm, A.; Kadas, L.; Hedlund, K.O.; Johansson, J.; Chapman, M.R.; *et al.* Uropathogenic *Escherichia coli* modulates immune responses and its curli fimbriae interact with the antimicrobial peptide LL-37. *PLoS Pathog.* **2010**, *6*, e1001010. [CrossRef] [PubMed]
188. Nagaoka, I.; Kuwahara-Arai, K.; Tamura, H.; Hiramatsu, K.; Hirata, M. Augmentation of the bactericidal activities of human cathelicidin CAP18/LL-37-derived antimicrobial peptides by amino acid substitutions. *Inflamm. Res.* **2005**, *54*, 66–73. [CrossRef] [PubMed]
189. Lysenko, E.S.; Gould, J.; Bals, R.; Wilson, J.M.; Weiser, J.N. Bacterial phosphorylcholine decreases susceptibility to the antimicrobial peptide LL-37/hCAP18 expressed in the upper respiratory tract. *Infect. Immun.* **2000**, *68*, 1664–1671. [CrossRef] [PubMed]
190. Tripathi, S.; Wang, G.; White, M.; Qi, L.; Taubenberger, J.; Hartshorn, K.L. Antiviral activity of the human cathelicidin, LL-37, and derived peptides on seasonal and pandemic influenza a viruses. *PLoS One* **2015**, *10*, e0124706. [CrossRef] [PubMed]
191. Barlow, P.G.; Svoboda, P.; Mackellar, A.; Nash, A.A.; York, I.A.; Pohl, J.; Davidson, D.J.; Donis, R.O. Antiviral activity and increased host defense against influenza infection elicited by the human cathelicidin LL-37. *PLoS ONE* **2011**, *6*, e25333. [CrossRef] [PubMed]
192. Tripathi, S.; Tecle, T.; Verma, A.; Crouch, E.; White, M.; Hartshorn, K.L. The human cathelicidin LL-37 inhibits influenza A viruses through a mechanism distinct from that of surfactant protein D or defensins. *J. Gen. Virol.* **2013**, *94*, 40–49. [CrossRef] [PubMed]
193. De Majumdar, S.; Yu, J.; Fookes, M.; McAteer, S.P.; Llobet, E.; Finn, S.; Spence, S.; Monahan, A.; Kissenpfennig, A.; Ingram, R.J.; *et al.* Elucidation of the rama regulon in *Klebsiella pneumoniae* reveals a role in LPS regulation. *PLoS Pathog.* **2015**, *11*, e1004627. [CrossRef] [PubMed]
194. Bergman, P.; Johansson, L.; Asp, V.; Plant, L.; Gudmundsson, G.H.; Jonsson, A.B.; Agerberth, B. *Neisseria gonorrhoeae* downregulates expression of the human antimicrobial peptide LL-37. *Cell. Microbiol.* **2005**, *7*, 1009–1017. [CrossRef] [PubMed]
195. Jones, A.; Georg, M.; Maudsdotter, L.; Jonsson, A.B. Endotoxin, capsule, and bacterial ttachment contribute to *Neisseria meningitidis* resistance to the human antimicrobial peptide LL-37. *J. Bacteriol.* **2009**, *191*, 3861–3868.
196. Bergsson, G.; Reeves, E.P.; McNally, P.; Chotirmall, S.H.; Greene, C.M.; Greally, P.; Murphy, P.; O'Neill, S.J.; McElvaney, N.G. LL-37 complexation with glycosaminoglycans in cystic fibrosis lungs inhibits antimicrobial activity, which can be restored by hypertonic saline. *J. Immunol.* **2009**, *183*, 543–551. [CrossRef] [PubMed]
197. Dean, S.N.; Bishop, B.M.; van Hoek, M.L. Susceptibility of *Pseudomonas aeruginosa* biofilm to alpha-helical peptides: D-enantiomer of LL-37. *Front. Microbiol.* **2011**, *2*. [CrossRef] [PubMed]
198. Dosler, S.; Karaaslan, E. Inhibition and destruction of *Pseudomonas aeruginosa* biofilms by antibiotics and antimicrobial peptides. *Peptides* **2014**, *62*, 32–37. [CrossRef] [PubMed]
199. Currie, S.M.; Findlay, E.G.; McHugh, B.J.; Mackellar, A.; Man, T.; Macmillan, D.; Wang, H.; Fitch, P.M.; Schwarze, J.; Davidson, D.J. The human cathelicidin LL-37 has antiviral activity against respiratory syncytial virus. *PLoS ONE* **2013**, *8*, e73659. [CrossRef] [PubMed]
200. Noore, J.; Noore, A.; Li, B. Cationic antimicrobial peptide LL-37 is effective against both extra- and intracellular *Staphylococcus aureus*. *Antimicrob. Agents Chemother.* **2013**, *57*, 1283–1290. [CrossRef] [PubMed]
201. Senyurek, I.; Paulmann, M.; Sinnberg, T.; Kalbacher, H.; Deeg, M.; Gutsmann, T.; Hermes, M.; Kohler, T.; Gotz, F.; Wolz, C.; *et al.* Dermcidin-derived peptides show a different mode of action than the cathelicidin LL-37 against *Staphylococcus aureus*. *Antimicrob. Agents Chemother.* **2009**, *53*, 2499–2509. [CrossRef] [PubMed]
202. Xiao, L.; Crabb, D.M.; Dai, Y.; Chen, Y.; Waites, K.B.; Atkinson, T.P. Suppression of antimicrobial peptide expression by ureaplasma species. *Infect. Immun.* **2014**, *82*, 1657–1665. [CrossRef] [PubMed]
203. Howell, M.D.; Jones, J.F.; Kisich, K.O.; Streib, J.E.; Gallo, R.L.; Leung, D.Y. Selective killing of vaccinia virus by LL-37: Implications for eczema vaccinatum. *J. Immunol.* **2004**, *172*, 1763–1767. [CrossRef] [PubMed]

204. Crack, L.R.; Jones, L.; Malavige, G.N.; Patel, V.; Ogg, G.S. Human antimicrobial peptides LL-37 and human beta-defensin-2 reduce viral replication in keratinocytes infected with varicella zoster virus. *Clin. Exp. Dermatol.* **2012**, *37*, 534–543. [CrossRef] [PubMed]
205. Laupland, K.B.; Ross, T.; Pitout, J.D.; Church, D.L.; Gregson, D.B. Community-onset urinary tract infections: A population-based assessment. *Infection* **2007**, *35*, 150–153. [CrossRef] [PubMed]
206. Kunin, C.M.; Polyak, F.; Postel, E. Periurethral bacterial flora in women. Prolonged intermittent colonization with *Escherichia coli*. *JAMA* **1980**, *243*, 134–139. [CrossRef] [PubMed]
207. Langlais, J.; Kan, F.W.; Granger, L.; Raymond, L.; Bleau, G.; Roberts, K.D. Identification of sterol acceptors that stimulate cholesterol efflux from human spermatozoa during *in vitro* capacitation. *Gamete Res.* **1988**, *20*, 185–201. [CrossRef] [PubMed]
208. Hamil, K.G.; Sivashanmugam, P.; Richardson, R.T.; Grossman, G.; Ruben, S.M.; Mohler, J.L.; Petrusz, P.; O'Rand, M.G.; French, F.S.; Hall, S.H. HE2beta and HE2gamma, new members of an epididymis-specific family of androgen-regulated proteins in the human. *Endocrinology* **2000**, *141*, 1245–1253. [PubMed]
209. Tollner, T.L.; Venners, S.A.; Hollox, E.J.; Yudin, A.I.; Liu, X.; Tang, G.; Xing, H.; Kays, R.J.; Lau, T.; Overstreet, J.W.; *et al.* A common mutation in the defensin DEFB126 causes impaired sperm function and subfertility. *Sci. Transl. Med.* **2011**, *3*. [CrossRef] [PubMed]
210. Tollner, T.L.; Yudin, A.I.; Treece, C.A.; Overstreet, J.W.; Cherr, G.N. Macaque sperm coating protein defb126 facilitates sperm penetration of cervical mucus. *Hum. Reprod.* **2008**, *23*, 2523–2534. [CrossRef] [PubMed]
211. Yudin, A.I.; Tollner, T.L.; Li, M.W.; Treece, C.A.; Overstreet, J.W.; Cherr, G.N. ESP13.2, a member of the beta-defensin family, is a macaque sperm surface-coating protein involved in the capacitation process. *Biol. Reprod.* **2003**, *69*, 1118–1128. [CrossRef] [PubMed]
212. Liu, Q.; Hamil, K.G.; Sivashanmugam, P.; Grossman, G.; Soundararajan, R.; Rao, A.J.; Richardson, R.T.; Zhang, Y.L.; O'Rand, M.G.; Petrusz, P.; *et al.* Primate epididymis-specific proteins: Characterization of ESC42, a novel protein containing a trefoil-like motif in monkey and human. *Endocrinology* **2001**, *142*, 4529–4539.
213. Yenugu, S.; Hamil, K.G.; Radhakrishnan, Y.; French, F.S.; Hall, S.H. The androgen-regulated epididymal sperm-binding protein, human beta-defensin 118 (defb118) (formerly esc42), is an antimicrobial beta-defensin. *Endocrinology* **2004**, *145*, 3165–3173. [CrossRef] [PubMed]
214. Yu, H.; Dong, J.; Gu, Y.; Liu, H.; Xin, A.; Shi, H.; Sun, F.; Zhang, Y.; Lin, D.; Diao, H. The novel human beta-defensin 114 regulates lipopolysaccharide (LPS)-mediated inflammation and protects sperm from motility loss. *J. Biol. Chem.* **2013**, *288*, 12270–12282. [CrossRef] [PubMed]
215. Diao, R.; Fok, K.L.; Chen, H.; Yu, M.K.; Duan, Y.; Chung, C.M.; Li, Z.; Wu, H.; Li, Z.; Zhang, H.; *et al.* Deficient human beta-defensin 1 underlies male infertility associated with poor sperm motility and genital tract infection. *Sci. Transl. Med.* **2014**, *6*. [CrossRef] [PubMed]
216. Li, P.; Chan, H.C.; He, B.; So, S.C.; Chung, Y.W.; Shang, Q.; Zhang, Y.D.; Zhang, Y.L. An antimicrobial peptide gene found in the male reproductive system of rats. *Science* **2001**, *291*, 1783–1785. [CrossRef] [PubMed]
217. Zhou, C.X.; Zhang, Y.L.; Xiao, L.; Zheng, M.; Leung, K.M.; Chan, M.Y.; Lo, P.S.; Tsang, L.L.; Wong, H.Y.; Ho, L.S.; *et al.* An epididymis-specific beta-defensin is important for the initiation of sperm maturation. *Nat. Cell Biol.* **2004**, *6*, 458–464. [CrossRef] [PubMed]
218. Diao, H.; Yu, H.G.; Sun, F.; Zhang, Y.L.; Tanphaichitr, N. Rat recombinant beta-defensin 22 is a heparin-binding protein with antimicrobial activity. *Asian J. Androl.* **2011**, *13*, 305–311. [CrossRef] [PubMed]
219. Mishra, B.; Lushnikova, T.; Wang, G. Small lipopeptides possess anti-biofilm capability comparable to daptomycin and vancomycin. *RSC Adv.* **2015**, *5*, 59758–59769. [CrossRef] [PubMed]
220. Mangoni, M.L.; Shai, Y. Short native antimicrobial peptides and engineered ultrashort lipopeptides: Similarities and differences in cell specificities and modes of action. *Cell. Mol. Life Sci.* **2011**, *68*, 2267–2280.
221. Makovitzki, A.; Avrahami, D.; Shai, Y. Ultrashort antibacterial and antifungal lipopeptides. *Proc. Natl. Acad. Sci. USA* **2006**, *103*, 15997–16002. [CrossRef] [PubMed]

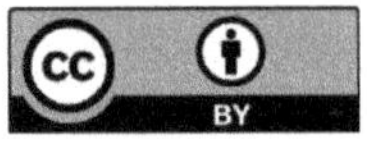

© 2016 by the authors. Licensee MDPI, Basel, Switzerland. This article is an open access article distributed under the terms and conditions of the Creative Commons Attribution (CC BY) license (http://creativecommons.org/licenses/by/4.0/).

MDPI AG
St. Alban-Anlage 66
4052 Basel, Switzerland
Tel. +41 61 683 77 34
Fax +41 61 302 89 18
http://www.mdpi.com

Pharmaceuticals Editorial Office
E-mail: pharmaceuticals@mdpi.com
http://www.mdpi.com/journal/pharmaceuticals

www.ingramcontent.com/pod-product-compliance
Lightning Source LLC
Chambersburg PA
CBHW051719210326
41597CB00032B/5537

* 9 7 8 3 0 3 8 4 2 4 6 2 8 *